Nursing Theories & Nursing Practice

Second Edition

Nursing Theories & Nursing Practice

SECOND EDITION

**Marilyn E. Parker,
PhD, RN, FAAN**

Quantum Foundation Center for Innovation in School
   and Community Well-Being
Christine E. Lynn College of Nursing
Florida Atlantic University
Boca Raton, Florida

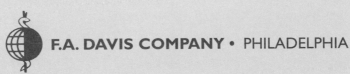

F.A. DAVIS COMPANY • PHILADELPHIA

F.A. Davis Company
1915 Arch Street
Philadelphia, PA 19103

Printed in the United States of America

Last digit indicates print number: 10 9 8 7 6 5 4 3 2 1

Acquisitions Editor: Joanne P. DaCunha, RN, MSN
Developmental Editor: Caryn Abramowitz
Project Editor: Kristin L. Kern
Cover Designer: Carolyn O'Brien

As new scientific information becomes available through basic and clinical research, recommended treat-ments and drug therapies undergo changes. The authors and publisher have done everything possible to make this book accurate, up to date, and in accord with accepted standards at the time of publication. The authors, editors, and publisher are not responsible for errors or omissions or for consequences from application of the book, and make no warranty, expressed or implied, in regard to the contents of the book. Any practice described in this book should be applied by the reader in accordance with professional standards of care used in regard to the unique circumstances that may apply in each situation. The reader is advised always to check product information (package inserts) for changes and new information re-garding dose and contraindications before administering any drug. Caution is especially urged when using new or infrequently ordered drugs.

Library of Congress Cataloging-in-Publication Data

Nursing theories and nursing practice / [edited by] Marilyn E. Parker—2nd ed.
    p. ; cm.
  Includes bibliographical references and index.
  ISBN 10: 0-8036-1196-X ISBN 13: 9780-8036-1196-2
   1. Nursing—Philosophy. 2. Nursing.
  [DNLM: 1. Nursing Theory—Biography. 2. Nurses—Biography. WY 86 N9737 2005]
I. Parker, Marilyn E.
  RT84.5.N8793 2005
  610.73′01—dc22   2005020396

Preface to the Second Edition

This book offers the perspective that nursing theory is essentially connected with nursing practice, research, education, and development. Nursing theories, regardless of complexity or abstraction, reflect nursing and are used by nurses to frame their thinking, action, and being in the world. As guides for nursing endeavors, nursing theories are practical in nature and facilitate communication with those being nursed as well as with colleagues, students, and persons practicing in related health and illness services. At the same time, all aspects of nursing are essential for developing and evolving nursing theory. It is hoped that these pages make clear the interrelations of nursing theory and various nursing endeavors and that the discipline and practice of nursing will thus be advanced.

This very special book is intended to honor the work of nursing theorists and nurses who use these theories in their day-to-day nursing care, by reflecting and presenting the unique contributions of eminent nursing thinkers and doers of our lifetimes. Our foremost nursing theorists have written for this book or their work has been described by nurses who have thorough knowledge of the theorist's work and who have a deep respect for the theorist as person, nurse, and scholar. Indeed, to the extent possible, contributing authors have been selected by theorists to write about their theoretical work. The pattern for each chapter was developed by each author or team of authors according to their individual thinking and writing styles, as well as the scientific perspectives of the chapter. This freedom of format has helped to encourage the latest and best thinking of contributing authors; several authors have shared the insight that in preparing a chapter for this book, their work has become more full and complete.

This book is intended to assist nursing students in undergraduate, master's, and doctoral nursing programs to explore and appreciate nursing theories and their use in nursing practice and scholarship. In addition and in response to calls from practicing nurses, this book is intended for use by those who desire to enrich their practice by the study of nursing theories and related illustrations of nursing practice and scholarship. The first section of the book provides an overview of nursing theory and a focus for thinking about evaluating and choosing nursing theory for use in nursing practice. An outline at the beginning of each chapter provides a map for the chapter. Selected points are highlighted in each chapter. An instructor's manual has been prepared for this book; it reflects the experiences of many who have both met the challenges and who have had such a good time teaching and learning nursing theory in undergraduate and graduate nursing programs.

The design of this book highlights work of nurses who were thinking and writing about nursing up to 50 years ago or more. Building then, as now, on the writings of Florence Nightingale, these nurse scholars have provided essential influences for the evolution of nursing theory. These influences can be seen in the theory presentations in the section of the book that includes the nursing theories that are most in use today. The last section of this book features theorists who initially developed nursing theories at the middle range, a conceptual model for nursing practice in community, and an emerging theory of technology in nursing. These contributing authors describe development processes and perspectives on their work, giving us a variety of views for the future as we move into the twenty-first century. Each chapter of the book includes both descriptions of a particular theory and the use of the theory in nursing practice, research, education, and administration.

For the latest and best thinking of some of nursing's finest scholars, all nurses who read and use this book will be grateful. For the continuing commitment of these scholars to our discipline and practice of nursing, we are all thankful. Continuing to learn and share what you love keeps the work and the love alive, nurtures the commitment, and offers both fun and frustration along the way. This has been illustrated in the enthusiasm for this book shared by many nursing theorists and contributing authors who have worked to create this book and by those who have added their efforts to make it live. For me, it has been a joy to renew friendships with colleagues who have joined me in preparing this book and to find new friends and colleagues as contributing authors.

Nursing Theories and Nursing Practice, now in the second edition, has roots in a series of nursing theory conferences held in South Florida beginning in 1989 and ending when efforts to cope with the aftermath of Hurricane Andrew interrupted the energy and resources needed for planning and offering the Fifth South Florida Nursing Theory Conference. Many of the theorists in this book addressed audiences of mostly practicing nurses at these conferences. Two books stimulated by those conferences and published by the National League for Nursing are *Nursing Theories in Practice* (1990) and *Patterns of Nursing Theories in Practice* (1993).

For me, even deeper roots of this book are found early in my nursing career, when I seriously considered leaving nursing for the study of pharmacy. In my fatigue and frustration, mixed with youthful hope and desire for more education, I could not answer the question "What is nursing?" and could not distinguish the work of nursing from other tasks I did every day. Why should I continue this work? Why should I seek degrees in a field that I could not define? After reflecting on these questions and using them to examine my nursing, I could find no one who would consider the questions with me. I remember being asked, "Why would you ask that question? You're a nurse; you must surely know what nursing is." Such responses, along with a drive for serious consideration of my questions, led me to the library. I clearly remember reading several descriptions of nursing that, I thought, could have just as well have been about social work or physical therapy. I then found nursing defined and explained in a book about education of practical nurses written by Dorothea Orem. During the weeks that followed, as I did my work of nursing in the hospital, I explored Orem's ideas about why people need nursing, nursing's purposes, and what nurses do. I found a fit of her ideas, as I understood them, with my practice, and I learned that I could go even further to explain and design nursing according to these ways of thinking about nursing. I discovered that nursing shared some knowledge and practices with other services, such as pharmacy and medicine, and I began to distinguish nursing from these related fields of practice. I decided to stay in nursing and made plans to study and work with Dorothea Orem. In addition to learning about nursing theory and its meaning in all we do, I learned from Dorothea that nursing is a unique discipline of knowledge and professional practice. In many ways, my earliest questions about nursing have guided my subsequent study and work. Most of what I have done in nursing has been a continuation of my initial experience of the interrelations of all aspects of nursing scholarship, including the scholarship that is nursing practice. Over the years, I have been privileged to work with many nursing scholars, some of whom are featured in this book. My love for nursing and my respect for our discipline and practice have deepened, and knowing now that these values are so often shared is a singular joy.

Many faculty colleagues and students continue to help me study nursing and have contributed to this book in ways I would never have adequate words to acknowledge. I have been fortunate to hold faculty appointments in universities where nursing theory has been honored and am especially fortunate today to be in a College of Nursing where faculty and students often ground our teaching, scholarship, and practice in nursing theory. I am grateful to my knowledgeable colleagues who reviewed and offered helpful suggestions for chapters of this book, and I am grateful to those who contributed as chapter authors. It is also our good fortune that many nursing theorists and other nursing scholars live in or willingly visit our lovely state of Florida.

During the preparation of the first edition of this book, nursing lost three of the theorists acclaimed in this book as essential influences on the evolution of nursing theory. Ernestine Wiedenbach died in the spring of 1998. As the book was being prepared for production, word came of the death of Dorothy Johnson. Hildegard Peplau died in March of 1999. Typical of their commitments to nursing, both Dorothy Johnson and Hildegard Peplau had told me of their interests in this project; they advised me on the authors they would like to have prepare the chapters on their theories and had asked to be given updates on our progress.

This book began during a visit with Joanne DaCunha, an expert nurse and editor for F. A. Davis Company, who has seen it to publication with what I believe is her love of nursing. I am grateful for her wisdom, kindness, and understanding of nursing. Caryn Abramowitz's respect for the purposes of this book and for the special contributions of the authors has been matched only by her fine attention to detail. Marguerite Purnell assisted with the first edition of this book, and Judy Czernda, a current doctoral student, has provided invaluable help with aspects of the second edition. I thank my husband, Terry Worden, for his abiding love and for always being willing to help, and my niece, Cherie Parker, who represents many nurses who inspire the work of this book.

Marilyn E. Parker
West Palm Beach, Florida

Nursing Theorists

Charlotte D. Barry, RN, PhD
Associate Professor
Christine E. Lynn College of Nursing
Florida Atlantic University
Boca Raton, Florida

Anne Boykin, RN, PhD
Dean and Professor
Christine E. Lynn College of Nursing
Florida Atlantic University
Boca Raton, Florida

Lydia Hall†

Virginia Henderson†

Dorothy Johnson*†

Imogene King*
Professor Emeritus
College of Nursing
University of South Florida
Tampa, Florida

Madeleine Leininger*, RN, PhD, CTN, FAAN
Professor Emeritus
College of Nursing
Wayne State University
Detroit, Michigan

Myra Levine†

Rozzano Locsin, RN, PhD
Professor
Christine E. Lynn College of Nursing
Florida Atlantic University
Boca Raton, Florida

Betty Neuman, RN, PhD, PLC, FAAN
Beverly, Ohio

Margaret Newman*
St. Paul, Minnesota

Florence Nightingale†

Dorothea E. Orem
Orem & Shields, Inc.
Savannah, Georgia

Ida Jean Orlando (Pelletier)*
Belmont, Massachusetts

Josephine Paterson*

Rosemarie Rizzo Parse, RN, PhD, FAAN
Founder and Editor, *Nursing Science Quarterly*
Professor and Niehoff Chair
Loyola University
Chicago, Illinois

Hildegard Peplau†

Marilyn E. Parker, RN, PhD, FAAN
Professor
Christine E. Lynn College of Nursing
Florida Atlantic University
Boca Raton, Florida

Marilyn Anne Ray, RN, PhD, CTN, CNAA
Professor
Christine E. Lynn College of Nursing
Florida Atlantic University
Boca Raton, Florida

Martha Rogers†

Sister Callista Roy, RN, PhD, FAAN
Professor of Nursing
Boston College
Boston, Massachusetts

Savina Schoenhofer, RN, PhD
Professor of Nursing
Alcorn State University
Natchez, Mississippi

Kristen Swanson, RN, PhD, FAAN
Professor
School of Nursing
University of Washington
Seattle, Washington

Jean Watson, PhD, RN, AHN–BC, FAAN
Distinguished Professor
Founder, Center for Human Caring
School of Nursing

University of Colorado Health Science Center
Denver, Colorado

Ernestine Wiedenbach†

Loretta Zderad*

†Deceased
*Retired

Contributing Authors

Patricia D. Aylward, RN, MSN
Manager, Training and Staff
    Development
Hospice of North Central Florida
Gainesville, Florida

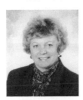

Sandra Schmidt Bunkers, RN, PhD, FAAN
Professor of Nursing
South Dakota State University
Brookings, South Dakota

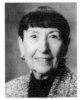

Nettie Birnbach, RN, EdD, FAAN
Professor Emeritus
College of Nursing
State University of New York at
    Brooklyn
Brooklyn, New York

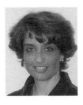

Debra A. Bournes, RN, PhD
Director of Nursing–New
    Knowledge and Innovation
University Health Network
Assistant Professor
University of Toronto
Toronto, Ontario, Canada

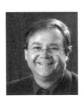

Howard Butcher, RN, PhD, APRN, BC
Assistant Professor
College of Nursing
University of Iowa
Iowa City, Iowa

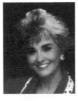

Marcia Dombro, RN, EdD
Chairperson, Continuing
    Professional/Community
    Education Alliance
Miami-Dade Community
    College
Miami, Florida

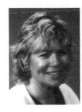

Lynne M. Hektor Dunphy, RN, PhD, FNP, CS
Professor
Christine E. Lynn College of
    Nursing
Florida Atlantic University
Boca Raton, Florida

Maureen Frey, RN, PhD
Nurse Researcher
Children's Hospital of Michigan
Detroit, Michigan

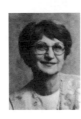

Theresa Gesse, RN, PhD
Professor
Founder and Director, Nurse
    Midwifery Program
School of Nursing
University of Miami
Miami, Florida

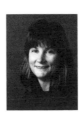

Shirley Countryman Gordon, RN, PhD
Associate Professor
Christine E. Lynn College of
    Nursing
Florida Atlantic University
Boca Raton, Florida

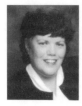

Bonnie Holaday, RN, DNS, FAAN
Professor of Nursing and in
   Institute of Family and
   Neighborhood Life
Clemson University
Clemson, South Carolina

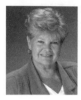

Marjorie Isenberg, RN, DNS, FAAN
Dean and Professor
College of Nursing
University of Arizona
Tuscon, Arizona

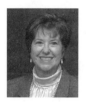

Mary Killeen, RN, PhD
Associate Professor
Department of Nursing
University of Michigan-Flint
Flint, Michigan

Susan Kleiman, PhD, RN, CS, NPP
Assistant Professor of Nursing
Lehman College
City University of New York
New York, New York

Danielle Linden, RN, MSN
Advanced Practice Nurse
Deerfield Beach, Florida

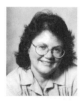

Violet Malinski, RN, PhD
Associate Professor
Hunter-Bellevue School of Nursing
City University of New York
New York, New York

Marilyn R. McFarland, RN, PhD
Adjunct Faculty
College of Nursing and Allied
   Health
Saginaw Valley State University
University Center, Michigan

Gail J. Mitchell, RN, PhD
Chief Nursing Officer
Sunnybrook Health Science Centre
Toronto, Ontario, Canada

Ann R. Peden, RN, DSN
Associate Professor
College of Nursing
University of Kentucky
Lexington, Kentucky

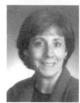

Margaret Dexheimer Pharris, RN, FAAN, PhD
Faculty, Adolescent Teaching
   Project
Assistant Director Sexual Assault
   Resource Service
School of Nursing
University of Minnesota
Minneapolis, Minnesota

Marguerite J. Purnell, PhD
Assistant Professor
Christine E. Lynn College of
   Nursing
Florida Atlantic University
Boca Raton, Florida

Maude Rittman, RN, PhD
Associate Chief of Nursing Service
   for Research
Gainesville Veteran's
   Administration Medical Center
Gainesville, Florida

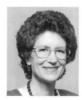

Karen Moore Schaeffer, RN, DNSc
Professor of Nursing
Temple University
College of Health Professions
Philadelphia, Pennsylvania

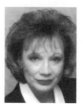

Christina Leibold Sieloff, RN, PhD
Assistant Professor
School of Nursing
Oakland University
Rochester, Michigan

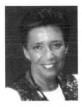

Theris A. Touhy, RN, ND, APRN, BC
Associate Professor
Christine E. Lynn College of
 Nursing
Florida Atlantic University
Boca Raton, Florida

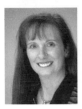

Marian C. Turkel, RN, PhD
Director of Professional Practice
 and Development
Northwestern Memorial Hospital
Faculty
University of Illinois at Chicago
College of Nursing
Chicago, Illinois

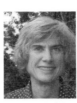

Terri Kaye Woodward, MSN
Holistic Clinical Nurse Specialist
The Children's Hospital
Denver, Colorado

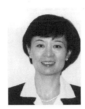

Lin Zhan, RN, PhD, FAAN
Professor and Director of the
 Nursing PhD Program
University of Massachusetts;
Lowell School of Health and
 Environment
Department of Nursing
Lowell, Massachusetts

Consultants

Catherine A. Andrews, PhD, RN
Assistant Professor
Edgewood College
Madison, Wisconsin

Sandy Forrest, PhD, RN
Department Chair and Professor
Mesa State College
Grand Junction, Colorado

Diana M.L. Newman, EdD, RN
Associate Professor
The University of Massachusetts Boston
Boston, Massachusetts

Martha Rogers, RN, MScN, EdD
Associate Professor and Associate Dean
York University
Toronto, Onatrio, Canada

Overview of Contents

SECTION I
Perspectives on Nursing Theory

An introduction to nursing theory includes: definitions of nursing theory, nursing theory and nursing knowledge, types of nursing theory, and nursing's need for theory. Choosing, analyzing, and evaluating nursing theory focuses on questions from practicing nurses about studying and using nursing theory, a guide for choosing a theory to study, and several frameworks for theory analysis and evaluation. A guide for the study of nursing theory for use in nursing practice is presented, along with questions for selecting theory for use in nursing administration and a chapter for evaluating nursing theory resources.

SECTION II
Evolution of Nursing Theory: Essential Influences

This section opens with a chapter on Florence Nightingale and a description of her profound influence on the discipline and practice of nursing. Subsequent chapters present major nursing theories that have both reflected and influenced nursing practice, education, research, and ongoing theory development in nursing during the last half of the twentieth century and into the new century.

SECTION III
Nursing Theory in Nursing Practice, Education, Research, and Administration

The major nursing theories in use today in the beginning of the twenty-first century are presented in this section. Most chapters about particular nursing theories are written by the theorists themselves. Some chapters are written by nurses with advanced knowledge about particular nursing theories; these authors have been acknowledged by specific theorists as experts in presenting their work. Each chapter also includes illustratrations of the use of the theory in nursing practice, research, education, or administration.

SECTION IV
Nursing Theory: Illustrating Processes of Development

This section includes four quite different chapters on processes and products of thinking about nursing theory and nursing practice. Each author writes about research and development of middle-range or nursing practice theory and about exploration of theory in the personal and professional contexts. The political and economic dimensions of one of the theories in contemporary nursing practice is illustrated.

INDEX

Contents

SECTION I

Perspectives on Nursing Theory

CHAPTER 1

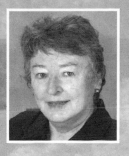

Marilyn E. Parker

Introduction to Nursing Theory

Marilyn E. Parker

$\mathcal{F}$lorence Nightingale taught us that nursing theories describe and explain what is and what is not nursing (Nightingale, 1859/1992). Today, knowledge development in nursing is taking place on several fronts, with a variety of scholarly approaches contributing to advances in the discipline. Nursing practice increasingly takes place in interdisciplinary community settings, and the form of nursing in acute care settings is rapidly changing. Various paradigms and value systems that express perspectives held by several groups within the discipline ground the knowledge and practice of nursing. Because the language of nursing is continually being formed and distinguished, it often seems confusing, as does any language that is new to the ears and eyes. Nurses who have active commitments to the work of the discipline, whether in nursing practice, research, education, or administration, play an essential role in the continuing development of nursing theory. This chapter offers an approach to understanding nursing theory within the context of nursing knowledge. It reviews the types of nursing theory and advances reasons why theory is so critical to nursing practice. The chapter closes with an invitation to share with contributing authors of this book their visions of nursing theory in the future.

Definitions of Nursing Theory

A *theory,* as a general term, is a notion or an idea that explains experience, interprets observation, describes relationships, and projects outcomes. Parsons (1949), often quoted by nursing theorists, wrote that theories help us know what we know and decide what we need to know. Theories are mental patterns or constructs created to help understand and find meaning from our experience, organize and articulate our knowing, and ask questions leading to new insights. As such, theories are

> *Theories are not discovered in nature but are human inventions.*

not discovered in nature but are human inventions. They are descriptions of our reflections, of what we observe, or of what we project and infer. For these reasons, theory and related terms have been defined and described in a number of ways according to individual experience and what is useful at the time. Theories, as reflections of understanding, guide our actions, help us set forth desired outcomes, and give evidence of what has been achieved. A theory, by traditional definition, is an organized, coherent set of concepts and their relationships to each other that offers descriptions, explanations, and predictions about phenomena.

Early writers about nursing theory brought definitions of theory from other disciplines to direct future work within nursing. Dickoff and James (1968, p. 198) define theory as a "conceptual system or framework invented for some purpose." Ellis (1968, p. 217) defined theory as "a coherent set of hypothetical, conceptual, and pragmatic principles forming a general frame of reference for a field of inquiry." McKay (1969, p. 394) asserted that theo-

ries are the capstone of scientific work and that the term refers to "logically interconnected sets of confirmed hypotheses." Barnum (1998, p. 1) later offers a more open definition of theory as a "construct that accounts for or organizes some phenomenon," and states simply that a nursing theory describes or explains nursing.

Definitions of theory emphasize various aspects of theory and demonstrate that even the conceptions of nursing theory are various and changing. Definitions of theory developed in recent years are more open and less structured than definitions created before the last decade. Not every nursing theory will fit every definition of what is a nursing theory. For purposes of nursing practice, a definition of nursing theory that has a focus on the meaning or possible impact of the theory on practice is desirable. The following definitions of theory are consistent with general ideas of theory in nursing practice, education, administration, or research.

- Theory is a set of concepts, definitions, and propositions that projects a systematic view of phenomena by designating specific interrelationships among concepts for purposes of describing, explaining, predicting, and/or controlling phenomena (Chinn & Jacobs, 1987, p. 71).
- Theory is a creative and rigorous structuring of ideas that projects a tentative, purposeful, and systematic view of phenomena (Chinn & Kramer, 2004, p. 268).
- Nursing theory is a conceptualization of some aspect of reality (invented or discovered) that pertains to nursing. The conceptualization is articulated for the purpose of describing, explaining, predicting, or prescribing nursing care (Meleis, 1997, p. 12).
- Nursing theory is an inductively and/or deductively derived collage of coherent, creative, and focused nursing phenomena that frame, give meaning to, and help explain specific and selective aspects of nursing research and practice (Silva, 1997, p. 55).

Nursing Theory in the Context of Nursing Knowledge

The notion of paradigm can be useful as a basis for understanding nursing knowledge. *Paradigm* is a global, general framework made up of assumptions about aspects of the discipline held by members to be essential in development of the discipline. The concept of paradigm comes from the work of Kuhn (1970, 1977), who used the term to describe models that guide scientific activity and knowledge development in disciplines. Kuhn set forth the view that science does not evolve as a smooth, regular, continuing path of knowledge development over time, but that there are periodic times of revolution when traditional thought is challenged by new ideas, and "paradigm shifts" occur. In addition, Kuhn's work has meaning for nursing and other practice disciplines because of his recognition that science is the work of a community of scholars in the context of society. Because paradigms are broad, shared perspectives held by members of the discipline, they are often called "worldviews." Paradigms and worldviews of nursing are subtle and powerful, permeating all aspects of the discipline and practice of nursing.

Kuhn's (1970, 1977) description of scientific development is particularly relevant to nursing today as new perspectives are being articulated, some traditional views are being strengthened, and some views are taking their places as part of our history.

> *As we continue to move away from the historical conception of nursing as a part of medical science, developments in the nursing discipline are directed by several new worldviews.*

As we continue to move away from the historical conception of nursing as a part of medical science, developments in the nursing discipline are directed by several new worldviews. Among these are fresh and innovative perspectives on person, nursing, and knowledge development. Changes in the nursing paradigm are being brought about by nursing scholars addressing disciplinary concerns based on values and beliefs about nursing as a human science, caring in nursing, and holistic nursing.

The literature offers additional ways to describe and understand nursing theory. Fawcett (1993, 2000) asserts that nursing theory is one component of a hierarchical structure of nursing knowledge development that includes metaparadigm, philosophy, conceptual models, nursing theory, and empirical indicators. These conceptual levels of knowledge development in nursing are interde-

pendent; each level of development is influenced by work at other levels. Walker and Avant (1995) describe the importance of relating theories that have been developed at these various levels of abstraction.

Theoretical work in nursing must be dynamic; that is, it must be continually in process and useful for the purposes and work of the discipline. It must be open to adapting and extending in order to guide nursing endeavors and to reflect development within nursing. Although there is diversity of opinion among nurses about terms used to describe theoretical development, the following discussion of types of theoretical development in nursing is offered as a context for further understanding nursing theory.

METAPARADIGM FOR NURSING

The metaparadigm for nursing is a framework for the discipline that sets forth the phenomena of interest and the propositions, principles, and methods of the discipline. The metaparadigm is very general and is intended to reflect agreement among members of the discipline about the field of nursing. This is the most abstract level of nursing knowledge and closely mirrors beliefs held about nursing. The metaparadigm offers a context for developing conceptual models and theories. Dialogue on the metaparadigm of nursing today is dynamic because of the range of considerations about what comprises the essence and form of nursing.

All nurses have some awareness of nursing's metaparadigm by virtue of being nurses. However, because the term may not be familiar, it offers no direct guidance for research and practice (Walker & Avant, 1995; Kim, 1997). Historically, the metaparadigm of nursing described concepts of person, environment, health, and nursing. Modifications and alternative concepts for this framework are being explored throughout the discipline (Fawcett, 2000). An example of alternative concepts is the work of Kim (1987, 1997), which sets forth four domains focusing on client, client-nurse encounters, practice, and environment. In recent years, increasing attention has been directed to the nature of nursing's relationship with the environment (Schuster & Brown, 1994; Kleffel, 1996). Newman, Sime, and Corcoran-Perry (1991, p. 3) propose that a single focus statement—"nursing is the study of caring in the human health experience"—guides the overall direction of the discipline. Reed (1995) challenges nurses to continue the dialogue about perspectives on knowledge development in the discipline. Higgins and Moore (2000) continue examination of levels of theoretical thinking in nursing and encourage recognition of the disciplinary strength of nursing.

NURSING PHILOSOPHY

Developments in the metaparadigm of nursing are accompanied by changes in statements of values and beliefs written as nursing philosophies. A philosophy comprises statements of enduring values and beliefs held by members of the discipline. These statements address the major concepts of the discipline, setting forth beliefs about what nursing is, how to think about and do nursing, the relationships of nursing, and the environment of nursing. Philosophical statements are practical guides for examining issues and clarifying priorities of the discipline. Nurses use philosophical statements to examine compatibility among personal, professional, organizational, and societal beliefs and values.

CONCEPTUAL MODELS OF NURSING

Conceptual models are sets of general concepts and propositions that provide perspectives on the major concepts of the metaparadigm, such as person, health and well-being, and the environment. Conceptual models also reflect sets of values and beliefs, as in philosophical statements and preferences for practice and research approaches. Fawcett (1993, 2000) points out that direction for research must be described as part of the conceptual model in order to guide development and testing of nursing theories. Conceptual models are less abstract than the metaparadigm and more abstract than theories, offering guidance (not distinct direction) to nursing endeavors. Conceptual models may also be called "conceptual frameworks" or "systems."

NURSING THEORIES

In general, nursing theory describes and explains the phenomena of interest to nursing in a systematic way in order to provide understanding for use in nursing practice and research. Theories are less abstract than conceptual models or systems, although they vary in scope and levels of abstraction. Grand theories of nursing are those general constructions about the nature and goals of nursing. Middle-range nursing theories point to practice and are useful in a defined set of nursing situations. Theories developed at the middle range include specific concepts and are less abstract than grand theories. At the next level, nursing practice theories address issues and questions in a particular practice setting in which nursing provides care for a specific population. In addition to considering the scope and levels of abstraction of nursing theories, they are also sometimes described by the content or focus of the theory, such as health promotion and caring and holistic nursing theories.

Types of Nursing Theory

Nursing theories have been organized into categories and types. George (2001) sets forth categories of theories according to the orientation of the theorist: nursing problems, interactions, general systems, and energy fields. Another view is that nursing theory forms a continuum of grand theories at one end and theories focused on practice at the other (Walker & Avant, 1995; Fitzpatrick, 1997). Meleis (1997) describes types of nursing theory based on their levels of abstraction and goal orientation. Barnum (1998) divides theories into those that *describe* and those that *explain* nursing phenomena. Types of nursing theories generally include grand theory, middle-range theory, and practice theory. These will be described here.

GRAND NURSING THEORY

Grand theories have the broadest scope and present general concepts and propositions. Theories at this level may both reflect and provide insights useful for practice but are not designed for empirical testing. This limits the use of grand theories for directing, explaining, and predicting nursing in particular situations. Theories at this level are intended to be pertinent to all instances of nursing.

Development of grand theories resulted from the deliberate effort of committed scholars who have engaged in thoughtful reflection on nursing practice and knowledge and on the many contexts of nursing over time. Nursing theorists who have worked at this level have had insights guided by nursing and related metaparadigms and sometimes have experienced leaps of knowing grounded in these insights. Although there is debate about which nursing theories are grand in scope, the following are usually considered to be at this level: Leininger's Theory of Culture Care Diversity and Universality, Newman's Theory of Health as Expanding Consciousness, Rogers' Science of Unitary Human Beings, Orem's Self-Care Deficit Nursing Theory, and Parse's Theory of Human Becoming. These theories are presented in the third section of this book.

MIDDLE-RANGE NURSING THEORY

Middle-range theory was proposed by Robert Merton (1968) in the field of sociology to provide theories that are both broad enough to be useful in complex situations and appropriate for empirical testing. Nursing scholars proposed using this level of theory because of the difficulty in testing grand theory (Jacox, 1974). Middle-range theories are more narrow in scope than grand theories and offer an effective bridge between grand theories and nursing practice. They present concepts and propositions at a lower level of abstraction and hold great promise for increasing theory-based research and nursing practice strategies.

The literature presents a growing number of reports of nurses' experiences of developing and using middle-range theory. A wide range of nursing practice situations and nursing issues are being addressed by middle-range theory. The methods used for developing middle-range theories are many and represent some of the most exciting work being published in nursing today. Many of these new theories are built on content from related disciplines and are brought into nursing practice and research (Lenz, Suppe, Gift, Pugh, & Milligan, 1995; Polk, 1997; Eakes, Burke, & Hainsworth, 1998). The literature also offers middle-range nursing theories that are directly related to grand theories of nursing (Olson & Hanchett, 1997; Ducharme, Ricard, Duquette, Levesque, & Lachance, 1998; Dunn, 2004). Reports of nursing theory developed at this level include implications for instrument development, theory testing through research, and nursing practice strategies. Illustrations of the process and

product of nursing theory developed at the middle range are presented in Section IV of this book.

NURSING PRACTICE THEORY

Nursing practice theory has the most limited scope and level of abstraction and is developed for use within a specific range of nursing situations. Theories developed at this level have a more direct impact on nursing practice than do theories that are more abstract. Nursing practice theories provide frameworks for nursing interventions and predict outcomes and the impact of nursing practice. At the same time, nursing questions, actions, and procedures may be described or developed as nursing practice theories. Ideally, nursing practice theories are interrelated with concepts from middle-range theories or may be deduced from theories at the middle range. Practice theories should also reflect concepts and propositions of more abstract levels of nursing theory. Theory developed at this level is also termed prescriptive theory (Dickoff, James, & Wiedenbach, 1968; Crowley, 1968), situation-specific theory (Meleis, 1997), and micro theory (Chinn & Kramer, 2004).

The day-to-day experience of nurses is a major source of nursing practice theory. The depth and complexity of nursing practice may be fully appreciated as nursing phenomena and relations among aspects of particular nursing situations are described and explained. Benner (1984) demon-

> *The day-to-day experience of nurses is a major source of nursing practice theory.*

strated that dialogue with expert nurses in practice is fruitful for discovery and development of practice theory. Research findings on various nursing problems offer data to develop nursing practice theories as nursing engages in research-based development of theory and practice. Nursing practice theory has been articulated using multiple ways of knowing through reflective practice (Johns & Freshwater, 1998). The process includes quiet reflection on practice, remembering and noting features of nursing situations, attending to one's own feelings, reevaluating the experience, and integrating new knowing with other experience (Gray & Forsstrom, 1991).

Nursing's Need for Nursing Theory

Nursing theories address the phenomena of interest to nursing, including the focus of nursing; the person, group, or population nursed; the nurse; the relationship of nurse and nursed; and the hoped-for goal or purposes of nursing. Based on strongly

> *Theories are patterns that guide the thinking about, being, and doing of nursing.*

held values and beliefs about nursing, and within contexts of various worldviews, theories are patterns that guide the thinking about, being, and doing of nursing. They provide structure for developing, evaluating, and using nursing scholarship and for extending and refining nursing knowledge through research. Nursing theories either implicitly or explicitly direct all avenues of nursing, including nursing education and administration. Nursing theories provide concepts and designs that define the place of nursing in health and illness care. Through theories, nurses are offered perspectives for relating with professionals from other disciplines who join with nurses to provide human services. Nursing has great expectations of its theories. At the same time, theories must provide structure and substance to ground the practice and scholarship of nursing and also be flexible and dynamic to keep pace with the growth and changes in the discipline and practice of nursing.

NURSING IS A DISCIPLINE

Nursing has taken its place as a discipline of knowledge that includes networks of facts, concepts, and approaches to inquiry. The discipline of nursing is also a community of scholars, including nurses in all nursing venues, who share a commitment to values, concepts, and processes to guide the

> *The discipline of nursing is a community of scholars, including nurses in all venues, where nursing occurs.*

thought and work of the discipline. The classic work of King and Brownell (1976) is consistent with thinking of nursing scholars about the discipline of nursing (Donaldson & Crowley, 1978; Meleis, 1977). These authors have set forth attributes of all disciplines. These have particular relevance for nursing and illustrate the need for nursing theory. The attributes of King and Brownell are used as a framework to address the need of the discipline for nursing theory. Each of the attributes is described next, from the perspective of the nursing discipline.

Expression of Human Imagination

Nursing theory is dependent on the imagination and questioning of nurses in practice and on their creativity to bring ideas of nursing theory into practice. In order to remain dynamic and useful, our discipline requires openness to new ideas and innovative approaches that grow out of members' reflections and insights.

Domain

A discipline of knowledge and professional practice must be clearly defined by statements of the *domain*—the theoretical and practical boundaries of that discipline and practice. The domain of nursing includes the phenomena of interest, problems to be addressed, main content and methods used, and roles required of the discipline's members (Kim, 1997; Meleis, 1997). The processes and practices claimed by members of the discipline community grow out of these domain statements. Nursing theories containing descriptions of nursing's domain may incorporate a statement of the discipline's focus. The focus may be set in statements about human, social, and ecological concerns addressed by nursing. The focus of the nursing discipline is a clear statement of social mandate and service used to direct the study and practice of nursing (Newman, Sime, & Corcoran-Perry, 1991).

Nightingale (1859/1992) may have led the call for domain and focus by distinguishing nursing from medicine and other services. Later, Donaldson and Crowley (1978) stated that a discipline has a special way of viewing phenomena and a distinct perspective that defines the work of the discipline. The call for clarity of focus continues in the current environment of nursing practice (Parse, 1997). Nursing theories set forth focus statements or definitions of the discipline and practice of nursing and direct thought and action to fulfill the unique purposes of nursing. This enhances autonomy, and accountability and responsibility are defined and supported. The domain of nursing is also called the "metaparadigm of nursing," as described in the previous section of this chapter.

Syntactical and Conceptual Structures

Syntactical and conceptual structures are essential to the discipline and are inherent in each of the nursing theories. The conceptual structure delineates the proper concerns of nursing, guides what is to be studied, and clarifies accepted ways of knowing and using content of the discipline. This structure is grounded in the metaparadigm and philosophies of nursing. The conceptual structure relates concepts within nursing theories, and it is from this structure that we learn what is and what is not nursing. The syntactical structures help nurses and other professionals understand the talents, skills, and abilities that must be developed within the community. This structure directs descriptions of data needed from research as well as evidence required to demonstrate the impact of nursing practice.

In addition, these structures guide nursing's use of knowledge, research, and practice approaches developed by related disciplines. It is only by being thoroughly grounded in the discipline's concepts, substance, and modes of inquiry that the boundaries of the discipline, however tentative, can be understood and possibilities for creativity across interdisciplinary borders can be created and explored.

Specialized Language and Symbols

As nursing theory has evolved, so has the need for concepts, language, and forms of data that reflect new ways of thinking and knowing in nursing. The complex concepts used in nursing scholarship and practice require language that can be used and understood. The language of nursing theory facilitates communication among members of the discipline. Expert knowledge of the discipline is often required for full understanding of the meaning of special terms.

Heritage of Literature and Networks of Communication

This attribute calls attention to the array of books, periodicals, artifacts, and aesthetic expressions, as well as audio, visual, and electronic media that have developed over centuries to communicate the nature and development of nursing. Conferences and other forums on every aspect of nursing and for nurses of all interests occur frequently throughout the world. Nursing organizations and societies also provide critical communication links. Nursing theories form the bases for many of the major contributions to the literature, conferences, societies, and other communication networks of the nursing discipline.

Tradition

The tradition and history of the nursing discipline is evident in study of nursing theories that have been developed over time. There is recognition that theories most useful today often have threads of connection with theoretical developments of past years. For example, many theorists have acknowledged the influence of Florence Nightingale and have acclaimed her leadership in influencing nursing theories of today. In addition, nursing has a rich heritage of practice. Nursing's practical experience and knowledge have been shared, transformed into content of the discipline, and are evident in the work of many nursing theorists (Gray & Pratt, 1991).

Values and Beliefs

Nursing has distinctive views of persons and strong commitments to compassionate and knowledgeable care of persons through nursing. Nurses often express their love and passion for nursing. Nurses in small groups and in larger nursing organizations express values, hopes, and dreams for the future of their discipline and offer recognition of and appreciation for achievements in the field. The statements of values and beliefs are expressed in the philosophies of nursing that are essential underpinnings of theoretical developments in the discipline.

Systems of Education

Nursing holds the stature and place of a discipline of knowledge and professional practice within institutions of higher education because of the grounding of articulated nursing theories that have set forth the unique contribution of nursing to human affairs. A distinguishing mark of any discipline is the education of future and current members of the community. Nursing theories, by setting directions for the substance and methods of inquiry for the discipline, provide the basis for nursing education and often the framework to organize nursing curricula.

NURSING IS A PROFESSIONAL PRACTICE

Closely aligned with attributes of nursing as a discipline previously described is consideration of nursing as a professional practice. Professional practice includes clinical scholarship and processes of nursing persons, groups, and populations who need the special human service that is nursing. The major reason for structuring and advancing nursing knowledge is for the sake of nursing practice.

> *The major reason for structuring and advancing nursing knowledge is for the sake of nursing practice.*

The primary purpose of nursing theories is to further the development and understanding of nursing practice. Theory-based research is needed in order to explain and predict nursing outcomes essential to the delivery of nursing care that is both humane and cost-effective (Gioiella, 1996). Because nursing theory exists to improve practice, the test of nursing theory is a test of its usefulness in professional practice (Fitzpatrick, 1997; Colley, 2003). The work of nursing theory is moving from academia into the realm of nursing practice. Chapters in the remaining sections of this book highlight use of nursing theories in nursing practice.

Nursing practice is both the source of and goal for nursing theory. From the viewpoint of practice, Gray and Forsstrom (1991) suggest that through use of theory, nurses find different ways of looking at and assessing phenomena, have rationale for their practice, and have criteria for evaluating outcomes. Recent studies reported in the literature affirm the importance of use of nursing theory to guide practice (Baker, 1997; Olson & Hanchett, 1997; Barrett, 1998; O'Neill & Kenny, 1998; Whitener, Cox, & Maglich, 1998). Further, these studies illustrate that nursing theory can stimulate creative thinking, facilitate communication, and clarify purposes and relationships of practice. The practicing nurse has an ethical responsibility to use the discipline's theoretical knowledge base, just as it is the nurse scholar's ethical responsibility to develop the knowledge base specific to nursing practice (Cody, 1997, 2003).

Integral to both the professional practice of nursing and nursing theory is the use of empirical indicators. These are developed to meet demands of clinical decision making in the context of rapidly changing needs for nursing and the knowledge required for the nursing practice. These indicators include procedures, tools, and instruments to determine the impact of nursing practice and are essential to research and management of outcomes of practice (Jennings & Staggers, 1998). Resulting data form the basis for improving quality of nursing care and influencing health-care policy. Empirical indicators, grounded carefully in nursing concepts, provide clear demonstration of the utility of nursing theory in practice, research, administration, and other nursing endeavors (Hart & Foster, 1998; Allison & McLaughlin-Renpenning, 1999). Fawcett (2000) has placed empirical indicators in the hierarchy of nursing knowledge and relates them to nursing theory when they are an outgrowth of particular aspects of nursing theories.

Meeting the challenges of systems of care delivery and interdisciplinary work demands practice from a theoretical perspective. Nursing's disciplinary focus is essential within an interdisciplinary environment (Allison & McLaughlin-Renpenning, 1999). Nursing actions reflect nursing concepts and thought. Careful, reflective, and critical thinking is the hallmark of expert nursing, and nursing theories should undergird these processes. Appreciation and use of nursing theory offer opportunity for successful collaboration with related disciplines and practices, and provide definition for nursing's overall contribution to health care. Nurses must know what they are doing, why they are doing what they are doing, what may be the range of outcomes of nursing, and indicators for measuring nursing's impact. These nursing theoretical frameworks serve in powerful ways as guides for articulating, reporting, and recording nursing thought and action.

One of the assertions referred to most often in the nursing theory literature is that theory is given birth in nursing practice and, following examination and refinement through research, must be returned to practice (Dickoff, James, & Wiedenbach, 1968). Within nursing as a practice discipline, nursing theory is stimulated by questions and curiosities arising from nursing practice. Development of nursing knowledge is a result of theory-based nursing inquiry. The circle continues as data, conclusions, and recommendations of nursing research are evaluated and developed for use in practice.

Nursing theory must be seen as practical and useful to practice, and the insights of practice must in turn continue to enrich nursing theory.

Nursing Theory and the Future

Nursing theory in the future will be more fully integrated with all domains of the discipline and practice of nursing. New and expanded nursing specialties, such as nursing informatics, call for development and use of nursing theory (Effken, 2003). New, more open and inclusive ways to theorize about nursing will be developed. These new ways will acknowledge the history and traditions of nursing but will move nursing forward into new realms of thinking and being. Gray and Pratt (1991, p. 454) project that nursing scholars will continue to develop theories at all levels of abstraction and that theories will be increasingly interdependent with other disciplines such as politics, economics, and aesthetics. These authors expect a continuing emphasis on unifying theory and practice that will contribute to the validation of the nursing discipline. Reed (1995) notes the "ground shifting" with reforming of philosophies of nursing science and calls for a more open philosophy, grounded in nursing's values, which connects science, philosophy, and practice. Theorists will work in groups to develop knowledge in an area of concern to nursing, and these phenomena of interest, rather than the name of the author, will define the theory (Meleis, 1992). Newman (2003) calls for a future in which we transcend competition and boundaries that have been constructed between nursing theories and instead appreciate the links among theories, thus moving toward a fuller, more inclusive and richer understanding of nursing knowledge.

Nursing's philosophies and theories must increasingly reflect nursing's values for understanding, respect, and commitment to health beliefs and practices of cultures throughout the world. It is im-

> *It is important to question to what extent theories developed and used in one major culture are appropriate for use in other cultures.*

portant to question to what extent theories developed and used in one major culture are appropriate for use in other cultures. To what extent must nurs-

ing theory be relevant in multicultural contexts? Despite efforts of many international scholarly societies, how relevant are our nursing theories for the global community? Can nursing theories inform us how to stand with and learn from peoples of the world? Can we learn from nursing theory how to come to know those we nurse, how to be with them, to truly listen and hear? Can these questions be recognized as appropriate for scholarly work and practice for graduate students in nursing? Will these issues offer direction for studies of doctoral students? If so, nursing theory will offer new ways to inform nurses for humane leadership in national and global health policy.

Perspectives of various time worlds in relation to present nursing concerns were described by Schoenhofer (1994). Faye G. Abdellah, one of nursing's finest international leaders, offers the advice that we must maintain focus on those we nurse (McAuliffe, 1998). Abdellah notes that nurses in other countries have often developed their systems of education, practice, and research based on learning from our mistakes. She further proposes an international electronic "think tank" for nurses around the globe to dialogue about nursing (McAuliffe, 1998). Such opportunities could lead nurses to truly listen, learn, and adapt theoretical perspectives to accommodate cultural variations. We must somehow come to appreciate the essence and beauty of nursing, just as Nightingale knew it to be. Perhaps it will be realized that the essence of nursing is universal and that only the ways of expressing nursing vary.

SUMMARY

One challenge of nursing theory is the perspective that theory is always in the process of developing and that, at the same time, it is useful for the purposes and work of the discipline. This may be seen as ambiguous or as full of possibilities. Continuing students of the discipline are required to study and know the basis for their contributions to nursing and to those we serve, while at the same time be open to new ways of thinking, knowing, and being in nursing. Exploring structures of nursing knowledge and understanding the nature of nursing as a discipline of knowledge and professional practice provides a frame of reference to clarify nursing theory. The wise study and use of nursing theory can be a helpful companion through the unfolding of this new millennium.

References

Allison, S. E., & McLaughlin-Renpenning, K. E. (1999). *Nursing administration in the 21st century: A self-care theory approach.* Thousand Oaks, CA: Sage Publications.

Baker, C. (1997). Cultural relativism and cultural diversity: Implications for nursing practice. *Advances in Nursing Science, 20*(1), 3–11.

Barnum, B. S. (1998). *Nursing theory: Analysis, application, evaluation* (5th ed.). Philadelphia: Lippincott.

Barrett, E. A. (1998). A Rogerian practice methodology for health patterning. *Nursing Science Quarterly, 11*(4), 136–138.

Benner, P. (1984). *From novice to expert: Excellence and power in clinical nursing practice.* New York: Addison-Wesley.

Chinn, P. (1994). *Developing substance: Mid-range theory in nursing.* Gaithersburg, MD: Aspen Publications.

Chinn, P., & Jacobs, M. (1987). *Theory and nursing: A systematic approach.* St. Louis: C. V. Mosby.

Chinn, P., & Kramer, M. (2004). *Integrated knowledge development in nursing.* St. Louis: C. V. Mosby.

Cody, W. K. (1997). Of tombstones, milestones, and gemstones: A retrospective and prospective on nursing theory. *Nursing Science Quarterly, 10*(1), 3–5.

Cody, W. K. (2003). Nursing theory as a guide to practice. *Nursing Science Quarterly, 16*(3), 225–231.

Colley, S. (2003). Nursing theory: Its importance to practice. *Nursing Standard, 17*(56), 33–37.

Crowley, D. (1968). Perspectives of pure science. *Nursing Research, 17*(6), 497–501.

Dickoff, J., & James, P. (1968). A theory of theories: A position paper. *Nursing Research, 17*(3), 197–203.

Dickoff, J., James, P., & Wiedenbach, E. (1968). Theory in a practice discipline. *Nursing Research, 17*(5), 415–435.

Donaldson, S. K., & Crowley, D. M. (1978). The discipline of nursing. *Nursing Outlook, 26*(2), 113–120.

Ducharme, F., Ricard, N., Duquette, A., Levesque, L., & Lachance, L. (1998). Empirical testing of a longitudinal model derived from the Roy Adaptation Model. *Nursing Science Quarterly, 11*(4), 149–159.

Dunn, K. S. (2004). Toward a middle-range theory of adaptation to chronic pain. *Nursing Science Quarterly, 17*(1), 78–84.

Eakes, G., Burke, M., & Hainsworth, M. (1998). Middle-range theory of chronic sorrow. *Image: Journal of Nursing Scholarship, 30*(2), 179–184.

Effken, J. A. (2003). An organizing framework for nursing informatics research. *Computers Informatics Nursing, 21*(6), 316–325.

Ellis, R. (1968). Characteristics of significant theories. *Nursing Research, 17*(3), 217–222.

Fawcett, J. (1993). *Analysis and evaluation of nursing theory.* Philadelphia: F. A. Davis Company.

Fawcett, J. (1999). *The relationship of theory and research* (2nd ed.). Philadelphia: F. A. Davis Company.

Fawcett, J. (2000). *Analysis and evaluation of contemporary nursing knowledge: Nursing models and nursing theories.* Philadelphia: F. A. Davis Company.

Fitzpatrick, J. (1997). Nursing theory and metatheory. In King, I., & Fawcett, J. (Eds.), *The language of nursing theory and metatheory.* Indianapolis, IN: Center Nursing Press.

George, J. (2001). *Nursing theories: The base for professional nursing practice.* Norwalk, CT: Appleton & Lange.

Gioiella, E. C. (1996). The importance of theory-guided research and practice in the changing health care scene. *Nursing Science Quarterly, 9*(2), 47.

Gray, J., & Forsstrom, S. (1991). Generating theory for practice: The reflective technique. In Gray, J., & Pratt, R. (Eds.). (1991). *Towards a discipline of nursing.* Melbourne: Churchill Livingstone.

Gray, J., & Pratt, R. (Eds.). (1991). *Towards a discipline of nursing.* Melbourne: Churchill Livingstone.

Hart, M., & Foster, S. (1998). Self-care agency in two groups of pregnant women. *Nursing Science Quarterly, 11*(4), 167–171.

Higgins, P. A., & Moore, S. M. (2000). Levels of theoretical thinking in nursing. *Nursing Outlook, 48*(4), 179–183.

Jacox, A. (1974). Theory construction in nursing: An overview. *Nursing Research, 23*(1), 4–13.

Jennings, B. M., & Staggers, N. (1998). The language of outcomes. *Advances in Nursing Science, 20*(4), 72–80.

Johns, C., & Freshwater, D. (1998). *Transforming nursing through reflective practice.* London: Oxford Science Ltd.

Kim, H. (1987). Structuring the nursing knowledge system: A typology of four domains. *Scholarly Inquiry for Nursing Practice: An International Journal, 1*(1), 99–110.

Kim, H. (1997). Terminology in structuring and developing nursing knowledge. In King, I., & Fawcett, J. (Eds.), *The language of nursing theory and metatheory.* Indianapolis, IN: Center Nursing Press.

King, A. R., & Brownell, J. A. (1976). *The curriculum and the disciplines of knowledge.* Huntington, NY: Robert E. Krieger Pub. Co.

Kleffel, D. (1996). Environmental paradigms: Moving toward an ecocentric perspective. *Advances in Nursing Science, 18*(4), 1–10.

Kuhn, T. (1970). *The structure of scientific revolutions* (2nd ed.). Chicago: University of Chicago Press.

Kuhn, T. (1977). *The essential tension: Selected studies in scientific tradition and change.* Chicago: University of Chicago Press.

Lenz, E., Suppe, F., Gift, A., Pugh, L., & Milligan, R. (1995). Collaborative development of middle-range theories: Toward a theory of unpleasant symptoms. *Advances in Nursing Science, 17*(3), 1–13.

McAuliffe, M. (1998). Interview with Faye G. Abdellah on nursing research and health policy. *Image: Journal of Nursing Scholarship, 30*(3), 215–219.

McKay, R. (1969). Theories, models and systems for nursing. *Nursing Research, 18*(5), 393–399.

Meleis, A. (1992). Directions for nursing theory development in the 21st century. *Nursing Science Quarterly, 5,* 112–117.

Meleis, A. (1997). *Theoretical nursing: Development and progress.* Philadelphia: Lippincott.

Merton, R. (1968). *Social theory and social structure.* New York: The Free Press.

Newman, M. (2003). A world of no boundaries. *Advances in Nursing Science, 26*(4), 240–245.

Newman, M., Sime, A., & Corcoran-Perry, S. (1991). The focus of the discipline of nursing. *Advances in Nursing Science, 14*(1), 1–6.

Nightingale, F. (1859/1992). *Notes on nursing: What it is and what it is not.* Philadelphia: Lippincott.

Olson, J., & Hanchett, E. (1997). Nurse-expressed empathy, patient outcomes, and development of a middle-range theory. *Image: Journal of Nursing Scholarship, 29*(1), 71–76.

O'Neill, D. P., & Kenny, E. K. (1998). Spirituality and chronic illness. *Image: Journal of Nursing Scholarship, 30*(3), 275–280.

Parse, R. (1997). Nursing and medicine: Two different disciplines. *Nursing Science Quarterly, 6*(3), 109.

Parsons, T. (1949). *Structure of social action.* Glencoe, IL: The Free Press.

Polk, L. (1997). Toward a middle-range theory of resilience. *Advances in Nursing Science, 19*(3), 1–13.

Reed, P. (1995). A treatise on nursing knowledge development for the 21st century: Beyond postmodernism. *Advances in Nursing Science, 17*(3), 70–84.

Schoenhofer, S. (1994). Transforming visions for nursing in the timeworld of *Einstein's Dreams. Advances in Nursing Science, 16*(4), 1–8.

Schuster, E., & Brown, C. (1994). *Exploring our environmental connections.* New York: National League for Nursing.

Silva, M. (1997). Philosophy, theory, and research in nursing: A linguistic journey to nursing practice. In King, I., & Fawcett, J. (Eds.), *The language of nursing theory and metatheory.* Indianapolis, IN: Center Nursing Press.

Walker, L., & Avant, K. (1995). *Strategies for theory construction in nursing.* Norwalk, CT: Appleton-Century-Crofts.

Whitener, L. M., Cox, K. R., & Maglich, S. A. (1998). Use of theory to guide nurses in the design of health messages for children. *Advances in Nursing Science, 20*(3), 21–35.

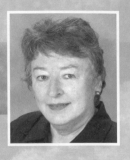

CHAPTER 2

Marilyn E. Parker

Studying Nursing Theory: Choosing, Analyzing, Evaluating

Marilyn E. Parker

$\mathcal{T}$he primary purpose for nursing theory is to advance the discipline and professional practice of nursing. One of the most urgent issues facing the

> *One of the most urgent issues facing the discipline of nursing is the artificial separation of nursing theory and practice.*

discipline of nursing is the artificial separation of nursing theory and practice. Nursing can no longer afford to see these endeavors as disconnected, belonging separately to either scholars or practitioners. The examination and use of nursing theories are essential for closing the gap between nursing theory and nursing practice. Nurses in practice have a responsibility to study and value nursing theories, just as nursing theory scholars must understand and appreciate the day-to-day practice of nursing.

When practicing nurses and nurse scholars work together, the discipline and practice of nursing benefit, and nursing service to our clients is enhanced. Examples in this book are plentiful as use of nursing theories in nursing practice is described and theory-based research to improve practice is highlighted. In addition, many of the nursing theorists in this book developed or refined their theories based on dialogue with nurses who shared descriptions of their practice. Examples from each section of this book include Ernestine Wiedenbach, Dorothea Orem, and Marilyn Ray.

The need to bridge the gap between nursing theory and practice is highlighted by considering a brief encounter during a question period at a conference. A nurse in practice, reflecting her experience, asked a nurse theorist, "What is the meaning of this theory to my practice? I'm in the real world! I want to connect—but how can connections be made between your ideas and my reality?" The nurse theorist responded by describing the essential values and assumptions of her theory. The nurse said, "Yes, I know what you are talking about. I just didn't know I knew it and I need help to use it in my practice" (Parker, 1993, p. 4). To remain current in the discipline, all nurses must be continuing students, must join in community to advance nursing knowledge and practice, and must accept their obligations to perform an ongoing investigation of nursing theories. Today, agencies that employ nurses are increasingly receiving recognition when

they acknowledge a nursing theory as a guiding framework for nursing practice. This provides excellent opportunity for nurses in practice and in administration to study, review, and evaluate nursing theories for use in practice. Communicating these reviews with the nursing theorists would be useful as a way to initiate dialogue among nurses and to form new bridges between the theory and practice of nursing.

This chapter discusses evaluating and selecting nursing theories for use in nursing: practice, education, administration, research, and development. Methods of analysis and evaluation of nursing theory set forth in the literature are presented. Although nursing theory is essential for all nursing, the main focus of theory analysis and evaluation in this chapter is the use of nursing theories in nursing practice. The chapter begins with responses to the questions: Why study nursing theory? What does the practicing nurse want from nursing theory?

Reasons for Studying Nursing Theory

Nursing practice is essential for developing, testing, and refining nursing theory. The everyday practice of nursing enriches nursing theory. When nurses are thinking about nursing, their ideas are about the content and structure of the discipline of nursing. Even if nurses do not conceptualize them in this way, their ideas are about nursing theory. The development of many nursing theories has been enhanced by reflection and dialogue about actual nursing situations. We might consider that as aspects of nursing theories are explored and refined in the day-to-day practice of nursing. Creative

> *Creative nursing practice is the direct result of ongoing theory-based thinking, decision making, and action of nurses.*

nursing practice is the direct result of ongoing theory-based thinking, decision making, and action of nurses. Nursing practice must continue to contribute to thinking and theorizing in nursing, just as nursing theory must be used to advance practice.

Nursing practice and nursing theory are guided by the same abiding values and beliefs. Nursing practice is guided by enduring values and beliefs as well as by knowledge held by individual nurses.

These values, beliefs, and knowledge echo those held by other nurses in the discipline, including nurse scholars and those who study and write about nursing's metaparadigm, philosophies, and theories. In addition, nursing theorists and nurses in practice think about and work with the same phenomena, including the person nursed, the actions and relationships in the nursing situation, and the context of nursing.

Many nurses practice according to ideas and directions from other disciplines, such as medicine, psychology, and public health. Historically, this is not uncommon to nursing and is deeply ingrained in the medical system, as well as in many settings in which nurses practice today. The depth and scope of the practice of nurses who follow notions about nursing held by other disciplines are limited to practices understood and accepted by those disciplines. Nurses who learn to practice from nursing perspectives are awakened to the challenges and opportunities of practicing nursing more fully and with a greater sense of autonomy, respect, and satisfaction for themselves and those they nurse. Nurses who practice from a nursing perspective approach clients and families in ways unique to nursing, they ask questions and receive and process information about needs for nursing differently, and they create nursing responses that are more wholistic and client-focused. These nurses learn to reframe their thinking about nursing knowledge and practice and are then able to bring knowledge from other disciplines into their practice—not to direct their practice, but in order to meet goals of nursing.

Nurses who understand nursing's theoretical base are free to see beyond immediate facts and delivery systems and are able to choose to bring the full range of health sciences and technologies into their practice. Nurses who study nursing theory realize that although no group actually owns ideas, disciplines do claim ideas for their use. In the same way, no group actually owns techniques, though disciplines do claim them for their practice. For example, before World War II, nurses rarely took blood pressure readings and did not give intramuscular injections. This was not because nurses were unable, but because they did not claim the use of these techniques to facilitate their nursing. Such a realization can also lead to understanding that the things nurses do that are often called nursing are not nursing at all. The techniques used by nurses, such as taking blood pressure readings and giving injections, are actually activities that give the nurse access to persons for nursing. Nursing theories inform the nurse about what nursing is and guide the use of other ideas and techniques for nursing purposes.

If nursing theory is to be useful—or practical—it must be brought into practice. At the same time, nurses can be guided by nursing theory in a full range of nursing situations. Nursing theory can change nursing practice: It provides direction for new ways of being present with clients, helps nurses realize ways of expressing caring, and provides approaches to understanding needs for nursing and designing care to address these needs. Chapters of this book affirm the use of nursing theory in practice and the study and assessment of theory for ultimate use in practice.

Questions from Practicing Nurses about Using Nursing Theory

Study of nursing theory may either precede or follow selection of a nursing theory for use in nursing practice. Analysis and evaluation of nursing theory are key ways to study theory. These activities are demanding and deserve the full commitment of nurses who undertake the work. Because it is understood that study of nursing theory is not a simple, short-term endeavor, nurses often question doing such work. The following questions about studying and using nursing theory have been collected from many conversations with nurses about nursing theory. These queries also identify specific issues that are important to nurses who consider study of nursing theory.

MY NURSING PRACTICE

- Does this theory reflect nursing practice as I know it? Can it be understood in relation to my nursing practice? Will it support what I believe to be excellent nursing practice?
- Is the theory specific to my area of nursing? Can the language of the theory help me explain, plan, and evaluate my nursing? Will I be able to use the terms to communicate with others?
- Can this theory be considered in relation to a wide range of nursing situations? How does it relate to more general views of nursing people in other settings?

- Will my study and use of this theory support nursing in my interdisciplinary setting?
- Will those from other disciplines be able to understand, facilitating cooperation?
- Will my work meet the expectations of patients and others? Will other nurses find my work helpful and challenging?

MY PERSONAL INTERESTS, ABILITIES, AND EXPERIENCES

- Is the study of nursing theories in keeping with my talents, interests, and goals? Is this something I want to do?
- Will I be stimulated by thinking about and trying to use this theory? Will my study of nursing be enhanced by use of this theory?
- What will it be like to think about nursing theory in nursing practice?
- Will my work with nursing theory be worth the effort?

RESOURCES AND SUPPORT

- Will this be useful to me outside the classroom?
- What resources will I need to understand more fully the terms of the theory?
- Will I be able to find the support I need to study and use the theory in my practice?

THE THEORIST, EVIDENCE, AND OPINION

- Who is the author of this theory? What is the background of nursing education and experience brought to this work by the theorist? Is the author an authoritative nursing scholar?
- How is the theorist's background of nursing education and experience brought to this work?
- What is the evidence that use of the theory may lead to improved nursing care? Has the theory been useful to guide nursing organizations and administrations? What about influencing nursing and health-care policy?
- What is the evidence that this nursing theory has led to nursing research, including questions and methods of inquiry? Did the theory grow out of nursing research reports? Out of nursing practice issues and problems?
- Does the theory reflect the latest thinking in nursing? Has the theory kept pace with the times in nursing? Is this a nursing theory for the future?

Choosing a Nursing Theory to Study

It is important to give adequate attention to selection of theories for study. Results of this decision will have lasting influences on one's nursing practice. It is not unusual for nurses who begin to work with nursing theory to realize their practice is changing and that their future efforts in the discipline and practice of nursing are markedly altered.

There is always some measure of hope mixed with anxiety as nurses seriously explore nursing theory for the first time. Individual nurses who practice with a group of colleagues often wonder how to select and study nursing theories. Nurses and nursing students in courses considering nursing theory have similar questions. Nurses in new practice settings designed and developed by nurses have the same concerns about getting started as do nurses in hospital organizations who want more from their nursing.

The following exercise is grounded in the belief that the study and use of nursing theory in nursing practice must have roots in the practice of the nurses involved. Moreover, the nursing theory used by particular nurses must reflect elements of practice that are essential to those nurses, while at the same time bringing focus and freshness to that practice. This exercise calls on the nurse to think about the major components of nursing, and calls forth the values and beliefs nurses hold most dear. In these ways, the exercise begins to parallel knowledge development reflected in the nursing metaparadigm and nursing philosophies described in Chapter 1. From this point on, the nurse is guided to connect nursing theory and nursing practice in the context of nursing situations.

An Exercise of Reflection for the Study of Nursing Theory

Select a comfortable, private, and quiet place to reflect and write. Relax by taking some deep, slow breaths. Think about the reasons you went into nursing in the first place. Bring your nursing practice into focus. Consider your practice today. Continue to reflect and, without being distracted, make notes so you won't forget your thoughts and feelings. If you are doing this exercise with a group of colleagues, try to wait until later to share your reflections, and only then as you wish to do so. When you have been still for a time and have taken the opportunity to reflect on your practice, you may proceed with the following questions. Continue to reflect and to make notes as you consider each question about your beliefs and values.

ENDURING VALUES

- What are the enduring values and beliefs that brought me to nursing?
- What beliefs and values keep me in nursing today?
- What are those values I hold most dear?
- What are the ties of these values to my personal values?
- How do my personal and nursing values connect with what is important to society?

NURSING SITUATIONS

Reflect on an instance of nursing in which you interacted with a person for nursing purposes. This can be a situation from your current practice or may be from your nursing in years past. Consider the purpose or hoped-for outcome of the nursing.

- Who was my patient as a person?
- What were the needs for nursing the person?
- Who was I as a person in the nursing situation?
- Who was I as a nurse in the situation?
- What was the interaction like between the patient and myself?
- What nursing responses did I offer to the needs of the patient?
- What other nursing responses might have been possible?
- What was the environment of the nursing situation?
- What about the environment was important to the needs for nursing and to my nursing responses?

CONNECTING VALUES AND THE NURSING SITUATION

Nursing can change when we consciously connect values and beliefs to nursing situations. Consider that values and beliefs are the basis for our nursing.

Briefly describe the connections of your values and beliefs with your chosen nursing situation.

- How are my values and beliefs reflected in the nursing situation?
- Are my values and beliefs in conflict in the situation?
- Do my values come to life in the nursing situation?
- Are my values frustrated?

VERIFYING AWARENESS AND APPRECIATION

In reflecting and writing about values and situations of nursing that are important to us, we often come to a fuller awareness and appreciation of nursing. Make notes about your insights. You might consider these initial notes the beginning of a journal in which you record your study of nursing theories and their use in nursing practice. This is a great way to follow your progress and is a source of nursing questions for future study. You may want to share this process and experience with your colleagues. These are ways to clarify and verify views about nursing and to seek and offer support for nursing values and situations that are critical to your practice. If you are doing this exercise in a group, share your essential values and beliefs with your colleagues.

MULTIPLE WAYS OF KNOWING AND REFLECTING ON NURSING THEORY

The previous reflective exercises offer guidance for knowing about values and nursing practice. Carper (1978) studied the nursing literature and described four essential patterns of knowing in nursing. Using the Phenix (1964) model of types of meaning, Carper described personal, empirical, ethical, and esthetic ways of knowing in nursing. Chinn and Kramer (2004) apply Carper's patterns of knowing to develop a framework for nursing knowledge. Additional patterns of knowing in nursing have been explored and described, and the initial four patterns have been the focus of much consideration in nursing (Ruth-Sahd, 2003; Leight, 2002; Thompson, 1999; Pierson, 1999; Boykin, Parker, & Schoenhofer, 1994; Parker, 2002). Chapter 4 of this text employs patterns of knowing to examine nursing theory resources.

To assist in the study of nursing theory, review the following descriptions of the Carper patterns of knowing, along with suggestions for use in the study of nursing theory.

- Personal knowing is about striving to know the self and to actualize authentic relationships between the nurse and the one nursed. Using this pattern of knowing in nursing, the client is not seen as an object but as a person moving toward fulfillment of potential (Carper, 1978). The nurse is also recognized as always learning and growing as a person and in professional practice. Reflecting on a person as a client and a person as a nurse in the nursing situation can enhance understanding of nursing practice and the centrality of relationships in nursing. These insights are useful for choosing and studying nursing theory.
- Empirical knowing in nursing is the most familiar of the ways of knowing to most nurses and nursing students. Empirical knowing concerns the science of nursing; the nurse uses empirical knowing to access data from nursing, from related disciplines, and from the client. Particular nursing situations may be influenced by many facts and theories from many sources and by many related facts about the person, family, and environment. The amount and quality of empirical knowing can guide selection of a nursing theory as a way to frame and use empirics for nursing purposes.
- Ethical knowing is increasingly important to the study and practice of nursing today. According to Carper (1978), ethics in nursing is the moral component guiding choices within the complexity of health care. Ethical knowing informs us of what is right, what is our obligation, what the nurse ought to do in this situation. Ethical knowing is essential in every action of the nurse in day-to-day nursing. These commitments of the nurse may be the focus of reflection and may be described as part of a nursing situation, guiding selection, and study of particular nursing theories.
- Esthetic knowing is described by Carper (1978) as the art of nursing. While nursing is often referred to as art, this aspect of nursing may not be as highly valued as the science and ethics of nursing. However, many nurses realize that esthetic knowing subsumes all other patterns of knowing, that the personal, empirical, and ethical knowing are combined in the fullness of esthetic knowing.
- It is the experience of these nurses that appreciation of wholeness, well-being, and a higher level of communication are part of esthetic knowing. Examples of this most complete knowing are frequent in nursing situations in which even momentary connection and genuine presence between the nursing and client is realized.
- Reflecting on the *experience* of nursing is primary in understanding esthetic knowing. Through such reflection, the nurse understands that nursing practice has in fact been *created,* that each instance of nursing is unique, and that outcomes of nursing cannot be precisely predicted. Nurses often express esthetic knowing through use of an art form, and thus recreate their esthetic knowing in new and unique ways. The student of nursing theory who has special appreciation for esthetic knowing may explore nursing theory that emphasizes presence and perhaps spirituality in the relationship of nurse and client.

USING INSIGHTS TO CHOOSE THEORY

The notes describing your experience will help in selecting a nursing theory to study and consider for guiding practice. You will want to answer these questions:

- What nursing theory seems consistent with the values and beliefs that guide my practice?
- What theories do I believe are consistent with my personal values and society's beliefs?
- What do I want from the use of nursing theory?
- Given my reflection on a nursing situation, do I want theory to support this description of my practice?
- Do I hope to use nursing theory to improve my experience of practice for myself and for my patients?

USING AUTHORITATIVE SOURCES

Use your questions and new insights to begin a literature search. Gather and use library resources, such as CINAHL. Search the Internet and use online resources for information on nursing theories and their use in practice, research, education, and administration. Join an online group dialogue about a particular nursing theory. You and your colleagues may seek consultation for assistance with analysis and evaluation of specific nursing theories.

USING A GUIDE TO SELECT A NURSING THEORY

This is the time to explore using the following guides for analysis and evaluation of nursing theory. Done individually or as a group, this is an additional opportunity to learn and to share. This is demanding work, but along with the challenge, this can also be fun, gratifying, and a good way to strengthen bonds with colleagues.

Analysis and Evaluation of Nursing Theory

It is important to understand definitions of nursing theory (as described in Chapter 1) before moving to theory analysis and evaluation. These definitions direct examination of structure, content, and purposes of theories. Although each of these definitions is adequate for study of any nursing theory, choose the definition that seems to best fit with your particular purpose for studing theory. For example, one of the definitions by Chinn and Jacobs (1987) or Chinn and Kramer (2004) may be chosen for using theory in research. The definition by Silva (1997) may be more appropriate for study of nursing theory for use in practice. Another way to think about this is to consider whether the definition of nursing theory in use fits the theory being analyzed and evaluated. Look carefully at the theory, read the theory as presented by the theorist, and read what others have written about the theory. The whole

> *The whole theory must be studied. Parts of the theory without the whole will not be fully meaningful and may lead to misunderstanding.*

theory must be studied. Parts of the theory without the whole will not be fully meaningful and may lead to misunderstanding.

Before selecting a guide for analysis and evalua-

tion, consider the level and scope of the theory, as discussed in the previous chapter. Is the theory a grand nursing theory? A philosophy? A middle-range nursing theory? A practice theory? Not all aspects of theory described in an evaluation guide will be evident in all levels of theory. For example, questions about the metaparadigm are probably not appropriate to use in analyzing middle-range theories. Whall (1996) recognizes this in offering particular guides for analysis and evaluation that vary according to three types of nursing theory: models, middle-range theories, and practice theories.

Theory analysis and evaluation may be thought of as one process or as a two-step sequence. It may be helpful to think of analysis of theory as necessary for adequate study of a nursing theory and evaluation of theory as the assessment of a theory's utility for particular purposes. Guides for theory evaluation are intended as tools to inform us about theories and to encourage further development, refinement, and use of theory. There are no guides for theory analysis and evaluation that are adequate and appropriate for every nursing theory.

Johnson (1974) wrote about three basic criteria to guide evaluation of nursing theory. These have continued in use over time and offer direction for guides in use today. These criteria state that the theory should:

- define the congruence of nursing practice with societal expectations of nursing decisions and actions;
- clarify the social significance of nursing, or the impact of nursing on persons receiving nursing; and
- describe social utility, or usefulness of the theory in practice, research, and education.

The following are outlines of the most frequently used guides for analysis and evaluation. These guides are components of the entire work about nursing theory of the individual nursing scholar and offer various interesting approaches to the study of nursing theory. Each guide should be studied in more detail than is offered in this introduction and should be examined in context of the whole work of the individual nurse scholar.

The approach to theory analysis set forth by Chinn and Kramer (2004) is to use guidelines for describing nursing theory that are based on their definition of theory that was presented in Chapter 1. The guidelines set forth questions that clarify the facts about aspects of theory: purpose, concepts, definitions, relationships, structure, assumptions, and scope. These authors suggest that the next step in the evaluation process is critical reflection about whether and how the nursing theory works. Questions are posed to guide this reflection:

• Is the theory clearly stated?
• Is it stated simply?
• Can the theory be generalized?
• Is the theory accessible?
• How important is the theory?

Fawcett (2000) developed a framework of questions that separates the activities of analysis and evaluation. Questions for analysis in this framework flow from the structural hierarchy of nursing knowledge proposed by Fawcett and defined in Chapter 1. The questions for evaluation guide examination of theory content and use for practical purposes. Following is a summary of the Fawcett (2000) framework.

For theory analysis, consideration is given to:

• scope of the theory
• metaparadigm concepts and propositions included in the theory
• values and beliefs reflected in the theory
• relation of the theory to a conceptual model and to related disciplines
• concepts and propositions of the theory

For theory evaluation, consideration is given to:

• significance of the theory and relations with structure of knowledge
• consistency and clarity of concepts, expressed in congruent, concise language
• adequacy for use in research, education, and practice
• feasibility to apply the theory in practical contexts

Meleis (1997) states that the structural and functional components of a theory should be studied prior to evaluation. The structural components are assumptions, concepts, and propositions of the theory. Functional components include descriptions of the following: focus, client, nursing, health, nurse-client interactions, environment, and nursing problems and interventions. After studying these dimensions of the theory, critical examination of these elements may take place, as summarized here:

• Relations between structure and function of the theory, including clarity, consistency, and simplicity
• Diagram of theory to further understand the theory by creating a visual representation
• Contagiousness, or adoption of the theory by a wide variety of students, researchers, and practitioners, as reflected in the literature
• Usefulness in practice, education, research, and administration
• External components of personal, professional, and social values, and significance

SUMMARY

Nursing theory, knowledge development through research, and nursing practice are closely linked and interrelated. In order to enhance both nursing practice and nursing theory, it is incumbent upon the practicing nurse to study theory, just as it is upon the theorist to study the practice of nursing. Considering a commitment to study nursing theory raises many questions from nurses about to undertake this important work. This chapter presented some of the questions worth considering before undertaking extensive study and deciding on a theory to guide practice. Analysis and evaluation of nursing theory are the main ways of studying nursing theory. Literature presents a number of different guides to analyzing and evaluating theory.

References

Boykin, A., Parker, M., & Schoenhofer, S. (1994). Aesthetic knowing grounded in an explicit conception of nursing. *Nursing Science Quarterly, 7*(4), 158–161.

Carper, B. A. (1978). Fundamental patterns of knowing in nursing. *Advances in Nursing Science, 1*(1), 13–23.

Chinn, P., & Jacobs, M. (1987). *Theory and nursing: A systematic approach.* St. Louis: C. V. Mosby.

Chinn, P., & Kramer, M. (2004). *Integrated knowledge development in nursing* (6th ed.). St. Louis: Mosby-Year Book.

Fawcett, J. (2000). *Analysis and evaluation of contemporary nursing knowledge.* Philadelphia: F. A. Davis.

Johnson, D. (1974). Development of theory: A requisite for nursing as a primary health profession. *Nursing Research, 23*(5), 372–377.

Leight, S. B. (2002). Starry night: Using story to inform aesthetic knowing in women's health nursing. *Journal of Advanced Nursing 37*(1), 108–114.

Meleis, A. (1997). *Theoretical nursing: Development and progress.* Philadelphia: Lippincott.

Parker, M. (1993). *Patterns of nursing theories in practice.* New York: National League for Nursing.

Parker, M. E. (2002). Aesthetic ways in day-to-day nursing. In Freshwater, D. (Ed.), *Therapeutic nursing: Improving patient care through self-awareness and reflection* (pp. 100–120). Thousand Oaks, CA: Sage Publications.

Phenix, P. H. (1964). *Realms of meaning.* New York: McGraw Hill.

Pierson, W. (1999). Considering the nature of intersubjectivity within professional nursing. *Journal of Advanced Nursing, 30*(2), 294–302.

Ruth-Sahd, L. A. (2003). Intuition: A critical way of knowing in a multicultural nursing curriculum. *Nursing Education Perspectives, 24*(3), 129–134.

Silva, M. (1997). Philosophy, theory, and research in nursing: A linguistic journey to nursing practice. In King, I., & Fawcett, J. (Eds.), *The language of nursing theory and metatheory.* Indianapolis, IN: Center Nursing Press.

Thompson, C. (1999). A conceptual treadmill: The need for 'middle ground' in clinical decision making theory in nursing. *Journal of Advanced Nursing, 30*(5), 1222–1229.

Whall, A. (1996). The structure of nursing knowledge: Analysis and evaluation of practice, middle-range, and grand theory. In Fitzpatrick, J., & Whall, A. (Eds.), *Conceptual models of nursing: Analysis and application* (3rd ed.). Stamford, CT: Appleton & Lange.

CHAPTER 3

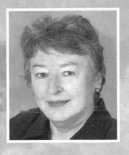

Marilyn E. Parker

Guides for Study of Theories for Practice and Administration

Marilyn E. Parker

$\mathcal{N}$urses, individually and in groups, are affected by rapid and dramatic change throughout health and medical systems. Nurses practice in increasingly diverse settings and often develop organized nursing practices through which accessible health care to communities can be provided. Community members may be active participants in selecting, designing, and evaluating the nursing they receive. Interdisciplinary practice is frequently the norm.

Theories and practices from related disciplines are brought to nursing to use for nursing purposes. The scope of nursing practice is continually being

> *The scope of nursing practice is continually being expanded to include additional knowledge and skills from related disciplines.*

23

expanded to include additional knowledge and skills from related disciplines, such as medicine and psychology. Although the majority of nurses practice in hospitals, an increasing number of nurses practice elsewhere in the community, taking the venue of their practice closer to those served by nursing.

Groups of nurses working together as colleagues to provide nursing often realize that they share the same values and beliefs about nursing. The study of nursing theories can clarify the purposes of nursing and facilitate building a cohesive practice to meet these purposes. Regardless of the setting of nursing practice, nurses may choose to study nursing theories together in order to design and articulate theory-based practice. The exercise in Chapter 2 is offered to facilitate this work.

This chapter offers guides for continuing study of nursing theory for use in nursing practice. Because many nurses are creating new practice organizations and settings, a guide for study of nursing theory for use in nursing administration has been developed. The guides are intended for use in conjunction with the overall study of nursing theory, including the methods of analysis and evaluation outlined in Chapter 2. The first guide is a set of questions for consideration in study and selection of a nursing theory for use in practice. The second guide is an outline of factors to consider when studying nursing theory for use in nursing organization and administration.

Responses to questions offered and points summarized in the guides may be found in nursing literature as well as in audiovisual and electronic resources. Primary source material, including the writing of nurses who are recognized authorities in specific nursing theories and the use of nursing theory, should be used. Subsequent chapters of this book offer such sources. Users of this guide are invited to examine each question carefully and add questions from other theory analysis and evaluation guides to meet their particular purposes.

Study of Theory for Nursing Practice

Four main questions have been developed and refined to facilitate study of nursing theories for use in nursing practice (Parker, 1993). These questions are intended to focus on concepts within the theories as well as on points of interest and general information about each theory. This guide was developed for use by practicing nurses and students in undergraduate and graduate nursing education programs. Many nurses and students have used these questions and have contributed to their continuing development. The guide may be used to study most of the nursing theories developed at all levels. It has been used to create surveys of nursing theories. An early motivation for developing this guide was the work by the Nursing Development Conference Group (1973).

A GUIDE FOR STUDY OF NURSING THEORY FOR USE IN PRACTICE

1 How is nursing conceptualized in the theory?

Is the focus of nursing stated?

- What does the nurse attend to when practicing nursing?
- What guides nursing observations, reflections, decisions, and actions?
- What does the nurse think about when considering nursing?
- What are illustrations of use of the theory to guide practice?

What is the purpose of nursing?

- What do nurses do when they are practicing nursing?
- What are exemplars of nursing assessments, designs, plans, and evaluations?
- What indicators give evidence of quality and quantity of nursing practice?
- Is the richness and complexity of nursing practice evident?

What are the boundaries or limits for nursing?

- How is nursing distinguished from other health and medical services?
- How is nursing related to other disciplines and services?
- What is the place of nursing in interdisciplinary settings?
- What is the range of nursing situations in which the theory is useful?

How can nursing situations be described?

- What are attributes of the one nursed?
- What are characteristics of the nurse?
- How can interactions of the nurse and the one nursed be described?
- Are there environmental requirements for the practice of nursing?

② **What is the context of the theory development?**

Who is the nursing theorist as person and as nurse?

- Why did the theorist develop the theory?
- What is the background of the theorist as nursing scholar?
- What are central values and beliefs set forth by the theorist?

What are major theoretical influences on this theory?

- What nursing models and theories influenced this theory?
- What are relationships of this theory with other theories?
- What nursing-related theories and philosophies influenced this theory?

What were major external influences on development of the theory?

- What were the social, economic, and political influences?
- What images of nurses and nursing influenced the theory?
- What was the status of nursing as a discipline and profession?

③ **Who are authoritative sources for information about development, evaluation, and use of this theory?**

Who are nursing authorities who speak about, write about, and use the theory?

- What are the professional attributes of these persons?
- What are the attributes of authorities, and how does one become one?

- Which other nurses should be considered authorities?

What major resources are authoritative sources on the theory?

- Books? Articles? Audiovisual media? Electronic media?
- What nursing societies share and support work of the theory?
- What service and academic programs are authoritative sources?

④ **How can the overall significance of the nursing theory be described?**

What is the importance of the nursing theory over time?

- What are exemplars of nursing theory use that structure and guide individual practice?
- Is the theory used to guide programs of nursing education?
- Is the theory used to guide nursing administration and organizations?
- Does published nursing scholarship reflect significance of the theory?

What is the experience of nurses who report consistent use of the theory?

- What is the range of reports from practice?
- Has nursing research led to further theory formulations?
- Has the theory been used to develop new nursing practices?
- Has the theory influenced design of methods of nursing inquiry?
- What has been the influence of the theory on nursing and health policy?

What are projected influences of the theory on nursing's future?

- How has nursing as a community of scholars been influenced?
- In what ways has nursing as a professional practice been strengthened?
- What future possibilities for nursing are open because of this theory?
- What will be the continuing social value of the theory?

Study of Theory for Nursing Administration

Literature on nursing delivery systems and administration have addressed the value of nursing theory for use in administration of nursing and healthcare organizations (Huckaby, 1991; Laurent, 2000; Walker, 1993; Young & Hayne, 1988). Nurses in group practice may seek to use a nursing theory that will not only guide their practice, but also provide visions for the organization and administration of their practice. A shared understanding of the focus of nursing can facilitate goal-setting and achievement as well as day-to-day communication among nurses in practice and administration. Allison and McLaughlin-Renpenning (1999) describe the need for a vision of nursing shared by all throughout health care and nursing organizations. These authors, using Orem's general Self-Care Deficit Nursing Theory (see Chapter 13), demonstrate that a theory of nursing can guide practice as well as the organization and administration.

The preceding guide for the study of nursing theories for use in nursing practice can be extended to consider essential aspects of nursing in organizations. The following questions are derived from components of a nursing administration model (Allison & McLaughlin-Renpenning, 1999). The questions are intended to guide descriptions of the nursing organization. Responses to these questions can be used to evaluate nursing theory for use in a nursing practice organization.

- What are purposes of the organization? Mission? Goals?
- What are the purposes of nursing? How do these purposes contribute to the purposes of the organization?
- How can the range of nursing situations be described? What is the population served?
- What nursing and related technologies are required for nursing?
- What are the projections for nursing situations and technological needs for the future?
- How is communication facilitated? In nursing? Among disciplines and services?
- How are services for those nursed coordinated?
- In what ways is nursing professional development achieved? Career advancement?
- How are research and development of nursing practice and theory advanced?

SUMMARY

This chapter has presented a guide designed for nurses to study nursing theory for use in practice. The guide is intended to accompany more general formats of analysis and evaluation of nursing theory. This guide provides additional evaluative components for nurses who are focusing on nursing practice. An additional set of questions is offered for nurses who are considering nursing organization and administration. These questions are intended to further guide the study of nursing theory for use in nursing organization and administration.

References

Allison, S. E., & McLaughlin-Renpenning, K. E. (1999). *Nursing administration in the 21st century: A self-care theory approach.* Thousand Oaks, CA: Sage Publications.

Huckaby, L. (1991). The role of conceptual frameworks in nursing practice, administration, education, and research. *Nursing Administration Quarterly, 15*(3), 17–28.

Laurent, C. L. (2000). A nursing theory for nursing leadership. *Journal of Nursing Management, 8,* 83–87.

Nursing Development Conference Group. (1973). *Concept formalization in nursing: Process and product.* Boston: Little, Brown & Co.

Parker, M. (1993). *Patterns of nursing theories in practice.* New York: National League for Nursing.

Walker, D. (1993). A nursing administration perspective on use of Orem's self-care nursing theory. In M. Parker (Ed.), *Patterns of nursing theories in practice* (pp. 253–263). New York: National League for Nursing.

Young, L., & Hayne, A. (1988). *Nursing administration: From concepts to practice.* Philadelphia: W. B. Saunders.

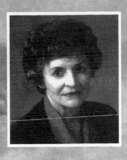

Marguerite J. Purnell

CHAPTER 4

Evaluating Nursing Theory Resources

Marguerite J. Purnell

Introduction

Never in human history have such vast quantities of information been so easily available. Within the brief space of a few decades, the acquisition, storage, and retrieval of information has been transformed from the realm of a labor-intensive manual process to that of a digital, multidimensional virtual medium. Societal thinking and language have been enriched by new technologies as well as the new meanings engendered by their processes and products.

Nursing exists on the cusp of continual change, with interfacing technological revolutions taking place in nursing education, practice, and research. The rapid advance and integration of technology has not only affected practice (Sparks, 1999), but has also affected ways in which nurses investigate, evaluate, think, and speak about practice (Turley, 1996).

Why Evaluate Resources for Nursing Inquiry and Research?

The value and reliability of any contribution to nursing knowledge is enhanced by the quality of the resources used. In the tactile, physical world of books, journals, and media recordings, emphasis rests upon evaluation of the author and contents of each resource. In the utilization of the Internet as a resource for "discovery" (Boyer, 1996, p. 3), another dimension requiring evaluation is realized: The host of the virtual environment, now ubiquitous and often fleeting, also must be identified, examined, and evaluated. Authorial responsibility and veracity in books and journals that are closely scrutinized and monitored by publishers, editors, and review boards may or may not be present when the owner of the Web site is an individual or group not subject to such review. Role-blurring between Web site author and owner is subtle yet insistent. The author of the Web pages, or the "webmaster," is most often another party hired to create and maintain the look of the Web site environment and is therefore not responsible for the content.

The explosion of available knowledge and accessible data has also created a paradox: The sheer volume of information has created a gap in the human ability to process and evaluate it (Jenkins, 2001). Finding relevant information is difficult (Sparks,

1998). Where does one begin? And if one begins, can the information that is often "here today and gone tomorrow" be relied upon as accurate and trustworthy? How can the information be evaluated? Given the complexity of data now available, can nursing theory resources even be evaluated across various types of media? Will the process be congruent with the theory and the values of the researcher?

Resources in nursing should be authoritative, accurate, and current and should be characterized by rich content. The guide for evaluation of theory resources presented within this chapter moves toward a realistic appraisal by the researcher of the applicability and utility of theory resources.

Theory as a Guiding Framework for Evaluation

Theory-based practice provides nurses with a perspective (Raudonis & Acton, 1997) and expresses the essential activity of nursing care in the enacting, adapting, and adding to the nursing human knowledge base. The framework for practice also becomes a framework for education, research, and administration (Boykin & Schoenhofer, 2001). A call for nursing is also a call for transforming knowledge and information; therefore, the response from nursing should be with clarity, conviction, and trustworthiness. In this way, nursing theory is integrated, lived out in the personhood of the nurse and continues to shape, guide, and focus the nurse in all activities. The consistent evaluation of resources is therefore an extension and affirmation of the values grounding the practice of nursing.

Ways of studying nursing are also becoming more creative and reflect rapid changes in technology and societal values. Publishers of educational media routinely complement traditional textbooks with the virtual world of Internet Web sites that offer sensate immersion in motion, color, and sound. Browsing on the Internet frequently results in traveling through a succession of hyperlinks that offer entertaining but specious information without traceable or verifiable sources. The thoughtful study of nursing theory, therefore, includes not only consideration of works contributed by the theorist, practitioners, and critics of the theory, but also the host media of the resource.

Explicit and implicit claims to truth and reality in electronic media cannot easily be disputed. To whom or what does one respond or carry concerns about the content? A framework of non-nursing values is engineered and deeply embedded in electronic information media. Conceptual frameworks in the nurse's mind provide the means of interfacing and transforming these values embedded in the electronic data bit (Carlton, Ryan, & Siktberg, 1998). The challenge for the nurse is to analyze,

> *The challenge for the nurse is to analyze, evaluate, and transform non-nursing values embedded in electronic media into a conceptual framework of human values that are realized in theory and actualized in practice.*

evaluate, and transform non-nursing values embedded in electronic media into a conceptual framework of human values that are realized in theory and actualized in practice.

The ubiquitous Web site—the most prolific and transient of electronic data or resource locators to which information seekers turn—is, for the most part, unregulated. It exists at the will of the Web site "owner." Claims of "authority" and ownership of those claims often cannot be traced or are not able to be proven. According to Hebda, Czar, and Mascara (1998), the authority of Web sites needs to be evaluated and validated, unless the source can be traced to a reputable institution such as in education or government.

Criteria for evaluating Internet Web pages abound (Harris, 1997; Howe, 2001; Tillman, 2003; Wilson, 2002). Methods and tools for evaluating and rating the quality of Web sites have been developed by a range of organizations (Rippen, 1999; Wilson, 2002). Wilson classifies these tools into five categories: codes of conduct, quality labels, user guides, filters, and third party certification. While these tools are generally applicable to health care and commercial Web sites, they do not directly address evaluation of the specialized content of nursing theory web pages.

In order to evaluate and substantiate resources for nursing inquiry, such as theorist home pages and nursing information Web sites, layers of electronic information must be peeled back to reveal those authoritative nurse scholars, scientists, and practitioners who are the sources of disseminated nursing knowledge. Since no two nursing information resources are exactly alike, guidelines for evaluation need to be flexible and adaptable.

The thoughtful nurse researcher should proceed flexibly in the research and evaluation process using "alternating rhythms" (Mayeroff, 1971, p. 21), focusing back and forth between wider and narrower frameworks to comprehend how one aspect is connected with the whole. Evaluation may be understood as alternating between two overlapping phases: The first phase is one in which technical design, organization, and aesthetic comportment of the Web site are considered in relation to the content. The second phase comprises focused evaluation on the reason for the Web site itself, that is, on the nursing theory and its preparation.

Can nurses be sure of what they know subjectively about theory resources? The response is clearly affirmative. Nurses know in many different ways, and when this knowing is recorded, shared, and confirmed, it becomes nursing knowledge. Understanding fundamental patterns of knowing in nursing is a way to begin the process of illuminating theory and research.

How Do You Know What You Know?

FUNDAMENTAL PATTERNS OF KNOWING

As you proceed in your search, you will experience several different patterns of knowing (Carper, 1975; Mueller, 1953; Phenix, 1964). Each pattern or realm describes different dimensions of the activity of knowing and, like "a range of colors" (Mueller, 1953, p. 33), provides a rich panorama of your talents and potential. These fundamental patterns of knowing are: personal, empiric, ethical, aesthetic (Carper, 1978), symbolic, and integrative (or synoptic) (Phenix, 1964). These patterns of knowing are fluid, recursive, and without discrete boundaries. You may be engaging in one or a blend of all the knowing patterns at the same time.

Personal Knowing

Personal knowing is understood as "the pattern most fundamental to understanding the meaning of health in terms of individual well-being" (Carper, 1975, p. 255). Personal knowing can broadly be described as subjective, concrete, direct, and existential and is relational to another human being. Phenix (1964) asserts that it "signifies relational insight or direct awareness" (p. 7) and interpersonal understanding. Personal knowing may be understood as a process of gradually comprehending meaning and unity in a set of particulars as you proceed through your search. You will experience personal knowing in conjunction with other patterns as you engage in your self-preparation and reflections prior to, during, and after your search.

Empirical Knowing

Empirical knowing relates to the science of nursing. According to Carper (1975), this type of knowing is "factual, descriptive and ultimately aimed at developing abstract and theoretical explanations. It is exemplary, discursively formulated, and publicly verifiable" (p. 254). You will be engaging in empirical knowing particularly when you recognize, assess, evaluate, and describe various aspects of the nursing theory resource.

Ethical Knowing

Ethics is the moral pattern of knowing that focuses on the primary principle of obligation and what ought to be done in the concept of service and respect for human life (Carper, 1978). The goals and actions of nursing, including your search, involve normative judgments of moral value. For example, your intention to undertake this search is guided by your ethical knowing that it *ought* to be done in order to increase critical nursing knowledge and thereby enhance human welfare.

Aesthetic Knowing

Aesthetic knowing is a perception of unity and resists expression into the discursive. Aesthetic knowing is *creative,* such as when it is combined with empirical knowing in the discovery and appreciation of theory. Aesthetic design is "controlled by perception of the balance, rhythm, proportion and unity of what is done in relation to the dynamic integration and articulation of the whole" (Carper, 1978, p. 255).

You will be engaging in aesthetic knowing when you evaluate the balance, organization, and harmony of the resource content. The immediate

> *You will be engaging in aesthetic knowing when you evaluate the balance, organization, and harmony of the resource content. The immediate visual appeal of the theory resource, whether or not it is pleasing, denotes aesthetic appreciation of beauty and organization.*

visual appeal of the theory resource, whether or not it is pleasing, denotes aesthetic appreciation of beauty and organization.

Symbolic Knowing

Symbolic knowing encompasses the realm of the abstract, the tacit, and profound knowing. Phenix (1964) states that symbolic systems constitute the most fundamental of all realms in that they must be used to express meanings of other realms.

Language and mathematics are included in the symbolic realms, as well as nondiscursive, symbolic forms used in all the arts and for the expression of feelings, values, ideals, rituals, and commitments. Symbolic forms are also indicated in signals, manners, and gestures and encompass experience and history.

You will be experiencing symbolic knowing when you engage in self-examination and reflection. Interpreting icons on the Internet, understanding the meaning of theory, and searching virtual media are also abstract ideas which you experientially know as symbolic of something greater.

Integrative (Synoptic) Knowing

Integrative (synoptic) knowing unites all knowledge and experience in the moment and creatively transforms it, providing a synopsis of meanings (Phenix, 1964). This critical way of knowing enables an individual to grow and change with the integration of knowledge.

As you analyze and summarize your findings, you will be integrating your experience, accumulated nursing knowledge, intuition, and knowing derived from your search to arrive at a unique conclusion about the nursing theory resource. Integrative knowing is linked to satisfaction. Therefore, as you begin your search, honor your unique and complex abilities and realize that you are able to articulate more than you had ever realized. Trust your knowing. When it is articulated and confirmed, it will be converted to nursing knowledge that can contribute to the knowledge base of nursing.

Preparing to Initiate a Search

BEGIN AT THE BEGINNING WITH YOURSELF

Organizing and purposefully attending to self before undertaking research affirms the intention and focus of your philosophical perspective. The-

> *Theoretical frameworks become blueprints for action.*

oretical frameworks become blueprints for action. Frustrations inherent in new methodologies, new technologies, and virtual information will be less able to deflect your nursing intention to uncover and integrate nursing knowledge if you are prepared. Attending to self in ways that are meaningful will quiet, focus, and center reflective inquiry.

CONNECTING WITH A COMPUTER

If you are new to computer searching of nursing literature, be prepared to spend many, many hours searching for information. When first becoming acquainted with the electronic world, be prepared to accept that you will forget where you are on this electronic highway. It takes practice and intense focus to remain on the elusive information trail. Forgive yourself if you accomplish little, and forgive the computer if you are "dropped" from a key theorist Web site and do not remember where it was. Practice self-care by becoming organized and

> *Practice self-care by becoming organized and exercise discipline by remaining within the parameters of your inquiry.*

exercise discipline by remaining within the parameters of your inquiry.

LINGERING IN THE LIBRARY

You may decide to go to the library and browse the shelves for ideas and inspiration. Seek the help of experts before you attempt the impossible and end up frustrated. Time spent browsing books and journals because they are interesting, yet irrelevant to your inquiry, also means that you will be reinitiating your search at another time.

AGING IN THE ARCHIVES

If you have identified a specific holding or collection that you wish to investigate in the library archives, engage the help of an archivist to clarify and expedite your search. A "hands-on" search of archived records involves painstaking handling, lengthy and careful perusing, and hours of time. Experiencing the spirit and feel of nursing history in tangible artifacts is enhanced by an unhurried examination. In your goal-directed endeavors to balance time, effort, and outcome, you may prefer to reserve time restricted activities to an electronic search.

BECOMING ORGANIZED

Becoming organized begins with thinking about the reason for your search, an estimation of the time involved, and the identification of the focus and scope of your inquiry. Following are questions and suggestions to guide your thoughts:

The Reason for Your Search

The reason for your search will influence your planning. Will your search be preparation for creation of a manuscript or will it be the beginning of formal research? Alternately, would you search simply because you would like to know more about a theorist or theory to apply to your practice?

Estimations of Time Involved

It is critical to decide how much time you realistically need to invest to successfully accomplish the search. Consult your planner and count the actual hours you have available and the days on which they are available. When is the absolute deadline for completing the search and for completing all research activities? Fill in blocks of time in your planner, building in a reserve of time in case you experience a problem with your computer or

> *Hint: If you are a beginning researcher, it is a good idea to double the amount of time you estimate you will need.*

browser. Hint: If you are a beginning researcher, it is a good idea to double the amount of time you estimate you will need.

Focus and Scope of Inquiry

Defining the focus of your search also helps assess the scope. For example, will your inquiry center on one particular theory or will your search include theory-based practice and research studies? Will you include critiques by other nurses and articles from other disciplines? What will you generally not include?

Wise Moves in Your Beginning Search

In your search for nursing theory resources, there is no need to "reinvent the wheel." Generally, you may be initiating searches in any or all of the following six areas:

1. Library online databases such as CINAHL (Cumulative Index of Nursing and Allied Health Literature): for books and journal articles accessible in full text or available by request from other libraries.
2. Library catalogs, bookshelves, and journal stacks: for books and journals not available in full text online.
3. References lists and bibliographies: from online database abstracts and full-text articles about theory with references that are "hot linked" directly to other related theory articles.
4. World Wide Web searches for nursing theory or theorists: through search engines such as Google, Yahoo, or Lycos.
5. Nursing theory "meta-sites" such as those listed in Table 4–1, which provides links directly to each theorist's Web site.
6. Comprehensive bibliographies: compiled within anthologies of nursing theories, such as in the one you are now reading.

A Search Example

As you reflect upon how to approach your preliminary search, you decide to begin with a survey of the nursing literature focusing on theory in CINAHL. You access your library from home and

Table 4–1	Select Nursing Theory Meta-sites and Directories

THE NURSING THEORY PAGE, HAHN SCHOOL OF NURSING AND HEALTH SCIENCE

http://www.sandiego.edu/nursing/theory
This nursing theory meta-site is clear, comprehensive, and well-maintained. It contains literature search tips, video and book resources, teaching tools, discussion forums, and related links to other nursing theory sites. Complementing the site is an article for researchers entitled "Searching Bibliographic Databases for Nursing Theory," with a contact address for author Margaret (Peg) Allen, MLS-AHIP.

A NURSING THEORY LINK PAGE, CLAYTON COLLEGE AND STATE UNIVERSITY, DEPARTMENT OF NURSING

http://healthsci.clayton.edu/eichelberger/nursing.htm
This rapidly growing meta-site contains links to newer and less well-known theory Web sites.

NURSING THEORY, COLLEGE OF NURSING AT VALDOSTA STATE UNIVERSITY

http://www.valdosta.edu/nursing/history_theory/theory.html
This meta-site contains links to the well-known "classic" nursing theorists.

NURSING THEORIES. NURSING ONLINE: RESOURCES FOR NURSING PROFESSION

http://www.nursing.iirt.net/theory.html
This smaller commercial site contains links to classic and less well-known theorists.

NURSING THEORIES A–Z. NURSES. INFO

http://www.nurses.info/nursing_theory.htm
This directory constitutes part of a commercial Web site and contains lists of nursing theorists classified by theory type. Also included are various professional services and discussion forums with lists of conferences and events.

enter CINAHL. You enter a word search for *nursing theory* and are dismayed to discover thousands of articles through which you would need to sift. Narrowing your search down further to an individual theory is productive, but you find that earlier works by nursing theorists are only abstracted and not available online in full text.

You would like to begin your search with primary references and realize that a time-saving strategy would be to locate the nurse theorist's home page on the Internet. You discover that nursing theory meta-sites provide links to the majority of nursing theory home pages and begin your journey through each home page. You discover that not all Web sites are created equal. Although some sites are exciting to visit, the information is less substantive, less scholarly, or less specific on some nursing theorist Web sites than on others. Given the multitude of Web sites, you wonder how you can distinguish which sites are the most valuable sources of information in the electronic domain. You also wonder about the credibility of Web site information that might be used as a scholarly, authoritative reference.

Unsubstantiated information worries you. It occurs to you that the information authority on some nursing theory Web sites may be tenuous and may constitute a weak link in your research methodology. You conclude that evaluation of nursing theory

> *Evaluation of nursing theory resources is of major importance in laying groundwork for consistent, credible, and authoritative research findings.*

resources is of major importance in laying groundwork for consistent, credible, and authoritative research findings. This is a good time to reflect, and

- clarify and adjust your expectations,
- clarify and adjust your needs, and
- clarify and adjust your methods.

There is little to show for your efforts except experience and rapidly accumulating wisdom. You decide that in addition to gaining more experience in literature searches, you need a way to distinguish credible and authoritative resources and to flexibly evaluate nursing theory resources across several types of media.

Using the Guide for Evaluating Theory (GET) Resources

Carefully consider the *GET Resources* in Table 4–2 and read each question. Choose as an exemplar for evaluation a Web site from a theorist in one of the chapters of this book. Begin evaluating this nursing theorist's Web site and as you thoughtfully consider each question, assess whether or not the information you gather from the resource meets the criteria. Make decisions based on your knowing. All

Table 4–2	**Guide for Evaluation of Theory Resources (GET Resources)**
Guiding Questions	**Evaluation**
REFLECTIONS ON AUTHORITY	**EVALUATION OF AUTHORITY**
Is the owner or author of this Web site or media resource the theory author?	Authoritative sources are known. Yes/No
	The owner/author is the theorist. Yes/No
Who are authoritative sources who speak, write about, and use this theory? Are they contributors to the content on this Web site or media?	Nursing authorities contribute to content. Yes/No
	Practitioners of nursing contribute to the content. Yes/No
What are the professional qualifications of these contributors? Have they written about this theory in other works not presented here?	Other organizations use, refer to, or maintain links to the content. Yes/No
What are other major resources on this theory that are authoritative? Books? Articles? Audiovisual media? Web sites?	**Evaluation of Authority:** **Acceptable/Not Acceptable**
What service and academic programs are authoritative sources?	
What nursing societies/organizations share and support the work of this theory? Do they also have a Web site?	

(Continued)

Table 4–2	**Guide for Evaluation of Theory Resources (GET Resources)** *(Continued)*

Guiding Questions	Evaluation
REFLECTIONS ON CONTENT	**EVALUATION OF CONTENT**
What is the purpose of the resource? Is it dedicated to the work of one theorist, or is it a meta-site for several? Is it a commercial or educational site?	Information presented is accurate. Yes/No
	Information is comprehensive and clear. Yes/No
Do authoritative sources show their credentials on the Web page or provide links to pages that do?	Information covers theory, practice, research, and administration. Yes/No
Does the resource provide information in a logical and easily accessible manner?	Information is current. Yes/No
	Bibliography included. Yes/No
Is there clear reference to source data, and are there specific HTML links to that data?	I found the information for which I was searching. Yes/No
Does the resource provide comprehensive, substantiated information? Is this information even in quality and quantity?	**Evaluation of Content:**
	Acceptable/Not Acceptable
Does the information cover nursing research, administration, and education?	
Is the information current? What evidence is presented to verify currency?	
Is an exhaustive bibliography provided?	
What information were you looking for that you did *not* find in this resource?	
REFLECTIONS ON THE WEB SITE OR MEDIA	
Is the Web site or media well maintained? Are you able to contact the webmaster from an onsite address?	The Web site/resource is easy to use and well organized. Yes/No
Is the Web site or media aesthetically pleasing?	The Web site/resource has unique characteristics. Yes/No
Are links clearly marked and active?	
Are you informed when you are seamlessly transferred to another Web site?	The Web site/resource is satisfying to visit. Yes/No
Are there fees or membership required to access the information you need?	I will recommend this resource to colleagues. Yes/No
What are unique characteristics of the Web site?	
This nursing theory resource will ground my inquiry as a credible, authoritative, and accurate source of information. Yes/No	
Reservations: _____	

questions may not apply to all Web sites and may be modified by the purpose of the Web site.

Reflective Preparations

Following are key reflective preparations that will help focus your activities:

- What do you want to know?
- What are your expectations of the resource?
- How complex do you expect the information to be?

- How comprehensive do you intend your analysis and evaluation to be?
- Will you share the results of your evaluation with colleagues?

When you have answered as many questions as you are able to, synthesize your findings. Compare your findings with other nursing theory resources and Web sites you have located and evaluated. Which resources and Web sites hold up under critical evaluation? Which can you use as a model?

Thoughts for Your Journey

Based on your thoughtful strategizing, expect your search and theory evaluation to yield surprising results. Nursing information resources are evolving, and Web sites or resources for new nursing theories are being continually developed. Regular evaluation of the resource each time that you wish to use it will ensure accuracy, credibility, currency, and trustworthiness of the information that contributes to your learning and scholarly practice. You are ultimately the one deciding the outcome of your evaluation and the influence of the resource on your research. Enjoy the journey!

> *Regular evaluation of the resource each time that you wish to use it will ensure accuracy, credibility, currency, and trustworthiness of the information that contributes to your learning and scholarly practice.*

References

Boyer, E. (1996). Clinical practice as scholarship. *Holistic Nursing Practice, 10*(3), 1–6.

Boykin, A., & Schoenhofer, S. O. (2001). *Nursing as caring: A model for transforming practice.* Sudbury, MA: Jones and Bartlett Publishers and National League for Nursing.

Carlton, K. H., Ryan, M. E., & Siktberg, L. L. (1998). Designing course for the Internet. *Nurse Educator, 23*(3), 45–50.

Carper, B. A. (1975). *Fundamental patterns of knowing in nursing.* Dissertation. Teachers College, Columbia University.

Carper, B. A. (1978). Fundamental patterns of knowing in nursing. *Advances in Nursing Science, 1*(1), 13–23.

Goldsborough, R. (2001). Finding "the best" websites. *RN, 64*(6), 19, 22.

Harris, R. (1997). Virtualsalt: Evaluating internet research sources. Accessed August 10, 2004. www.virtualsalt.com/evalu8it.htm.

Hebda, T., Czar, P., & Mascara, C. (1998). *Handbook of informatics for nurses and health care professionals.* Menlo Park, CA: Addison-Wesley.

Howe, W. Walt's navigating the net forum: Evaluating quality. Accessed Web site August 10, 2004. www.walthowe.com/navnet/quality.html.

Jenkins, D. (2001). User beware of information on the Internet. *Clinical Nurse Specialist, 15*(4), 162–163.

Mayeroff, M. (1971). *On caring.* New York: HarperPerennial.

Mueller, G. E. (1953). *Dialectic: A way into and with philosophy.* NY: Bookman Assoc.

Phenix, P. H. (1964). *Realms of meaning.* New York: McGraw Hill.

Raudonis, B. M., & Acton, G. J. (1997). Theory-based nursing practice. *Journal of Advanced Nursing, 26*, 138–145.

Rippen, H. E. (1999). White paper: Criteria for assessing the quality of health information on the Internet (working draft). *Mitretek Systems, Health Information Policy Institute (HITI), and Agency for Health Care Policy and Research (AHCPR).* Accessed August 10, 2004. http://hitiweb.mitretek.org/docs/criteria.html.

Sparks, S., & Rizzolo, M. A. (1998). World Wide Web search tools. *Image: Journal of Nursing Scholarship, 30*(2), 161–171.

Tillman, H. N. (2003). Evaluating quality on the net. Accessed website August 10, 2004. www.hopetillman.com/findqual.html.

Turley, J. (1996). Nursing decision making and the science of the concrete. *Holistic Nursing Practice, 11*(1), 6–14.

Wilson, P. (2002). How to find the good and avoid the bad and ugly: A short guide to tools for rating the quality of health information on the internet. *British Medical Journal, 324*(7337), 598–600.

Evolution of Nursing Theory: Essential Influences

CHAPTER 5

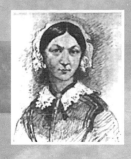

Florence Nightingale

Florence Nightingale's Legacy of Caring and Its Applications

Lynne M. Hektor Dunphy

Introducing the Theorist

Florence Nightingale transformed a "calling from God" and an intense spirituality into a new social role for women: that of nurse. Her caring was a public one. "Work your true work," she wrote, "and you will find God within you" (Woodham-Smith, C. 1983, p. 74). A reflection on this statement appears in a well-known quote from *Notes on Nursing* (1859/1992): "Nature [i.e., the manifestation of God] alone cures ... what nursing has to do ... is put the patient in the best condition for nature to act upon him" (Macrae, 1995, p. 10). Although Nightingale never defined human care or caring in *Notes on Nursing,* there is no doubt that her life in nursing exemplified and personified an ethos of caring. Jean Watson (1992, p. 83), in the 1992 commemorative edition of *Notes on Nursing,* observed, "Although Nightingale's feminine-based caring-healing model has transcended time and is prophetic for this century's health reform, the model is yet to truly come of age in nursing or the health care system." Boykin and Dunphy in a reflective essay (2002) extend this thinking and relate Nightingale's life, rooted in compassion and caring, as an exemplar of justice-making (p. 14). *Justice-making* is understood as a manifestation of compassion and caring, "for it is our actions that brings about justice" (p. 16).

This chapter reiterates Nightingale's life from the years 1820 to 1860, delineating the formative influences on her thinking and providing historical context for her ideas about nursing as we recall them today. Part of what follows is a well-known tale; yet it remains a tale that is irresistible, casting an age-old spell on the reader, like the flickering shadow of Nightingale and her famous lamp in the dark and dreary halls of the Barrack Hospital, Scutari, on the outskirts of Constantinople, circa 1854 to 1856. And it is a tale that still carries much relevance for nursing practice today.

Early Life and Education

A profession, a trade, a necessary occupation, something to fill and employ all my faculties, I have always felt essential to me, I have always longed for, consciously or not. ... The first thought I can remember, and the last, was nursing work. ...

—**Florence Nightingale, cited in Cook (1913, p. 106)**

Nightingale was born in 1820 in Florence, Italy—the city she was named for. The Nightingales were on an extended European tour, begun in 1818 shortly after their marriage. This was a common journey for those of their class and wealth. Their first daughter, Parthenope, had been born in the city of that name in the previous year.

A legacy of humanism, liberal thinking, and love of speculative thought was bequeathed to Nightingale by her father. His views on the education of women were far ahead of his time. W. E. N., her father William's nickname, undertook the education of both his daughters. Florence and her sister studied music; grammar; composition; modern languages; Ancient Greek and Latin; constitutional history and Roman, Italian, German, and Turkish history; and mathematics (Barritt, 1973).

From an early age, Florence exhibited independence of thought and action. The sketch (Figure 5–1) of W. E. N. and his daughters was done by Nightingale's beloved aunt, Julia Smith. It is Parthenope, the older sister, who clutches her father's hand and Florence who, as described by her aunt, "independently stumps along by herself" (Woodham-Smith, 1983, p. 7).

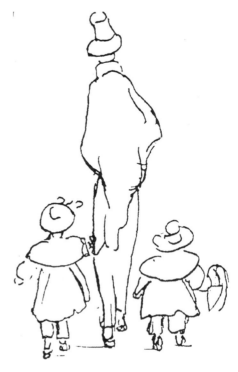

FIGURE 5–1 This sketch of W.E.N. and his daughters was done by one of his wife Fanny's sisters, Julia Smith. *From Woodham-Smith, p. 9, permission of Sir Henry Verney, Bart.*

Travel also played a part in Nightingale's education. Eighteen years after Florence's birth, the Nightingales and both daughters made an extended tour of France, Italy, and Switzerland between the years of 1837 and 1838 and later to Egypt and Greece (Sattin, 1987). From there, Nightingale visited Germany, making her first acquaintance with Kaiserswerth, a Protestant religious community that contained the Institution for the Training of Deaconesses, with a hospital school, penitentiary, and orphanage. A Protestant pastor, Theodore Fleidner, and his young wife had established this community in 1836, in part to provide training for women deaconesses (Protestant "nuns") who wished to nurse. Nightingale was to return there in 1851 against much family opposition to stay from July through October, participating in a period of "nurses training" (Cook, Vol. I, 1913; Woodham-Smith, 1983).

Life at Kaiserswerth was spartan. The trainees were up at 5 A.M., ate bread and gruel, and then worked on the hospital wards until noon. Then they had a 10-minute break for broth with vegetables. Three P.M. saw another 10-minute break for tea and bread. They worked until 7 P.M., had some broth, and then Bible lessons until bed. What the Kaiserswerth training lacked in expertise it made up for in a spirit of reverence and dedication. Florence wrote, "The world here fills my life with interest and strengthens me in body and mind" (Huxley, 1975).

In 1852, Nightingale visited Ireland, touring hospitals and keeping notes on various institutions along the way. Nightingale took two trips to Paris in 1853, hospital training again was the goal, this time with the sisters of St. Vincent de Paul, an order of nursing sisters. In August 1853, she accepted her first "official" nursing post as superintendent of an "Establishment for Gentlewomen in Distressed Circumstances during Illness," located at 1 Harley Street, London. After six months at Harley Street, Nightingale wrote in a letter to her father: "I am in the hey-day of my power" (Nightingale, cited in Woodham-Smith, 1983, p. 77).

By October 1854, larger horizons beckoned.

Spirituality

Today I am 30—the age Christ began his Mission. Now no more childish things, no more vain things, no more love, no more marriage. Now, Lord let me think

only of Thy will, what Thou willest me to do. O, Lord, Thy will, Thy will....

— **Florence Nightingale, private note, 1850, cited in Woodham-Smith (1983, p. 130)**

By all accounts, Nightingale was an intense and serious child, always concerned with the poor and the ill, mature far beyond her years. A few months before her seventeenth birthday, Nightingale recorded in a personal note dated February 7, 1837, that she had been called to God's service. What that service was to be was unknown at that point in time. This was to be the first of four such experiences that Nightingale documented.

The fundamental nature of her religious convictions made her service to God, through service to

> *The fundamental nature of her religious convictions made her service to God, through service to humankind, a driving force in her life.*

humankind, a driving force in her life. She wrote: "The kingdom of Heaven is within; but we must make it without" (Nightingale, private note, cited in Woodham-Smith, 1983).

It would take 16 long and torturous years, from 1837 to 1853, for Nightingale to actualize her calling to the role of nurse. This was a revolutionary choice for a woman of her social standing and position, and her desire to nurse met with vigorous family opposition for many years. Along the way, she turned down proposals of marriage, potentially, in her mother's view, "brilliant matches," such as that of Richard Monckton Milnes. However, her need to serve God and to demonstrate her caring through meaningful activity proved stronger. She did not think that she could be married and also do God's will.

Calabria and Macrae (1994) note that for Nightingale there was no conflict between science and spirituality; actually, in her view, science is necessary for the development of a mature concept of God. The development of science allows for the concept of one perfect God who regulates the universe through universal laws as opposed to random happenings. Nightingale referred to these laws, or the organizing principles of the universe, as "Thoughts of God" (Macrae, 1995, p. 9). As part of God's plan of evolution, it was the responsibility of human beings to discover the laws inherent in the universe and apply them to achieve well-being. In *Notes on Nursing* (1860/1969, p. 25), she wrote:

> God lays down certain physical laws. Upon his carrying out such laws depends our responsibility (that much abused word). . . . Yet we seem to be continually expecting that He will work a miracle—i.e. break his own laws expressly to relieve us of responsibility.

Influenced by the Unitarian ideas of her father and her extended family, as well as by the more traditional Anglican church she attended, Nightingale remained for her entire life a searcher of religious truth, studying a variety of religions and reading widely. She was a devout believer in God. Nightingale wrote: "I believe that there is a Perfect Being, of whose thought the universe in eternity is the incarnation" (Calabria & Macrae, 1994, p. 20). Dossey (1998) recasts Nightingale in the mode of "religious mystic." However, to Nightingale, mystical union with God was not an end in itself but was the source of strength and guidance for doing one's work in life. For Nightingale, service to God was service to humanity (Calabria & Macrae, 1994, p. xviii).

In Nightingale's view, nursing should be a search for the truth; it should be a discovery of God's laws of healing and their proper application. This is what she was referring to in *Notes on Nursing* when she wrote about the Laws of Health, as yet unidentified. It was the Crimean War that provided the stage for her to actualize these foundational beliefs, rooting forever in her mind certain "truths." In the Crimea, she was drawn closer to those suffering injustice. It was in the Barracks Hospital of Scutari that Nightingale acted justly and responded to a call for nursing from the prolonged cries of the British soldiers (Boykin and Dunphy, 2002, p. 17).

War

I stand at the altar of those murdered men and while I live I fight their cause.

—Nightingale, cited in Woodham-Smith (1983)

Nightingale had powerful friends and had gained prominence through her study of hospitals and health matters during her travels. When Great Britain became involved in the Crimean War in 1854, Nightingale was ensconced in her first official nursing post at 1 Harley Street. Britain had joined France and Turkey to ward off an aggressive Russian advance in the Crimea (Figure 5–2). A successful advance of Russia through Turkey could threaten the peace and stability of the European continent.

The first actual battle of the war, the Battle of Alma, was fought in September 1854. It was written of that battle that it was a "glorious and bloody victory." The best technology of the times, the telegraph, was to have an effect on what was to follow. In prior wars, news from the battlefields trickled home slowly. However, the telegraph enabled war correspondents to telegraph reports home with rapid speed. The horror of the battlefields was relayed to a concerned citizenry. Descriptions of wounded men, disease, and illness abounded. Who was to care for these men? The French had the Sisters of Charity to care for their sick and wounded. What were the British to do? (Woodham-Smith, 1983; Goldie, 1987).

The minister of war was Sidney Herbert, Lord Herbert of Lea, who was the husband of Liz Herbert; both were close friends of Nightingale. Herbert had an innovative solution: appoint Miss Nightingale and charge her to head a contingent of nurses to the Crimea to provide help and organization to the deteriorating battlefield situation. It was a brave move on the part of Herbert. Medicine and war were exclusively male domains. To send a woman into these hitherto uncharted waters was risky at best. But, as is well known, Nightingale was no ordinary woman, and she more than rose to the occasion. In a passionate letter to Nightingale, requesting her to accept this post, Herbert wrote:

> Your own personal qualities, your knowledge and your power of administration, and among greater things, your rank and position in society, give you advantages in such a work that no other person possesses. (Dolan, 1971, p. 2)

At the same time, such that their letters actually crossed, Nightingale wrote to Herbert, offering her services. Accompanied by 38 handpicked "nurses" who had no formal training, she arrived on November 4, 1854, to "take charge" and did not return to England until August 1856.

Biographer Woodham-Smith and Nightingale's own correspondence, as cited in a number of sources (Cook, 1913; Huxley, 1975; Goldie, 1987; Summers, 1988; Vicinus & Nergaard, 1990), paint the most vivid picture of the experiences that

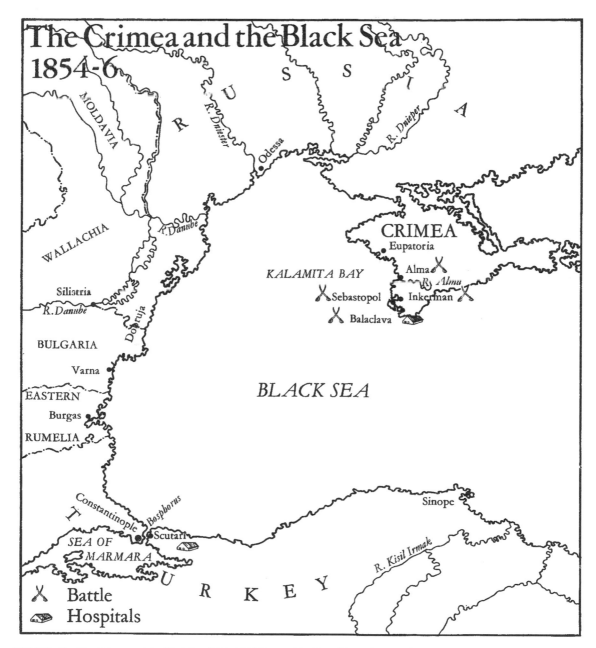

FIGURE 5–2   The Crimea and the Black Sea, 1854–1856. *Designed by Manuel Lopez Parras in Elspeth Huxley, Florence Nightingale (1975), p. 998, G. P. Putnam's Sons, New York.*

Nightingale sustained there, experiences that cemented her views on disease and contagion, as well as her commitment to an environmental approach to health and illness:

> The filth became indescribable. The men in the corridors lay on unwashed floors crawling with vermin. As the Rev. Sidney Osborne knelt to take down dying messages, his paper became thickly covered with lice.

There were no pillows, no blankets; the men lay, with their heads on their boots, wrapped in the blanket or greatcoat stiff with blood and filth which had been their sole covering for more than a week...[S]he [Miss Nightingale] estimated...there were more than 1000 men suffering from acute diarrhea and only 20 chamber pots.... [T]here was liquid filth which floated over the floor an inch deep. Huge wooden tubs stood in the halls and corridors for the men to use. In this filth lay the men's food—Miss Nightingale saw the skinned carcass of a sheep lie in a ward all night . . . the stench from the hospital could be smelled *outside* the walls (Woodham-Smith, 1983).

Upon her arrival in the Crimea, the immediate priority of Nightingale and her small band of nurses was not in the sphere of medical or surgical nursing as currently known; rather, their order of business was *domestic management*. This is evidenced in the following exchange between Nightingale and one of her party as they approached Constantinople: "Oh, Miss Nightingale, when we land don't let there be any red-tape delays, let us get straight to nursing the poor fellows!" Nightingale's reply: "The strongest will be wanted at the wash tub" (Cook, 1913; Dolan, 1971).

Although the bulk of this work continued to be done by orderlies after Nightingale's arrival (with the laundry farmed out to the soldiers' wives), it was accomplished under Nightingale's eagle eye: "She insisted on the huge wooden tubs in the wards being emptied, standing [obstinately] by the side of each one, sometimes for an hour at a time, never scolding, never raising her voice, until the orderlies gave way and the tub was emptied" (Cook, 1913; Summers, 1988; Woodham-Smith, 1983).

Nightingale set up her own extra "diet kitchen." Small portions, helpings of such things as arrowroot, port wine, lemonade, rice pudding, jelly, and beef tea, whose purpose was to tempt and revive the appetite, were provided to the men. It was therefore a logical sequence from cooking to feeding, from administering food to administering medicines. Because no antidote to infection existed at this time, the provision—by Nightingale and her nurses—of cleanliness, order, encouragement to eat, feeding, clean bed linen, clean bodies, and clean wards, was essential to recovery (Summers, 1988).

Mortality rates at the Barrack Hospital in Scutari fell. In February, at Nightingale's insistence, the prime minister had sent to the Crimea a sanitary commission to investigate the high mortality rates. Beginning their work in March, they described the conditions at the Barrack Hospital as "murderous." Setting to work immediately, they opened the channel through which the water supplying the hospital flowed, where a dead horse was found. The commission cleared "556 handcarts and large baskets full of rubbish . . . 24 dead animals and 2 dead horses buried." In addition, they flushed and

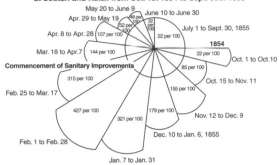

FIGURE 5–3 Diagram by Florence Nightingale showing declining mortality rates. *From Cohen, I. B. (1981). Florence Nightingale: The passionate statistician. Scientific American, 250(3): 128–137.*

cleansed sewers, limewashed walls, tore out shelves that harbored rats, and got rid of vermin. The commission, Nightingale said, "saved the British Army." Miss Nightingale's anticontagionism was sealed as the mortality rates began showing dramatic declines (Rosenberg, 1979).

Figure 5–3 illustrates Nightingale's own hand-drawn "coxcombs" (as they were referred to), as Nightingale, being always aware of the necessity of documenting outcomes of care, kept copious records of all sorts (Cook, 1913; Rosenberg, 1979; Woodham-Smith, 1983).

Florence Nightingale possessed *moral authority*, so firm because it was grounded in caring and was in a larger mission that came from her spirituality. For Miss Nightingale, spirituality was a much broader, more unitive concept than that of religion. Her spirituality involved the sense of a presence higher than human presence, the divine intelligence that creates, sustains, and organizes the universe, and an awareness of our inner connection to this higher reality. Through this inner connection flows creative endeavors and insight, a sense of purpose and direction. For Miss Nightingale, spirituality was intrinsic to human nature and was the deepest, most potent resource for healing. Nightingale was to write in *Suggestions for Thought* (Calabria & Macrae, 1994, p. 58) that "human consciousness is tending to become what God's consciousness is—to become One with the consciousness of God." This progression of consciousness to unity with the divine was an evolutionary view and not typical of either the Anglican or Unitarian views of the time (Rosenberg, 1979;

Welch, 1986; Widerquist, 1992; Slater, 1994; Calabria & Macrae, 1994; Macrae, 1995).

There were four miles of beds in the Barrack Hospital at Scutari, a suburb of Constantinople. A letter to the *London Times* dated February 24, 1855, reported the following:

> When all the medical officers have retired for the night and silence and darkness have settled upon those miles of prostrate sick, she may be observed, alone with a little lamp in her hand, making her solitary rounds (Kalisch & Kalisch, 1987).

In April 1855, after having been in Scutari for six months, Florence wrote to her mother, "[A]m in sympathy with God, fulfilling the purpose I came into the world for" (Woodham-Smith, 1983, p. 97). Henry Wadsworth Longfellow authored "Santa Filomena" to commemorate Miss Nightingale.

> Lo! In That House of Misery
> A lady with a lamp I see
> Pass through the glimmering gloom
> And flit from room to room
> And slow as if in a dream of bliss
> The speechless sufferer turns to kiss
> Her shadow as it falls
> Upon the darkening walls
> As if a door in heaven should be
> Opened and then closed suddenly
> The vision came and went
> The light shone and was spent.
> A lady with a lamp shall stand
> In the great history of the land
> A noble type of good
> Heroic womanhood
>
> *(Longfellow, cited in Dolan, 1971, p. 5).*

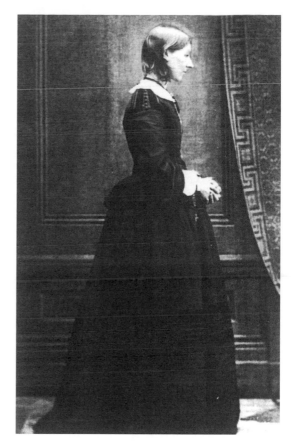

FIGURE 5–4 A rare photograph of Florence taken on her return from the Crimea. Although greatly weakened by her illness, she refused to accept her friends' advice to rest, and pressed on relentlessly with her plans to reform the army medical services. *From Elspeth Huxley, Florence Nightingale (1975), p. 139, G. P. Putnam's Sons, New York.*

Miss Nightingale slipped home quietly, arriving at Lea Hurst in Derbyshire on August 7, 1856, after 22 months in the Crimea and after sustained illness from which she was never to recover; after ceaseless work; and after witnessing suffering, death, and despair that would haunt her for the remainder of her life. Her hair was shorn; she was pale and drawn (Figure 5–4). She took her family by surprise. The next morning, a peal of the village church bells and a prayer of Thanksgiving were, her sister wrote, "'all the innocent greeting' except for those provided by the spoils of war that had proceeded her— a one-legged sailor boy, a small Russian orphan, and a large puppy found in some rocks near Balaclava. All England was ringing with her name,

but she had left her heart on the battlefields of the Crimea and in the graveyards of Scutari" (Huxley, 1975, p. 147).

Introducing the Theory

In watching disease, both in private homes and public hospitals, the thing which strikes the experienced observer most forcefully is this, that the symptoms or the sufferings generally considered to be inevitable and incident to the disease are very often not symptoms of the disease at all, but of something quite different—of the want of fresh air, or light, or of warmth, or of quiet, or of cleanliness, or of

punctuality and care in the administration of diet, of each or of all of these.
—Florence Nightingale, *Notes on Nursing* (1860/1969, p. 8)

The Medical Milieu

To gain a better understanding of Nightingale's ideas on nursing, one must enter the peculiar world of nineteenth-century medicine and its views on health and disease. Considerable new medical knowledge had been gained by 1800. Gross anatomy was well known; chemistry promised to throw light on various body processes. Vaccination against smallpox existed. There were some established drugs in the pharmacopoeia: cinchona bark, digitalis, and mercury. Certain major diseases, such as leprosy and the bubonic plague had almost disappeared. The crude death rate in western Europe was falling, largely related to decreasing infant mortality as a result of improvement in hygiene and standard of living (Ackernecht, 1982; Shyrock, 1959).

Yet physicians at the turn of the century, in 1800, still had only the vaguest notion of diagnosis. Speculative philosophies continued to dominate medical thought, although inroads and assaults continued to be made that eventually gave way to a new outlook on the nature of disease: from belief in general states common to all illnesses to an understanding of disease-specificity resultant symptomatology. It was this shift in thought—a paradigm shift of the first order—that gave us the triumph of twentieth-century medicine, with all its attendant glories and concurrent sterility.

The eighteenth century was host to two major traditions or paradigms in the healing arts: one based on "empirics" or "experience," trial and error, with an emphasis on curative remedies; the other based on Hippocratic notions and learning. Evidence of both these trends persisted into the nineteenth century and can be found in Nightingale's philosophy.

Consistent with the speculative and philosophical nature of her superior education (Barritt, 1973), Nightingale, like many of the physicians of her time, continued to emphatically disavow the reality of specific states of disease. She insisted on a view of sickness as an "adjective," not a substantive noun. Sickness was not an "entity" somehow separable from the body. Consistent with her more holistic view, sickness was an aspect or quality of the body as a whole. Some physicians, as she phrased it, taught that diseases were like cats and dogs, distinct species necessarily descended from other cats and dogs. She found such views misleading (Nightingale, 1860/1969).

At this point in time, in the mid-nineteenth century, there were two competing theories regarding the nature and origin of disease. One view was known as "contagionism," postulating that some diseases were communicable, spread via commerce and population migration. The strategic consequences of this explanatory model was *quarantine,* and its attendant bureaucracy aimed at shutting down commerce and trade to keep disease away from noninfected areas. To the new and rapidly emerging merchant classes, quarantine represented government interference and control (Ackernecht, 1982; Arnstein, 1988).

The second school of thought on the nature and origin of disease, of which Nightingale was an ardent champion, was known as "anticontagionism." It postulated that disease resulted from local environmental sources and arose out of "miasmas"—clouds of rotting filth and matter, activated by a variety of things such as meteorologic conditions (note the similarity to elements of water, fire, air, and earth on humors); the filth must be eliminated from *local* areas to prevent the spread of disease. Commerce and "infected" individuals were left alone (Rosenberg, 1979).

William Farr, another Nightingale associate and avid anticontagionist, was Britain's statistical superintendent of the General Register Office. Farr categorized epidemic and infectious diseases as *zygomatic,* meaning pertaining to or caused by the process of fermentation. The debate as to whether fermentation was a chemical process or a "vitalistic" one had been raging for some time (Swazey & Reed, 1978). The familiarity of the process of fermentation helps to explain its appeal. Anyone who had seen bread rise could immediately grasp how a minute amount of some contaminating substance could in turn "pollute" the entire atmosphere, the very air that was breathed. What was at issue was the *specificity* of the contaminating substance. Nightingale, and the anticontagionists, endorsed the position that a "sufficiently intense level of atmospheric contamination could induce both endemic and epidemic ills in the crowded hospital wards [with particular configurations of environmental circumstances determining which]" (Rosenberg, 1979).

Anticontagionism reached its peak prior to the political revolutions of 1848; the resulting wave of conservatism and reaction brought contagionism back into dominance, where it remained until its reformulation into the germ theory in the 1870s. Leaders of the contagionists were primarily high-ranking military physicians, politically united. These divergent worldviews accounted in some part for Nightingale's clashes with the military physicians she encountered during the Crimean War.

Given the intellectual and social milieu in which Nightingale was raised and educated, her stance on contagionism seems preordained and logically consistent. Likewise, the eclectic religious philosophy she evolved contained attributes of the philosophy of Unitarianism with the fervor of Evangelicalism, all based on an organic view of humans as part of nature. The treatment of disease and dysfunction was inseparable from the nature of man as a whole, and likewise, the environment. And all were linked to God.

The emphasis on "atmosphere" (or "environment") in the Nightingale model is consistent with the views of the "anticontagionists" of her time. This worldview was reinforced by Nightingale's Crimean experiences, as well as her liberal and progressive political thought. Additionally, she viewed all ideas as being distilled through a distinctly *moral* lens (Rosenberg, 1979). As such, Nightingale was typical of a number of her generation's intellectuals. These thinkers struggled to come to grips with an increasingly complex and changing world order and frequently combined a language of two disparate realms of authority: the moral realm and the emerging scientific paradigm that has assumed dominance in the twentieth century. Traditional religious and moral assumptions were garbed in a mantle of "scientific objectivity," often spurious at best, but more in keeping with the increasingly rationalized and bureaucratic society accompanying the growth of science.

The Feminist Context of Nightingale's Caring

I have an intellectual nature which requires satisfaction and that would find it in him. I have a passionate nature which requires satisfaction and that would find it in him. I have a moral, an active nature which requires satisfaction and that would not find it in his life.

—Florence Nightingale, private note, 1849, cited in Woodham-Smith (1983, p. 51)

Florence Nightingale wrote the following tortured note upon her final refusal of Richard Monckton Milnes's proposal of marriage: "I know I could not bear his life," she wrote, "that to be nailed to a continuation, an exaggeration of my present life without hope of another would be intolerable to me—that voluntarily to put it out of my power ever to be able to seize the chance of forming for myself a true and rich life would seem to be like suicide" (Nightingale, personal note cited in Woodham-Smith, 1983, p. 52). For Miss Nightingale there was no compromise. Marriage and pursuit of her "mission" were not compatible. She chose the mission, a clear repudiation of the mores of her time, which were rooted in the time-honored role of family and "female duty."

The census of 1851 revealed that there were 365,159 "excess women" in England, meaning women who were not married. These women were viewed as redundant, as described in an essay about the census entitled, "Why Are Women Redundant?" (Widerquist, 1992, p. 52). Many of these women had no acceptable means of support, and Nightingale's development of a suitable occupation for women, that of nursing, was a significant historical development and a major contribution by Nightingale to women's plight in the nineteenth century. However, in other ways, her views on women and the question of women's rights were quite mixed.

Notes on Nursing: What It Is and What It Is Not (1859/1969) was written not as a manual to teach

> *Notes on Nursing: What It Is and What It Is Not (1859/1969) was written not as a manual to teach nurses to nurse, but rather to help all women to learn how to nurse.*

nurses to nurse, but rather to help all women to learn how to nurse. Nightingale believed all women required this knowledge in order to take proper care of their families during times of sickness and to promote health—specifically what Nightingale referred to as "the health of houses," that is, the "health" of the environment, which she espoused. Nursing, to her, was clearly situated within the context of female duty.

In *Ordered to Care: The Dilemma of American Nursing* (1987, p. 43), historian Susan Reverby traces contemporary conflicts within the nursing profession back to Nightingale herself. She asserts that Nightingale's ideas about female duty and authority, along with her views on disease causality, brought about an independent field—that of nursing—that was separate, and in the view of Nightingale, equal, if not superior, to that of medicine. But this field was dominated by a female hierarchy and insisted on both deference and loyalty to the physician's authority. Reverby sums it up as follows: "Although Nightingale sought to free women from the bonds of familial demand, in her nursing model she rebound them in a new context."

Does the record support this evidence? Was Nightingale a champion for women's rights or a regressive force? As noted earlier, the answer is far from clear.

The shelter for all moral and spiritual values, threatened by the crass commercialism that was flourishing in the land, as well as the spirit of critical inquiry that accompanied this age of expanding scientific progress, was agreed upon: the home. All considered this to be a "sacred place, a Temple" (Houghton, 1957, p. 343). And who was the head of this home? Woman. Although the Victorian family was patriarchal in nature, in that women had virtually no economic and/or legal rights, they nonetheless yielded a major *moral* role (Houghton, 1957; Perkins, 1987; Arnstein, 1988).

There was hostility on the part of men as well as on the part of some women to women's emancipation. Many intelligent women—for example, Beatrice Webb, George Eliot, and, at times, Nightingale herself—viewed their sex's emancipation with apprehension. In Nightingale's case, the best word might be "ambivalence." There was a fear of weakening women's moral influence, coarsening the feminine nature itself.

This stance is best equated with *cultural feminism,* defined as a belief in inherent gender differences. Women, in contrast to men, are viewed as morally superior, the holders of family values and continuity; they are refined, delicate, and in need of

protection. This school of thought, important in the nineteenth century, used arguments for women's suffrage such as the following: "[W]omen must make themselves felt in the public sphere because their *moral* perspective would improve corrupt masculine politics." In the case of Nightingale, these cultural feminist attitudes "made her impatient with the idea of women seeking rights and activities just because men valued these entities." (Campbell & Bunting, 1990, p. 21).

Nightingale had chafed at the limitations and restrictions placed on women, especially "wealthy" women with nothing to do: "What these [women] suffer—even physically—from the want of such work no one can tell. The accumulation of nervous energy, which has had nothing to do during the day, makes them feel every night, when they go to bed, as if they were going mad...." Despite these vivid words, authored by Nightingale (1852/1979) in the fiery polemic "Cassandra," which was used as a rallying cry in many feminist circles, her view of the solution was measured. Her own resolution, painfully arrived at, was to break from her family and actualize her caring mission, that of nurse. One of the many results of this was that a useful occupation for other women to pursue was founded. Although Nightingale approved of this occupation outside of the home for other women, certain other occupations—that of doctor, for example—she viewed with hostility and as inappropriate for women. Why should these women not be nurses or nurse midwives, a far superior calling in Nightingale's view than that of a medicine "man" (Monteiro, 1984)?

Welch (1990) terms Nightingale a "Christian feminist" on the eve of her departure to the Crimea. She returned even more skeptical of women. Writing to her close friend Mary Clarke Mohl, she described women that she worked with in the Crimea as being incompetent and incapable of independent thought (Woodham-Smith, 1983; Welch, 1990). According to Palmer (1977), by this time in her life, the concerns of the British people and the demands of service to God took precedence over any concern she had ever had about women's rights.

In other words, Nightingale, despite the clear freedom in which she lived her own life, nonetheless genderized the nursing role, leaving it rooted in nineteenth-century morality. Nightingale is seen constantly trying to improve the existing order and to work within that order; she was above all a reformer, seeking to improve the existing order, not to change the terrain radically.

In Nightingale's mind, the specific "scientific" activity of nursing hygiene was the central element in health care, without which medicine and surgery would be ineffective:

> The Life and Death, recovery or invaliding of patients generally depends not on any great and isolated act, but on the unremitting and thorough performance of every minute's practical duty. (Nightingale, 1860/1969)

This "practical duty" was the work of women, and the conception of the proper division of labor resting upon work demands internal to each respective "science," nursing and medicine, obscured the professional inequality. The later successes of medical science heightened this inequity. The scientific grounding espoused by Nightingale for nursing was ephemeral at best, as later nineteenth-century discoveries proved much of her analysis wrong, although nonetheless powerful. Much of her strength was in her rhetoric; if not always logically consistent, it certainly was morally resonant (Rosenberg, 1979).

Despite exceptional anomalies, such as women physicians, what Nightingale effectively accomplished was a genderization of the division of labor in health care: male physicians and female nurses. This appears to be a division that Nightingale supported. Because this "natural" division of labor was rooted in the family, women's work outside the home ought to resemble domestic tasks and complement the "male principle" with the "female." Thus, nursing was left on the shifting sands of a soon-outmoded "science"; the main focus of its authority grounded in an equally shaky moral sphere, also subject to change and devaluation in an increasingly secularized, rationalized, and technological twentieth century.

Nightingale failed to provide institutionalized nursing with an autonomous future, on an equal parity with medicine. She did, however, succeed in providing women's work in the public sphere, establishing for numerous women an identity and source of employment. Although that public identity grew out of women's domestic and nurturing roles in the family, the conditions of a modern society required public as well as private forms of care. It is questionable whether more could

have been achieved at that point in time (King, 1988).

A woman, Queen Victoria, presided over the age: "Ironically, Queen Victoria, that panoply of family happiness and stubborn adversary of female independence, could not help but shed her aura upon single women." The queen's early and lengthy widowhood, her "relentlessly spreading figure and commensurately increasing empire, her obstinate longevity which engorged generations of men and the collective shocks of history, lent an epic quality to the lives of solitary women" (Auerbach, 1982, pp. 120–121). Both Nightingale and the queen saw themselves as working through men, yet their lives added new, unexpected, and powerful dimensions to the myth of Victorian womanhood, particularly that of a woman alone and in command (Auerbach, 1982, pp. 120–121).

Nightingale's clearly chosen spinsterhood repudiated the Victorian family. Her unmarried life provides a vision of a powerful life lived on her own terms. This is not the spinsterhood of convention—one to be pitied, one of broken hearts—but a *radically* new image. She is freed from the trivia of family complaints and scorns the feminist collectivity; yet in this seemingly solitary life, she finds union not with one man but with all men, personified by the British soldier.

Lytton Strachey's well-known evocation of Nightingale, iconoclastic and bold, is perhaps closest to the decidedly masculine imagery she selected to describe herself, as evidenced in this imaginary speech to her mother written in 1852:

> Well, my dear, you don't imagine with my "talents," and my "European reputation" and my "beautiful letters" and all that, I'm going to stay dangling around my mother's drawing room all my life! ... [Y]ou must look upon me as your vagabond son ... I shan't cost you nearly as much as a son would have done, or had I married. You must consider me married or a son. (Woodham-Smith, 1983, p. 66)

Ideas about Nursing

Every day sanitary knowledge, or the knowledge of nursing, or in other words, of how to put the constitution in such a state as that it will have no disease, or that it can recover from disease, takes a higher place.

—**Florence Nightingale,** *Notes on Nursing*
(1860/1969), Preface

Evelyn R. Barritt, professor of nursing, suggested that nursing became a science when Nightingale identified her laws of nursing, also referred to as the laws of health, or nature (Barritt, 1973). The remainder of all nursing theory may be viewed as mere branches and "acorns," all fruit of the roots of Nightingale's ideas. Early writings of Nightingale, compiled in *Notes on Nursing: What It Is and What It Is Not* (1860/1969), provided the earliest systematic perspective for defining nursing. According to Nightingale, analysis and application of universal "laws" would promote well-being and relieve the suffering of humanity. This was the goal of nursing.

As noted by the caring theorist Madeline Leininger, Nightingale never defined human care or caring in Nightingale's *Notes on Nursing* (1859/1992, p. 31), and she goes on to wonder if Nightingale considered "components of care such as comfort, support, nurturance, and many other care constructs and characteristics and how they would influence the reparative process." Although Nightingale's conceptualizations of nursing, hygiene, the laws of health, and the environment never explicitly identify the construct of caring, an underlying ethos of care and commitment to others echoes in her words and, most importantly, resides in her actions and the drama of her life.

Nightingale did not theorize in the way we are accustomed to today. Patricia Winstead-Fry (1993), in a review of the 1992 commemorative edition of Nightingale's *Notes on Nursing* (1859/1992, p. 161), states: "Given that theory is the interrelationship of concepts which form a system of propositions that can be tested and used for predicting practice, Nightingale was not a theorist. None of her major biographers present her as a theorist. She was a consummate politician and health care reformer." Her words and ideas, contextualized in the earlier portion of this chapter, ring differently than those of the other nursing theorists you will study in this book. However, her underlying ideas continue to be relevant and, some would argue, prescient.

Karen Dennis and Patricia Prescott (1985) note that including Nightingale among the nurse theorists has been a recent development. They make the case that nurses today continue to incorporate in their practice the insight, foresight, and, most important, the clinical acumen of Nightingale's century-old vision of nursing. As part of a larger study, they collected a large base of descriptions from both nurses and physicians describing "good"

nursing practice. Over 300 individual interviews were subjected to content analysis; categories were named inductively and validated by four members of the project staff, separately.

Noting no marked differences in the descriptions obtained from either the nurses or physicians, the authors report that despite their independent derivation, the categories that emerged during the study bore a striking resemblance to nursing practice as described by Nightingale: prevention of illness and promotion of health, observation of the sick, and attention to physical environment. Also referred to by Nightingale as the "health of houses," this physical environment included ventilation of both the patient's rooms and the larger environment of the "house": light, cleanliness, and the taking of food; attention to the interpersonal milieu, which included variety; and not indulging in superficialities with the sick or giving them false encouragement.

The authors note that "the words change but the concepts do not" (Dennis & Prescott, 1985, p. 80). In keeping with the tradition established by Nightingale, they note that nurses continue to foster an interpersonal milieu that focuses on the person, while manipulating and mediating the environment to "put the patient in the best condition for nature to act upon him" (Nightingale, 1860/1969, p. 133).

Afaf I. Meleis (1997), nurse scholar, does not compare Nightingale to contemporary nurse theorists; nonetheless, she refers to her frequently. Meleis states that it was Nightingale's conceptualization of environment as the focus of nursing activity and her deemphasis of pathology, emphasizing instead the "laws of health" (as yet unknown), that were the earliest differentiation of nursing and medicine. Meleis (1997, pp. 114–116) describes Nightingale's concept of nursing as including "the proper use of fresh air, light, warmth, cleanliness, quiet, and the proper selection and administration of diet, all with the least expense of vital power to the patient." These ideas clearly had evolved from Nightingale's observations and experiences. The art of observation was identified as an important nursing function in the Nightingale model. And this observation was what should form the basis for nursing ideas. Meleis speculates on how differently the theoretical base of nursing might have evolved if we had continued to consider extant nursing practice as a source of ideas.

Pamela Reed and Tamara Zurakowski (1983/1989, p. 33) call the Nightingale model "visionary." They state: "At the core of all theory development activities in nursing today is the tradition of Florence Nightingale." They also suggest four major factors that influenced her model of nursing: religion, science, war, and feminism, all of which are discussed in this chapter.

The assumptions in the following section were identified by Victoria Fondriest and Joan Osborne (1994).

NIGHTINGALE'S ASSUMPTIONS

1. Nursing is separate from medicine.
2. Nurses should be trained.
3. The environment is important to the health of the patient.
4. The disease process is not important to nursing.
5. Nursing should support the environment to assist the patient in healing.
6. Research should be utilized through observation and empirics to define the nursing discipline.
7. Nursing is both an empirical science and an art.
8. Nursing's concern is with the person in the environment.
9. The person is interacting with the environment.
10. Sick and well are governed by the same laws of health.
11. The nurse should be observant and confidential.

The goal of *nursing* as described by Nightingale is assisting the patient in his or her retention of "vital powers" by meeting his or her needs, and

> *The goal of nursing as described by Nightingale is assisting the patient in his or her retention of "vital powers" by meeting his or her needs, and thus, putting the patient in the best condition for nature to act upon (Nightingale, 1860/1969).*

thus, putting the patient in the best condition for nature to act upon (Nightingale, 1860/1969). This must not be interpreted as a "passive state," but rather one that reflects the patient's capacity for self-healing facilitated by nurses' ability to create an environment conducive to health. The focus of this nursing activity was the proper use of fresh air, light, warmth, cleanliness, quiet, proper selection and administration of diet, monitoring the patient's expenditure of energy, and observing. This activity was directed toward the environment and the patient (see Nightingale's Assumptions).

Health was viewed as an additive process, the result of environmental, physical, and psychological factors, not just the absence of disease. Disease was the reparative process of the body to correct a problem and could provide an opportunity for spiritual growth. The laws of health, as defined by Nightingale, were those to do with keeping the person, and the population, healthy. This was dependent upon proper environmental control—for example, sanitation. The environment was what the nurse manipulated. It included those physical elements external to the patient. Nightingale isolated five environmental components essential to an individual's health: clean air, pure water, efficient drainage, cleanliness, and light.

> *Nightingale isolated five environmental components essential to an individual's health: clean air, pure water, efficient drainage, cleanliness, and light.*

The *patient* is at the center of the Nightingale model, which incorporates a holistic view of the person as someone with psychological, intellectual, and spiritual components. This is evidenced in her acknowledgment of the importance of "variety." For example, she wrote of "the degree . . . to which the nerves of the sick suffer from seeing the same walls, the same ceiling, the same surroundings" (Nightingale, 1860/1969). Likewise, her chapter on "chattering hopes and advice" illustrates an astute grasp of human nature and of interpersonal relationships. She remarked upon the spiritual component of disease and illness, and she felt they could present an opportunity for spiritual growth. In this, all persons were viewed as equal.

A *nurse* was defined as any woman who had "charge of the personal health of somebody," whether well, as in caring for babies and children, or sick, as an "invalid" (Nightingale, 1860/1969). It was assumed that all women, at one time or another in their lives, would nurse. Thus, all women needed to know the laws of health. Nursing proper, or "sick" nursing, was both an art and a science and required organized, formal education to care for those suffering from disease. Above all, nursing was "service to God in relief of man"; it was a "calling" and "God's work" (Barritt, 1973). Nursing activities served as an "art form" through which spiritual development might occur (Reed & Zurakowski, 1983/1989). All nursing actions were guided by the nurses' *caring*, which was guided by underlying ideas about God.

Consistent with this caring base is Nightingale's views on *nursing as an art and a science*. Again, this was a reflection of the marriage, essential to Nightingale's underlying worldview, of science and spirituality. On the surface, these might appear to be odd bedfellows; however, this marriage flows directly from Nightingale's underlying religious and philosophic views, which were operationalized in her nursing practice. Nightingale was an empiricist, valuing the "science" of observation with the intent of use of that knowledge to better the life of humankind. The application of that knowledge required an artist's skill, far greater than that of the painter or sculptor:

> Nursing is an art; and if it is to be made an art, it requires as exclusive a devotion, as hard a preparation, as any painter's or sculptor's work; for what is the having to do with dead canvas or cold marble, compared with having to do with the living body—the Temple of God's spirit? It is one of the Fine Arts; I had almost said, the finest of the Fine Arts. (Florence Nightingale, cited in Donahue, 1985, p. 469)

Nursing is an art; and if it is to be made an art, it requires as exclusive a devotion, as hard a preparation, as any painter's or sculptor's work; for what is the having to do with dead canvas or cold marble, compared with having to do with the living body—the Temple of God's spirit? It is one of the Fine Arts; I had almost said, the finest of the Fine Arts.

Nightingale's ideas about nursing health, the environment, and the person were grounded in experience; she regarded one's sense *observations* as the

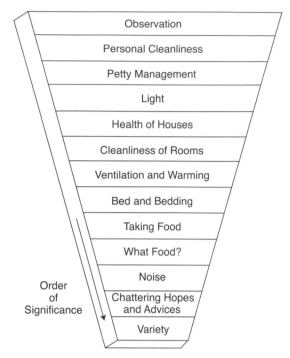

FIGURE 5–5 Perspective on Nightingale's 13 canons. *Illustration developed by V. Fondriest, RN, BSN, and J. Osborne, RN, C BSN in October 1994.*

only reliable means of obtaining and verifying knowledge. Theory must be reformulated if inconsistent with empirical evidence. This experiential knowledge was then to be transformed into empirically based generalizations, an inductive process, to arrive at, for example, the laws of health. Regardless of Nightingale's commitment to empiricism and experiential knowledge, her early education and religious experience also shaped this emerging knowledge (Hektor, 1992).

According to Nightingale's model, nursing contributes to the ability of persons to maintain and restore health directly or indirectly through managing the environment. The person has a key role in his or her own health, and this health is a function of the interaction between person, nurse, and environment. However, neither the person nor the environment is discussed as influencing the nurse (Figure 5–5).

Although it is difficult to describe the interrelationship of the concepts in the Nightingale model, Figure 5–6 is a schema that attempts to delineate this. Note the prominence of "observation" on the outer circle (important to all nursing functions)

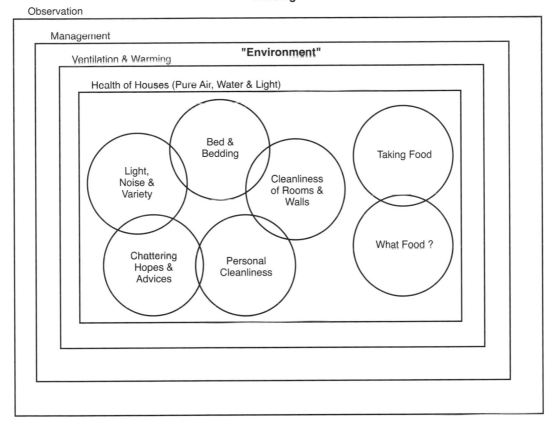

FIGURE 5–6   Nightingale's model of nursing and the environment. *Illustration developed by V. Fondriest, RN, BSN, and J. Osborne, RN, C BSN.*

and the interrelationship of the specifics of the interventions, such as "bed and bedding" and "cleanliness of rooms and walls," that go into making up the "health of houses" (Fondriest & Osborne, 1994).

Nightingale's Legacy

Philip and Beatrice Kalisch (1987, p. 26) describe the popular and glorified images that arose out of the portrayals of Florence Nightingale during and after the Crimean War—that of nurse as self-sacrificing, refined, virginal, and an "angel of mercy," a far less threatening image than one of educated and skilled professional nurses. They attribute nurses' low pay to the perception of nursing as a "calling," a way of life for devoted women with private means, such as Florence Nightingale

(Kalisch & Kalisch, 1987, p. 20). Well over 100 years later, the amount of scholarship on Nightingale provides a more realistic portrait of a complex and brilliant woman. To quote Auerbach (1982) and Strachey (1918), "a demon, a rebel . . ."

Florence Nightingale's legacy of caring and the activism it implies is carried on in nursing today. There is a resurgence and inclusion of concepts of spirituality in current nursing practice and a delineation of nursing's caring base that in essence began with the nursing life of Florence Nightingale. Nightingale's caring, as demonstrated in this chapter, extended beyond the individual patient, beyond the individual person. She herself said that the specific business of nursing was the least important of the functions into which she had been forced in the Crimea. Her caring encompassed a broadened sphere—that of the British Army and, indeed, the entire British Commonwealth.

SUMMARY

The unique aspects of Florence Nightingale's personality and social position, combined with historical circumstances, laid the groundwork for the evolution of the modern discipline of nursing. Are the challenges and obstacles that we face today any more daunting than what confronted Nightingale when she arrived in the Crimea in 1854? Nursing for Florence Nightingale was what we might call today her "centering force." It allowed her to express her spiritual values as well as enabled her to fulfill her needs for leadership and authority. As historian Susan Reverby noted, today we are challenged with the dilemma of how to practice our integral values of caring in an unjust health-care system that does not value caring. Let us look again to Florence Nightingale for inspiration, for she remains a role model par excellence on the transformation of values of caring into an *activism* that could potentially transform our current health-care system into a more humanistic and *just* one. Her activism situates her in the context of justice-making. *Justice-making* is understood as a manifestation of compassion and caring, for it is actions that bring about justice (Boykin & Dunphy, 2002, p. 16). Florence Nightingale's legacy of connecting caring with activism can then truly be said to continue.

References

Ackernecht, E. (1982). *A short history of medicine.* Baltimore: Johns Hopkins University Press.

Arnstein, W. (1988). *Britain: Yesterday and today.* Lexington, MA: D. C. Heath & Co.

Auerbach, N. (1982). *Women and the demon: The life of a Victorian myth.* Cambridge, MA: Harvard University Press.

Barritt, E. R. (1973). Florence Nightingale's values and modern nursing education. *Nursing Forum, 12,* 7–47.

Boykin, A., & Dunphy, L. M. (2002). Justice-making: Nursing's call. *Policy, Politics, & Nursing Practice, 3,* 14–19.

Bunting, S., & Campbell, J. (1990). Feminism and nursing: An historical perspective. *Advances in Nursing Science, 12,* 11–24.

Calabria, M., & Macrae, J. (Eds.). (1994). *Suggestions for thought by Florence Nightingale: Selections and commentaries.* Philadelphia: University of Pennsylvania Press.

Cohen, I. B. (1981). Florence Nightingale: The passionate statistician. *Scientific American, 250*(3): 128–137.

Cook, E. T. (1913). *The life of Florence Nightingale* (Vols. 1–2). London: Macmillan.

Dennis, K. E., & Prescott, P. A. (1985). Florence Nightingale: Yesterday, today and tomorrow. *Advances in Nursing Science, 7*(2), 66–81.

Dolan, J. (1971). *The grace of the great lady.* Chicago: Medical Heritage Society.

Donahue, P. (1985). *Nursing: The finest art.* St. Louis: Mosby.

Dossey, B. (1998). Florence Nightingale: A 19th century mystic. *Journal of Holistic Nursing, 16*(2), 111–164.

Erickson, E. (1950). *Childhood and society.* New York: W. W. Norton & Co., Inc.

Erikson, E. (1958). *Young man Luther.* New York: W. W. Norton & Co., Inc.

Erikson, E. (1974). *Dimensions of a new identity.* New York: W. W. Norton & Co., Inc.

Firestone, S. (1971). *The dialectic of sex.* New York: Bantam Books.

Fondriest, V., & Osborne, J. (1994). A theorist before her time? Presentation, NGR 5110, Nursing Theory and Advanced Practice Nursing, School of Nursing, Florida International University, N. Miami, FL.

Goldie, S. (1987). *I have done my duty: Florence Nightingale in the Crimean War, 1854–1856.* Iowa City: University of Iowa Press.

Hektor, L. M. (1984). *Florence Nightingale, 1837–1853: Identity, crisis and resolution.* Unpublished master's thesis. Hunter-Bellevue School of Nursing, New York, NY.

Hektor, L. M. (1992). *Nursing, science, and gender: Florence Nightingale and Martha E. Rogers.* Unpublished doctoral dissertation, University of Miami.

Houghton, W. (1957). *The Victorian frame of mind.* New Haven, CT: Yale University Press.

Huxley, E. (1975). *Florence Nightingale.* New York: G. P. Putnam's Sons.

Kalisch, P. A., & Kalisch, B. J. (1987). *The changing image of the nurse.* Menlo Park, CA: Addison-Wesley.

King, M. G. (1988). Gender: A hidden issue in nursing's professionalizing reform movement. Boston: Boston University School of Nursing. In *Strategies for Theory Development V,* March 10–12.

Macrae, J. (1995). Nightingale's spiritual philosophy and its significance for modern nursing. *Image: Journal of Nursing Scholarship, 27,* 8–10.

Meleis, A. I. (1997). *Theoretical nursing: Development and progress* (3rd ed.). Philadelphia: J. B. Lippincott.

Monteiro, L. (1984). On separate roads: Florence Nightingale and Elizabeth Blackwell. *Signs: Journal of Women in Culture & Society, 9,* 520–533.

Newman, Margaret A. (1972). Nursing's theoretical evolution. *Nursing Outlook, 20,* 449–453.

Nightingale, F. (1852/1979). *Cassandra,* with an introduction by Myra Stark. Westbury, NY: Feminist Press.

Nightingale, F. (1859). *Notes on nursing: What it is and what it is not.* London: Harrison & Sons.

Nightingale, F. (1859/1992). *Notes on nursing: Commemorative edition with commentaries by contemporary nursing leaders.* Philadelphia: J. B. Lippincott.

Nightingale, F. (1860). *Suggestions for thought to searchers after religious truths* (Vols. 2–3). London: George E. Eyre & William Spottiswoode.

Nightingale, F. (1860/1969). *Notes on nursing: What it is and what it is not.* New York: Dover.

Palmer, I. S. (1977). Florence Nightingale: Reformer, reactionary, research. *Nursing Research, 26,* 84–89.

Perkins, J. (1987). *Women and marriage in nineteenth century England.* Chicago: Lyceum Books, Inc.

Quinn, V., & Prest, J. (Eds.). (1981). *Dear Miss Nightingale: A selection of Benjamin Jowett's letters to Florence Nightingale, 1860–1893.* Oxford: Clarendon Press.

Reed, P. G., & Zurakowski, T. L. (1983/1989). Nightingale: A visionary model for nursing. In Fitzpatrick, J., & Whall, A. (Eds.), *Conceptual models of nursing: Analysis and application.* Bowie, MD: Robert J. Brady.

Reverby, S. M. (1987). *Ordered to care: The dilemma of American nursing (1865–1945).* New York: Cambridge University Press.

Rosenberg, C. (1979). *Healing and history.* New York: Science History Publications.

Sattin, A. (Ed.). (1987). *Florence Nightingale's letters from Egypt: A journey on the Nile, 1849–1850.* New York: Weidenfeld & Nicolson.

Shyrock, R. (1959). *The history of nursing.* Philadelphia: W. B. Saunders & Co.

Slater, V. E. (1994). The educational and philosophical influences on Florence Nightingale, an enlightened conductor. *Nursing History Review, 2,* 137–152.

Strachey, L. (1918). *Eminent Victorians: Cardinal Manning, Florence Nightingale, Dr. Arnold, General Gordon.* London: Chatto & Windus.

Summers, A. (1988). *Angels and citizens: British women as military nurses, 1854–1914.* London: Routledge & Kegan Paul.

Swazey, J., & Reed, K. (1978). Louis Pasteur: Science and the application of science. In Swazey, J., & Reed, K. (Eds.), *Today's medicine, tomorrow's science.* U.S. Government Printing Office: DHEW Pub. No. NIH 78–244. Washington, DC: U.S. Government Printing Office.

Vicinus, M., & Nergaard, B. (Eds.). (1990). *Ever yours, Florence Nightingale: Selected letters.* Cambridge, MA: Harvard University Press.

Watson, J. (1992). Commentary. In *Notes on nursing: What it is and what it is not* (pp. 80–85). Commemorative edition. Philadelphia: J. B. Lippincott.

Welch, M. (1986). Nineteenth-century philosophic influences on Nightingale's concept of the person. *Journal of Nursing History, 1*(2), 3–11.

Welch, M. (1990). Florence Nightingale: The social construction of a Victorian feminist. *Western Journal of Nursing Research, 12,* 404–407.

Widerquist, J. G. (1992). The spirituality of Florence Nightingale. *Nursing Research, 41,* 49–55.

Winstead-Fry, P. (1993). Book review: *Notes on nursing: What it is and what it is not.* Commemorative edition. *Nursing Science Quarterly, 6*(3), 161–162.

Woodham-Smith, C. (1983). *Florence Nightingale.* New York: Atheneum 97.

Bibliography

Aiken, C. A. (1915). *Lessons from the life of Florence Nightingale.* New York: Lakeside.

Aldis, M. (1914). *Florence Nightingale.* New York: NOPHN.

Andrews, M. R. (1929). *A lost commander.* Garden City, NY: Doubleday.

Baly, M. E. (1986). *Florence Nightingale: The nursing legacy.* New York: Methuen.

Bishop, W. J. (1962). *A bio-bibliography of Florence Nightingale.* London: Dawson's of Pall Mall.

Boyd, N. (1982). *Three Victorian women who changed their world.* New York: Oxford.

Bullough, V., Bullough, B., & Stanton, M. (Eds.). (1990). *Florence Nightingale and her era: A collection of new scholarship.* New York: Garland Publishing.

Cope, Z. (1958). *Florence Nightingale and the doctors.* Philadelphia: J. B. Lippincott.

Cope, Z. (1961). *Six disciples of Florence Nightingale.* New York: Pitman.

Davies, C. (1980). *Rewriting nursing history.* London: Croom Helm.

Donahue, P. (1985). *Nursing: The finest art.* St. Louis, MO: Mosby.

French, Y. (1953). *Six great Englishwomen.* London: H. Hamilton.

Goldsmith, M. L. (1937). *Florence Nightingale: The woman and the legend.* London: Hodder & Stoughton.

Gordon, R. (1979). *The private life of Florence Nightingale.* New York: Atheneum.

Haldale, E. (1931). *Mrs. Gaskell and her friends.* New York: Appleton.

Herbert, R. G. (1981). *Florence Nightingale: Saint, reformer or rebel?* Melbourne: F. L. Krieger.

Nash, R. (1937). *A sketch for the life of Florence Nightingale.* London: Society for Promoting Christian Knowledge.

Newtown, M. E. (1949). *Florence Nightingale's philosophy of life and education.* Unpublished doctoral dissertation, Stanford University, School of Education, Stanford, CA.

Nightingale, F. (1911). *Letters from Miss Florence Nightingale on health visiting in rural districts.* London: King.

Nightingale, F. (1954). *Selected writings.* Compiled by Lucy R. Seymer. New York: Macmillan.

Nightingale, F. (1974). *Letters of Florence Nightingale in the History of Nursing Archive.* Boston: Boston University Press.

Nightingale, F. (1976). *Notes on hospitals.* New York: Gordon.

O'Malley, I. B. (1931). *Life of Florence Nightingale, 1820–1856.* London: Butterworth.

Pollard, E. (1902). *Florence Nightingale: The wounded soldiers' friend.* London: Partridge.

Rosenberg, C. (Ed.). (1989). *Florence Nightingale on hospital reform.* New York: Garland Publishing.

Selanders, L. C. (1993). *Florence Nightingale: An environmental adaptation theory.* Newbury Park, CA: Sage Publications.

Seymer, L. R. (1951). *Florence Nightingale.* New York: Macmillan.

Smith, F. B. (1982). *Florence Nightingale: Reputation and power.* New York: St. Martin's.

Tooley, S. A. (1905). *The life of Florence Nightingale.* New York: Macmillan.

Woodsey, A. H. (1950). *A century of nursing.* New York: Putnam.

Wren, D. (1949). *They enriched humanity: Adventurers of the 19th century.* London: Skilton.

PERIODICALS

Address given at fiftieth anniversary of founding by Florence Nightingale of first training school for nurses at St. Thomas's Hospital, London, England. *American Journal of Nursing, 11,* 331–361.

Agnew, L. R. (1958). Florence Nightingale: Statistician. *American Journal of Nursing, 58,* 644.

Baly, M. (1986). Shattering the Nightingale myth. *Nursing Times, 82*(24), 16–18.

Baly, M. E. (1969). Florence Nightingale's influence on nursing today. *Nursing Times, 65,* 1–4.

Barker, E. R. (1989). Caregivers as casualties: War experiences and the postwar consequences for both Nightingale-and-Vietnam-era nurses. *Western Journal of Nursing Research, 11,* 628–631.

Bishop, W. J. (1957a). Florence Nightingale bibliography. *International Nursing Review, 4,* 64.

Bishop, W. J. (1957b). Florence Nightingale letters. *American Journal of Nursing, 57,* 607.

Blanchard, J. R. (1939). Florence Nightingale: A study in vocation. *New Zealand Nursing Journal, 32,* 193–197.

Boylen, J. O. (1974). The Florence Nightingale–Mary Stanley controversy: Some unpublished letters. *Medical History, 18*(2), 186–193.

Brow, E. J. (1954). Florence Nightingale and her international influence. *International Nursing Review, 1,* 17–19.

Clayton, R. E. (1974). How men may live and not die in India: Florence Nightingale. *Australian Nurses Journal, 2,* 10–11.

Collins, W. J. (1945). Florence Nightingale and district nursing. *Nursing Mirror, 81,* 74.

Cope, Z. (1960). Florence Nightingale and her nurses. *Nursing Times, 56,* 597.

Dunbar, V. M. (1954). Florence Nightingale's influence on nursing education. *International Nursing Review, 1,* 17–23.

Extracts from letters from the Crimea. (1932). *American Journal of Nursing, 32,* 537–538.

Fink, L. G. (1934). Catholic influences in the life of Florence Nightingale. *Hospital Progress, 15,* 482–489.

Florence Nightingale as a leader in the religious and civic thought of her time. (1936). *Hospitals, 10,* 78–84.

Florence Nightingale bibliography. (1956). *Nursing Research, 5,* 87.

Florence Nightingale's letter. (1932*). Nursing Times, 28,* 699.

Florence Nightingale's letter of advice to Bellevue. (1911). *American Journal of Nursing, 11,* 361–364.

Grier, B., & Grier, M. (1978). Contributions of the passionate statistician (Florence Nightingale). *Research in Nursing and Health, 1*(3), 103–109.

Gropper, E. I. (1990). Florence Nightingale: Nursing's first environmental theorist. *Nursing Forum, 25*(3), 30–33.

Hektor, L. M. (1994). Florence Nightingale and the women's movement. Friend or foe? *Nursing Inquiry, 1*(1), 38–45.

Iveson-Iveson, J. (1983). Nurses in society: A legend in the breaking (Florence Nightingale). *Nursing Mirror, 156*(19), 26–27.

Jones, H. W. (1940). Some unpublished letters of Florence Nightingale. *Bulletin of the History of Medicine, 8,* 1389–1396.

Kerling, N. J. (1976). Letters from Florence Nightingale. *Nursing Mirror, 143*(1), 68.

Konstatinova, M. (1923). In the cradle of nursing. *American Journal of Nursing, 24,* 47–49.

Kopf, E. W. (1978). Florence Nightingale as statistician. *Research in Nursing and Health, 1*(3), 93–102.

Levine, M. E. (1963). Florence Nightingale: The legend that lives. *Nursing Forum, 2,* 24.

Loane, S. F. (1911). Florence Nightingale and district nursing. *American Journal of Nursing, 11,* 383–384.

Mackie, T. T. (1942). Florence Nightingale and tropical and military medicine. *American Journal of Tropical Medicine, 22,* 1–8.

McCarthy, D. O., Ouimet, M. E., & Daun, J. M. (1991). Shades of Florence Nightingale: Potential impact of noise stress on wound healing. *Holistic Nursing Practice, 5*(4), 39–48.

McDonald, L. (Ed.). (2003–200_). The collected works of Florence Nightingale, Vols. I–XVI projected. Vols I–VI available as of May 2004. Waterloo, Canada: Wilford Laurier University Press.

Florence Nightingale: An introduction to her life and family (Vol. I).

Florence Nightingale's spiritual journey: Biblical annotations, sermons and journal notes (Vol. II).

Florence Nightingale's theology: Essays, letters and journal notes (Vol. III).

Florence Nightingale on mysticism and Eastern religions (Vol. IV).

Florence Nightingale on society and politics, philosophy, science, education and literature (Vol. V).

Florence Nightingale on public health care (Vol. VI).

Florence Nightingale's European travel (Vol. VII).

Florence Nightingale's suggestions for thought (Vol. VIII).

Florence Nightingale on medicine, midwifery and prostitution (Vol. IX).

Florence Nightingale and the foundation of professional nursing (Vols. X–XI).

Florence Nightingale and public health care in India (Vols. XII–XIII).

Florence Nightingale and the Crimean War (Vol. XIV).

Florence Nightingale on war and militarism (Vol. XV).

Florence Nightingale and hospital reform (Vol. XVI).

Monteiro, L. (1972). Research into things past: Tracking down one of Miss Nightingale's correspondents. *Nursing Research, 21,* 526–529.

Monteiro, L. A. (1985a). Florence Nightingale on public health nursing. *American Journal of Public Health, 75,* 181–186.

Monteiro, L. A. (1985b). Response in anger: Florence Nightingale on the importance of training for nurses. *Journal of Nursing History, 1*(1), 11–18.

Nagpal, N. (1985). Florence Nightingale: A multifaceted personality. *Nursing Journal of India, 76,* 110–114.

Newton, M. E. (1952). Florence Nightingale's concept of clinical teaching. *Nursing World, 126,* 220–221.

Notting, M. A. (1927). Florence Nightingale as a statistician. *Public Health Nursing, 19,* 207–209.

Noyes, C. D. (1931). Florence Nightingale: Sanitarian and hygienist. *Red Cross Courier, 10,* 41, 42.

Oman, C. (1950). Florence Nightingale as seen by two biographers. *Nursing Mirror, 92,* 30–31.

Palmer, I. S. (1976). Florence Nightingale and the Salisbury incident. *Nursing Research, 25*(5), 370–377.

Palmer, I. S. (1983a). Florence Nightingale: The myth and the reality. *Nursing Outlook, 79,* 40–42.

Palmer, I. S. (1983b). Nightingale revisited. *Nursing Outlook, 31*(4), 229–233.

Parker, P. (1977). Florence Nightingale: First lady of administrative nursing. *Supervisor Nurse, 8,* 24–25.

Pearce, E. C. (1954). The influence of Florence Nightingale on the spirit of nursing. *International Nursing Review, 1,* 20–22.

Pope, D. S. (1995). Music, noise and the human voice in the nurse-patient environment. *Image Journal of Nursing Scholarship, 27,* 291–295.

Rajabally, M. (1994). Florence Nightingale's personality: A psychoanalytic profile. *International Journal of Nursing Studies, 31*(3), 269–278.

Richards, L. (1920). Recollections of Florence Nightingale. *American Journal of Nursing, 20,* 649.

Richards, L. (Ed.). (1934). Letters of Florence Nightingale. *Yale Review, 24,* 326–347.

Ross, M. (1954). Miss Nightingale's letters. *American Journal of Nursing, 53,* 593–594.

Scovil, E. R. (1911). Personal recollections of Florence Nightingale. *American Journal of Nursing, 11,* 365–368.

Seymer, L. R. (1951). Florence Nightingale at Kaiserwerth. *American Journal of Nursing, 51,* 424–426.

Seymer, L. R. (1970). Nightingale nursing school: 100 years ago. *American Journal of Nursing, 60,* 658.

Seymer, S. (1979). The writings of Florence Nightingale. *Nursing Journal of India, 70*(5), 121, 128.

Showalter, E. (1981). Florence Nightingale's feminist complaint: Women, religion, and suggestions for thought. *Signs, 5.*

Sparacino, P. S. A. (1994). Clinical practice: Florence Nightingale: A CNS role model. *Clinical Nurse Specialist, 8*(2), 64.

Thomas, S. P. (1993). The view from Scutari: A look at contemporary nursing. *Nursing Forum, 28*(2), 19–24.

White, F. S. (1923). At the gate of the temple. *Public Health Nursing, 15,* 279–283.

Whittaker, E., & Oleson, V. L. (1967). Why Florence Nightingale? *American Journal of Nursing, 67,* 2338.

Widerquist, J. G. (1992). The spirituality of Florence Nightingale. *Nursing Research, 41,* 499–555.

Woodham-Smith, Mrs. C. (1947). Florence Nightingale as a child. *Nursing Mirror, 85,* 91–92.

Woodham-Smith, Mrs. C. (1952). Florence Nightingale revealed. *American Journal of Nursing, 52,* 570–572.

Woodham-Smith, Mrs. C. (1954). The greatest Victorian. *Nursing Times, 50,* 737–741.

Yeates, E. L. (1962). The Prince Consort and Florence Nightingale. *Nursing Mirror, 113,* iii–iv.

Florence Nightingale at Embley in 1857: pencil drawing of her by G. Scharf. This was one of the most active and fruitful periods of her life, but as happened so often, she reacted with symptoms of nervous distress. From Elspeth Huxley: *Florence Nightingale* (1975), p. 139, G. P. Putnam's Sons, New York.

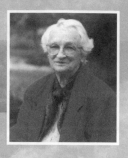

Hildegard E. Peplau

CHAPTER 6

PART ONE: Hildegard E. Peplau's Process of Practice-Based Theory Development and Its Applications

Ann R. Peden

Introducing the Theorist

Hildegard Peplau was an outstanding leader and pioneer in psychiatric nursing whose career spanned seven decades. A review of the events in her life also serves as an introduction to the history of modern psychiatric nursing. With the publication of *Interpersonal Relations in Nursing* in 1952, Peplau provided a framework for the practice of psychiatric nursing that would result in a paradigm shift in this field of nursing. Prior to this, patients were viewed as objects to be observed. Peplau taught that patients were not objects but were subjects and that psychiatric nurses must participate with the patients, engaging in the nurse-patient relationship. This was a revolutionary idea. Although *Interpersonal Relations in Nursing* was not well received when it was first published in 1952, it has since been reprinted (1988) and translated into at least six languages.

Hildegard Peplau entered nursing for practical reasons, seeing it as a way to leave home and have an occupation. As she adapted to nursing school, she made the conscious decision that if she was going to be a nurse, then she would be a good one (Peplau, 1998).

Peplau served as the college head nurse and later as executive officer of the Health Service at Bennington College, Vermont. While working there as a nurse, she began taking courses that would lead to a bachelor of arts degree in interpersonal psychology. Dr. Eric Fromm was one of her teachers at Bennington. An experience while working in the Health Service served to pique Peplau's interest in psychiatric nursing. A young student with symptoms of schizophrenia came to the clinic seeking help. Peplau did not know what to do for her. The student left Bennington to receive treatment and returned to complete her education later. The successful recovery of this young woman was a positive experience for Peplau.

Upon graduation from Bennington, Peplau joined the Army Nurse Corps. She was assigned to the School of Military Neuropsychiatry in England. This experience introduced her to the psychiatric problems of soldiers at war and allowed her to work with many great psychiatrists. After the war, Peplau attended Columbia University on the GI Bill and earned her master's in psychiatric-mental health nursing.

After her graduation in 1948, Peplau was invited to remain at Columbia and teach in their master's program. She immediately searched the library for books to use with students, but she found very few. At that time, the psychiatric nurse was viewed as a companion to patients, someone who would play games and take walks but talk about nothing substantial. In fact, nurses were instructed not to talk to patients about their problems, thoughts, or feelings. Peplau began teaching at Columbia, knowing that she wanted to change the education and practice of psychiatric nursing. There was no direction for what to include in graduate nursing programs. She took educational experiences from psychiatry and psychology and adapted them to nursing education. Peplau described this as a time of "innovation or nothing."

Her goal was to prepare nurse psychotherapists, referring to this training as "talking to patients" (Peplau, 1960, 1962). She arranged clinical experiences for her students at Brooklyn State Hospital, the only hospital in the New York City area that would take them. At the hospital, students were assigned to back wards, working with the most chronic and severely ill patients. Each student met twice weekly with the same patient, for a session lasting one hour. According to Peplau, the nurses resisted this practice tremendously and thought this was an awful thing to do (Peplau, 1998). Using carbon paper, verbatim notes were taken during the session. Students then met individually with Peplau to go over the interaction in detail. Through this process, both Peplau and her students began to learn what was helpful and what was harmful in the interaction.

In 1955, Peplau left Columbia to teach at Rutgers, where she began the Clinical Nurse Specialist program in psychiatric–mental health nursing. The students were prepared as nurse psychotherapists, developing expertise in individual, group, and family therapies. Peplau required of her students "unflinching self-scrutiny," examining their own verbal and nonverbal communication and its effects on the nurse-patient relationship. Students were encouraged to ask, "What message am I sending?"

In 1956, Peplau began spending her summers touring the country, offering week-long clinical workshops in state hospitals. This activity was instrumental in teaching interpersonal theory and the importance of the nurse-patient relationship to psychiatric nurses. The workshops also provided a forum from which Peplau could promote advanced education for psychiatric nurses. Her belief that psychiatric nurses must have advanced degrees encouraged large numbers of psychiatric nurses to seek master's degrees and eventual certification as psychiatric–mental health clinical specialists.

During her career as a nursing educator, a total of 100 students had the opportunity to study with Peplau. These students have become leaders in psychiatric nursing. Many have gone on to earn doctoral degrees, becoming psychoanalysts, writing prolifically in the field of psychiatric nursing, and entering and influencing the academic world. Their influence has resulted in the integration of the nurse-patient relationship and the concept of anxiety into the culture of nursing. In 1974, Peplau retired from Rutgers. This allowed her more time to

devote to the larger profession of nursing. Throughout her career, Peplau actively contributed to the American Nurses' Association (ANA) by serving on various committees and task forces. She is the only person who has been both the executive director and president of ANA. Peplau served on the ANA committee that wrote the Social Policy Statement. For the first time in nursing's history, nursing had a phenomenological focus—human responses.

Peplau held 11 honorary degrees. In 1994, she was inducted into the American Academy of Nursing's Living Legends Hall of Fame. She was named one of the 50 great Americans by *Marquis Who's Who* in 1995. In 1997, Peplau received the Christiane Reiman Prize, nursing's most prestigious award. In 1998, she was inducted into the ANA Hall of Fame.

Internationally, Peplau was an advisor to the World Health Organization (WHO); she was a

THE EXPERIENCE OF A SECOND-GENERATION PEPLAU STUDENT

In 1987, I began doctoral study at the University of Alabama at Birmingham. At that time, Dr. Elizabeth Morrison was assigned as my faculty advisor and chaired my dissertation committee. Dr. Morrison is one of the 100 students who studied directly with Peplau and is a Peplau scholar. Peplau described her as "a professor's delight: intelligent, responsible, responsive, career-oriented and always cheerful… she has taken her own career and further professional development seriously and has contributed greatly to the advancement of the profession" (Peplau, personal communication, September 16, 1998). After Dr. Morrison's graduation from Rutgers, she maintained a relationship with Peplau and has tested Peplau's theory in practice (Morrison, 1992; Morrison, Shealy, Kowalski, LaMont, & Range, 1996).

While beginning work on my dissertation, I began to read the writings of Peplau more carefully. Like most psychiatric nurses, I applied her interpersonal theory in my clinical practice. I had actually been taught interventions developed by Peplau as an undergraduate nursing student in psychiatric nursing. However, like many nurses educated before the 1980s, I was not told that a theorist named Peplau was guiding my practice. This I discovered after graduating from my baccalaureate program, when I began to read Peplau's work, especially her writings on anxiety and hallucinations (Peplau, 1952, 1962). In the course of reading her work with the "eye" of a doctoral student, I discovered her paper on theory development that had been presented at the first Nursing Theory Conference in 1969. In that paper, Peplau (1989a) described the process of practice-based theory development. Reading this work was very exciting. In the paper, Peplau described a methodology for developing theory in practice. This will be described more completely later in this chapter.

As my dissertation proposal developed, Dr. Morrison encouraged me to send it to Peplau for her to read. This idea made me extremely anxious, but Dr. Morrison persisted. She had talked to Peplau and Peplau said that she would be glad to read my proposal. This began a correspondence with Peplau that continued for years, until her death in 1999. She enriched my professional life, and I am honored that she was interested in what I thought and what I was doing. When considering the link between Peplau, Elizabeth Morrison, and me, I consider myself a second-generation student of Peplau. From the beginning of her research career, Peplau provided guidance, direction, and feedback—answering many questions, sharing resources, and providing contacts with other psychiatric nurse researchers. She shared her knowledge and expertise with countless numbers of psychiatric nurses. In fact, this has been a hallmark of her professional life—sharing, developing, and responding to nurses as they sought knowledge.

member of their First Nursing Advisory Committee and contributed to WHO's first paper on psychiatric nursing. She served as a consultant to the Pan-American Health Association, and she served two terms on the International Council of Nurses' Board of Directors. Even after her retirement, she continued to mentor nurses in many countries.

Hildegard Peplau died in March 1999 at her home in Sherman Oaks, California.

Introducing the Theory

In 1969, at the first Nursing Theory Conference, Hildegard Peplau proposed a research methodology to guide "development of knowledge from observations in nursing situations" (Peplau, 1989a, p. 22). Peplau asserted that nursing was an applied science and that nurses used established knowledge for beneficial purposes. According to Peplau (1988, p. 12), nurses not only "use the knowledge that 'producing scientists' publish," but they, in practice, create the context whereby this knowledge is transformed into nursing knowledge, linking nursing processes with nursing practice (Reed, 1996).

> *Peplau urged nurses to use nursing situations as a source of observations from which unique nursing concepts could be derived.*

Peplau urged nurses to use nursing situations as a source of observations from which unique nursing concepts could be derived. Practice provided the context for initiating and testing nursing theory. To direct nurses in the development of practice-based theory, Peplau (1989a) proposed a three-step process that would assist in this pursuit.

OBSERVATIONS

Theory development begins with observations made in practice. In the first step, the nurse observes a phenomenon, which is then named, categorized, or classified. The nurse relies on an already existing body of knowledge from which to derive the name of the concept or phenomenon. By relying on existing literature to assist in naming the concept, further information about the concept is gained. Included in this step are the continuing

clinical observations of the nurse who seeks regularities in the phenomenon.

Peplau (1952) identified several methods of observation, including participant observation, spectator observation, and interviewer and random observation. Participant observation, in which the nurse observes while participating, yields the most valuable clinical knowledge. This includes the recording of observations of both self and the other in order to analyze the interpersonal process. Peplau identified the participant-observer as one of the characteristic roles of the professional nurse (Peplau, 1989b). Validation of the nurse's observations, either with other professionals or with patients, is encouraged, in order to decrease observer bias (Peplau, 1989c). A nurse enters clinical situations with "theoretical understanding, personal bias, and previously acquired nursing knowledge" (Reed, 1996, p. 31).

SORTING AND CLASSIFICATION

In the second step of the process, the nurse sorts and classifies information about the phenomenon. Decoding, subdividing data, categorizing data, identifying layers of meaning at different levels of abstraction, and applying a conceptual framework to explain the phenomenon may occur as a means of interpreting observations (Peplau, 1989b). At that time, a structure for obtaining more information about the phenomenon emerges. Further observation or interviewing leads to a clearer, more explicit description of the phenomenon or concept. The nurse works to identify all of the behaviors associated with the concept. Included in this step is the collection of information about patterns or processes that accompany the phenomenon.

Using Peplau's process, clinical data are collected via observation and interview. Verbatim recordings of interactions with patients are examined for regularities. The nurse, as the interviewer, assists the patient in providing a thorough description of the concept or process. Peplau (1989d) offered interview techniques that encouraged description; for example: "Describe one time that you were ... "; "Describe one example ... "; "Say more about that ... "; and "Fill in the details about that experience" (Peplau, 1989d, pp. 221–222). Only by thorough description of the concept or process can the nurse assure that all of the behaviors associated with the process are identified.

INTERVENTIONS

The last step of the process leads to the development of interventions. Peplau viewed nursing interventions as those that "assisted patients in gaining interpersonal and intellectual competencies evolved through the nurse-patient relationship" (O'Toole & Welt, 1989, p. 351). Useful interventions are derived and tested (Peplau, 1989c).

Peplau used this process to study clinical phenomena. Both she and her students collected verbatim recordings of interactions with patients. These recordings were examined for regularities. Similar-looking data were then transcribed onto 3-by-5-inch index cards, which were then sorted, classified, and counted. As early as 1948, Peplau's students at Teachers College (Columbia University) were asked to make carbon copies of their interactions with patients. Peplau studied these and noticed that the students could not talk in a friendly way until the patients had said "I need you" or "I like you." Her analysis of similar nurse-patient interactions led to her theory of anxiety and subsequently to nursing interventions to decrease anxiety (O'Toole & Welt, 1989).

PART TWO

Applications

Peplau's work has had remarkable influence on nursing practice and education as we know it today and on development of later nursing theories. One of her major contributions to nursing was reinforcing nurses' awareness of the knowledge-rich content of practice. The next part of this chapter reviews in depth Peplau's practice-based process as applied to a set of four related research studies. It then discusses future applications of Peplau's work.

RESEARCH

Peplau's process of practice-based theory development has directed a program of research in the area of depression in women (Peden, 1998). Beginning with the identification of a clinical phenomenon—women recovering from depression—and culminating in the testing of an intervention to reduce

> *Beginning with the identification of a clinical phenomenon—women recovering from depression—and culminating in the testing of an intervention to reduce negative thinking in depressed women, Peplau's process of practice-based theory development has provided direction and structure for four studies.*

negative thinking in depressed women, Peplau's process of practice-based theory development has provided direction and structure for four studies.

The treatment of depression had been studied extensively. Nevertheless, a thorough description of the recovery process of women with depression was not reflected in the literature. The identification of a clinical phenomenon and a review of available information related to that phenomenon were the first steps in Peplau's process.

In the second step, researchers conducted a descriptive, exploratory study (Peden, 1993). Seven women who were recovering from depression were interviewed, and a process of recovering was described. Peplau assisted in the design of the semistructured interview guide (personal communication, December 14, 1990). Verbatim transcripts of the audiotaped interviews were analyzed. The process of recovering was initiated by a crisis or "turning point" experience. It continued with professional support and the support of friends and family. Recovering, according to the participants, required determination, work over time, and a series of successes that enhanced self-esteem and maintained balance. The process was dynamic, occurring in a nonserial order, with back-and-forth movement among the categories and phases. It was internal and ongoing. This study raised many questions and provided further direction for study. While participating in the interviews, the women shared strategies or techniques that facilitated recovering (Peden, 1994). These included cognitive skills, positive self-talk, and use of affirmations. They also identified negative thinking as the most difficult symptom to overcome.

Follow-up Study

Continuing in step two of the process, a follow-up study (Peden, 1996) was conducted a year later to further describe the recovery process of women who had been depressed. No new phases of the recovering process were identified. Interventions that assisted patients in recovering instilled hope were psychoeducational in nature, included cognitive interventions that change thinking styles, and provided for individualized treatment.

Peden's study (1996) concluded with the realization that more information was needed on the symptom of negative thinking. To understand a phenomenon, one must analyze its etiology, its cause, its meaning, and any clues to successful intervention (Peplau, 1989c). At the suggestion of Peplau (personal communication, January 16, 1993), work began, returning to the first step of the process to gather more information about the symptom of negative thinking.

Negative Thinking

A qualitative study (Peden, 2000) was designed to describe the nature or inherent quality of negative thoughts, their content or subject matter, and the origins of the negative thoughts experienced by women with major depression. The participants also shared strategies they used to manage the negative thoughts. The sample consisted of six women with a diagnosis of major depression who were experiencing or had experienced negative thoughts and were willing to talk about the experiences. The women participated in a series of six group interviews, the purpose of which was to elicit negative views/thoughts held by the group participants. The group interviews focused on the women's life experiences, views of self and significant others, lifestyles, and past experiences.

Researchers examined transcripts for regularities (Peplau, 1989b) and developed a coding guide. Codes were derived from available literature and were based on recommendations from Peplau (personal communication, January 16, 1993) and other codes that emerged from the initial review of the data. Codes included negative thinking related to self, negative thinking related to significant others, interactions with significant others, and developing view of self. After coding the data, researchers looked for recurring themes (Peplau, 1989a).

For the six women who participated in the study, the negative thoughts had their origins in childhood. Common childhood experiences included suppression of emotion, restrictive parenting, learning to be passive, lack of praise or compliments, high parental expectations, stifled communication, and lack of emotional support. The

negative thoughts focused primarily on self, being different, disappointing self and others, not being perfect, and always failing. The women described their self-talk as constant, negative, and demeaning. They identified various means of managing the negative thoughts. Once again, the use of affirmations, positive self-talk, and learning to change thinking were identified as reducing negative thinking. Steps one and two of the process of practice-based theory development had provided direction for moving into the third step, design of an intervention.

Testing an Intervention

A six-week group intervention was designed specifically to incorporate cognitive-behavioral techniques to assist in reducing negative thinking in depressed women. As described earlier, thought stopping and positive self-talk (or affirmations) were identified as key strategies in reducing negative thoughts. The intervention was designed using specific content from Gordon and Tobin's (1991) *Insight* program, Copeland's (1992) *The Depression Workbook,* and the investigator's own clinical experiences with depressed women. Affirmations, direct actions, thought stopping, and information on distorted thinking styles were introduced to the group members. Guided by Peplau's (1952) theory of interpersonal nursing, the introduction of cognitive-behavioral techniques did not occur until the second group session. The focus of the first week was on enhancing the development of the nurse-patient relationship to decrease anxiety, increase trust and security within the group, and lay the foundation for the intervention.

To pilot-test the intervention, 13 women with a diagnosis of major depression were randomly assigned either to a control or to an experimental group. All subjects were under psychiatric care in an outpatient clinic and receiving antidepressant medication. The experimental group participated in the six-week cognitive-behavioral group intervention for one hour per week. The control group continued with routine psychiatric care.

Pre- and post-test measures were collected on depression using the Beck Depression Inventory (BDI) (Beck, Ward, Mendelson, Mock, & Erbaugh, 1961) and on negative thinking using the Crandall Cognitions Inventory (Crandall & Chambless, 1986) and the Automatic Thoughts Questionnaire (Hollon & Kendall, 1980). Feedback from the five participants in the experimental group indicated that the intervention was beneficial. There were more significant decreases from pretest to post-test in the experimental group in negative thoughts and depressive symptoms and an increase in self-esteem than in the control group. Although the sample size was small, the intervention had a significant positive effect on depression.

Testing the Intervention with At-Risk Women

Upon recommendation of Peplau (personal communication, January 16, 1993), the intervention was tested on at-risk college women to determine if it had preventive effects (Peden, Hall, Rayens, & Beebe, 2000a, 2000b). A randomized controlled prevention trial was conducted to test the efficacy of a cognitive-behavioral group intervention in reducing negative thinking and depressive symptoms and enhancing self-esteem in a sample of 92 college women ages 18 to 24. Depression risk status was determined by scores on the Center for Epidemiologic Studies—Depression Scale (CES-D) (Radloff, 1977) and the BDI (Beck et al., 1961).

As they were enrolled, the participants were randomly assigned to either the control or experimental groups. Those participants assigned to the experimental group participated in the six-week cognitive-behavioral group intervention. Data on self-esteem, depressive symptoms, and negative thinking were collected from both groups at one month, at six months, and at eighteen months after the intervention to assess the interventions' long-term effects (Peden, Hall, Rayens, & Beebe, 2001).

The intervention did have a positive effect on depressive symptoms, negative thinking, and self-esteem in a group of at-risk college women. Reducing negative thinking in at-risk individuals may decrease the risk for depression. The intervention has also been tested with low-income single mothers who were identified as being at-risk for depression (Peden, Hall, Rayens, & Grant, in press). Plans are underway to continue to test the intervention with other at-risk groups to continue to gather further support for its preventive effects.

THE FUTURE

Study of Peplau's work is very timely. In 1969 she proposed using practice as the basis for theory de-

velopment. At that time it was a radical idea. Now the trend is to return to practice for knowledge development. Peplau used clinical situations to derive theories inductively and then tested them in clinical practice. She also applied existing social science theories to nursing phenomena, combining induction (observation and classification) with deduction (the application of known concepts and processes to data). This provided a creative, nonlinear approach to the formation of ideas.

She also proposed the linkage of qualitative and quantitative methods. Using her methodology, the nurse would begin with an in-depth look at a phenomenon, which would evolve into a quantitative study testing an intervention directed at the phenomenon. These ideas, proposed during the positivist period of nursing, were highly revolutionary. It is unlikely that Peplau's contemporaries would have embraced her process of practice-based theory development. In fact, the debates related to knowledge development in nursing and the accompanying quantitative/qualitative rift did not occur until the 1980s. However, as nursing has come to recognize practice knowledge as one of the ways of knowing, researchers may return to Peplau's ideas offered at the first Nursing Theory Conference (Peplau, 1969) for direction.

SUMMARY

Peplau's process of practice-based theory development came at a time in nursing when grand theories were being developed and theoretical nursing was highly valued. These theories are now being criticized as too broad and too remote from nursing to be applied. Now, nurses are returning to practice for knowledge development. Peplau, always ahead of her time, provided an "approach to knowledge development through the scholarship of practice; nursing knowledge is developed in practice as well as for practice" (Reed, 1996, p. 29). Peplau used observations in clinical situations as the basis for hypotheses and interventions that were then tested in clinical practice. She also applied existing theories from the social sciences to nursing phenomena:

> The process of combining induction (observation and classification) with deduction (the application of known concepts and processes to

data) provides a creative nonlinear approach to the formation of ideas, one that uses the data of practice, as well as extant theories as the basis of those formulations. (O'Toole & Welt, 1989, p. 355)

Peplau's methodology also linked qualitative and quantitative methods. After a qualitative, in-depth look at a phenomenon, a quantitative study would be developed to test an intervention directed at the phenomenon. Peplau's ideas and approach to nursing were highly revolutionary at the time; few of her contemporaries openly embraced her process of practice-based theory development. It was not until the 1980s that nursing scholars debated approaches to knowledge development in nursing, and a rift developed among advocates of quantitative versus qualitative approaches.

The use of Peplau's process of practice-based theory development as a research methodology has provided the structure for developing research in the area of depression in women. The identification of a clinical problem and an in-depth look at its etiology, patterns, and processes directed the design and testing of an intervention. As interventions were tested and supported in clinical research, the findings were reported to support the growing body of psychiatric nursing knowledge.

References

Beck, A. T., Ward, C. H., Mendelson, M., Mock, L., & Erbaugh, J. (1961). An inventory for measuring depression. *Archives of General Psychiatry, 4*, 561–571.

Copeland, M. E. (1992). *The depression workbook*. Oakland, CA: New Harbinger.

Crandell, C. J., & Chambless, D. L. (1986). The validation of an inventory for measuring depressive thoughts: The Crandell Cognitions Inventory. *Behavioral Research and Theory, 24*, 402–411.

Gordon, V., & Tobin, M. (1991). *Insight: A cognitive enhancement program for women*. Available from Verona Gordon, University of Minnesota, Minneapolis.

Hollon, S. D., & Kendall, P. C. (1980). Cognitive self-statements in depression: Development of an automatic thoughts questionnaire. *Cognitive Theory and Research, 4*, 383–395.

Morrison, E. G. (1992). Inpatient practice: An integrated framework. *Journal of Psychosocial Nursing and Mental Health Services, 30*(1), 26–29.

Morrison, E. G., Shealy, A. H., Kowalski, C., LaMont, J., & Range,

B. A. (1996). Work roles of staff nurses in psychiatric settings. *Nursing Science Quarterly, 9*, 17–21.

O'Toole, A., & Welt, S. R. (1989). *Interpersonal theory in nursing practice: Selected works of Hildegard Peplau*. New York: Springer.

Peden, A. (1993). Recovering in depressed women: Research with Peplau's theory. *Nursing Science Quarterly, 6*(3), 140–146.

Peden, A. R. (1994). Up from depression: Strategies used by women recovering from depression. *Journal of Psychiatric and Mental Health Nursing, 2*, 77–84.

Peden, A. R. (1996). Recovering from depression: A one-year follow-up. *Journal of Psychiatric and Mental Health Nursing, 3*, 289–295.

Peden, A. R. (1998). The evolution of an intervention: The use of Peplau's process of practice-based theory development. *Journal of Psychiatric and Mental Health Nursing, 5*(3), 173–178.

Peden, A. R. (2000). Negative thoughts of depressed women. *Journal of the American Psychiatric Nurses Association, 6*, 41–48.

Peden, A. R., Hall, L. A., Rayens, M. K., & Beebe, L. L. (2000a). Reducing negative thinking decreases the risk of depressive symptoms in college women. *The Journal of Nursing Scholarship, 32*, 145–151.

Peden, A. R., Hall, L. A., Rayens, M. K., & Beebe, L. L. (2000b). Negative thinking mediates the effect of self-esteem on depressive symptoms in college women. *Nursing Research, 4*, 201–207.

Peden, A. R., Hall, L. A., Rayens, M. K., & Beebe, L. L. (2001). Preventing depression in high-risk college women: A report of an 18-month follow-up. *Journal of American College Health, 4*, 299–308.

Peden, A. R., Hall, L. A., Rayens, M. K., & Grant, E. (in press). Negative thinking and the mental health of low-income single mothers. *Journal of Nursing Scholarship*.

Peplau, H. E. (1952). *Interpersonal relations in nursing*. New York: G. P. Putnam's Sons. (English edition reissued as a paperback in 1988 by Macmillan Education Ltd., London.)

Peplau, H. E. (1960). Talking with patients. *American Journal of Nursing, 60*, 964–967.

Peplau, H. E. (1962). The crux of psychiatric nursing. *American Journal of Nursing, 62*, 50–54.

Peplau, H. E. (1988). The art and science of nursing: Similarities, differences and relations. *Nursing Science Quarterly, 1*, 8–15.

Peplau, H. E. (1989a). Theory: The professional dimension. In O'Toole, A., & Welt, S. R. (Eds.), *Interpersonal theory in nursing practice: Selected works of Hildegard Peplau* (pp. 21–30). New York: Springer.

Peplau, H. E. (1989b). Interpersonal relations: The purpose and characteristics of professional nursing. In O'Toole, A., & Welt, S. R. (Eds.), *Interpersonal theory in nursing practice: Selected works of Hildegard Peplau* (pp. 42–55). New York: Springer.

Peplau, H. E. (1989c). Interpretation of clinical observations. In O'Toole, A., & Welt, S. R. (Eds.), *Interpersonal theory in nursing practice: Selected works of Hildegard Peplau* (pp. 149–163). New York: Springer.

Peplau, H. E. (1989d). Investigative counseling. In O'Toole, A., & Welt, S. R. (Eds.), *Interpersonal theory in nursing practice: Selected works of Hildegard Peplau* (pp. 205–229). New York: Springer.

Peplau, H. E. (1998). *Life of an angel: Interview with Hildegard Peplau (1998)*. Hatherleigh Co. Audiotape available from the American Psychiatric Nurses Association. www.apna.org/items.htm

Radloff, L. S. (1977). The CES-D Scale: A self-report depression scale for research in the general population. *Applied Psychological Measurement, 1,* 385–401.

Reed, P. G. (1996). Transforming practice knowledge into nursing knowledge: A revisionist analysis of Peplau. *Image, 28,* 29–33.

Sills, G. (1998). Peplau and professionalism: The emergence of the paradigm of professionalization. *Journal of Psychiatric and Mental Health Nursing, 5*(3), 167–172.

Van Survellan, G. M., & Dull, L. V. (1981). Group psychotherapy for depressed women: A model. *Journal of Psychosocial Nursing, 19,* 25–31.

Bibliography

Armstrong, M., & Kelly, A. (1993). Enhancing staff nurses' interpersonal skills: Theory to practice. *Clinical Nurse Specialist, 7*(6), 313–317.

Armstrong, M., & Kelly, A. (1995). More than the sum of their parts: Martha Rogers and Hildegard Peplau. *Archives of Psychiatric Nursing, 9*(1), 40–44.

Barker, P. (1993). The Peplau legacy: Hildegard Peplau. *Nursing Times, 89*(11), 48–51.

Barker, P. (1998). The future of the theory of interpersonal relations: A personal reflection on Peplau's legacy. *Journal of Psychiatric and Mental Health Nursing, 5*(3), 213–220.

Beeber, L. S. (1998). Treating depression through the nurse-client relationship. *Nursing Clinics of North America, 33,* 153–172.

Beeber, L. S. (2000). Hildahood: Taking the interpersonal theory of nursing to the neighborhood. *Journal of the American Psychiatric Nurses Association, 6,* 49–55.

Beeber, L. S., & Bourbonniere, M. (1998). The concept of interpersonal pattern in Peplau's theory of nursing. *Journal of Psychiatric and Mental Health Nursing, 5*(3), 187–192.

Beeber, L. S., & Caldwell, C. L. (1996). Pattern integrations in young depressed women: Parts I–II. *Archives of Psychiatric Nursing, 10,* 151–164.

Beeber, L. S., & Charlie, M. L. (1998). Depressive symptom reversal for women in a primary care setting: A pilot study. *Archives of Psychiatric Nursing, 12,* 247–254.

Burd, S. F. (1963). The development of an operational definition using the process of learning as a guide. In Burd, S. F., & Marshall, A. (Eds.), *Some clinical approaches to psychiatric nursing.* New York: Macmillan.

Burton, G. (1958). Personal, impersonal, and interpersonal relations. Cited in Smoyak, S. A., & Rouslin, S. (Eds.), *A collection of classics in psychiatric nursing literature.* Thorofare, NJ: Charles B. Slack.

Buswell, C. (1997). A model approach to care of a patient with alcohol problems. *Nursing Times, 93,* 34–35.

Chambers, M. (1998). Interpersonal mental health nursing: Research issues and challenges. *Journal of Psychiatric and Mental Health Nursing, 5*(3), 203–212.

Comley, A. (1994). A comparative analysis of Orem's self-care model and Peplau's interpersonal theory. *Journal of Advanced Nursing, 20*(4), 755–760.

Dennis, S. (1996). Implementing a nursing model for ward-based students. *Nursing Standard, 11,* 33–35.

Doncliff, B. (1994). Putting Peplau to work. *Nursing New Zealand, 2*(1), 20–22.

Douglass, J. L., Sowell, R. L., & Phillips, K. D. (2003). Using Peplau's theory to examine the psychosocial factors associated with HIV-infected women's difficulty in taking their medications. *Journal of Theory Construction, 7*(1), 10–17.

Feely, M. (1997). Using Peplau's theory in nurse-patient relations. *International Nursing Review, 44,* 115–120.

Field, W. E., Jr. (Ed.). (1979). *The psychotherapy of Hildegard E. Peplau.* New Braunfels, TX: PSF Publications.

Forchuk, C. (1993). *Hildegard E. Peplau: Interpersonal Nursing.* Newbury Park, CA: Sage.

Forchuk, C. (1994). The orientation phase of the nurse-client relationship: Testing Peplau's theory. *Journal of Advanced Nursing, 20*(3), 532–537.

Forchuk, C., & Dorsay, J. (1995). Hildegard Peplau meets family systems nursing: Innovation in theory-based practice. *Journal of Advanced Nursing, 21*(1), 110–115.

Forchuk, C., Jewell, J., Schofield, R., Sircelj, M., & Valledor, T. (1998). From hospital to community: Bridging therapeutic relationships. *Journal of Psychiatric and Mental Health Nursing, 5*(3), 197–202.

Forchuk, C., & Reynolds, W. (2001). Clients' reflections on relationships with nurses: Comparisons from Canada and Scotland. *Journal of Psychiatric and Mental Health Nursing, 9,* 45–51.

Forchuk, C., Westwell, J., Martin, A., Azzapardi, W. B., Kosterewa-Tolman, D., & Hux, M. (1998). Factors influencing movement of chronic psychiatric patients from the orientation to the working phase of the nurse-client relationship on an inpatient unit. *Perspectives in Psychiatric Care, 34,* 36–44.

Forchuk, C., Westwell, J., Martin, M., Bamber-Azzaparadi, W., Kosterewa-Tolman, D., & Hux, M. (2000). The developing nurse-client relationship: Nurses' perspectives. *Journal of the American Psychiatric Nurses Association, 6,* 3–10.

Fowler, J. (1994). A welcome focus on a key relationship: Using Peplau's model in palliative care. *Professional Nurse, 10*(3), 194–197.

Fowler, J. (1995). Taking theory into practice: Using Peplau's model in the care of patients. *Professional Nurse, 10*(4), 226–230.

Garrett, A., Manuel, D., & Vincent, C. (1976). Stressful experiences identified by student nurses. *Journal of Nursing Education, 15*(6), 9–21.

Gauthier, P. (2000). Use of Peplau's Interpersonal Relations Model to counsel people with AIDS. *Journal of the American Psychiatric Nurses Association, 6,* 119–125.

Gregg, D. E. (1978). Hildegard E. Peplau: Her contributions. *Perspective in Psychiatric Care, 16*(3), 118–121.

Hall, K. (1994). Peplau's model of nursing: Caring for a man with AIDS. *British Journal of Nursing, 3*(8), 418–422.

Hays, D. (1961). Teaching a concept of anxiety. *Nursing Research, 10*(2), 108–113.

Hofling, C. K., & Leininger, M. M. (1960). Basic psychiatric concepts in nursing. Cited in Smoyak, S. A., & Rouslin, S. (Eds.) (1982). *A collection of classics in psychiatric nursing literature.* Thorofare, NJ: Charles B. Slack.

Iveson, J. (1982). A two-way process . . . theories in nursing practice . . . Peplau's nursing model. *Nursing Mirror, 155* (18), 52.

Jacobson, G. A. (1999). Parenting processes: A descriptive study using Peplau's theory. *Nursing Science Quarterly, 12,* 240–244.

Jewell, J. A., & Sullivan, E. A. (1996). Application of nursing theories in health education. *Journal of the American Psychiatric Nurses Association, 2,* 79–85.

Jones, A. (1995). Utilizing Peplau's psychodynamic theory for stroke patient care. *Journal of Clinical Nursing, 4*(1), 49–54.

Jones, A. (1996). The value of Peplau's theory for mental health nursing. *British Journal of Nursing, 5,* 877–881.

Keda, A. (1970). From Henderson to Orlando to Wiedenbach: Thoughts on completion of translation of basic principles of clinical nursing. *Comprehensive Nursing Quarterly, 5*(1), 85–94.

Kelley, S. J. (1996). "It's just me, my family, and my nurse . . . oh, yeah, and Nintendo: Hildegard Peplau's day with kids with cancer. *Journal of the American Psychiatric Nurses Association, 2,* 11–14.

LaMonica, E. (1981). Construct validity of an empathy instrument. *Research in Nursing and Health, 4,* 389–400.

Lego, S. (1980). The one-to-one nurse-patient relationship. *Perspectives in Psychiatric Care, 18*(2), 67–89. (Reprinted from *Psychiatric nursing 1946–1974: A report on the state of the art,* American Journal of Nursing Co.)

Lego, S. (1998). The application of Peplau's theory to group psychotherapy. *Journal of Psychiatric and Mental Health Nursing, 5*(3), 193–196.

Marshall, J. (1963). Dr. Peplau's strong medicine for psychiatric nurses. *Smith, Kline & French Reporter, 7,* 11–14.

McCarter, P. (1980). New statement defines scope of practice: Discussion with Dr. Lane and Dr. Peplau. *American Nurse, 12*(4), 1, 8, 24.

Methven, D., & Schlotfeldt, R. M. (1962). The social interaction inventory. *Nursing Research, 11*(2), 83–88.

Muff, J. (1996). Images of life on the verge of death: Dream and drawing of people with AIDS. *Perspectives in Psychiatric Care, 32,* 10–22.

Nursing Theories Conference Group. J. B. George, Chairperson. (1980). *Nursing theories: The base for professional nursing practice* (pp. 73–89). Englewood Cliffs, NJ: Prentice-Hall.

Olson, T. (1996). Fundamental and special: The dilemma of psychiatric-mental health nursing. *Archives of Psychiatric Nursing, 10,* 3–15.

Orlando, I. (1961). The dynamic nurse-patient relationship. Cited by Smoyak, S. A., & Rouslin, S. (Eds.) (1982). *A collection of classics in psychiatric nursing literature.* Thorofare, NJ: Charles B. Slack.

Osborne, O. (1984). Intellectual traditions in psychiatric nursing. *Journal of Psychosocial Nursing, 22*(1), 27–32.

Peplau, H. E. (1964). *Basic principles of patient counseling* (2nd ed.). Philadelphia: Smith, Kline, & French Laboratories.

Price, B. (1998). Explorations in body image care: Peplau and practice knowledge. *Journal of Psychiatric and Mental Health Nursing, 5*(3), 179–186.

Reynolds, W. J. (1997). Peplau's theory in practice. *Nursing Science Quarterly, 10,* 168–170.

Schafer, P., & Middleton, J. (2001). Examining Peplau's pattern integrations in long-term care. *Rehabilitation Nursing, 26,* 292–297.

Sills, G. M. (1977). Research in the field of psychiatric nursing, 1952–1977. *Nursing Research, 28*(3), 201–207.

Sills, G. M. (1978). Hildegard E. Peplau: Leader, practitioner, academician, scholar, and theorist. *Perspectives in Psychiatric Care, 16*(3), 122–128.

Slevin, E. (1996). Interpreting problematic behavior in people with learning disabilities. *British Journal of Nursing, 5,* 610–612, 625–627.

Smoyak, S. A., & Rouslin, S. (Eds.). (1982). *A collection of classics in psychiatric nursing literature.* Thorofare, NJ: Charles B. Slack.

Spring, F. E., & Turk, H. (1962, Fall). A therapeutic behavior scale. *Nursing Research, 11*(4), 214–218.

Thelander, B. L. (1997). The psychotherapy of Hildegard Peplau in the treatment of people with serious mental illness. *Perspectives in Psychiatric Care, 33,* 24–32.

Thomas, M. D., Baker, J. M., & Estes, N. J. (1970). Anger: A tool for developing self-awareness. *American Journal of Nursing, 70*(12), 2586–2590.

Topf, M., & Dambacher, B. (1979). Predominant source of interpersonal influence in relationships between psychiatric patients and nursing staff. *Research in Nursing and Health, 2*(1), 35–43.

Usher, K. J., & Arthur, D. (1997). Nurses and neuroleptic medication: Applying theory to a working relationship with clients and their families. *Journal of Psychiatric & Mental Health Nursing, 4,* 117–123.

Yamashita, M. (1997). Family caregiving: Application of Newman's and Peplau's theories. *Journal of Psychiatric & Mental Health Nursing, 4,* 401–405.

OTHER SOURCES

Arnold, W., & Nieswiadomy, R. (1993). Peplau's theory with an emphasis on anxiety. In Ziegler, S. M. (Ed.), *Theory-directed nursing practice.* New York: Springer.

Forchuk, C. (1993). *Hildegard E. Peplau: Interpersonal nursing theory.* Newbury Park, CA: Sage.

BOOK CHAPTERS

Peplau, H. E. (1969). Theory: The professional dimension. In Norris, C. (Ed.), *Proceedings of the first nursing theory conference* (March 21–28). Kansas City: University of Kansas Medical Center, Department of Nursing Education.

Peplau, H. E. (1987). Nursing science: A historical perspective. In Parse, R. (Ed.), *Nursing science: Major paradigms, theories, critiques.* Philadelphia: W. B. Saunders.

JOURNAL ARTICLES

Peplau, H. E. (1951). Toward new concepts in nursing and nursing education. *American Journal of Nursing, 52*(12), 722–724.

Peplau, H. E. (1952). The psychiatric nurses' family group. *American Journal of Nursing, 52*(12), 1475–1477.

Peplau, H. E. (1953). The nursing team in psychiatric facilities. *Nursing Outlook, 1*(2), 90–92.

Peplau, H. E. (1953). Themes in nursing situations: Power. *American Journal of Nursing, 52*(10), 1221–1223.

Peplau, H. E. (1953). Themes in nursing situations: Safety. *American Journal of Nursing, 53*(11), 1343–1346.

Peplau, H. E. (1955). Loneliness. *American Journal of Nursing, 55*(12), 1476–1481.

Peplau, H. E. (1956). Present day trends in psychiatric nursing. *Neuropsychiatry, 111*(4), 190–204.

Peplau, H. E. (1956). An undergraduate program in psychiatric nursing. *Nursing Outlook, 4,* 400–410.

Peplau, H. E. (1957). What is experiential teaching? *American Journal of Nursing, 57*(7), 884–886.

Peplau, H. E. (1958). Educating the nurse to function in psychiatric services. In *Nursing personnel for mental health programs* (pp. 37–42). Atlanta: Southern Regional Educational Board.

Peplau, H. E. (1960). Anxiety in the mother-infant relationship. *Nursing World, 134*(5), 33–34.

Peplau, H. E. (1960). A personal responsibility: A discussion of anxiety in mental health. *Rutgers Alumni Monthly,* March, 14–16.

Peplau, H. E. (1963). Interpersonal relations and the process of adaptations. *Nursing Science, 1*(4), 272–279.

Peplau, H. E. (1964). Psychiatric nursing skills and the general hospital patient. *Nursing Forum, 3*(2), 28–37.

Peplau, H. E. (1965). The heart of nursing: Interpersonal relations. *Canadian Nurse, 61*(4), 273–275.

Peplau, H. E. (1965). Specialization in professional nursing. *Nursing Science, 3*(4), 268–287.

Peplau, H. E. (1966). Trends in nursing and nursing education. *NJSNA News Letter, 22*(3), 17–27.

Peplau, H. E. (1967). Interpersonal relations and the work of the industrial nurse. *Industrial Nurse Journal, 15*(10), 7–12.

Peplau, H. E. (1967). The work of psychiatric nurses. *Psychiatric Opinion, 4*(1), 5–11.

Peplau, H. E. (1968). Psychotherapeutic strategies. *Perspectives in Psychiatric Care, 6*(6), 264–289.

Peplau, H. E. (1969). Professional closeness as a special kind of involvement with a patient, client, or family group. *Nursing Forum, 8*(4), 342–360.

Peplau, H. E. (1970). Professional closeness as a special kind of involvement with a patient, client or family group. *Comprehensive Nurse Quarterly, 5*(3), 66–81.

Peplau, H. E. (1971). Communication in crisis intervention. *Psychiatric Forum, 2,* 1–7.

Peplau, H. E. (1972). The independence of nursing. *Imprint, 9,* 11.

Peplau, H. E. (1972). The nurse's role in health care delivery systems. *Pelican News, 28,* 12–14.

Peplau, H. E. (1974). Creativity and commitment in nursing. *Image: Journal of Nursing Scholarship, 6,* 3–5.

Peplau, H. E. (1974). Is health care a right? Affirmative response. *Image: Journal of Nursing Scholarship, 7,* 4–10.

Peplau, H. E. (1974). Talking with patients. *Comprehensive Nursing Quarterly, 9*(3), 30–39.

Peplau, H. E. (1975). An open letter to a new graduate. *Nursing Digest, 3,* 36–37.

Peplau, H. E. (1975). Interview with Dr. Peplau: Future of nursing. *Japanese Journal of Nursing, 39*(10), 1046–1050.

Peplau, H. E. (1977). The changing view of nursing. *International Nursing Review, 24,* 43–45.

Peplau, H. E. (1978). Psychiatric nursing: Role of nurses and psychiatric nurses. *International Nursing Review, 25,* 41–47.

Peplau, H. E. (1980). The psychiatric nurses: Accountable? To whom? For what? *Perspectives in Psychiatric Care, 18,* 128–134.

Peplau, H. E. (1982). Some reflections on earlier days in psychiatric nursing. *Journal of Psychosocial Nursing Mental Health Services, 20,* 17–24.

Peplau, H. E. (1987). American Nurses' Association social policy statement: Part I. *Archives of Psychiatric Nursing, 1*(5), 301–307.

Peplau, H. E. (1987). Tomorrow's world. *Nursing Times, 83,* 29–33.

Peplau, H. E. (1989). Future direction in psychiatric nursing from the perspective of history. *Journal of Psychosocial Nursing, 27*(2), 18–28.

Peplau, H. E. (1992). Interpersonal relations: A theoretical framework for application in nursing practice. *Nursing Science Quarterly, 5*(1), 13–18.

Peplau, H. E. (1995). Hildegard Peplau in a conversation with Mark Welch, Part I. *Nursing Inquiry, 2*(1), 53–56.

Peplau, H. E. (1995). Hildegard Peplau in a conversation with Mark Welch, Part II. *Nursing Inquiry, 2*(2), 115–116.

Peplau, H. E. (1996). Commentary. *Archives of Psychiatry Nursing, 10*(1), 14–15.

Peplau, H. E. (1996). Encounters along a career line. *Journal of the American Psychiatric Nurses Association, 2,* 36.

Peplau, H. E. (1997). The ins and outs of psychiatric-mental health nursing and the American Nurses' Association. *Journal of the American Psychiatric Nurses Association, 3,* 10–16.

Peplau, H. E. (1997). Is health care a right? *Image, 29,* 220–224.

Peplau, H. E. (1997). Peplau's theory of interpersonal relations. *Nursing Science Quarterly, 10,* 162–167.

INTERVIEWS

Peplau, H. E. (1985). Help the public maintain mental health. *Nursing Success Today, 2*(5), 30–34.

Peplau, H. E. (1985). The power of the dissociative state. *Journal of Psychosocial Nursing, 23*(8), 31–33.

CHAPTERS AND PAMPHLETS

Peplau, H. E. (1956). *The yearbook of modern nursing.* New York: G. P. Putnam's Sons.

Peplau, H. E. (1959). Principles of psychiatric nursing. In *American Handbook of Psychiatry* (Vol. 2). New York: Basic Books.

Peplau, H. E. (1962). Will automation change the nurse, nursing, or both? *Technical innovations in health care: Nursing implications* (Pamphlet 5). New York: American Nurses' Association.

Peplau, H. E. (1963). Counseling in nursing practice. In Harms, E., & Schreiber, P. (Eds.), *Handbook of counseling techniques.* New York: Pergamon.

Peplau, H. E. (1967). Psychiatric nursing. In Freedman, A. M., & Kaplan, A. I. (Eds.), *Comprehensive textbook of psychiatry.* New York: Williams & Wilkins.

Peplau, H. E. (1968). Operational definitions and nursing practice. In Zderad, L. T., & Belcher, H. C. (Eds.), *Developing behavioral concepts in nursing.* Atlanta: Southern Regional Education Board.

Peplau, H. E. (1969). Pattern perpetuation in schizophrenia. In Sankar, D. (Ed.), *Schizophrenia: Current concepts and research.* Hicksville, NY: PJD Publications.

Peplau, H. E. (1992). Notes on Nightingale. In Nightingale, F. (1859/1992), *Notes on nursing: What it is, and what it is not.* Philadelphia: J. B. Lippincott.

Peplau, H. E. (1995). Another look at schizophrenia from a nursing standpoint. In *Psychiatric Nursing 1946 to 1994: A report on the state of the art*. St. Louis: Mosby.

Peplau, H. E. (1995). Preface. In *Psychiatric nursing 1946 to 1994: A report on the state of the art*. St. Louis: Mosby.

THESES

Peplau, H. E. (1953). *An exploration of some process elements which restrict or facilitate instructor-student interaction in a classroom, Type B*. Doctoral Project, Teachers College, Columbia University, New York.

CHAPTER 7

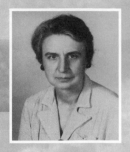

Ernestine Wiedenbach

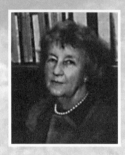

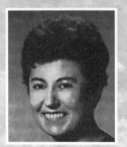

Virginia A. Henderson   *Ida Jean Orlando (Pelletier)*

PART ONE: Twentieth-Century Nursing
Wiedenbach, Henderson, and Orlando's Theories and Their Applications

Theresa Gesse & Marcia Dombro, Shirley C. Gordon, Maude R. Rittman

Introducing the Theorists

Ernestine Wiedenbach, Virginia Henderson, and Ida Jean Orlando are three of the most important influences on nursing theory development of the twentieth century. Indeed, their work continues to ground nursing thought in the new century. The work of each of these nurse scholars was based on nursing practice, and today some of this work might be referred to as practice theories. Concepts and terms they first used are heard today around the globe.

This chapter provides a brief overview of each of these three important twentieth-century nursing theorists. The content of this chapter is based on work from scholars who have studied or worked with these theorists and who wrote chapters about each for *Nursing Theories and Nursing Practice* 1st edition. To the extent possible, content written by each of the identified authors is used. For a wealth of additional information on these nurses, scholars, researchers, thinkers, writers, practitioners, and educators, please consult the reference and bibliography sections at the end of this chapter.

ERNESTINE WIEDENBACH

Wiedenbach was born in 1900 in Germany to an American mother and a German father who migrated to the United States when Ernestine was a child. She received a bachelor of arts degree from Wellesley College in 1922. She graduated from Johns Hopkins School of Nursing in 1925 (Nickel, Gesse, & MacLaren, 1992.). After completing a master of arts at Columbia Univeristy in 1934, she became a professional writer for the *American Journal of Nursing* and played a critical role in the recruitment of nursing students and military nurses during World War II. At age 45, she began her studies in nurse-midwifery. Wiedenbach's roles as practitioner, teacher, author and theorist were consolidated as a member of the Yale University School of Nursing where Yale colleagues William Dickoff and Patricia James encouraged her development of prescriptive theory (Dickoff, James & Wiedenbach, 1968). Even after her retirement in 1966, she and her lifelong friend Caroline Falls offered informal seminars in Miami, always reminding students and faculty of the need for clarity of purpose, based on reality. She even continued to use her gift for writing to transcribe books for the blind, including a Lamaze childbirth manual, which she prepared on her Braille typewriter. Ernestine Wiedenbach died in April 1998 at the age of 98 (Gesse & Dombro, 1992, p. 70–71).

IDA JEAN ORLANDO

Ida Jean Orlando was born in 1926 in New York. Her nursing education began at New York Medical College School of Nursing where she received a diploma in nursing. In 1951 she received a bachelor of science degree in public health nursing from St. John's University in Brooklyn, New York, and in 1954 she completed a master's degree in nursing from Columbia University. Orlando's early nursing practice experience included obstetrics, medicine, and emergency room nursing. Her first book, *The Dynamic Nurse-Patient Relationship: Function, Process and Principles* (1961), was based on her research and blended nursing practice, psychiatric–mental health nursing, and nursing education. It was published when she was director of the graduate program in mental health and psychiatric nursing at Yale University School of Nursing.

Orlando's theoretical work is both practice and research-based and was funded by the National Institute of Mental Health to improve education of nurses about concepts and interpersonal relationships. The method of her study was qualitative and inductive, using naturalistic inquiry methods. As a consultant at McLean Hospital in Belmont, Massachusetts, Orlando continued to study nursing practice and developed a training program and nursing service department based on her theory. From evaluation of this program, she published her second book, *The Discipline and Teaching of Nursing Process* (Orlando, 1972; Rittman, 1991).

VIRGINIA HENDERSON

Born in Kansas City, Missouri, in 1897, Virginia Henderson was the fifth of eight children. With two of her brothers serving in the armed forces during World War I and in anticipation of a critical shortage of nurses, Virginia Henderson entered the Army School of Nursing at Walter Reed Army Hospital. It was there that she began to question the regimentalization of patient care and the concept of nursing as ancillary to medicine (Henderson, 1991).

She described her introduction to nursing as a "series of almost unrelated procedures, beginning with an unoccupied bed and progressing to aspiration of body cavities" (Henderson, 1991, p. 9). It was also at Walter Reed Army Hospital that she met Annie W. Goodrich, the dean of the School of Nursing. Henderson admired Goodrich's intellectual abilities and stated: "Whenever she visited our unit, she lifted our sights above techniques and routine" (Henderson, 1991, p. 11). Henderson credited Goodrich with inspiring her with the "ethical significance of nursing" (Henderson, 1991, p. 10).

As a member of society during a war, Henderson considered it a privilege to care for sick and wounded soldiers (Henderson, 1960). This experience forever influenced her ethical understanding of nursing and her appreciation of the importance and complexity of the nurse-patient relationship.

She continued to explore the nature of nursing as her student experiences exposed her to different ways of being in relationship with patients and their families. For instance, a pediatric experience as a student at Boston Floating Hospital introduced Henderson to patient-centered care in which nurses were assigned to patients instead of tasks, and warm nurse-patient relationships were encouraged (Henderson, 1991). Following a summer spent with the Henry Street Visiting Nurse Agency in New York City, Henderson began to appreciate the importance of getting to know the patients and their environments. She enjoyed the less formal visiting nurse approach to patient care and became skeptical of the ability of hospital regimes to alter patients' unhealthy ways of living upon returning home (Henderson, 1991). She entered Teachers College at Columbia University, earning her baccalaureate degree in 1932 and her master's degree in 1934. She continued at Teachers College as an instructor and associate professor of nursing for the next 20 years.

Virginia Avenel Henderson presented her definition of the nature of nursing in a era when few nurses had ventured into describing the complex phenomena of modern nursing. Henderson wrote about nursing the way she lived it: focusing on what nurses do, how nurses function, and on nursing's unique role in health care. Her works are beautifully written in jargon-free, everyday language. Her search for a definition of nursing ultimately influenced the practice and education of nursing

around the world. Her pioneer work in the area of identifying and structuring nursing knowledge has provided the foundation for nursing scholarship for generations to come.

Introducing the Theories

Virginia Henderson, sometimes known as the modern day Florence Nightingale, developed the definition of nursing that is most well known internationally. Ernestine Wiedenbach gave us new ways to think about nursing practice and nursing scholarship, introducing us to the ideas of: (1) nursing as a professional practice discipline, and (2) nursing practice theory. Ida Jean Orlando was perhaps the first nurse to use qualitative research methods and was the first to articulate nursing concepts based on both her practice and her research. Each of these nurses helped us focus on the patient, instead of on the tasks to be done, and to plan care to meet needs of the person. Each of these women emphasized caring based on the perspective of the individual being cared for—through observing, communicating, designing, and reporting. Each was concerned with the unique aspects of nursing practice and scholarship and with the essential question of, "What is nursing?"

WIEDENBACH

Initial work on Wiedenbach's prescriptive theory is presented in her article in the *American Journal of Nursing* (1963) and her book, *Meeting the Realities in Clinical Teaching* (1969). Her explanation of prescriptive theory is that: "Account must be

> *"Account must be taken of the motivating factors that influence the nurse not only in doing what she does but also in doing it the way she does it with the realities that exist in the situation in which she is functioning."*

taken of the motivating factors that influence the nurse not only in doing what she does but also in doing it the way she does it with the realities that exist in the situation in which she is functioning." (Wiedenbach, 1970, p. 2.) Three ingredients essential to the prescriptive theory are:

1. *The nurse's central purpose in nursing is the nurse's professional commitment.* For Wiedenbach, the central purpose in nursing is to motivate the individual and/or facilitate his efforts to overcome the obstacles that may interfere with his ability to respond capably to the demands made of him by the realities in his situation (Wiedenbach, 1970, p. 4). She emphasized that the nurse's goals are grounded in the nurse's philosophy, that "those beliefs and values that shape her attitude toward life, toward fellow human beings and toward herself." The three concepts that epitomize the essence of such a philosophy are: (1) reverence for the gift of life; (2) respect for the dignity, autonomy, worth, and individuality of each human being; and (3) resolution to act dynamically in relation to one's beliefs (Wiedenbach, 1970, p. 4). She recognized that nurses have different values and various commitments to nursing and that to

> **To formulate one's purpose in nursing is a "soul-searching experience."**

formulate one's purpose in nursing is a "soul-searching experience." She encouraged each nurse to undergo this experience and be "willing and ready to present your central purpose in nursing for examination and discussion when appropriate" (Wiedenbach, 1970, p. 5).

2. *The prescription indicates the broad general action that the nurse deems appropriate to fulfillment of her central purpose.* The nurse will have thought through the kind of results to be sought and will take action to obtain these results, accepting accountability for what she does and for the outcomes of her action. Nursing action, then, is deliberate action that is mutually understood and agreed upon and that is both patient-directed and nurse-directed (Wiedenbach, 1970, p. 5).

3. *The realities are the aspects of the immediate nursing situation that influence the results the nurse achieves through what she does* (Wiedenbach, 1970, p. 3). These include the physical, psychological, emotional, and spiritual factors in which nursing action occurs. Within the situation are these components:

   • The Agent, who is the nurse supplying the nursing action;

• The Recipient, or the patient receiving this action or on whose behalf the action is taken;
• The Framework, comprised of situational factors that affect the nurse's ability to achieve nursing results;
• The Goal, or the end to be attained through nursing activity on behalf of the patient;
• The Means, the actions and devices through which the nurse is enabled to reach the goal.

ORLANDO

Nursing is responsive to individuals who suffer or anticipate a sense of helplessness; it is focused on the process of care in an immediate experience; it is concerned with providing direct assistance to individuals in whatever setting they are found for the purpose of avoiding, relieving, diminishing or curing the individual's sense of helplessness. (Orlando, 1972)

The essence of Orlando's theory, the Dynamic Nurse-Patient Relationship, reflects her beliefs that practice should be based on needs of the patient and that communication with the patient is essential to understanding needs and providing effective nursing care. Following is an overview of the major components of Orlando's work.

1. *The nursing process* includes identifying needs of patients, responses of the nurse, and nursing action. The nursing process, as envisioned and practiced by Orlando, is not the linear model often taught today, but is more reflexive and circular and occurs during encounters with patients.

2. *Understanding the meaning* of patient behavior is influenced by the nurse's perceptions, thoughts, and feelings. It may be validated through communication between nurse and patient. Patients experience distress when they cannot cope with unmet needs. Nurses use direct and indirect observations of patient behavior to discover distress and meaning.

3. *Nurse-patient interactions* are unique, complex, and dynamic processes. Nurses help patients express and understand the meaning of behavior. The basis for nursing action is the distress experienced and expressed by the patient.

4. *Professional nurses* function in an independent role from physicians and other health-care providers.

HENDERSON

While working on the 1955 revision of the *Textbook of the Principles and Practice of Nursing,* Henderson focused on the need to be clear about the function of nurses. She opened chapter one with the following question: What is nursing and what is the function of the nurse? (Harmer & Henderson, 1955, p. 1). Henderson believed this question was fundamental to anyone choosing to pursue the study and practice of nursing.

Definition of Nursing

Her often-quoted definition of nursing first appeared in the fifth edition of *Textbook of the Principles and Practice of Nursing* (Harmer & Henderson, 1955, p. 4):

> Nursing is primarily assisting the individual (sick or well) in the performance of those activities contributing to health or its recovery (or to a peaceful death), that he would perform unaided if he had the necessary strength, will, or knowledge. It is likewise the unique contribution of nursing to help people be independent of such assistance as soon as possible.

In presenting her definition of nursing, Henderson hoped to encourage others to develop their own working concept of nursing and nursing's unique function in society. She believed the definitions of the day were too general and failed to differentiate nurses from other members of the health team, which led to the following questions: "What is nursing that is not also medicine, physical therapy, social work, etc.?" and "What is the unique function of the nurse?" (Harmer & Henderson, 1955, p. 4).

Based on Henderson's definition, and after coining the term "basic nursing care," Henderson identified 14 components of basic nursing care that reflect needs pertaining to personal hygiene and healthful living, including helping the patient carry out the physician's therapeutic plan (Henderson, 1960; 1966, pp. 16–17):

1. Breathe normally
2. Eat and drink adequately
3. Eliminate body wastes
4. Move and maintain desirable postures
5. Sleep and rest
6. Select suitable clothes—dress and undress
7. Maintain body temperature within normal range by adjusting clothing and modifying the environment
8. Keep the body clean and well groomed and protect the integument
9. Avoid dangers in the environment and avoid injuring others
10. Communicate with others in expressing emotions, needs, fears, or opinions
11. Worship according to one's faith
12. Work in such a way that there is a sense of accomplishment
13. Play or participate in various forms of recreation
14. Learn, discover, or satisfy the curiosity that leads to normal development and health and use the available health facilities.

PART TWO

Applications

WIEDENBACH

"The practice of clinical nursing is goal directed, deliberately carried out and patient centered"

> *"The practice of clinical nursing is goal directed, deliberately carried out and patient centered."*

(Wiedenbach, 1964, p. 23). Figure 7–1 represents a spherical model that depicts the "experiencing individual" as the central focus (Wiedenbach, 1964). This model and detailed charts were later edited and published in *Clinical Nursing: A Helping Art* (Wiedenbach, 1964).

In a paper entitled "A Concept of Dynamic Nursing" (Wiedenbach, 1962, p. 7), she described the model as follows:

> In its broadest sense, Practice of Dynamic Nursing may be envisioned as a set of concentric circles, with the experiencing individual in the circle at its core. Direct service, with its three components, identification of the individual's experienced need for help, ministration of help needed, and validation that the help provided fulfilled its purpose, fills the circle adjacent to the core. The next circle holds the essential concomitants of direct service: coordination, i.e., charting, recording, reporting, and conferring;

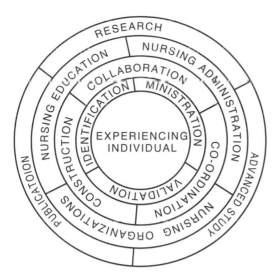

FIGURE 7–1 Professional Nursing practice focus and components. *Reprinted with permission from the Wiedenbach Reading Room (1962), Yale University School of Nursing.*

consultation, i.e., conferencing, and seeking help or advice; and collaboration, i.e., giving assistance or cooperation with members of other professional or nonprofessional groups concerned with the individual's welfare. The content of the fourth circle represents activities which are essential to the ultimate well-being of the experiencing individual, but only indirectly related to him: nursing education, nursing administration and nursing organizations. The outermost circle comprises research in nursing, publication and advanced study, the key ways to progress in every area of practice.

Wiedenbach's nursing practice application of her prescriptive theory was evident in her practice examples. These often related to general basic nursing procedures and to maternity nursing practice. In discussing the practice and process of nursing, she stated:

> The focus of Practice is the experiencing individual, i.e., the individual for whom the nurse is caring, and the way he and only he perceived his condition or situation. For example, a mother had a red vaginal discharge on her first postpartum day. The doctor had recognized it as lochi, a normal concomitant of the phenomenon of involution, and had left an order for her to be up and move about. Instead of trying to get up, the mother remained, immobile in her bed. The nurse who wanted to help her out of bed expressed surprise at the mother's unwilling to do so, when she seemed to be progressing so well. The mother explained that she had a red discharge, and this to her

was evidence of onset of hemorrhage. This terrified her and made her afraid to move. Her sister, she added, had hemorrhaged and almost lost her life the day after she had her baby two years ago. The nurse expressed her understanding of the mother's fear, but then encouraged her to compare her current experience with that of her sister. When the mother tried to do this, she recognized gross differences, and accepted the nurse's explanation of the origin of the discharge. The mother then voiced her relief, and validated it by getting out of bed without further encouragement (Wiedenbach, 1962, pp. 6–7).

Wiedenbach considered nursing a "practical phenomenon" that involved action. She believed that this was necessary to understand the theory that underlies the "nurse's way of nursing." This involved "knowing what the nurse wanted to accomplish, how she went about accomplishing it, and in what context she did what she did" (Wiedenbach, 1970, p. 1058). Realizing her early efforts to link theory, practice, and merit, and to include these also in nursing education, Wiedenbach stated:

> May each of you spark nurses in and of the future, to make theory a conscious part of their practice. The opportunity you have to do this is exciting! And it is rewarding, for, by helping nurses to uncover the theory that underlies their practice, you are paving the way for them to render a finer quality of service to the patient, and to gain a deepened sense of fulfillment for themselves (Wiedenbach, 1970, p. 15).

ORLANDO

Orlando's theoretical work was based on analysis of thousands of nurse-patient interactions to describe major attributes of the relationship. Based on this work, her later book provided direction for understanding and using the nursing process (Orlando, 1972). This has been known as the first theory of nursing process and has been widely used in nursing education and practice in the United States and across the globe. Orlando considered her overall work to be a theoretical framework for the practice of professional nursing, emphasizing the essentiality of the nurse-patient relationship. Orlando's theoretical work reveals and bears witness to the essence of nursing as a practice discipline.

While there is little evidence in the literature that Orlando's theory has been directly used in nursing practice, it is highly probable that nurses familiar with her writing used her work to guide or more fully understand their practice. During the 1960s, several studies were published that explored nursing practice issues. These works focused on patients' complaints of pain (Barron, 1966; Bochnak, 1963), incidence of post-operative vomiting (Dumas & Leonard, 1963), patient admission processes (Elms & Leonard, 1966), nurses' responses to expressed patient needs (Gowan & Morris, 1964), and the effects of patient assistance with planning nursing procedure administration (Tryson, (1963).

The most important contribution of Orlando's theoretical work is what it says about the values underpinning the nursing practice. Inherent in this theory is a strong statement: What transpires between the patient and the nurse is of the highest value. The true worth of her nursing theory is that it clearly states what nursing is or should be today. Regardless of the changes in the health-care system, the human transaction between the nurse and the patient in any setting holds the greatest value, not only for nursing, but also for society at large. Orlando's theory can serve as a philosophy as well as a theory, because it is the foundation upon which our profession has been built. With all of the benefits that modern technology and modern health care bring—and there are many—we need to pause and ask the question "What is at risk in health care today"? The answer to that question may lead to reconsideration of the value of Orlando's theory as perhaps the critical link for enhancing relationships between nursing and patient today (Rittman, 2001).

HENDERSON

Based on the assumption that nursing has a unique function, Henderson believed that nursing independently initiates and controls activities related to basic nursing care. Relating the conceptualization of basic care components with the unique functions of nursing provided the initial groundwork for introducing the concept of independent nursing practice. In her 1966 publication, *The Nature of Nursing,* Henderson stated: "It is my contention that the nurse is, and should be legally, an independent practitioner and able to make independent judgments as long as he, or she, is not diagnosing, prescribing treatment for disease, or making a prognosis, for these are the physician's functions" (Henderson, 1966, p. 22).

Furthermore, Henderson believed that functions pertaining to patient care could be categorized as nursing and non-nursing. She believed that limiting nursing activities to "nursing care" was a useful method of conserving professional nurse power (Harmer & Henderson, 1955). She defined non-nursing functions as those that are not a service to the person (mind and body) (Harmer & Henderson, 1955). For Henderson, examples of non-nursing functions included ordering supplies, cleaning and sterilizing equipment, and serving food (Harmer & Henderson, 1955).

At the same time, Henderson was not in favor of the practice of assigning patients to lesser trained workers on the basis of complexity level. For Henderson, "all 'nursing care' . . . is essentially complex because it involves constant adaptation of procedures to the needs of the individual" (Harmer & Henderson, 1955, p. 9).

As the authority on basic nursing care, Henderson believed that the nurse has the responsibility to assess the needs of the individual patient, help individuals meet their health needs, and/or provide an environment in which the individual can perform activities unaided. It is the nurse's role, according to Henderson, "to 'get inside the patient's skin' and supplement his strength, will or knowledge according to his needs" (Harmer & Henderson, 1955, p. 5). Conceptualizing the nurse as a substitute for the patient's lack of necessary will, strength, or knowledge to attain good health and to complete or make the patient whole, highlights the complexity and uniqueness of nursing.

Based on the success of *Textbook of the Principles and Practice of Nursing* (fifth edition), Henderson was asked by the International Council of Nurses (ICN) to prepare a short essay that could be used as a guide for nursing in any part of the world. Despite Henderson's belief that it was difficult to promote a universal definition of nursing, *Basic Principles of Nursing Care* (Henderson, 1960) became an international sensation. To date, it has been published in 29 languages and is referred to as the twentieth-century equivalent of Florence Nightingale's *Notes on Nursing.* After visiting countries worldwide, she concluded that nursing varied from country to country and that rigorous attempts to define it have been unsuccessful, leaving the "nature of nursing" largely an unanswered question (Henderson, 1991).

Henderson's definition of nursing has had a lasting influence on the way nursing is practiced around the globe. She was one of the first nurses to articulate that nursing had a unique function yielding a valuable contribution to the health care of individuals. In writing reflections on the nature of nursing, Henderson (1966) states that her concept of nursing anticipates universally available health care and a partnership among doctors, nurses, and other health-care workers.

Library Research and Development

Henderson has been heralded as the greatest advocate for nursing libraries worldwide. Following the completion of her revised text in 1955, Henderson moved to Yale University. It was here that she began what would become a distinguished career in library science research.

Of all her contributions to nursing, Virginia Henderson's work on the identification and control of nursing literature is perhaps her greatest. In the 1950s there was an increasing interest on the part of the profession to establish a research basis for the nursing practice. It was also recognized that the body of nursing knowledge was unstructured and therefore inaccessible to practicing nurses and educators. Henderson encouraged nurses to become active in the work of classifying nursing literature.

Virginia Henderson remained a strong advocate for nursing resource development throughout her lifetime. In 1990, the Sigma Theta Tau International Library was named in her honor. Henderson insisted that if the library was to bear her name, the electronic networking system would have to advance the work of staff nurses by providing them with current, jargon-free information wherever they were based (McBride, 1997).

SUMMARY

Among other theorists featured in the section II of this book, Wiedenbach, Henderson, and Orlando introduced nursing theory to us in the mid-twentieth century. Each of these nurses looked at their nursing and explored nurse-patient interactions using nursing practice as the basis for their thought and for their published scholarship. These nurse theorists defined the ways nursing is thought about, practiced, and researched, both in the U.S. and around the world. Perhaps most importantly, each of these nurse theorists stated

and responded to the question "What is nursing?" Their responses helped all who followed to understand that the one nursed is person, not object, and that the relationship of nurse and patient is valuable to all.

References

Barron, M. A. (1966). The effects varied nursing approaches have on patients' complaints of pain. *Nursing Research, 15*(1), 90–91.

Bochnak, M. A. (1963). The effect of an automatic and deliberative process of nursing activity on the relief of patients' pain: A clinical experiment. *Nursing Research, 12*(3), 191–193.

Dickoff, J., James, P., & Wiedenbach, E. (1968). Theory in a practice discipline. *Nursing Research, 14*(5).

Dumas, R. G., & Leonard, R. C. (1963). The effect of nursing on the incidence of post-operative vomiting. *Nursing Research, 12*(1), 12–15.

Elms, R. R., & Leonard, R. C. (1966). The effects of nursing approaches during admission. *Nursing Research, 15*(1), 39–48.

Gesse, T., & Dombro, M. (1991). Ernestine Wiedenbach clinical nursing: A helping art. In M. Parker, *Nursing theories and nursing practice* (1st ed), (pp. 69–84). Philadelphia: FA Davis.

Gesse, T., & Dombro, M. (2001). Ernestine Wiedenbach clinical nursing: A helping art. In M. Parker, *Nursing theories and nursing practice* (pp. 69–84). Philadelphia: FA Davis.

Gordon, S. C. (2001). Virginia Avenel Henderson definition of nursing. In Parker, M., *Nursing theories and nursing practice* (pp. 143–149). Philadelphia: FA Davis.

Gowan, N. I., & Morris, M. (1964). Nurses' responses to expressed patient needs. *Nursing Research, 13*(1), 68–71.

Harmer, B., & Henderson, V. A. (1955). *Textbook of the principles and practice of nursing.* New York: Macmillan.

Henderson, V. A. (1960). *Basic principles of nursing care.* Geneva: International Council of Nurses.

Henderson, V. A. (1966). *The nature of nursing.* New York: The National League for Nursing Press.

Henderson, V. A. (1991). *The nature of nursing: Reflections after 25 years.* New York: The National League for Nursing Press.

Kim, H. S. (1983). *The nature of theoretical thinking in nursing.* Norwalk, CT: Appleton-Century-Crofts.

McBride, A. B. (Narrator). (1997). Celebrating Virginia Henderson (video). Available from Center for Nursing Press, 550 West North Street, Indianapolis, IN 46202.

Nickel, S., Gesse, T., & MacLaren, A. (1992). Her professional legacy. *Journal of Nurse Midwifery, 3*(161).

Orlando, I. J. (1961/1990). *The dynamic nurse-patient relationship: Function, process and principles.* New York: National League for Nursing (reprinted from 1961 edition). New York: G. P. Putnam's Sons.

Orlando, I. J. (1972). *The discipline and teaching of nursing process: An evaluative study.* New York: G. P. Putnam's Sons.

Rittman, M. R. (1991). Ida Jean Orlando (Pelletier)—the dynamic nurse-patient relationship. In M. Parker, *Nursing theories and nursing practice* (pp. 125–130). Philadelphia: FA Davis.

Tryson, P. A. (1963). An experiment of the effect of patients' participation in planning the administration of a nursing procedure. *Nursing Research, 12*(4), 262–265.

Wiedenbach, E. (1962). *A concept of dynamic nursing: Philosophy, purpose, practice and process.* Paper presented at the Conference on Maternal and Child Nursing, Pittsburgh, PA. Archives, Yale University School of Nursing, New Haven, CT.

Wiedenbach, E. (1963). The helping art of nursing. *American Journal of Nursing, 63*(11).

Wiedenbach, E. (1964). *Clinical nursing: A helping art.* New York: Springer.

Wiedenbach, E. (1969). *Meeting the realities in clinical teaching.* New York: Springer.

Wiedenbach, E. (1970). *A systematic inquiry: Application of theory to nursing practice.* Paper presented at Duke University, Durham, NC (author's personal files).

Bibliography

WIEDENBACH BIBLIOGRAPHY

BOOKS

Wiedenbach, E. (1958/1967). *Family centered maternity nursing* (2nd ed. rev.). New York: Putnam.

Wiedenbach, E. (1972/1977). Maternity nursing today. In *The nursing process in maternity nursing* (2nd ed. rev). New York: McGraw Hill Publishing.

Wiedenbach, E., & Falls, C. (1978). *Communication: Key to effective nursing.* New York: Tiresias Press.

JOURNAL ARTICLES

Wiedenbach, E. (1940). Toward educating 130 million people—A history of the Nursing Information Bureau. *American Journal of Nursing, 40,* January, 13–18.

Wiedenbach, E. (1942). Overcoming mental barriers—A true story. *American Journal of Nursing, 42,* November, 1247–1252.

Wiedenbach, E. (1949). Childbirth as mothers say they like it. *Public Health Nursing, 51,* August, 417–426.

Wiedenbach, E. (1960). Nurse-midwifery . . . Purpose, practice and opportunity. *Nursing Outlook, 8,* May, 256–259.

Wiedenbach, E. (1962). Contributions of nurse-midwifery to maternity care today. *Bulletin of the American College of Nurse Midwives, 8,* Summer.

Wiedenbach, E. (1965). Family nurse practitioner for maternal and child care. *Nursing Outlook, 13,* December.

Wiedenbach, E. (1968). Genetics and the nurse. *Bulletin of the American College of Nurse-Midwifery, 13*(5), May, 8–13.

Wiedenbach, E. (1968). Nurse's role in family planning. *Nursing Clinics of North America, 3*(6), June, 355–365.

Wiedenbach, E. (1970). Nurses' wisdom in nursing theory. *American Journal of Nursing, 70,* May, 1057–1062.

Wiedenbach, E., Dickoff, J., & James, P. (1968). Theory in a practice discipline. Part 1. *Nursing Research 17*(5), September–October, 415–437.

Wiedenbach, E., Dickoff, J., & James, P. (1968). Theory in a practice discipline. Part II. *Nursing Research 17*(6), November–December, 545–554.

Wiedenbach, E., & Thomas, H. (1954). Support during labor. *Journal of the American Medical Association, 156*(9), September, 3–10.

UNPUBLISHED MANUSCRIPTS

Wiedenbach, E. (1961). *Growth and development of the nurse-midwifery program at Yale.* Unpublished manuscript, Yale University School of Nursing.

Wiedenbach, E. (1962). Professional nursing practice—focus and components. Unpublished manuscript, Yale University School of Nursing, New Haven, CT.

Wiedenbach, E. (1963). *Suggested statement of philosophy.* Unpublished manuscript, Yale University School of Nursing, New Haven, CT.

Wiedenbach, E. (1965). *Emergency maternal and newborn care.* Paper presented to the Connecticut State Council on Civil Defense Nursing, December 2, 1965. Yale University School of Nursing, New Haven, CT.

Wiedenbach, E. (1965). *Interpretation of elements in evaluation functional ability.* Unpublished manuscript, Yale University School of Nursing, New Haven, CT.

Wiedenbach, E. (1965). *Qualities and competencies students are expected to acquire.* Unpublished manuscript, Yale University School of Nursing, New Haven, CT.

Wiedenbach, E. (1966). *Functions of the professional nurse and the impact of nursing education.* Paper presented at the South Ohio League for Nursing, January 26, Cincinnati, OH.

Wiedenbach, E. (1969). *The meaning of theory to clinical practice.* Paper presented at the University of Colorado School of Nursing, October 27, Denver, CO.

UNPUBLISHED DOCUMENTS

Nickel, S. (1981a). A historical nursing review: The life and career contributions of Ernestine Wiedenbach. Unpublished thesis, University of Miami, Coral Gables, FL.

Nickel, S. (1981b). Audio-visual taped interview with Ernestine Wiedenbach, Tape 1, October 20, 1980; Tape 2, February 2, 1981; Tape 3, May 22, 1981. Copy in University of Miami School of Nursing Archives, Coral Gables, FL.

Wiedenbach, E. (1981). Audio-visual taped interview with Ernestine Wiedenbach. February 14, 1981. University of Miami School of Nursing Archives, Coral Gables, FL.

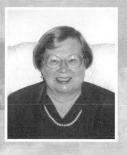

Dorothy Johnson

CHAPTER 8

PART ONE: Dorothy Johnson's Behavioral System Model and Its Applications

Bonnie Holaday

Introducing the Theorist

Dorothy Johnson's earliest publications pertained to what knowledge base nurses needed for nursing care (Johnson, 1959, 1961). Throughout her career, Johnson stressed that nursing had a unique, independent contribution to health care that was distinct from "delegated medical care." Johnson was one of the first "grand theorists" to present her views as a conceptual model. Her model was the first to provide both a guide to understanding and a guide to action. These two ideas—understanding seen first as a holistic, behavioral system process mediated by a complex framework and second as an active process of encounter and response—are central to the work of other theorists who followed her lead and developed conceptual models for nursing practice.

Dorothy Johnson was born on August 21, 1919, in Savannah, Georgia. She received her associate of arts degree from Armstrong Junior College in Savannah, Georgia, in 1938 and her bachelor of science in nursing degree from Vanderbilt University in 1942. She practiced briefly as a staff nurse at the Chatham-Savannah Health Council before attending Harvard University, where she received her master of public health (MPH) in 1948. She began her academic career at Vanderbilt University School of Nursing. A call from Lulu Hassenpplug, dean of the School of Nursing, enticed her to go to the University of California at Los Angeles (UCLA) in 1949. She served there as an assistant, associate, and professor of pediatric nursing until her retirement in 1978. She passed away in 1999.

During her academic career, Dorothy Johnson addressed issues related to nursing practice, nursing education, and nursing science. While she was a pediatric nursing advisor at the Christian Medical College School of Nursing in Vellare, South India, she wrote a series of clinical articles for the *Nursing Journal of India* (Johnson, 1956, 1957). She worked with the California Nurses' Association, the National League for Nursing, and the American Nurses' Association to examine the role of the clinical nurse specialist, the scope of nursing practice, and the need for nursing research. She also completed a Public Health Service–funded research project ("Crying as a Physiologic State in the Newborn Infant") in 1963 (Johnson & Smith, 1963). The foundations of her model and her beliefs about nursing are clearly evident in these early publications.

Introducing the Theory

Johnson has noted that her theory, the Johnson Behavioral System Model (JBSM), evolved from philosophical ideas, theory and research, her clinical background, and many years of thought, discussions, and writing (Johnson, 1968). She cited a number of sources for her theory. From Florence Nightingale came the belief that nursing's concern is a focus on the person rather than the disease. Systems theorists (Buckley, 1968; Chin, 1961; Parsons & Shils, 1951; Rapoport, 1968; and Von Bertalanffy, 1968) were all sources for her model. Johnson's background as a pediatric nurse is also evident in the development of her model. In her

papers, Johnson cited developmental literature to support the validity of a behavioral system model (Ainsworth, 1964; Crandal, 1963; Gerwitz, 1972; Kagan, 1964; and Sears, Maccoby, & Levin, 1954). Johnson also noted that a number of her subsystems had biological underpinnings.

Johnson's theory and her related writings reflect her knowledge about both development and general systems theories. The combination of nursing, development, and general systems introduces into the rhetoric about nursing theory development some of the specifics that make it possible to test hypotheses and conduct critical experiments.

FIVE CORE PRINCIPLES

Johnson's model incorporates five core principles of system thinking: wholeness and order, stabilization, reorganization, hierarchic interaction, and

> *Johnson's model incorporates five core principles of system thinking: wholeness and order, stabilization, reorganization, hierarchic interaction, and dialectical contradiction.*

dialectical contradiction. Each of these general systems principles has analogs in developmental theories that Johnson used to verify the validity of her model (Johnson, 1980, 1990). Wholeness and order provide the basis for continuity and identity, stabilization for development, reorganization for growth and/or change, hierarchic interaction for discontinuity, and dialectical contradiction for motivation. Johnson conceptualized a person as an open system with organized, interrelated, and interdependent subsystems. By virtue of subsystem interaction and independence, the whole of the human organism (system) is greater than the sum of its parts (subsystems). Wholes and their parts create a system with dual constraints: Neither has continuity and identity without the other.

The overall representation of the model can also be viewed as a behavioral system within an environment. The behavioral system and the environment are linked by interactions and transactions. We define the person (behavioral system) as being comprised of subsystems and the environment as being comprised of physical, interpersonal (e.g., father, friend, mother, sibling), and sociocultural (e.g., rules and mores of home, school, country, and other cultural contexts) components that supply the sustenal imperatives (Grubbs, 1980; Holaday, 1997; Johnson, 1990; Meleis, 1991).

Wholeness and Order

The developmental analogy of wholeness and order is continuity and identity. Given the behavioral system's potential for plasticity, a basic feature of the system is that both continuity and change can exist across the life span. The presence of or potentiality for at least some plasticity means that the key way of casting the issue of continuity is not a matter of deciding what exists for a given process or function of a subsystem. Instead, the issue should be cast in terms of determining patterns of interactions among levels of the behavioral system that may promote continuity for a particular subsystem at a given point in time. Johnson's work infers that continuity is in the relationship of the parts rather than in their individuality. Johnson (1990) noted that at the psychological level, attachment (affiliative) and dependency are examples of important specific behaviors that change over time while the representation (meaning) may remain the same. Johnson stated: "[D]evelopmentally, dependence behavior in the socially optimum case evolves from almost total dependence on others to a greater degree of dependence on self, with a certain amount of interdependence essential to the survival of social groups" (1990, p. 28). In terms of behavioral system balance, this pattern of dependence to independence may be repeated as the behavioral system engages in new situations during the course of a lifetime.

Stabilization

Stabilization or behavioral system balance is another core principle of the JBSM. Dynamic systems respond to contextual changes by either a homeostatic or homeorhetic process. Systems have a set point (like a thermostat) that they try to maintain by altering internal conditions to compensate for changes in external conditions. Human thermoregulation is an example of a homeostatic process that is primarily biological but is also behavioral (turning on the heater). Narcissism or the use of attribution of ability or effort are behavioral homeostatic processes we use to interpret activities so they are consistent with our mental organization.

From a behavioral system perspective, homeor-

rhesis is a more important stabilizing process than is homeostatis. In homeorrhesis, the system stabilizes around a trajectory rather than a set point. A toddler placed in a body cast may show motor lags when the cast is removed but soon shows age-appropriate motor skills. An adult newly diagnosed with asthma who does not receive proper education until a year after diagnosis can successfully incorporate the material into her daily activities. These are examples of homeorhetic processes or self-righting tendencies that can occur over time.

What we as nurses observe as development or adaptation of the behavioral system is a product of stabilization. When a person is ill or threatened with illness, he or she is subject to biopsychosocial perturbations. The nurse, according to Johnson (1980, 1990), acts as the external regulator and monitors patient response, looking for successful adaptation to occur. If behavioral system balance returns, there is no need for intervention. If not, the nurse intervenes to help the patient restore behavioral system balance. It is hoped that the patient matures and with additional hospitalizations the previous patterns of response have been assimilated and that there are few disturbances.

Reorganization

Adaptive reorganization occurs when the behavioral system encounters new experiences in the environment that cannot be balanced by existing system mechanisms. Adaptation is defined as change that permits the behavioral system to maintain its set points best in new situations. To the extent that the behavioral system cannot assimilate the new conditions with existing regulatory mechanisms, accommodation must occur either as a new relationship between subsystems or by the establishment of a higher order or different cognitive schema (set, choice). The nurse acts to provide conditions or resources essential to help the accommodation process, may impose regulatory or control mechanisms to stimulate or reinforce certain behaviors, or may attempt to repair structural components (Johnson, 1980).

The difference between stabilization and reorganization is that the latter involves change or evolution. A behavioral system is embedded in an environment, but it is capable of operating independently of environmental constraints through the process of adaptation. The diagnosis of a chronic illness, the birth of a child, or the development of a healthy lifestyle regimen to prevent problems in later years are all examples where accommodation not only promotes behavioral system balance, but also involves a developmental process that results in the establishment of a higher order or more complex behavioral system.

Hierarchic Interaction

Each behavioral system exists in a context of hierarchical relationships and environmental relationships. From the perspective of general systems theory, a behavioral system that has the properties of wholeness and order, stabilization, and reorganization will also demonstrate a hierarchic structure (Buckley, 1968). Hierarchies, or a pattern of relying on particular subsystems, lead to a degree of stability. A disruption or failure will not destroy the whole system but leads instead to a decomposition to the next level of stability.

The judgment that a discontinuity has occurred is typically based on a lack of correlation between assessments at two points of time. For example, one's lifestyle prior to surgery is not a good fit postoperatively. These discontinuities can provide opportunities for reorganization and development.

Dialectical Contradiction

The last core principle is the motivational force for behavioral change. Johnson (1980) described these as drives and noted that these responses are developed and modified over time through maturation, experience, and learning. A person's activities in the environment lead to knowledge and development. However, by acting on the world, each person is constantly changing it and his or her goals, and therefore changing what he or she needs to know. The number of environmental domains that the person is responding to include the biological, psychological, cultural, familial, social, and physical setting. The person needs to resolve (maintain behavioral system balance of) a cascade of contradictions between goals related to physical status, social roles, and cognitive status when faced with illness or the threat of illness. Nurses' interventions during these periods can make a significant difference in the lives of the persons involved. Behavioral system balance is restored and a new level of development is attained.

Johnson's model is unique, in part, because it takes from both general systems and developmental theories. One may analyze the patient's response in terms of behavioral system balance, and, from a developmental perspective ask, "Where did this come from and where is it going?" The developmental component necessitates that we identify and understand the processes of stabilization and sources of disturbances that lead to reorganization. These need to be evaluated by age, gender, and culture. The combination of systems theory and development identifies "nursing's unique social mission and our special realm of original responsibility in patient care" (Johnson, 1990, p. 32).

MAJOR CONCEPTS OF THE MODEL

Next, we review the model as a behavioral system within an environment.

Person

Johnson conceptualized a nursing client as a behavioral system. The behavioral system is orderly, repetitive, and organized with interrelated and interdependent biological and behavioral subsystems. The client is seen as a collection of behavioral subsystems that interrelate to form the behavioral

> *The client is seen as a collection of behavioral subsystems that interrelate to form the behavioral system.*

system. The system may be defined as "those complex, overt actions or responses to a variety of stimuli present in the surrounding environment that are purposeful and functional" (Auger, 1976, p. 22). These ways of behaving form an organized and integrated functional unit that determines and limits the interaction between the person and environment and establishes the relationship of the person to the objects, events, and situations in the environment. Johnson (1980, p. 209) considered such "behavior to be orderly, purposeful and predictable; that is, it is functionally efficient and effective most of the time, and is sufficiently stable and recurrent to be amenable to description and exploration."

Subsystems

The parts of the behavioral system are called *subsystems*. They carry out specialized tasks or functions needed to maintain the integrity of the whole behavioral system and manage its relationship to the environment. Each of these subsystems has a set of behavioral responses that is developed and modified through motivation, experience, and learning.

Johnson identified seven subsystems. However, in this author's operationalization of the model, as in Grubbs (1980), I have included eight subsystems. These eight subsystems and their goals and functions are described in Table 8–1. Johnson noted that these subsystems are found cross-culturally and across a broad range of the phylogenetic scale.

She also noted the significance of social and cultural factors involved in the development of the subsystems. She did not consider the seven subsystems as complete, because "the ultimate group of response systems to be identified in the behavioral system will undoubtedly change as research reveals new subsystems or indicated changes in the structure, functions, or behavioral groupings in the original set" (Johnson, 1980, p. 214).

Table 8–1	**The Subsystems of Behavior**

ACHIEVEMENT SUBSYSTEM

Goal	Mastery or control of self or the environment
Function	To set appropriate goals
	To direct behaviors toward achieving a desired goal
	To perceive recognition from others
	To differentiate between immediate goals and long-term goals
	To interpret feedback (input received) to evaluate the achievement of goals

AFFILIATIVE SUBSYSTEM

Goal	To relate or belong to someone or something other than oneself; to achieve intimacy and inclusion
Function	To form cooperative and interdependent role relationships within human social systems
	To develop and use interpersonal skills to achieve intimacy and inclusion
	To share
	To be related to another in a definite way
	To use narcissistic feelings in an appropriate way

AGGRESSIVE/PROTECTIVE SUBSYSTEM

Goal	To protect self or others from real or imagined threatening objects, persons, or ideas; to achieve self-protection and self-assertion
Function	To recognize biological, environmental, or health systems that are potential threats to self or others
	To mobilize resources to respond to challenges identified as threats
	To use resources or feedback mechanisms to alter biological, environmental, or health input or human responses in order to diminish threats to self or others
	To protect one's achievement goals
	To protect one's beliefs
	To protect one's identity or self-concept

DEPENDENCY SUBSYSTEM

Goal	To obtain focused attention, approval, nurturance, and physical assistance; to maintain the environmental resources needed for assistance; to gain trust and reliance
Function	To obtain approval, reassurance about self
	To make others aware of self
	To induce others to care for physical needs
	To evolve from a state of total dependence on others to a state of increased dependence on the self
	To recognize and accept situations requiring reversal of self-dependence (dependence upon others)
	To focus on another or oneself in relation to social, psychological, and cultural needs and desires

(Continued on the following page)

Table 8-1	**The Subsystems of Behavior–** *(Continued)*

ELIMINATIVE SUBSYSTEM

Goal   To expel biological wastes; to externalize the internal biological environment

Function   To recognize and interpret input from the biological system that signals readiness for waste excretion

To maintain physiological homeostasis through excretion

To adjust to alterations in biological capabilities related to waste excretion while maintaining a sense of control over waste excretion

To relieve feelings of tension in the self

To express one's feelings, emotions, and ideas verbally or nonverbally

INGESTIVE SUBSYSTEM

Goal   To take in needed resources from the environment to maintain the integrity of the organism or to achieve a state of pleasure; to internalize the external environment

Function   To sustain life through nutritive intake

To alter ineffective patterns of nutritive intake

To relieve pain or other psychophysiological subsystems

To obtain knowledge or information useful to the self

To obtain physical and/or emotional pleasure from intake of nutritive or nonnutritive substances

RESTORATIVE SUBSYSTEM

Goal   To relieve fatigue and/or achieve a state of equilibrium by reestablishing or replenishing the energy distribution among the other subsystems; to redistribute energy

Function   To maintain and/or return to physiological homeostasis

To produce relaxation of the self system

SEXUAL SUBSYSTEM

Goal   To procreate, to gratify or attract; to fulfill expectations associated with one's sex; to care for others and to be cared about by them

Function   To develop a self-concept or self-identity based on gender

To project an image of oneself as a sexual being

To recognize and interpret biological system input related to sexual gratification and/or procreation

To establish meaningful relationships in which sexual gratification and/or procreation may be obtained

Source: Based on J. Grubbs (1980). An interpretation of the Johnson behavioral system model. In J. P. Riehl & C. Roy (Eds.), *Conceptual models for nursing practice* (2nd ed., pp. 217–254). New York: Appleton-Century-Crofts; D. E. Johnson (1980). The behavioral system model for nursing. In J. P. Riehl & C. Roy (Eds.), *Conceptual models for nursing practice* (2nd ed., pp. 207–216). New York: Appleton-Century-Crofts; D. Wilkie (1987). *Operationalization of the JBSM.* Unpublished paper. University of California, San Francisco; and B. Holaday (1972). *Operationalization of the JBSM.* Unpublished paper. University of California, Los Angeles.

Each subsystem has functions that serve to meet the conceptual goal. Functional behaviors are those activities carried out to meet these goals. These behaviors may vary with each individual, depending on the person's age, sex, motives, cultural values, social norms, and self-concepts. In order for the subsystem goals to be accomplished, behavioral system structural components must meet functional requirements of the behavioral system.

Each subsystem is composed of at least four structural components that interact in a specific pattern. These parts are goal, set, choice, and action. The goal of a subsystem is defined as the desired result or consequence of the behavior. The basis for the goal is a universal drive whose existence can be supported by scientific research. In general, the drive of each subsystem is the same for all people, but there are variations among individuals (and within individuals over time) in the specific objects or events that are drive-fulfilling, in the value placed on goal attainment, and in drive strength. With drives as the impetus for the behavior, goals can be identified and are considered universal.

Behavioral set is a predisposition to act in a certain way in a given situation. The behavioral set represents a relatively stable and habitual behavioral pattern of responses to particular drives or stimuli. It is learned behavior and is influenced by knowledge, attitudes, and beliefs. Set contains two components: perseveration and preparation. Perseveratory set refers to consistent tendency to react to certain stimuli with the same pattern of behavior. The preparatory set is contingent upon the function of the perseveratory set. The preparatory set functions to establish priorities for attending or not attending to various stimuli.

The conceptual set is an additional component to the model (Holaday, 1982). It is a process of ordering that serves as the mediating link between stimuli from the preparatory and perseveratory sets. Here attitudes, beliefs, information, and knowledge are examined before a choice is made. There are three levels of processing—an inadequate conceptual set, a developing conceptual set, and a sophisticated conceptual set.

The third and fourth components of each subsystem are choice and action. Choice refers to the individual's repertoire of alternative behaviors in a situation that will best meet the goal and attain the desired outcome. The larger the behavioral repertoire of alternative behaviors in a situation, the more adaptable is the individual. The fourth structural component of each subsystem is the observable action of the individual. The concern is with the efficiency and effectiveness of the behavior in goal attainment. Actions are any observable responses to stimuli.

For the eight subsystems to develop and maintain stability, each must have a constant supply of functional requirements (sustenal imperatives). The concept of functional requirements tends to be confined to conditions of the system's survival, and it includes biological as well as psychosocial needs. The problems are related to establishing the types of functional requirements (universal versus highly specific) and finding procedures for validating the assumptions of these requirements. It also suggests a classification of the various states or processes on the basis of some principle and perhaps the establishment of a hierarchy among them. The Johnson model proposes that, for the behavior to be maintained, it must be protected, nurtured, and stimulated: It requires protection from noxious stimuli that threaten the survival of the behavioral system; nurturance, which provides adequate input to sustain behavior; and stimulation, which contributes to continued growth of the behavior and counteracts stagnation. A deficiency in any or all of these functional requirements threatens the behavioral system as a whole, or the effective functioning of the particular subsystem with which it is directly involved.

Environment

Johnson referred to the internal and external environment of the system. She also referred to the interaction between the person and the environment and to the objects, events, and situations in the environment. She also noted that there are forces in the environment that impinge on the person and to which the person adjusts. Thus, the environment consists of all elements that are not a part of the individual's behavioral system but influence the system and can serve as a source of sustenal imperatives. Some of these elements can be manipulated by the nurse to achieve health (behavioral system balance or stability) for the patient. Johnson provided no other specific definition of the environment, nor did she identify what she considered internal versus external environment. But much can be inferred from her writings, and system theory also provides additional insights into the environment component of the model.

The external environment may include people, objects, and phenomena that can potentially permeate the boundary of the behavioral system. This external stimulus forms an organized or meaningful pattern that elicits a response from the individual. The behavioral system attempts to maintain equilibrium in response to environmental factors by assimilating and accommodating to the forces that impinge upon it. Areas of external environment of interest to nurses include the physical settings, people, objects, phenomena, and psychosocial-cultural attributes of an environment.

Johnson provided detailed information about the internal structure and how it functions. She also noted that "[i]llness or other sudden internal or external environmental change is most frequently responsible for system malfunction" (Johnson, 1980, p. 212). Such factors as physiology, temperament, ego, age and related developmental capacities, attitudes, and self-concept are general regulators that may be viewed as a class of internalized intervening variables that influence set, choice, and action. They are key areas for nursing assessment. For example, a nurse attempting to respond to the needs of an acutely ill hospitalized six-year-old would need to know something about the developmental capacities of a six-year-old, and about self-concept and ego development, to understand the child's behavior.

Health

Johnson viewed health as efficient and effective functioning of the system and as behavioral system balance and stability. Behavioral system balance and stability are demonstrated by observed behavior that is purposeful, orderly, and predictable. Such behavior is maintained when it is efficient and effective in managing the person's relationship to the environment.

Behavior changes when efficiency and effectiveness are no longer evident or when a more optimal level of functioning is perceived. Individuals are said to achieve efficient and effective behavioral functioning when their behavior is commensurate with social demands, when they are able to modify their behavior in ways that support biologic imperatives, when they are able to benefit to the fullest extent during illness from the physician's knowledge and skill, and when their behavior does not reveal unnecessary trauma as a consequence of illness (Johnson 1980, p. 207).

Behavior system imbalance and instability are not described explicitly but can be inferred from the following statement to be a malfunction of the behavioral system:

> The subsystems and the system as a whole tend to be self-maintaining and self-perpetuating so long as conditions in the internal and external environment of the system remain orderly and predictable, the conditions and resources necessary to their func-tional requirements are met, and the interrelationships among the subsystems are harmonious. If these conditions are not met, malfunction becomes apparent in behavior that is in part disorganized, erratic, and dysfunctional. Illness or other sudden internal or external environmental change is most frequently responsible for such malfunctions. (Johnson 1980, p. 212)

Thus, Johnson equates behavioral system imbalance and instability with illness. However, as Meleis

(1991) has pointed out, we must consider that illness may be separate from behavioral system functioning. Johnson also referred to physical and social health, but did not specifically define wellness. Just as the inference about illness may be made, it may be inferred that wellness is behavioral system balance and stability, as well as efficient and effective behavioral functioning.

Nursing and Nursing Therapeutics

Nursing is viewed as "a service that is complementary to that of medicine and other health professions, but which makes its own distinctive contribution to the health and well-being of

> **Nursing is viewed as "a service that is complementary to that of medicine and other health professions, but which makes its own distinctive contribution to the health and well-being of people."**

people." Johnson (1980, p. 207) distinguished nursing from medicine by noting that nursing views the patient as a behavioral system, and medicine views the patient as a biological system. In her view, the specific goal of nursing action is "to restore, maintain, or attain behavioral system balance and stability at the highest possible level for the individual" (Johnson, 1980, p. 214). This goal may be expanded to include helping the person achieve an optimal level of balance and functioning when this is possible and desired.

The goal of the system's action is behavioral system balance. For the nurse, the area of concern is a behavioral system threatened by the loss of order and predictability through illness or the threat of illness. The goal of nurses' action is to maintain or restore the individual's behavioral system balance and stability or to help the individual achieve a more optimal level of balance and functioning.

Johnson did not specify the steps of the nursing process but clearly identified the role of the nurse as an external regulatory force. She also identified questions to be asked when analyzing system functioning, and she provided diagnostic classifications to delineate disturbances and guidelines for interventions.

Johnson (1980) expected the nurse to base judgments about behavioral system balance and stability on knowledge and an explicit value system. One important point she made about the value system is that "given that the person has been provided with an adequate understanding of the potential for and means to obtain a more optimal level of behavioral functioning than is evident at the present time, the final judgment of the desired level of functioning is the right of the individual" (Johnson, 1980, p. 215).

The source of difficulty arises from structural and functional stresses. Structural and functional problems develop when the system is unable to meet its own functional requirements. As a result of the inability to meet functional requirements, structural impairments may take place. In addition, functional stress may be found as a result of structural damage or from the dysfunctional consequences of the behavior. Other problems develop when the system's control and regulatory mechanisms fail to develop or become defective.

The model differentiates four diagnostic classifications to delineate these disturbances. A disorder originating within any one subsystem is classified as either an insufficiency, which exists when a subsystem is not functioning or developed to its fullest capacity due to inadequacy of functional requirements, or as a discrepancy, which exists when a behavior does not meet the intended conceptual goal. Disorders found between more than one subsystem are classified either as an incompatibility, which exists when the behaviors of two or more subsystems in the same situation conflict with each other to the detriment of the individual, or as dominance, which exists when the behavior of one subsystem is used more than any other, regardless of the situation or to the detriment of the other subsystems. This is also an area where Johnson believed additional diagnostic classifications would be developed. Nursing therapeutics deal with these three areas.

The next critical element is the nature of the interventions the nurse would use to respond to the behavioral system imbalance. The first step is a thorough assessment to find the source of the difficulty or the origin of the problem. There are at least three types of interventions that the nurse can use to bring about change. The nurse may attempt to repair damaged structural units by altering the individual's set and choice. The second would be for the nurse to impose regulatory and control measures. The nurse acts outside the patient environment to provide the conditions, resources, and

controls necessary to restore behavioral system balance. The nurse also acts within and upon the external environment and the internal interactions of the subsystem to create change and restore stability. The third, and most common, treatment modality is to supply or to help the client find his or her own supplies of essential functional requirements. The nurse may provide nurturance (resources and conditions necessary for survival and growth; the nurse may train the client to cope with new stimuli and encourage effective behaviors), stimulation (provision of stimuli that brings forth new behaviors or increases behaviors, that provides motivation for a particular behavior, and that provides opportunities for appropriate behaviors), and protection (safeguarding from noxious stimuli, defending from unnecessary threats, and coping with a threat on the individual's behalf). The nurse and the client negotiate the treatment plan.

PART TWO

Applications

Fundamental to any professional discipline is the development of a scientific body of knowledge that can be used to guide its practice. JBSM has served as a means for identifying, labeling, and classifying phenomena important to the nursing discipline. Nurses have used the JBSM model since the early 1970s, and the model has demonstrated its ability to provide: a medium for theoretical growth; organization for nurses' thinking, observations, and interpretations of what was observed; a systematic structure and rationale for activities; direction to the search for relevant research questions; solutions for patient care problems; and, finally, criteria to determine if a problem has been solved.

RESEARCH

Stevenson and Woods state: "Nursing science is the domain of knowledge concerned with the adaptation of individuals and groups to actual or potential health problems, the environments that influence health in humans and the therapeutic interventions that promote health and affect the consequences of illness" (1986, p. 6). This position focuses efforts in nursing science on the expansion of knowledge about clients' health problems and nursing therapeutics. Nurse researchers have demonstrated the usefulness of Johnson's model in a clinical practice in a variety of ways. The majority of the research focuses on clients' functioning in terms of maintaining or restoring behavioral system balance, understanding the system and/or subsystems by focusing on the basic sciences, or focusing on the nurse as an agent of action who uses the JBSM to gather diagnostic data or to provide care that influences behavioral system balance.

Dr. Anayis Derdiarian's research program involves both the client and the nurse as agents of action. Derdiarian's early research tested an instrument designed to measure and describe, using the JBSM perspective, the perceived behavioral changes of cancer patients (Derdiarian, 1983; Derdiarian & Forsythe, 1983). The research was based on Johnson's premise that illness is a noxious stimulus that affects the behavioral system balance. The results demonstrated by the instrument possessed content validity, strong internal consistency, and thus strong reliability. A later study (Derdiarian, 1988) explained the effects of the variables of age, site, and stage of cancer on "set" behaviors of the Johnson model's eight behavioral subsystems. The study also served to further validate her instrument.

These studies were important for two reasons. First, Derdiarian examined the impact of three moderator variables on set behavior. The measure can be taken as an indicator of the construct of "behavioral set." The construct was defined by a network of relations that were tied to observables and were therefore empirically testable. This validation study linked a particular measure, the Derdiarian Behavioral System Model (DBSM), to the more general theoretical construct, "behavioral set," that was embedded in the JBSM's more comprehensive theoretical network.

The results indicated significant differences in some mean factor scores in the subsystems among the groups stratified by age, site of cancer, and stage of cancer. Therefore, this study extended the development of the "nomological network" (Cronbach & Meehl, 1955) of the Johnson model. It provided evidence that the measure exhibited, at least in part, the network of relations derived from the theory of the construct. It also elaborated the nomological network by increasing the definiteness of the components of the model (e.g., connections between the moderator variables, behavioral set, and subsystem behaviors). The linking of instrument behaviors to a more general attribute provided not only an evidential basis for interpreting the process underlying the instrument scores, but also a basis for inferring researchable implications of the scores from the broader network of the construct's meaning. A further test of the instrument (Derdiarian & Schobel, 1990) indicated a rank order among the subsystems' response frequency counts as well as among their importance values. Derdiarian also found that changes in the aggressive/protective subsystem made both direct and indirect effects on changes in other subsystems (Derdiarian, 1990).

Derdiarian also examined the nurse as an action agent within the practice domain. She focused on the nurses' assessment of the patient using the DBSM and the effect of using this instrument on the quality of care (Derdiarian, 1990, 1991). This approach expanded the view of nursing knowledge from exclusively client based to knowledge about the context and practice of nursing that is model based. The results of these studies found a significant increase in patient and nurse satisfaction when the DBSM was used. Derdiarian also found that a model-based, valid, and reliable instrument could improve the comprehensiveness and the quality of assessment data, the method of assessment, and the quality of nursing diagnosis, interventions, and outcomes.

Derdiarian's body of work reflects the complexity of nursing's knowledge as well as the strategic problem-solving capabilities of the JBSM. Her article (Derdiarian, 1991) demonstrated the clear relationship between Johnson's theory and nursing practice.

Other nurse researchers have demonstrated the utility of Johnson's model for clinical practice. Coward and Wilke (2000) used the JBSM to examine cancer pain control behaviors. D'Huyvetter (2000) found that defining trauma as a disease, and approaching it within the context of the JBSM, helps the practitioner develop effective interventions.

Lewis and Randell (1990) used the JBSM to identify the most common nursing diagnoses of hospitalized geopsychiatric patients. They found that 30 percent of the diagnoses were related to the achievement subsystem. They also found that the JBSM was more specific than NANDA (North

---

Box 8–1 **Author's Research Highlighted**

My program of research has examined normal and atypical patterns of behavior of children with a chronic illness and the behavior of their parents and has examined the interrelationship between the children and the environment. My goal was to determine the causes of instability within and between subsystems (e.g., breakdown in internal regulatory or control mechanisms) and to identify the source of problems in behavioral system balance.

My first study (Holaday, 1974) compared the achievement behavior of chronically ill and healthy children. The study showed that chronically ill children differed in attributional tendencies when compared with healthy children and showed that the response patterns differed within the chronically ill group when compared to certain dimensions (e.g., gender, age at diagnosis). Males and children diagnosed at birth attributed both success and failure to the presence or absence of ability and little to effort. This is a pattern found in children with low achievement needs. The results indicated behavioral system imbalance and focused my attention on interventions directed toward set, choice, and action.

The next series of studies used the concept of "behavioral set" and examined how mothers and their chronically ill infants interacted (Holaday, 1981, 1982, 1987). Patterns of maternal response provided information related to the setting of the "set goal" or behavioral set; that is, the degree of proximity and speed of maternal response. Mothers with chronically ill infants rarely did not respond to a cry indicating a narrow behavioral set. Further analysis of the data led to the identification of a new structural component of the model-conceptual set. A person's conceptual set was defined as an organized cluster of cognitive units that were used to interpret the content information from the preparatory and perseveratory sets. A conceptual set may differ both in the number of cognitive units involved and in the degree of organization exhibited. The various cognitive units that make up a conceptual set may vary in complexity depending on the situation. Three levels of conceptual set have been identified, ranging from a very simple to a complex "set" with a high degree of connectedness between multiple perspectives (Holaday, 1982). Thus, the conceptual set functions as an information collection and processing unit. Examining a person's set, choice, and conceptual set offered a way to examine issues of individual cognitive patterns and its impact on behavioral system balance.

The most recent study (Holaday, Turner-Henson, & Swan, 1997) drew from the knowledge gained from previous studies. This study viewed the JBSM as holistic, in that it assumed that all part processes—biological, physical, psychological, and sociocultural—are interrelated; developmental, in that it assumed that development proceeds from a relative lack of differentiation toward a goal of differentiation and hierarchic integration of organismic functioning; and system-oriented, in that a unit of analysis was the person in the environment where the person's physical and/or biological (e.g., health), psychological, interpersonal, and sociocultural levels of organization are operative and interrelated with the physical, interpersonal, and sociocultural levels of organization in the environment. Our results indicate that it was possible to determine the impact of a lack of functional requirements on a child's actions and to identify behavioral system imbalance and the need for specific types of nursing intervention.

The goal of my research program has been to describe the relations both among and within the subsystems that make up the integrated whole and to identify the type of nursing interventions that restore behavioral system balance.

American Nursing Diagnosis Association) diagnoses, which demonstrated considerable overlap. Poster, Dee, and Randell (1997) found the JBSM was an effective framework to use to evaluate patient outcomes.

EDUCATION

Johnson's model was used as the basis for undergraduate education at the UCLA School of Nursing. The curriculum was developed by the fac-

ulty; however, no published material is available that describes this process. Texts by Wu (1973) and Auger (1976) extended Johnson's model and provided some idea of the content of that curriculum. Later, in the 1980s, Harris (1986) described the use of Johnson's theory as a framework for UCLA's curriculum. The Universities of Hawaii, Alaska, and Colorado also used the JBSM as a basis for their undergraduate curricula.

Loveland-Cherry and Wilkerson (1983) analyzed Johnson's model and concluded that the model could be used to develop a curriculum. The primary focus of the program would be the study of the person as a behavioral system. The student would need a background in systems theory and in the biological, psychological, and sociological sciences.

NURSING PRACTICE AND ADMINISTRATION

Johnson has influenced nursing practice because she enabled nurses to make statements about the links between nursing input and health outcomes for clients. The model has been useful in practice because it identifies an end product (behavioral system balance), which is nursing's goal. Nursing's

> *Nursing's specific objective is to maintain or restore the person's behavioral system balance and stability, or to help the person achieve a more optimum level of functioning.*

specific objective is to maintain or restore the person's behavioral system balance and stability, or to help the person achieve a more optimum level of functioning. The model provides a means for identifying the source of the problem in the system. Nursing is seen as the external regulatory force that acts to restore balance (Johnson, 1980).

One of the best examples of the model's use in practice has been at the University of California, Los Angeles, Neuropsychiatric Institute (UCLA—NPI). Auger and Dee (1983) designed a patient classification system using the JBSM. Each subsystem of behavior was operationalized in terms of critical adaptive and maladaptive behaviors. The behavioral statements were designed to be measurable, relevant to the clinical setting, observable, and specific to the subsystem. The use of the model has had a major impact on all phases of the nursing process, including a more systematic assessment process, identification of patient strengths and problem areas, and an objective means for evaluating the quality of nursing care (Dee & Auger, 1983).

The early works of Dee and Auger lead to further refinement in the patient classification system. Behavioral indices for each subsystem have been further operationalized in terms of critical adaptive and maladaptive behaviors. Behavioral data is gathered to determine the effectiveness of each subsystem (Dee & Randell, 1989; Dee, 1990).

The scores serve as an acuity rating system and provide a basis for allocating resources. These resources are allocated based on the assigned levels of nursing intervention, and resource needs are calculated based on the total number of patients assigned according to levels of nursing interventions and the hours of nursing care associated with each of the levels (Dee & Randell, 1989) (see Table 8–2). The development of this system has provided nursing administration with the ability to identify the levels of staff needed to provide care (licensed vocational nurse versus registered nurse), bill patients for actual nursing care services, and identify nursing services that are absolutely necessary in times of budgetary restraint. Recent research has demonstrated the importance of a model-based nursing database in medical records (Poster, Dee, & Randell, 1997) and the effectiveness of using a model to identify the characteristics of a large hospital's managed behavioral health population in relation to observed nursing care needs, level of patient functioning on admission and discharge, and length of stay (Dee, Van Servellen, & Brecht, 1998).

The work of Vivien Dee and her colleagues has demonstrated the validity and usefulness of the JBSM as a basis for clinical practice within a healthcare setting. From the findings of their work, it is clear that the JBSM established a systematic framework for patient assessment and nursing interventions, provided a common frame of reference for all practitioners in the clinical setting, provided a framework for the integration of staff knowledge about the clients, and promoted continuity in the delivery of care. These findings should be generalizable to a variety of clinical settings.

Table 8-2 Nursing Staffing Budget Unit: 2-South.

SHIFT	ACTUAL NO. PATIENTS	LEVELS OF NURSING INTERVENTIONS				#STL	PATIENT HOURS	—TOTAL COST—			—COST PER PATIENT—		
		I	II	III	IV			BUDGET	ACTUAL	VAR	BUDGET	ACTUAL	VAR
N	12.3	1.5	7.1	3.5	0.1	2.49	1.65	181734	54156	27578	40.2	35.2	5.0
D	12.0	1.2	7.3	3.4	0.2	4.24	2.91	358208	338014	20194	79.1	79.6	−0.4
E	12.2	1.2	7.3	3.6	0.1	3.82	2.55	183008	270855	−87847	40.4	61.9	−21.5
					Totals	10.55	7.11	722950	763025	−40075	159.7	176.7	−16.9

Source: V. Dee & B. Randell (1989). *NPH Patient Classification System: A theory-based nursing practice model for staffing.* Paper presented at the UCLA Neuropsychiatric Institute and Hospital.

SUMMARY

The Johnson Behavioral System Model captures the richness and complexity of nursing. While the perspective presented here is embedded in the past, there remains the potentiality for the theory's further development and the uncovering and shaping of significant research problems that have both theoretical and practical value. There are a variety of problem areas worthy of investigation that are suggested by the JBSM assumptions and from previous studies. Some examples include examining the levels of integration (biological, psychological, and sociocultural) within and between the subsystems. For example, a study could examine the way a person deals with the transition from health to illness with the onset of asthma. There is concern with the relations between one's biological system (e.g., unstable, problems breathing), one's psychological self (e.g., achievement goals, need for assistance, self-concept), self in relation to the physical environment (e.g., allergens, being away from home), and transactions related to the sociocultural context (e.g., attitudes and values about the sick). The study of transitions (e.g., the onset of puberty, menopause, death of a spouse, onset of acute illness) also represents a treasury of open problems for research with the JBSM. Findings obtained from these studies will provide not only an opportunity to revise and advance the theoretical conceptualization of the JBSM, but will also provide information about nursing interventions. The JBSM approach leads us to seek common organizational parameters in every scientific explanation and does so using a shared language about nursing and nursing care.

References

Ainsworth, M. (1964). Patterns of attachment behavior shown by the infant in interactions with mother. *Merrill-Palmer Quarterly, 10,* 51–58.

Auger, J. (1976). *Behavioral systems and nursing.* Englewood Cliffs, NJ: Prentice-Hall.

Auger, J., & Dee, V. (1983). A patient classification system based on the Behavioral Systems Model of Nursing: Part 1. *Journal of Nursing Administration, 13*(4), 38–43.

Buckley, W. (Ed.). (1968). *Modern systems research for the behavioral scientist.* Chicago: Aldine.

Chin, R. (1961). The utility of system models and developmental models for practitioners. In Benne, K., Bennis, W., & Chin, R. (Eds.), *The planning of change.* New York: Holt.

Coward, D. D., & Wilke, D. J. (2000). Metastatic bone pain: Meanings associated with self-report and management decision making. *Cancer Nursing, 23*(2), 101–108.

Crandal, V. (1963). Achievement. In Stevenson, H. W. (Ed.), *Child psychology.* Chicago: University of Chicago Press.

Cronbach, L. J., & Meehl, P. (1955). Construct validity in psychological tests. *Psychological Bulletin, 52,* 281–301.

Dee, V. (1990). Implementation of the Johnson Model: One hospital's experience. In Parker, M. (Ed.), *Nursing theories in practice* (pp. 33–63). New York: National League for Nursing.

Dee, V., & Auger, J. (1983). A patient classification system based on the Behavioral System Model of Nursing: Part 2. *Journal of Nursing Administration, 13*(5), 18–23.

Dee, V., & Randell, B. P. (1989). *NPH patient classification system: A theory based nursing practice model for staffing.* Paper presented at the UCLA Neuropsychiatric Institute, Los Angeles, CA.

Dee, V., Van Servellen, G., & Brecht, M. (1998). Managed behavioral health care patients and their nursing care problems, level of functioning and impairment on discharge. *Journal of the American Psychiatric Nurses Association, 4*(2), 57–66.

Derdiarian, A. K. (1983). An instrument for theory and research development using the behavioral systems model for nursing: The cancer patient. *Nursing Research, 32,* 196–201.

Derdiarian, A. K. (1988). Sensitivity of the Derdiarian Behavioral Systems Model Instrument to age, site and type of cancer: A preliminary validation study. *Scholarly Inquiring for Nursing Practice, 2,* 103–121.

Derdiarian, A. K. (1990). The relationships among the subsystems of Johnson's Behavioral System Model. *Image, 22,* 219–225.

Derdiarian, A. (1991). Effects of using a nursing model-based instrument on the quality of nursing care. *Nursing Administration Quarterly, 15*(3), 1–16.

Derdiarian, A. K., & Forsythe, A. B. (1983). An instrument for theory and research development using the behavioral systems model for nursing: The cancer patient. Part II. *Nursing Research, 3,* 260–266.

Derdiarian, A. K., & Schobel, D. (1990). Comprehensive assessment of AIDS patients using the behavioral systems model for nursing practice instrument. *Journal of Advanced Nursing, 15,* 436–446.

D'Huyvetter, C. (2000). The trauma disease. *Journal of Trauma Nursing, 7*(1), 5–12.

Gerwitz, J. (Ed.). (1972). *Attachment and dependency.* Englewood Cliffs, NJ: Prentice-Hall.

Grubbs, J. (1980). An interpretation of the Johnson behavioral system model. In Riehl, J. P., & Roy, C. (Eds.), *Conceptual models for nursing practice* (pp. 217–254). New York: Appleton-Century-Crofts.

Harris, R. B. (1986). Introduction of a conceptual model into a fundamental baccalaureate course. *Journal of Nursing Education, 25,* 66–69.

Holaday, B. (1972). Unpublished operationalization of the Johnson Model. University of California, Los Angeles.

Holaday, B. (1974). Achievement behavior in chronically ill children. *Nursing Research, 23,* 25–30.

Holaday, B. (1981). Maternal response to their chronically ill infants' attachment behavior of crying. *Nursing Research, 30,* 343–348.

Holaday, B. (1982). Maternal conceptual set development: Identifying patterns of maternal response to chronically ill infant crying. *Maternal Child Nursing Journal, 11,* 47–59.

Holaday, B. (1987). Patterns of interaction between mothers and their chronically ill infants. *Maternal Child Nursing Journal, 16,* 29–45.

Holaday, B. (1997). Johnson's behavioral system model in nursing practice. In Alligood, M., & Marriner-Tomey, A. (Eds.), *Nursing theory: Utilization and application* (pp. 49–70). St. Louis: Mosby-Year Book.

Holaday, B., Turner-Henson, A., & Swan, J. (1997). The Johnson Behavioral System Model: Explaining activities of chronically ill children. In Hinton-Walker, P., & Newman, B. (Eds.), *Blueprint for use of nursing models: Education, research, practice, and administration* (pp. 33–63). New York: National League for Nursing.

Johnson, D. E. (1956). A story of three children. *The Nursing Journal of India, XLVII*(9), 313–322.

Johnson, D. E. (1957). Nursing care of the ill child. *The Nursing Journal of India, XLVIII*(1), 12–14.

Johnson, D. E. (1959). The nature and science of nursing. *Nursing Outlook, 7,* 291–294.

Johnson, D. E. (1961). The significance of nursing care. *American Journal of Nursing, 61,* 63–66.

Johnson, D. E. (1968). *One conceptual model of nursing.* Unpublished lecture. Vanderbilt University.

Johnson, D. E. (1980). The behavioral system model for nursing. In Riehl, J. P., & Roy, C. (Eds.), *Conceptual models for nursing practice* (2nd ed., pp. 207–216). New York: Appleton-Century-Crofts.

Johnson, D. E. (1990). The Behavioral System Model for Nursing. In Parker, M. E. (Ed.), *Nursing theories in practice* (pp. 23–32). New York: National League for Nursing.

Johnson, D. E., & Smith, M. M. (1963). *Crying as a physiologic state in the newborn infant.* Unpublished research report, PHS Grant NV–00055–01 (formerly GS–9768).

Kagan, J. (1964). Acquisition and significance of sex role identity. In Hoffman, R., & Hoffman, G. (Eds.), *Review of child development research.* New York: Russell Sage Foundation.

Lewis, C., & Randell, R. B. (1990). Alteration in self-care: An instance of ineffective coping in the geriatric patient. In Carroll-Johnson, R. M. (Ed.), *Classification of nursing diagnosis: Proceedings of the 9th conference.* Philadelphia: J. B. Lippincott.

Loveland-Cherry, C., & Wilkerson, S. (1983). Dorothy Johnson's behavioral system model. In Fitzpatrick, J., & Whall, A. (Eds.), *Conceptual models of nursing: Analysis and application.* Bowie, MD: Robert J. Brady.

Meleis, A. I. (1991). *Theoretical nursing: Development and progress.* Philadelphia: J. B. Lippincott.

Parsons, T., & Shils, E. A. (Eds.). (1951). *Toward a general theory of action: Theoretical foundations for the social sciences.* New York: Harper & Row.

Poster, E. C., Dee, V., & Randell, B. P. (1997). The Johnson Behavioral Systems Model as a framework for patient outcome evaluation. *Journal of the American Psychiatric Nurses Association, 3*(3), 73–80.

Rapoport, A. (1968). Forward to modern systems research for the behavior scientist. In Buckley, W. (Ed.), *Modern systems research for the behavioral scientist.* Chicago: Aldine.

Sears, R., Maccoby, E., & Levin, H. (1954). *Patterns child rearing.* White Plains, NY: Row & Peterson.

Stevenson, J. S., & Woods, N. F. (1986). Nursing science and contemporary science: Emerging paradigms. In *Setting the agenda for year 2000: Knowledge development in nursing* (pp. 6–20). Kansas City, MO: American Academy of Nursing.

Von Bertalanffy, L. (1968). *General systems theory: Foundations, development, application.* New York: George Braziller.

Wilkie, D. (1987). Unpublished operationalization of the Johnson model. University of California, San Francisco.

Wu, R. (1973). *Behavior and illness.* Englewood Cliffs, NJ: Prentice-Hall.

CHAPTER 9

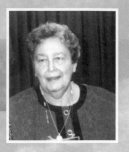

Myra Levine

PART ONE: Myra Levine's Conservation Model and Its Applications

Karen Moore Schaefer

Introducing the Theorist

Myra Levine has been called a Renaissance woman—highly principled, remarkable, and committed to what happens to the patients' quality of life. She was a daughter, sister, wife, mother, friend, educator, administrator, student of humanities, scholar, enabler, and confidante. She was amazingly intelligent, opinionated, quick to respond, loving, caring, trustworthy, and global in her vision of nursing. She lives on in the author's heart, as I hope she will in yours as you learn about her and the model she unknowingly created to develop nursing knowledge.

Levine was born in Chicago and was raised with a sister and a brother with whom she shared a close, loving relationship (Levine, 1988b). She was also very fond of her father, who was a hardware man. He was often ill and frequently hospitalized with gastrointestinal problems. She thinks that this might have been why she had such a great interest in nursing. Levine's mother was a strong woman who kept the home filled with love and warmth. She was very supportive of Levine's choice to be a nurse. "[My mother] probably knew as much about nursing as I did" (Levine, 1988b) because she was devoted to caring for her father when he was ill.

Levine began attending the University of Chicago but chose to attend Cook County School of Nursing when she could no longer afford the university. Being in nursing school was a new experience for her; she called it a "great adventure" (Levine, 1988b). She received her diploma from Cook County in 1944. She later received her bachelor of science degree from the University of Chicago in 1949 and her master of science in nursing from Wayne State University in 1962.

Aside from her husband and children, education was Levine's primary interest, although she had clinical experience in the operating room and in oncology nursing. She was a civilian nurse at the Gardiner General Hospital, director of nursing at Drexel Home in Chicago, clinical instructor at Bryan Memorial Hospital in Lincoln, Nebraska, and administrative supervisor at University of Chicago Clinics and Henry Ford Hospital in Michigan. She was chairperson of clinical nursing at Cook County School of Nursing and a faculty member at Loyola University, Rush University, and University of Illinois. She was a visiting professor at Tel Aviv University in Israel and Recanti School of Nursing at Ben Gurion University of the Negev in Beer Sheeva, Israel. She was professor emeritus in Medical Surgical Nursing, University of Chicago, a charter fellow of the American Association of Nurses (FAAN), and a member of Sigma Theta Tau International, from which she received the Elizabeth Russell Belford Award as distinguished educator. She received an honorary doctorate from Loyola University in 1992.

Introducing the Theory

F. A. Davis Company published the first edition of Myra Levine's textbook *Introduction to Clinical Nursing* in 1969 and the second and last editions in 1973. In discussing the first edition of her book,

Levine (1969a, p. 39) said: "I decided against using 'holistic' in favor of 'organismic,' largely because the term 'holistic' had been appropriated by pseudoscientists endowing it with the mythology of transcendentalism. I used 'holism' in the second edition in 1973 because I realized it was too important to be abandoned to the mystics. I believed that it was the proper description of the way the internal environment and the external environment were joined in the real world." In the introduction to the second edition, she wrote:

> There is something very final about a printed page, and yet books do have a life all their own. They gather life from the use to which they are put, and when they succeed in communicating among many individuals in many places, then their intent is most truly served. The most remarkable fact about the first edition of this book has been the exchange of interests that has resulted from the willingness with which its readers and users have communicated with its author. (Levine, 1973, p. vii)

This passage suggests that Levine's original book (1969b) provided a model to teach medical surgical nursing and created a dialogue among colleagues about the plan itself. The text has continued to create dialogue about the art and science of nursing with ongoing research serving as a testament to its value (Delmore, 2003; Mefford, 1999).

FOUNDATIONS OF CLINICAL NURSING

Levine's original reason for writing the book was to find a way to teach the foundations of nursing that would focus on nursing and was organized in such a way that nursing students would learn the skill as well as the rationale for the skill. She felt that too often the focus was on skill and not on the reasons why the skill is performed. She felt that nursing research was generally ignored. Her intent was to bring practice and research together to establish nursing as an applied science. The book was used as a beginning nursing text by Levine and many of her colleagues.

The first chapter of her text was entitled, "Introduction to Patient Centered Nursing Care," a model of care delivery that is now acclaimed to be the answer to cost-effective delivery of health-care services today. She believed that patient-centered care was "individualized nursing care" (Levine, 1973, p. 23). She discussed the theory of causation, a unified theory of health and disease, the meaning of the conservation principles, the hospital as environment, and patient-centered intervention. The nursing care chapters in her text focus on nursing care of the patient with:

1. failure of the nervous system;
2. failure of the integration resulting from hormonal imbalance;
3. disturbance of homeostasis: fluid and electrolyte imbalance;
4. disturbance of homeostasis: nutritional needs;
5. disturbance of homeostasis: systemic oxygen needs;
6. disturbance of homeostasis: cellular oxygen needs;
7. disease arising from aberrant cellular growth;
8. inflammatory problems; and
9. holistic response.

Her way of organizing the material was a shift from teaching nursing based on the disease model. Her final chapter on the holistic response represented a major shift away from disease to the systems way of thinking. Informed by other disciplines, she discussed the integrated system, the interaction of systems creating the sense of well-being, energy exchange at the organismic level and at the cellular level, perception of self, the affect of space on self-perception, and the circadian rhythm.

As Levine wrote her book, major changes took place in the curriculum at Cook County Hospital

---

Box 9–1 **Influences on the Conservation Model**

Levine used the inductive method to develop her model. She "borrowed" information from other disciplines while retaining the basic structure of nursing in the model (Levine, 1988a). As she continued to write about her model, she integrated information from other sciences and increasingly cited personal experiences as evidence of her work's validity. The following is a list of the influences in the development of her philosophy of nursing and the Conservation Model.

1. Levine indicated that Florence Nightingale, through her focus on observation (Nightingale, 1859) provided great attention to energy conservation and recognized the need for structural integrity. Levine relates Nightingale's discussion of social integrity to Nightingale's concern for sanitation, which she says implies an interaction between the person and the environment.
2. Irene Beland influenced Levine's thinking about nursing as a compassionate art and rigid intellectual pursuit (Levine, 1988b). Levine also credited Beland (1971) for the theory of specific causation and multiple factors.
3. Feynman (1965) provided support for Levine's position that conservation was a natural law, arguing that the development of theory cannot deny the importance of natural law (Levine, 1973).
4. Bernard (1957) is recognized for his contribution in the identification of the interdependence of bodily functions (Levine, 1973).
5. Levine (1973) emphasized the dynamic nature of the internal milieu, using Waddington's (1968) term "homeophoresis."
6. Use of Bates's (1967) formulation of the external environment as having three levels of factors (perceptual, operational, and conceptual), challenging the integrity of the individual, helped to emphasize the complexity of the environment.
7. The description of illness is based on Wolf's (1961) description of disease as adaptation to noxious environmental forces.
8. Selye's (1956) definition of "stress" is included in Levine's (1989c) description of her organismic stress response as "being recorded over time and . . . influenced by the accumulated experience of the individual" (p. 30).
9. The perceptual organismic response incorporates Gibson's (1966) work on perception as a mediator of behavior. His identification of the five perceptual systems, including hearing, sight, touch, taste, and smell, contributed to the development of the perceptual response.
10. The notion that individuals seek to defend their personhood is grounded in Goldstein's (1963) explanation of soldiers who, despite brain injury, sought to cling to some semblance of self-awareness.
11. Dubos's (1965) discussion of the adaptability of the organism helped support Levine's explanation that adaptation occurs within a range of responses.
12. Levine's personal experiences influenced her thinking in several ways. When hospitalized, she said, "the experience of wholeness is universally acknowledged" (Levine, 1996, p. 39).

(Levine, 1988b). She and her colleagues began to focus on the importance of nursing research and taught perception, sleep, distance (space), and periodicity as a factor in health and disease. See the "Influences on the Conservation Model" that follows.

THE COMPOSITION OF THE CONSERVATION MODEL

As an organizing framework for nursing practice, the goal of the Conservation Model is to promote

> *The goal of the Conservation Model is to promote adaptation and maintain wholeness using the principles of conservation.*

adaptation and maintain wholeness using the principles of conservation. The model guides the nurse to focus on the influences and responses at the organismic level. The nurse accomplishes the goals of the model through the conservation of energy, structure, and personal and social integrity (Levine, 1967). Interventions are provided in order to improve the patient's condition (therapeutic) or to promote comfort (supportive) when change in the patient's condition is not possible. The outcomes of the interventions are assessed through the organismic response.

Although Levine identified two concepts critical to the use of her model—adaptation and wholeness—conservation is fundamental to the outcomes expected when the model is used. Conservation is therefore handled as the third major concept of the model. Using the model in practice requires that the nurse understand the commonplaces (Barnum, 1994) of health, person, environment, and nursing.

Components

Before delving into the inner workings of Levine's model, it is necessary to understand its components.

Adaptation

Adaptation is the process of change, and conservation is the outcome of adaptation. Adaptation is the process whereby the patient maintains integrity within the realities of the environment (Levine, 1966, 1989a). Adaptation is achieved through the "frugal, economic, contained, and controlled use of environmental resources by the individual in his or her best interest" (Levine, 1991, p. 5). In her view:

The environmental "fit" that underscores successful adaptation suggests that every species has fixed patterns of response uniquely designed to ensure success in essential life activities, demonstrating that adaptation is both historical and specific. However, tremendous opportunities for individual accommodations are locked into the gene structure of each species; every individual is one of a kind. (p. 5)

Every individual has a unique range of adaptive responses. These responses will vary based on heredity, age, gender, or challenges of an illness experience. For example, the response to weakness of the cardiac muscle is an increased heart rate, dilation of the ventricle, and thickening of the myocardial muscle. While the responses are the same, the timing and the manifestation of the organismic response (e.g., pulse rate) will be unique for each individual.

Redundancy, history, and specificity characterize adaptation. These characteristics are "rooted in history and awaiting the specific circumstances to which they respond" (Levine, 1991, p. 6). The genetic structure develops over time and provides the foundation for these responses. Specificity, while sharing traits with a species, has individual potential that creates a variety of adaptation outcomes. For example, diabetes has a genetic component, which explains the fundamental decrease in sugar metabolism. However, the organismic responses vary (renal perfusion, blood vessel integrity), for example, based on genetic alterations, age, gender, and therapeutic management techniques.

Redundancy represents the fail-safe options available to the individual to ensure continued adaptation. Levine (1991) believed that health is dependent on the ability to select from redundant options. She hypothesized that aging may be the result of the failure of redundant systems. If this is the case, then survival is dependent on redundant options, which are often challenged and limited by illness, disease, and aging. When the compensatory response to cardiac disease is no longer able to maintain an adequate blood flow to vital organs during activity, survival becomes increasingly difficult. Adaptation represents the accommodation between the internal and external environments.

Conservation

Conservation is the product of adaptation and is a common principle underlying many of the basic

> *Conservation is the product of adaptation and is a common principle underlying many of the basic sciences. Conservation is critical to understanding an essential element of human life.*

sciences. Conservation is critical to understanding an essential element of human life:

> Implicit in the knowledge of conservation is the fact of wholeness, integrity, unity—all of the structures that are being conserved . . . conservation of the integrity of the person is essential to ensuring health and providing the strength to confront disability . . . the importance of conservation in the treatment of illness is precisely focused on the reclamation of wholeness, of health. . . . Every nursing act is dedicated to the conservation, or "keeping together," of the wholeness of the individual. (Levine, 1991, p. 3)

Individuals are continuously defending their wholeness to keep together the life system. Individuals defend themselves in constant interaction with their environment, choosing the most economic, frugal, and energy-sparing options that safeguard their integrity. Conservation seeks to achieve a balance of energy supply and demand that is within the unique biological capabilities of the individual (Schaefer, 1991a).

Maintaining the proper balance involves the nursing intervention coupled with the patient's participation to assure the activities are within the safe limits of the patient's ability to participate. Although energy cannot be directly observed, the consequences of energy exchanges are predictable, recognizable, and manageable (Levine, 1973, 1991).

Wholeness

Wholeness is based on Erikson's (1964) description of wholeness as an open system: "Wholeness emphasizes a sound, organic, progressive mutuality between diversified functions and parts within an entirety, the boundaries of which are open and fluid" (p. 63). Levine (1973) stated that "the unceasing interaction of the individual organism with its environment does represent an 'open and fluid' system, and a condition of health, wholeness, exists when the interaction or constant adaptations to the environment, permit ease—the assurance of integrity . . . in all the dimensions of life" (p. 11). This continuous dynamic, open interaction between the internal and external environment provides the basis for holistic thought, the view of the individual as whole.

Health, Person, Environment, and Nursing

Health and disease are patterns of adaptive change. From a social perspective, health is the ability to function in social roles. Health is culturally determined: "[I]t is not an entity, but rather a definition imparted by the ethos and beliefs of the groups to which the individual belongs" (personal communication, February 21, 1995). Health is an individual

> *Health is an individual response that may change over time in response to new situations, new life challenges, and aging, or in response to social, political, economic, and spiritual factors. Health is implied to mean unity and integrity. The goal of nursing is to promote health.*

response that may change over time in response to new situations, new life challenges, and aging, or in response to social, political, economic, and spiritual factors. Health is implied to mean unity and integrity. The goal of nursing is to promote health. Levine (1991) clarified what she meant by health as:

> the avenue of return to the daily activities compromised by ill health. It is not only the insult or the injury that is repaired but the person himself or herself. . . . It is not merely the healing of an afflicted part. It is rather a return to self hood, where the encroachment of the disability can be set aside entirely, and the individual is free to pursue once more his or her own interests without constraint. (p. 4)

In all of life's challenges, individuals will constantly attempt to attain, retain, maintain, or protect their integrity (health, wholeness, and unity).

To Levine, the holistic person is a thinking being who is aware of the past and oriented to the future. The wholeness (integrity) of the individual demands that the "individual life has meaning only in the context of social life" (Levine, 1973, p. 17). The person responds to change in an integrated, sequential, yet singular fashion while in constant interaction with the environment. Levine (1996) defined "the person" as a spiritual being, quoting Genesis 1:27: "And God created man in his own image, in the image of God created He him. Male and female created He them.... Sanctity of life is manifested in everyone. The holiness of life itself [testifies] to its spiritual reality" (p. 40). "Person" can be an individual, a family, or a community.

Levine's (1968a, 1968b, 1973) discussion of the person includes recognition that the person is defined to a certain degree based on the boundaries defined by Hall (1966) as "personal space." Levine rejected the notion that energy can be manipulated and transferred from one human to another as in therapeutic touch. Yet a person is affected by the presence of another relative to his or her personal space boundaries. Admittedly, some of this is defined based on cultural ethos, yet what is it about the "bubble" that results in a specific organismic response? It may be that the energy involved in the interaction is not clearly defined. Scientists are challenged to examine this. Levine encouraged creativity such as therapeutic touch but rejected activities that are not scientifically sound.

The *environment* completes the wholeness of the individual. The individual has both an internal and external environment. The internal environment combines the physiological and pathophysiological aspects of the individual and is constantly challenged by the external environment.

The external environment includes those factors that impinge on and challenge the individual. The environment as described by Levine (1973) was adapted from the following three levels of environment identified by Bates (1967).

The *perceptual* environment includes aspects of the world that individuals are able to seize or interpret through the senses. The individual "seeks, selects, and tests information from the environment in the context of his [her] definition of himself [herself], and so defends his [her] safety, his [her] identity, and in a larger sense, his [her] purpose" (Levine, 1971, p. 262).

The *operational* environment includes factors that may physically affect individuals but are not directly perceived by them, such as radiation, microorganisms, and pollution.

The *conceptual* environment includes the cultural patterns characterized by spiritual existence and mediated by language, thought, and history. Factors that affect behavior—such as norms, values, and beliefs—are also part of the conceptual environment.

Nursing is "human interaction" (Levine, 1973, p. 1). "The nurse enters into a partnership of human experience where sharing moments in time—some

trivial, some dramatic—leaves its mark forever on each patient" (Levine, 1977, p. 845). The goal of nursing is to promote adaptation and maintain wholeness (health). The goal is accomplished through the use of the conservation principles: energy, structure, personal, and social.

The Model

Energy conservation is dependent on the free exchange of energy with the internal and external environment to maintain the balance of energy supply and demand. Conservation of structural integrity is dependent on an intact defense system (immune system) that supports healing and repair to preserve the structure and function of the whole being.

The conservation of personal integrity acknowledges the individual as one who strives for recognition, respect, self-awareness, humanness, self-hood, and self-determination. The conservation of social integrity recognizes the individual as a social being who functions in a society that helps to establish boundaries of the self. The value of the individual is recognized, but it is also recognized that the individual resides within a family, a community, a religious group, an ethnic group, a political system, and a nation (Levine, 1973).

The outcome of nursing involves the assessment of organismic responses. The nurse is responsible for responding to a request for health care and for recognizing altered health and the patient's organismic response to altered health. An organismic response is a change in behavior or change in the level of functioning during an attempt to adapt to the environment. The organismic responses are intended to maintain the patient's integrity. According to Levine (1973), the levels of organismic response include:

1. *Response to fear (flight/fight response).* This is the most primitive response. It is the physiological and behavioral readiness to respond to a sudden and unexpected environmental change; it is an instantaneous response to real or imagined threat.
2. *Inflammatory response.* This is the second level of response intended to provide for structural integrity and the promotion of healing. Both are defenses against noxious stimuli and the initiation of healing.
3. *Response to stress.* This is the third level of response, which is developed over time and influenced by each stressful experience encoun-

tered by the patient. If the experience is prolonged, the stress can lead to damage to the systems.

4. *Perceptual response.* This is the fourth level of response. It involves gathering information for the environment and converting it to a meaningful experience.

The organismic responses are redundant in the sense that they coexist. The four responses help individuals protect and maintain their integrity. They are integrated by their cognitive abilities, the wealth of previous experiences, the ability to define relationships, and the strength of their adaptive abilities.

Nurses use the scientific process and creative abilities to provide nursing care to the patient (Schaefer, 1998). The nursing process incorporates these abilities, thereby improving the care of the patient (see Table 9–1).

PHILOSOPHICAL NOTES

ASSUMPTIONS AND VALUES OF THE CONSERVATION MODEL

① The person is viewed as a holistic being: "The experience of wholeness is the foundation of all human enterprises" (Levine, 1991, p. 3).

Table 9–1	Use of the Nursing Process According to Levine
Process	**Application of the Process**
Assessment	Collection of provocative facts through observation and interview of challenges to the internal and external environments.
	The nurse observes the patient for organismic responses to illness, reads medical reports, evaluates results of diagnostic studies, and talks with patients and their families (support persons) about their needs for assistance. The nurse assesses for physiological and pathophysiological challenges to the internal environment and the factors in the perceptual, operational, and conceptual levels of the external environment that challenge the individual.
*Trophicognosis**	Nursing diagnosis that gives the provocative facts meaning.
	The nurse arranges the provocative facts in a way that provides meaning to the patient's predicament. A judgment is the trophicognosis.**
Hypotheses	Direct the nursing interventions with the goal of maintaining wholeness and promoting adaptation. Nurses seek validation of the patients' problems with the patients or support persons. The nurses then propose hypotheses about the problems and the solutions, such as: Eight glasses of water a day will improve bowel evacuation. These become the plan of care.
Interventions	Test the hypotheses.
	Nurses use hypotheses to direct care. The nurse tests proposed hypotheses. Interventions are designed based on the conservation principles: conservation of energy, structural integrity, person integrity, and social integrity. Interventions are not imposed but are determined to be mutually acceptable. The expectation is that this approach will maintain wholeness and promote adaptation.
Evaluation	Observation of organismic response to interventions.
	The outcome of hypothesis testing is evaluated by assessing for organismic response that means the hypotheses are supported or not supported. Consequences of care are either therapeutic or supportive: therapeutic measures improve the sense of well-being; supportive measures provide comfort when the downward course of illness cannot be influenced. If the hypotheses are not supported, the plan is revised and new hypotheses are proposed.

*The novice nurse may use the conservation principles at this point to assist with the organization of the provocative facts. The expert nurse integrates this into the environmental assessments.

**Trophicognosis is a nursing care judgment arrived at through the use of the scientific process (Levine, 1965). The scientific process is used to make observations and select relevant data to form hypothetical statements about the patients' predicaments (Schaefer, 1991a).

Source: "Levine's Nursing Process Using Critical Thinking." In M. R. Alligood & A. Marriner-Tomey (Eds.). (1997). *Nursing theory: Utilization and application.* St. Louis: Mosby. Revised and used with permission of Mosby.

2 Human beings respond in a singular yet integrated fashion.

3 Each individual responds wholly and completely to every alteration in his or her life pattern.

4 Individuals cannot be understood out of the context of their environment.

5 "Ultimately, decisions for nursing care are based on the unique behavior of the individual patient. . . . A theory of nursing must recognize the importance of unique detail of care for a single patient within an empiric framework which successfully describes the requirements of all patients" (Levine, 1973, p. 6).

6 "Patient-centered care means individualized nursing care. It is predicated on the reality of common experience: every man is a unique individual, and as such requires a unique constellation of skills, techniques, and ideas designed specially for him" (Levine, 1973, p. 23).

7 "Every self-sustaining system monitors its own behavior by conserving the use of resources required to define its unique identity" (Levine, 1991, p. 4).

8 The nurse is responsible for recognizing the state of altered health and the patient's organismic response to altered health.

9 Nursing is a unique contributor to patient care (Levine, 1988a).

10 The patient is in an altered state of health (Levine, 1973). A patient is one who seeks health care because of a desire to remain healthy or one who identifies a known or possible risk behavior.

11 A guardian-angel activity assumes that the nurse accepts responsibility and shows concern based on knowledge that makes it possible to decide on the patient's behalf and in his [or her] best interest (Levine, 1973).

Values

1 All nursing actions are moral actions.

2 Two moral imperatives are the sanctity of life and the relief of suffering.

3 Ethical behavior "is the day-to-day expression of one's commitment to other persons and the ways in which human beings relate to one another in their daily interactions" (Levine, 1977, p. 846).

4 A fully informed individual should make decisions regarding life and death in advance of the situations. These decisions are not the role of the health-care providers or families (Levine, 1989b).

5 Judgments by nurses or doctors about quality of life are inappropriate and should not be used as a basis for the allocation of care (Levine, 1989b).

6 "Persons who require the intensive interventions of critical care units enter with a contract of trust. To respect trust . . . is a moral responsibility" (Levine, 1988b, p. 88).

PART TWO

Applications

The model's universality is supported by the model's use in a variety of situations and patients' conditions across the life span. A growing body of research is providing support for the development of scientific knowledge related to the model.

USE OF THE CONSERVATION MODEL IN PRACTICE

The model has been used to guide patient care in settings such as critical care (Brunner, 1985; Langer, 1990; Littrell & Schumann, 1989; Lynn-McHale & Smith, 1991; Tribotti, 1990), acute care (Foreman, 1989, 1991, 1996; Molchany, 1992; Schaefer, 1991a; Schaefer & Shober-Potylycki, 1993; Schaefer, Swavely, Rothenberger, Hess, & Willistin, 1996), emergency room (Pond & Taney, 1991), primary care (Pond, 1991), in the operating room (Crawford-Gamble, 1986), long-term/extended care (Cox, 1991), homeless (Pond, 1991), and in the community (Dow & Mest, 1997; Pond, 1991).

This model has been used with a variety of patients across the life span, including the neonate (Mefford, 1999; Tribotti, 1990), infant (Newport, 1984; Savage & Culbert, 1989), young child (Dever, 1991), pregnant woman (Roberts, Fleming, & (Yeates) Giese, 1991), young adult (Pasco & Halupa,

1991), long-term ventilator patient (Higgins, 1998; Delmore, 2003), and older adult and elderly patients (Cox, 1991; Foreman, 1991, 1996; Hirschfeld, 1976), including the frail elderly patient (Happ, personal communication, January 31, 1995; Roberts, Brittin, Cook, & deClifford, 1994).

The model has been used as a framework for wound care (Cooper, 1990), managing respiratory illness (Dow & Mest, 1997; Roberts, Brittin, Cook, & deClifford, 1994), managing sleep in the patient with a myocardial infarction (Littrell & Schumann, 1989), developing nursing diagnoses (MacLean, 1989; Taylor, 1989), practicing enterostomal therapy (Neswick, 1997), assessing for changes in bladder function in posthysterectomy women (O'Laughlin, 1986). It has also been used for developing plans of care for women with chronic illness (Schaefer, 2002), care of intravenous sites (Dibble, Bostrom-Ezrati, & Rizzuto, 1991), skin care (Burd et al., 1994), developing day room admission (Clark, Fraaza, Schroeder, & Maddens, 1995), and care of patients undergoing treatment for cancer (Webb, 1993), and as an approach to the assessment and design of interventions to support staff nurses through change (Jost, 2000). Universities and colleges are considering continued and new use of the model as the framework for undergraduate (Grindley & Paradowski, 1991) and graduate programs (Schaefer, 1991b).

Current work on the model is in process in the areas of community health. The following is a brief summary of beginning clarification of the model's use in community-based care.

Modified for Use in Community-Based Care

The principles of community health nursing that are fundamental to community-based care can be practiced in any setting. This discussion focuses on community-based care using Levine's Conservation Model to provide a foundation for the future of nursing practice and to dispel the myth that the model is inappropriate for the community.

The focus of health in the community is based on the assumption that community-based care is often informed by the one-on-one care provided to individuals. Using Levine's Conservation Model, community was initially defined as "a group of people living together within a larger society, sharing common characteristics, interests, and location"

(*National League for Nursing Self Study Report,* 1978). Clark (1992) provides examples of the use of the conservation principles with the individual, family, and community as a testament to the model's flexibility/universality.

The approach to community begins with the collection of facts and a thorough community assessment (provocative facts). The internal environment assessment directs the nurse to examine the patterns of health and disease among the people of the community and their use of programs available to promote a healthy community. The assessment of the external environment directs the nurse to examine the perceptual, operational, and conceptual levels of the environment in which the people live. The perceptual environment incorporates those factors that are processed by the senses. On a community basis these factors might include an assessment of:

1. how the media affects the health of the people;
2. how the quality of the air influences health patterns and housing development;
3. the availability of nutritious and affordable foods throughout the community;
4. noise pollution; and
5. relationships among the community's subcultures.

The operational environment would encourage a more detailed assessment of the factors in the environment that affect the individual's health but are not perceived by the people. These might include surveillance of communicable diseases, assessment for the use of toxins in industry, disposal of waste products, consideration for exposure to radiation from electrical lines, and examination of buildings for asbestos, lead, and radon.

The conceptual environment focuses the assessment on the ethnic and cultural patterns in the community. An assessment of types of houses of worship and health-care settings might be included. In this area, the effect of the communities external to the one being assessed would be addressed in order to determine factors that may influence the function of the target community.

The novice nurse will benefit from using the conservation principles to guide continued assessment to assure a thorough understanding of the community. When considering energy conservation, areas to assess might include:

1. Hours of employment
2. Water supply
3. Community budget
4. Food sources

An assessment of structural integrity might include:

1. City planning
2. Availability of resources
3. Transportation
4. Traffic patterns
5. Public services

Assessment of personal integrity might include:

1. Community identity
2. Mission of the government
3. Political environment

Assessment of the social integrity might include:

1. Recreation
2. Social services
3. Opportunities for employment

See Table 9–2, Levine's Conservation Model—Nursing Process in the Community

USE OF THE CONSERVATION MODEL IN RESEARCH

"Nurses are constantly testing what they propose will work in their practice based on what they know" (Schaefer, 1991a, p. 45). This continuous testing expands what is known about practice and offers new insights to improve the practice of nursing. Levine (1973) maintained that research is critical to the development of a scientifically sound body of knowledge for nursing. She felt that the conservation principles offer an approach to nursing that is scientific, research oriented, and universal in practice. She said that research should focus on the maintenance of wholeness and the interaction between the internal and external environments of the individuals (Levine, 1978). For the purpose of discovery, and contrary to the notion of

Table 9–2	**Levine's Conservation Model—Nursing Process in the Community**
Process	**Application of the Process**
Assessment	Collection of provocative facts through observation and interview.
	The nurse uses observation, review of census data, statistics, data from community member interviews, and so on to collect provocative facts about the community. Use of windshield assessments or other formally developed community assessments are helpful in the collection of data.
Trophicognosis	Community diagnosis.
	The nurse organizes that data in such a way as to provide meaning. A judgment or trophicognosis is made.
Hypotheses	Directs the nurse to provide interventions that will promote adaptation and maintain wholeness of the community.
	In discussion with the community members, the nurse validates her judgments about the community's predicament. The nurse then proposes hypotheses about the problems and solutions, such as: Providing shelter to abused women will reduce the morbidity associated with continuous uninterrupted abuse.
Interventions	Test the hypotheses.
	Nurses use the hypotheses to direct the plan of care for the community. The nurse tests the proposed hypotheses to try to remedy the predicament. The nurses select the most appropriate solutions with the help of the community members. Interventions are based on the conservation principles of energy, structural integrity, personal integrity, and social integrity. The shelter for abused women provides for structural integrity of the community while preserving the energy, personal, and social integrity of the women who choose shelter.
Evaluation	Observation of organismic response to interventions.
	The outcome of hypothesis testing is evaluated by assessing for organismic response. For example, an expected outcome of shelters for abused women might be a reduction in emergency room visits for injury resulting from suspected abuse or an increase in the number of women who are able to remove themselves from an abusive relationship.

wholeness, Levine supported the testing of variables that represent a single integrity. For example, Lane and Winslow (1987) focused on energy conservation, whereas Roberts, Fleming, and (Yeates) Giese (1991) focused on energy conservation and structural integrity. To be true to the model, investigators can explain their findings within the framework and consider how the findings support the goal of promoting adaptation and maintaining wholeness.

Because the model supports understanding and description, both qualitative and quantitative approaches are appropriate to develop the model and theories derived from the model. The qualitative approach helps to explain how the patient experiences the challenges to their internal and external environments. The quantitative approach helps to test the relationships between the variables, and, in some cases, provides for the testing of causal models. These predictive models help clinicians alter the environments to promote adaptation and maintain wholeness.

Combining qualitative and quantitative (mixed methods) approaches to the study concepts using Levine's model helps to preserve the art and the science of nursing. Interactions with patients are both predictive and creative. Qualitative research helps to provide a way for the nurses to repeatedly share the creative aspects of their work. Qualitative data helps to explain the quantitative data and provides a more holistic perspective regarding the data experience.

Several investigators have contributed significant research to the support and expansion of the Conservation Model as a model for nursing practice. Theories developed from the model will provide propositions from which hypotheses can be developed and tested. Following is a summary of several of the conclusions of research using the Conservation Model as a framework.

1. Responding to involuntary urges was as efficient as, and resulted in less perineal damage than, sustained breath holding during the second stage of labor (Yeates & Roberts, 1984). There were no differences in the mean duration of the second stage of labor between the two groups.

2. Interventions that are employed as a course of routine rather than based on individual needs actually increase the physiological burden of healing following birth and act as a significant threat to the psychological adjustments of the postpartum period (Fleming, 1988).

3. Conservation of energy can be maintained by placing the infant skin to skin on the mother's chest, covered with a warm blanket (Newport, 1984).

4. Ludington (1990) found that simple skin-to-skin contact was effective in reducing activity and state-related energy expenditure in the newborn of 34 to 36 weeks' gestation.

5. There is no significant difference in energy expenditure between basin, tub, or shower bathing 5 to 17 days postmyocardial infarction (Winslow, Lane, & Gaffney, 1985). The differences that did exist were related more to subject variability than the type of bathing. The experimental group had significantly lower oxygen consumption than did the control group.

6. Age, arterial pressure on bypass, and body temperature on the first and third postoperative days best predicts delirious patients (Foreman, 1989). Acutely confused patients were differentiated best from those not confused by 10 variables representing all four conservation principles.

7. Higgens (1998) found that fatigue was present in ventilator patients 100 percent of the time and that fatigue and depression were significantly correlated. Despite the fact that sleep disturbances were present and nutrition was compromised, there were no significant relationships with fatigue.

8. Schaefer's (1991b; Schaefer & Shober-Potylcki, 1993) research supports the finding that the experience of fatigue in congestive heart failure is an experience that affects one's whole sense of being.

9. Mefford (1999) developed a theory of health promotion for preterm infants derived from Levine's Conservation Model. She examined the relationship of nursing caregiving to health outcomes of infants. Although the proposed models were not supported, findings revealed that an increase in the level of consistency of nursing caregiving decreased the age at which health was achieved, and an increase in the level of consistency in nursing caregiving also reduced resource utilization.

Winslow (personal communication, October 14, 1993) indicated that an important outcome of her studies of bathing and toileting was that hospitalized patients had a significantly lower oxygen consumption during these activities than did healthy subjects. Patients moved more slowly and deliberately than did the healthy subjects. Consistent with Levine's (1973, p. 7) notion that we "reduce activity to that which is absolutely necessary," patients seem to reduce activity on their own to promote healing. Levine (1989) later stated that:

> The conservation of energy is clearly evident in the very sick, whose lethargy, withdrawal, and self-concern are manifested while, in its wisdom, the body is spending its energy resource on the processes of healing. (p. 332)

Many of the studies using the Conservation Model as the basis for the investigation are single studies or are the beginnings of research program development. There is no replication and little consistency in how the variables are measured. The results of the studies are therefore not sufficient to change nursing practice but they do cluster in two areas that, with continued study, could have a major influence on how nurses practice.

In general, the studies support that energy can be conserved with nursing interventions and can be measured through the assessment of organismic responses. Patients inherently conserve their own energy when confronted with environmental challenges. The second important finding is that attention to the conservation principles explains the organismic response of confusion (delirium) better than does any single principle alone. This supports the assumption that using the conservation principles to guide interventions will promote adaptation and maintain wholeness.

Investigators are encouraged to continue their excellent work with Levine's model. New investigators are encouraged to consider the Conservation Model as a basis for study and to test the propositions developed from the theories discussed later in this chapter. It is only with continued research that a scientific basis for nursing will be developed.

USE OF THE CONSERVATION MODEL IN THE TWENTY-FIRST CENTURY

Nurses of the future will continue to build on the basic principles of nursing established by Florence Nightingale (1859). Nightingale was a visionary woman who knew that nurses should be prepared professionals in institutions of higher education. Levine continued in this tradition and focused a great deal of her professional career on preparing advanced practice nurses as clinical nurse specialists. Levine's Conservation Model and the theories developed from the model provide a basis for the future of professional nursing. The model includes a method for assessment; identification of problems; development of a hypothesis about the problem; the identification, selection, and application of an intervention; and an evaluation of the response. The interventions are provided based on the assumption that if the intervention attends to the conservation of energy, structural, personal and social integrities, the patient will return to wholeness (health). Health is a goal for individuals, families, communities, and populations at large. From a global perspective, "health for all" is an appropriate metaphor. Wholeness is universally understood. The model includes three major concepts that are critical to understanding the health-care delivery systems of the future: adaptation, wholism (health), and conservation (balance of energy supply and demand within the capabilities of the patient [organization, community, and universe]).

> *The model includes three major concepts that are critical to understanding the health-care delivery systems of the future: adaptation, wholism (health), and conservation (balance of energy supply and demand within the capabilities of the patient [organization, community, and universe]).*

The Conservation Model provides the conceptual basis for the development of three theories: the theory of conservation, the theory of redundancy, and the theory of therapeutic intention.

About theory, Levine said:

1. "The serious study of any discipline requires a theoretical baseline which gives it substance and meaning" (1969a, p. xi).
2. "The essential science concepts develop the rationale [for nursing actions], using ideas from all areas of knowledge that contribute to the development of the nursing process in the specific area of the model" (cited in Fawcett, 1995, p. 136).

3. Nursing theory should define the boundaries of nursing.

4. "Nursing theory is too important an enterprise to be undertaken without the strictest rules of scientific discovery and explanation.... It is the researcher who should challenge the cherished ideas and find the data that will support or refute the theorist's claims. The practitioner must provide the ultimate test of relevance to the theorist's work. Unless the theory can be interpreted by the nurse who reaches the patient wherever nursing is practiced, theory will remain a questionable entity ... theory should teach nurses what they are" (1988a, pp. 20–21).

5. It is essential that concepts that are shared from other disciplines are accurately reproduced and used appropriately (1996). The sharing of concepts from other disciplines has enhanced nursing scholarship and provided nurses with the knowledge and skills to provide holistic care.

6. "At every level where theory is taught ... the content of courses in nursing theory ought to excite what Brunner (1985) called the effective surprise, where the combination of recognition and discovery adds new dimensions to nursing practice" (1995, p. 12).

7. "[I]t is imperative that there be a variety [of nursing theories]—for there is no global theory of nursing that fits every situation" (1995, p. 13).

8. "Not everything that is accepted as theory now can—nor should—survive, but 'serious intellectual inquiry' will create new theories, and nursing can only prosper when it does" (1995, p. 14).

In summary, Levine proposed that nursing theory is an adjunctive science, that it provides for the development of the intellectual component of nursing essential for understanding the why of nursing actions, is tested through use by practitioners, is not universal in the sense that there is no one global theory of nursing that will fit all situations, and should be refined and further developed by new researchers. She noted that some theories might be time limited and new theories would be developed. Levine's work continues to encourage the intellectual pursuits of "her" students. We learn and grow as we continue to review and reinterpret her work in preparation for the future of nursing.

Alligood (1997) first made the Theory of Conservation explicit. The Theory of Conservation is rooted in the concept of conservation and is based on the assumption that all nursing actions are conservation principles (Levine, 1973). Conservation is natural law that is fundamental to many basic sciences. The purpose of conservation is "to keep together," which means "to maintain a proper balance between active nursing interventions coupled with patient participation on the one hand and the safe limits of the patients' abilities to participate on the other" (Levine, 1973, p. 13). The Theory of Conservation is based on the universal principle of conservation, which provides the foundation for the conservation principles in the model. Conservation assures wholeness, integrity, and unity.

The conservation principles form the major propositions (Levine, 1973, pp. 13, 444, and 446):

1. The individual is always within an environment milieu, and the consequences of his awareness of his environment persistently influence his behavior at any given moment.

2. The individual protects and defends himself within his environment by gaining all the information he can about it.

3. The nurse participates actively in every patient's environment, and much of what she does supports his adaptations as he struggles in the predicament of illness.

4. Even in the presence of disease, the organism responds wholly to the environment interaction in which it is involved, and a considerable element of nursing care is devoted to restoring the symmetry of response—symmetry that is essential to the well-being of the organism (Levine, 1969b, p. 98).

The Theory of Therapeutic Intention was developed to provide a way to organize nursing interventions out of the biological realities that nurses had to confront (Fawcett, 1995). The biological realities faced by nurses include areas of concern that focus on living organisms; their structure, form, function, behavior, growth, and development; and relationships to their environment and organisms like and unlike themselves. Given the biological realities of health, illness, and disease, nurses are organizing interventions across the life span, in a variety of settings, and based on the principles drawn from nursing and other disciplines (epidemiology, psychology, sociology, theology, etc.). The Theory of Therapeutic Intention is directly related to the biological realities. Therefore, the guiding assumptions for this theory are:

1. Conservation is the outcome of adaptation.
2. Change associated with therapeutic intervention results in adaptation.
3. The proper application of conservation (conservation principles) results in the restoration of health.
4. Activities directed toward the preservation of health include health promotion, surveillance, illness prevention, and follow-up activities.

According to Fawcett (2000), Levine identified the following goals of the theory of therapeutic intention:

1. Support the integrated healing and optimal restoration of structure and function [by supporting and enhancing] the natural response to disease. This goal can be reached if the nurse caring for a patient with burns changes dressing as ordered, provides medication to reduce the pain associated with treatment, offers complementary pain-reducing techniques, listens carefully to the concerns the patient may have regarding self related to scarring from the burns, refers to appropriate counseling, and works closely with the family or support persons to maintain connections for the patient.
2. Provide support for a failing autoregulatory portion of the integrated system (e.g., medical/surgical treatments).
3. Restore individual integrity and well-being (e.g., work with children with ADHD—attention deficit hyperactivity disorder).
4. Provide supportive measures to assure comfort and promote human concern when therapeutic measures are not possible (e.g., care of the dying).
5. Balance a toxic risk against the threat of disease (e.g., nurses who facilitate immunization).
6. Manipulate diet and activity to correct metabolic imbalances and to stimulate physiological processes (e.g., care of the anorexic young woman).
7. Reinforce or antagonize usual response to create a therapeutic change (e.g., enhance pain relief with music therapy).

The expected outcome of therapeutic intentions would be a therapeutic response measured by the organismic change (e.g., adaptation resulting in conservation).

The theory of redundancy is grounded in the concept of adaptation. Change is the process of adaptation and conservation is the outcome of adaptation. The theory of redundancy assumes that there are fail-safe options available in the physiological, anatomical, and psychological responses of individuals who are employed in the development of patient care. The body has more than one way for its function to be accomplished. It involves a series of adaptive responses (cascade of integrated responses—simultaneous, not separate) available when the stability of the organism is challenged (Schaefer, 1991b). The selection of an option rests with the knowledge of the health-care provider in consultation with the patient. When redundant choices are lost, survival becomes difficult and ultimately fails for lack of fail-safe options—either those that the patient possesses (e.g., two lungs) or those that can be employed on his or her behalf (e.g., medications or a pacemaker) (Levine, 1991).

SUMMARY

Levine's notion of the environment as complex provides an excellent basis for continuing to develop an improved understanding of the environment. Studying the interactions between the external and the internal environment will provide for a better understanding of adaptation. This focus will provide for additional information about the challenges in the external environment and how they change over time. It is important that we understand the changes that occur and how the person who adapted before now changes the adaptive response in order to maintain balance or integrity. This adaptive response will inform the organismic response. With an improved repertoire of organismic responses, we can test how to predict these responses, hence assure that the responses that are adaptive will occur. This is said with the understanding that nurses recognize when the goal is to maintain comfort only (e.g., supportive interventions).

Moving to a more global perspective, the environment as defined according to Levine

(1973) provides nurses with the opportunity to enhance their understanding of it and to provide interventions for communities that suffer from environmental disasters. An assessment of the internal environment's response to the challenge of the external environment (e.g., destruction from hurricanes) will immediately identify the altered health status of the community and the community needs. An assessment of the external environment will provide an understanding of the changes occurring due to the assault on the internal environment and a more detailed assessment of the perceptive, organismic, and conceptual levels of the environmental challenges. There is no question that this approach to describing, defining, and planning for environmental challenges will identify (1) the perceptual challenges, (2) the organismic challenges that may not be immediately known to the residents (e.g., pollution of air and water), and (3) the conceptual issues that increase the nurses' awareness of the social, political, and economic impact on the predicament. This provides the nurses with the opportunity to develop a political agenda and perhaps design public policy that might improve interventions in the context of a disaster. The Conservation Model has the components needed to provide nurses with a global perspective of the environment.

The practice of nurses and advanced practice nurses is changing rapidly to keep up with the current speed of health-care system changes. Levine's Conservation Model provides an approach that educates good nurses and provides a foundation for their practice, whatever the role or the setting. Nurse practitioners, case managers, program planners, nurse midwives, nurse anesthetists, and nurse entrepreneurs are encouraged to test the model as a basis for improving and guiding their practice. Whatever the results, they should publish them to assure the continued development of the art and science of nursing. Levine will applaud their efforts.

Theory is the poetry of science. The poet's words are familiar, each standing alone, but brought together they sing, they astonish, they teach. The theorist offers a fresh vision, familiar concepts brought together in bold, new designs. . . . The theorist and poet seek excitement in the sudden insights that make ordinary experience extraordinary, but theory caught in the intellectual exercises of the academy becomes alive only when it is made a true instrument of persuasion. (Levine, 1995, p. 14)

References

Alligood, M. R. (1997). Models and theories: Critical thinking structures. In Alligood, M. R., & Marriner-Tomey, A. (Eds.), *Nursing theory: Utilization and application* (pp. 31–45). St. Louis: Mosby.

Barnum, B. J. S. (1994). *Nursing theory: Analysis, application, evaluation* (4th ed.). Philadelphia: J. B. Lippincott.

Bates, M. (1967). A naturalist at large. *Natural History, 76,* 8–16.

Beland, I. (1971). *Clinical nursing: Pathophysiological and psychological implications* (2nd ed.). New York: Dover.

Bernard, C. (1957). *An introduction to the study of experimental medicine.* New York: Dover.

Bruner, J. (1979). *On knowing: Essays for the left hand.* New York: Argenaemun.

Brunner, M. (1985). A conceptual approach to critical care nursing using Levine's model. *Focus on Critical Care, 12*(2), 39–44.

Burd, C., Olson, B., Langemo, D., Hunter, S., Hanson, D., Osowki, K. F., & Sauvage, T. (1994). Skin care strategies in a skilled nursing home. *Journal of Gerontological Nursing, 20*(11), 28–34.

Clark, L. R., Fraaza, V., Schroeder, S., & Maddens, M. E. (1995). Alternative nursing environments: Do they affect hospital outcomes? *Journal of Gerontological Nursing, 21*(11), 32–38.

Clark, M. J. (1992). *Nursing in the community.* Norwalk, CT: Appleton & Lange.

Cooper, D. H. (1990). Optimizing wound healing: A practice within nursing's domain. *Nursing Clinics of North America, 25*(1), 165–180.

Cox, R. A. Sr. (1991). A tradition of caring: Use of Levine's model in long-term care. In Schaefer, K. M., & Pond, J. B. (Eds.), *The conservation model: A framework for nursing practice* (pp. 179–197). Philadelphia: F. A. Davis.

Crawford-Gamble, P. E. (1986). An application of Levine's conceptual model. *Perioperative Nursing Quarterly, 2*(1), 64–70.

Deiriggi, P. M., & Miles, K. E. (1995). The effects of waterbeds on heart rate in preterm infants . . . including a commentary by White-Traut, R. C. *Scholarly Inquiry for Nursing Practice, 9*(3), 245–262.

Delmore, B. A. (2003). Fatigue and prealbumin levels during the weaning process in long-term ventilated patients (Doctoral dissertation, New York University, 2003). *Dissertation Abstracts International,* 64-05B, 2127.

Dever, M. (1991). Care of children. In Schaefer, K. M., & Pond, J. B. (Eds.), *The conservation model: A framework for nursing practice* (pp. 71–83). Philadelphia: F. A. Davis.

Dibble, S. L., Bostrom-Ezerati, J., & Ruzzuto, C. (1991). Clinical predictors of intravenous site symptoms. *Research in Nursing & Health, 14*, 413–420.

Dow, J. S., & Mest, C. G. (1997). Psychosocial interventions for patients with chronic obstructive pulmonary disease. *Home-Healthcare-Nurse, 15*(6), 414–420.

Dubos, R. (1965). *Man adapting.* New Haven: Yale University Press.

Erickson, E. H. (1964). *Insight and responsibility.* New York: W. W. Norton & Co.

Fawcett, J. (1995) *Conceptual models of nursing* (3rd ed.). Philadelphia: F. A. Davis.

Fawcett, J. (2000). *Analysis and evaluation of contemporary nursing knowledge: Nursing models and theories.* Philadelphia: F. A. Davis.

Feynman, R. (1965). *The character of physical law.* Cambridge, MA: MIT Press.

Fleming, N. (1988). Comparison of women with different perineal conditions after childbirth. *Dissertation Abstracts International, 48*, 2924B. Microfilm No. 8728762.

Foreman, M. D. (1989). Confusion in the hospitalized elderly: Incidence, onset, and associated factors. *Research in Nursing & Health, 12*(1), 21–29.

Foreman, M. D. (1991). Conserving cognitive integrity of the hospitalized elderly. In Schaefer, K. M., & Pond, J. B. (Eds.), *The conservation model: A framework for nursing practice* (pp. 133–150). Philadelphia: F. A. Davis.

Foreman, M. D. (1996). *The evolution of delirium.* Abstract. Midwest Nursing Research Society. Kansas City, MO.

Gibson, J. E. (1966). *The senses considered as perceptual systems.* Boston: Houghton Mifflin.

Goldstein, K. (1963). *The organism.* Boston: Beacon Press.

Grindley, J., & Paradowski, M. B. (1991). Developing an undergraduate program using Levine's model. In Schaefer, K. M., & Pond, J. B. (Eds.), *The conservation model: A framework for nursing practice* (pp. 199–208). Philadelphia: F. A. Davis.

Hall, E. (1966). *The hidden dimension.* Garden City, NY: Doubleday.

Happ, M. B., Williams, C. C., Strumpf, N. E., & Burger, S. G. (1996). Individualized care for frail elderly: *Theory and Practice, Journal of Gerontological Nursing, 22*(3), 7–14.

Higgins, P. A. (1998). Patients' perception of fatigue while undergoing long-term mechanical ventilation: Incidence and associated factors. *Heart and Lung: Journal of Acute and Critical Care, 27*(3), 177–183.

Hirschfeld, M. H. (1976). The cognitively impaired older adult. *American Journal of Nursing, 76*, 1981–1984.

Jost, S. G. (2000). An assessment and intervention strategy for managing staff needs during change. *Journal of Nursing Administration, 30*(1), 34–40.

Lane, L. D., & Winslow, E. H. (1987). Oxygen consumption, cardiovascular response, and perceived exertion in healthy adults during rest, occupied bedmaking, and unoccupied bedmaking activity. *Cardiovascular Nursing, 23*(6), 31–36.

Langer, V. S. (1990). Minimal handling protocol for the intensive care nursery. *Neonatal Network, 9*(3), 23–27.

Levine, M. E. (1965). Trophicognosis: An alternative to nursing diagnosis. *ANA Regional Clinical Conferences, 2*, 55–70.

Levine, M. E. (1966). Adaptation and assessment: A rationale for nursing intervention. *American Journal of Nursing, 66*, 2450–2453.

Levine, M. E. (1967). The four conservation principles of nursing. *Nursing Forum, 6*, 45–59.

Levine, M. E. (1968a). Knock before entering personal space bubbles (Part I). *Chart, 65*(1), 58–62.

Levine, M. E. (1968b). Knock before entering personal space bubbles (Part II). *Chart, 65*(2), 82–84.

Levine, M. E. (1969a). *Introduction to clinical nursing.* Philadelphia: F. A. Davis.

Levine, M. E. (1969b). The pursuit of wholeness. *American Journal of Nursing, 69*, 93–98.

Levine, M. E. (1971). Holistic nursing. *Nursing Clinics of North America, 6*(2), 253–263.

Levine, M. E. (1973). *Introduction to clinical nursing* (2nd ed.). Philadelphia: F. A. Davis.

Levine, M. E. (1977). Nursing ethics and the ethical nurse. *American Journal of Nursing, 77*(5), 845–849.

Levine, M. E. (1978). Cancer chemotherapy: A nursing model. *Nursing Clinics of North America, 13*(2), 271–280.

Levine, M. E. (1982a). Bioethics of cancer nursing. *Rehabilitation Nursing, 7*, 27–31, 41.

Levine, M. E. (1982b). The bioethics of cancer nursing. *Journal of Enterostomal Therapy, 9*, 11–13.

Levine, M. E. (1988a). Antecedents from adjunctive disciplines: Creation of nursing theory. *Nursing Science Quarterly, 1*(1), 16–21.

Levine, M. E. (1988b). Myra Levine. In Schoor, T. M., & Zimmerman, A. (Eds.), *Making choices, taking chances: Nurse leaders tell their stories* (pp. 215–228). St. Louis: C. V. Mosby.

Levine, M. E. (1989a). The conservation model: Twenty years later. In Riehl-Sisca, J. P. (Ed.), *Conceptual models for nursing practice* (pp. 325–337). Norwalk, CT: Appleton & Lange.

Levine, M. E. (1989b). Ration or rescue: The elderly in critical care. *Critical Care Nursing, 12*(1), 82–89.

Levine, M. E. (1989c). The ethics of nursing rhetoric. *Image: Journal of Nursing Scholarship, 21*(1), 4–5.

Levine, M. E. (1989d). Beyond dilemma. *Seminars in Oncology Nursing, 5*, 124–128.

Levine, M. E. (1991). The conservation model: A model for health. In Schaefer, K. M., & Pond, J. B. (Eds.), *The conservation model: A framework for nursing practice* (pp. 1–11). Philadelphia: F. A. Davis.

Levine, M. E. (1992). Nightingale redux. In Barnum, B. S. (Ed.), *Nightingale's notes on nursing.* Philadelphia: J. B. Lippincott.

Levine, M. E. (1995). The rhetoric of nursing theory. *Image: Journal of Nursing Scholarship, 27*(2), 11–14.

Levine, M. E. (1996). The conservation principles: A retrospective. *Nursing Science Quarterly, 9*(1), 38–41.

Littrell, K., & Schumann, L. (1989). Promoting sleep for the patient with a myocardial infarction. *Critical Care Nurse, 9*(3), 44–49.

Ludington, S. M. (1990). Energy conservation during skin-to-skin contact between premature infants and their mothers. *Heart & Lung, 19*(5), 445–451.

Lynn-McHale, D. J., & Smith, A. (1991). Comprehensive assessment of families of the critically ill. In Leske, J. S. (Ed.), *AACN clinical issues in critical care nursing* (pp. 195–209). Philadelphia: J. B. Lippincott.

MacLean, S. L. (1989). Activity intolerance: Cues for diagnosis. In Carroll-Johnson, R. M. (Ed.), *Classification proceedings of the Eighth Annual Conference of North American Nursing*

Diagnosis Association (pp. 320–327). Philadelphia: J. B. Lippincott.

Mid-Year Convocation: Loyola University, Chicago. The Conferring of Honorary Degrees by R. C. Baumhart. Candidate for the degree of Doctor of Humane Letters, 1992, p. 6.

Molchany, C. A. (1992). Ventricular septal and free wall rupture complicating acute MI. *Journal of Cardiovascular Nursing, 6*(4), 38–45.

National League for Nursing Self Study Report. (1978). Allentown College of St. Francis de Sales, Department of Nursing.

Neswick, R. S. (1997). Myra E. Levine: A theoretical basis for ET nursing. *Professional Practice, 24*(1), 6–9.

Newport, M. A. (1984). Conserving thermal energy and social integrity in the newborn. *Western Journal of Nursing Research, 6*(2), 175–197.

Nightingale, F. (1859). *Notes on nursing: What it is, and what it is not.* London: Harrison & Sons.

O'Laughlin, K. M. (1986). Change in bladder function in the woman undergoing radical hysterectomy for cervical cancer. *Journal of Obstetric, Gynecologic and Neonatal Nursing, 15*(5), 380–385.

Pasco, A., & Halupa, D. (1991). Chronic pain management. In Schaefer, K. M., & Pond, J. B. (Eds.), *The conservation model: A framework for nursing practice* (pp. 101–117). Philadelphia: F. A. Davis.

Pond, J. B. (1991). Ambulatory care of the homeless. In Schaefer, K. M., & Pond, J. B. (Eds.), *The conservation model: A framework for nursing practice* (pp. 167–178). Philadelphia: F. A. Davis.

Pond, J. B., & Taney, S. G. (1991). Emergency care in a large university emergency department. In Schaefer, K. M., & Pond, J. B. (Eds.), *The conservation model: A framework for nursing practice* (pp. 151–166). Philadelphia: F. A. Davis.

Roberts, J. E., Fleming, N., & (Yeates) Giese, D. (1991). Perineal integrity. In Schaefer, K. M., & Pond, J. B. (Eds.), *The conservation model: A framework for nursing practice* (pp. 61–70). Philadelphia: F. A. Davis.

Roberts, K. L., Brittin, M., Cook, M., & deClifford, J. (1994). Boomerang pillows and respiratory capacity. *Clinical Nursing Research, 3*(2), 157–165.

Roberts, K. L., Brittin, M., & deClifford, J. (1995). Boomerang pillows and respiratory capacity in frail elderly women. *Clinical Nursing Research, 4*(4), 465–471.

Savage, T. A., & Culbert, C. (1989). Early interventions: The unique role of nursing. *Journal of Pediatric Nursing, 4*(5), 339–345.

Schaefer, K. M. (1991a). Levine's conservation principles and research. In Schaefer, K. M., & Pond, J. B. (Eds.), *The conservation model: A framework for nursing practice* (pp. 45–59). Philadelphia: F. A. Davis.

Schaefer, K. M. (1991b). Care of the patient with congestive heart failure. In Schaefer, K. M., & Pond, J. B. (Eds.), *The conservation model: A framework for nursing practice* (pp. 119–132). Philadelphia: F. A. Davis.

Schaefer, K. M. (2002). Levine's conservation model in practice. In Alligood, M. R., & Marriner-Tomey, A. (Eds.), *Nursing theory: Utilization and application* (pp. 197–217). St. Louis: Mosby.

Schaefer, K. M., & Pond, J. B. (1994). Levine's conservation model as a guide to nursing practice. *Nursing Science Quarterly, 7*(2), 53–54.

Schaefer, K. M., & Shober-Potylycki, M. J. (1993). Fatigue associated with congestive heart failure: Use of Levine's Conservation Model. *Journal of Advanced Nursing, 18,* 260–268.

Schaefer, K. M., Swavely, D., Rothenberger, C., Hess, S., & Willistin, D. (1996). Sleep disturbances post coronary artery bypass surgery. *Progress in Cardiovascular Nursing, 11*(1), 5–14.

Schaefer, K., Artigue, G., Foli, K., Johnson, T., Tomey, A., Poat, M., Poppa, L., Woeste, R., & Zoretich, S. (1998). Myra Estrin Levine: The Conservation Model. In Tomey, A. M., & Alligood, M. R. (Eds.), *Nursing theorists and their work* (4th ed., pp. 195–206). St. Louis: Mosby.

Selye, H. (1956). *The stress of life.* New York: McGraw-Hill.

Taylor, J. W. (1989). Levine's conservation principles: Using the model for nursing diagnosis in a neurological setting. In Riehl-Sisca, J. P. (Ed.), *Conceptual models for nursing practice* (3rd ed., pp. 349–358). Norwalk, CT: Appleton & Lange.

Tribotti, S. (1990). Admission to the neonatal intensive care unit: Reducing the risks. *Neonatal Network, 8*(4), 17–22.

Waddington, C. H. (Ed.). (1968). *Towards a theoretical biology: I. Prolegomena.* Chicago: Aldine.

Webb, H. (1993). Holistic care following palliative Hartmann's procedure. *British Journal of Nursing, 2*(2), 128–132.

Winslow, E. H., Lane, L. D., & Gaffney, F. A. (1985). Oxygen consumption and cardiovascular response in patients and normal adults during in-bed and out-of-bed toileting. *Journal of Cardiac Rehabilitation, 4,* 348–354.

Wolf, S. (1961). Disease as a way of life: Neural integration in systemic pathology. *Perspectives on Biological Medicine, 5,* 288–303.

Yeates, D. A., & Roberts, J. E. (1984). A comparison of two bearing-down techniques during the second stage of labor. *Journal of Nurse Midwifery, 29,* 3–11.

Bibliography

Bunting, S. M. (1988). The concept of perception in selected nursing theories. *Nursing Science Quarterly, 1*(4), 39–44.

Fawcett, J., Brophy, S. F., Rather, M. L., & Ross, J. (1997). Commentary about Levine's *On creativity in nursing. Image: Journal of Nursing Scholarship, 29*(3), 218–219.

Fawcett, J., Tulman, L., & Samarel, N. (1995). Enhancing function in life transitions and serious illness. *Advanced Practice Nursing, 1*(3), 50–57.

Flaskerud, J. H., & Halloran, E. J. (1980). Areas of agreement in nursing theory development. *Advances in Nursing Sciences, 3*(1), 1–17.

Frauman, A. C., & Rasch, R. T. R. (1995). Myra Levine, At last a clear voice of reason [Letter to the editor]. *Image: Journal of Nursing Scholarship, 27,* 262.

Griffith-Kenney, J. W., & Christensen, P. (1986). *Nursing process: Application of theories, frameworks, and models* (pp. 6, 24–25). St. Louis: Mosby.

Hall, K. V. (1979). Current trends in the use of conceptual frameworks in nursing education. *Journal of Nursing Education, 18*(4), 26–29.

Leonard, M. K. (1990). Myra Estrin Levine. In George, J. B. (Ed.), *Nursing theories: The base for professional nursing practice* (pp. 181–192). Englewood Cliffs, NJ: Prentice-Hall.

Levine, E. B., & Levine, M. E. (1965). Hippocrates, father of nursing, too? *American Journal of Nursing, 65*(12), 86–88.

Levine, M. E. (1963). Florence Nightingale: The legend that lives. *Nursing Forum, 2*(4), 24–35.

Levine, M. E. (1964a). Not to startle, though the way were deep. *Nursing Science, 3*(1), 58–67.

Levine, M. E. (1964b). There need be no anonymity. *First, 18*(9), 4.

Levine, M. E. (1965a). The professional nurse and graduate education. *Nursing Science, 3,* 206–214.

Levine, M. E. (1965b). Trophicognosis: An alternative to nursing diagnosis. *ANA Regional Clinical Conferences, 2,* 55–70.

Levine, M. E. (1967a). Medicine-nursing dialogue belongs at patient's bedside. *Chart, 64*(5), 136–137.

Levine, M. E. (1967b). This I believe about patient-centered care. *Nursing Outlook, 15,* 53–55.

Levine, M. E. (1967c). For lack of love alone. *Accent, 39*(7), 179–202.

Levine, M. E. (1968). The pharmacist in the clinical setting: A nurse's viewpoint. *American Journal of Hospital Pharmacy, 25*(4), 168–171.

Levine, M. E. (1969a). Nursing in the 21st century. *National Student Association.*

Levine, M. E. (1969b). Constructive student power. *Chart, 66*(2), 42FF.

Levine, M. E. (1969c). Small hospital—Big nursing (Part I). *Chart, 66,* 265–269.

Levine, M. E. (1969d). Small hospital—Big nursing (Part II). *Chart, 66,* 310–315.

Levine, M. E. (1970a). Dilemma. *ANA Clinical Conferences,* 338–342.

Levine, M. E. (1970b). Symposium on a drug compendium: View of a nursing educator. *Drug Information Bulletin,* 133–135.

Levine, M. E. (1970c). Breaking through the medications mystique. Published simultaneously in *American Journal of Nursing, 70*(4), 799–803; and *Amercian Journal of Hospital Pharmacy, 27*(4), 294–299.

Levine, M. E. (1971a). Consider the implications for nursing in the use of physician's assistant. *Hospital Topics, 49,* 60–63.

Levine, M. E. (1971b). The time has come to speak of health care. *AORN Journal, 13,* 37–43.

Levine, M. E. (1971c). *Renewal for nursing.* Philadelphia: F. A. Davis.

Levine, M. E. (1971d). Nursing grand rounds: Congestive heart failure. *Nursing '72, 2,* 18–23.

Levine, M. E. (1972a). Nursing educators—An alienating elite? *Chart, 69*(2), 56–61.

Levine, M. E. (1972b). Nursing grand rounds: Complicated care of CVA. *Nursing '72, 2*(3), 3–34.

Levine, M. E. (1972c). Nursing grand rounds: Insulin reactions in a brittle diabetic. *Nursing '72, 2*(5), 6–11.

Levine, M. E. (1972d). Issues in rehabilitation: The quadriplegic adolescent. *Nursing '72, 2,* 6.

Levine, M. E. (1972e). Nursing grand rounds: Severe trauma. *Nursing '72, 2*(9), 33–38.

Levine, M. E. (1972f). Benoni. *American Journal of Nursing, 12*(3), 466–468.

Levine, M. E. (1973a). A letter from Myra. *Chart, 70*(9). (Also in *Israel Nurses' Journal,* December 1973, in English and Hebrew.)

Levine, M. E. (1973b). On creativity in nursing. *Image: Journal of Nursing Scholarship, 3*(3), 15–19.

Levine, M. E. (1974). The pharmacist's clinical role in interdisciplinary care: A nurse's viewpoint. *Hospital Formulary Management, 9,* 47.

Levine, M. E. (1975). On creativity in nursing. *Nursing Digest, 3,* 38–40.

Levine, M. E. (1976). On the nursing ethic and the negative command. *Proceedings of the Intensive Conference, Faculty of the University of Illinois Medical Center.* Philadelphia, PA: Society for Health and Human Values.

Levine, M. E. (1977a). History of nursing in Illinois. *Proceedings of the Bicentennial Workshop of the University of Illinois College of Nursing.* Chicago, IL: University of Illinois Press.

Levine, M. E. (1977b). Primary nursing: Generalist and specialist education. *Proceedings of the American Academy of Nursing,* Kansas City, MO: American Nurses Association.

Levine, M. E. (1978a). Kapklvoo and nursing, too (editorial). *Research in Nursing and Health, 1*(2), 51.

Levine, M. E. (1978b). Does continuing education improve practice? *Hospitals, 52*(21), 138–140.

Levine, M. E. (1979). Knowledge base required by generalized and specialized nursing practice. *ANA Publication* (G–127), 57–69.

Levine, M. E. (1980). The ethics of computer technology in health care. *Nursing Forum, 19*(2), 193–198.

Levine, M. E. (1984a). A conceptual model for nursing: The four conservation principles. *Proceedings from Allentown College of St. Francis de Sales.*

Levine, M. E. (1984b). *Myra Levine.* Paper presented at the Nurse Theorist Conference, Edmonton, Alberta, Canada (cassette recording).

Levine, M. E. (1985a). What's right about rights? In Carmi, A., & Schneider, S. (Eds.), *Proceedings of the First International Congress of Nursing Law and Ethics.* Berlin: Springer Verlag.

Levine, M. E. (1985b). [Review of the book *Magic Bullets.*] *Oncology Nursing Forum, 12,* 101–102.

Levine, M. E. (1985c, August). *Myra Levine.* Paper presented at the conference on Nursing Theory in Action, Edmonton, Alberta, Canada (cassette recording).

Levine, M. E. (1988). What does the future hold for nursing? 25th Anniversary Address, 18th District. *Illinois Nurses Association Newsletter, XXIV*(6), 1–4.

Levine, M. E. (1990). Conservation and integrity. In Parker, M. (Ed.), *Nursing theories in practice* (pp. 189–201). New York: National League for Nursing.

Levine, M. E. (1994). Some further thought on nursing rhetoric. In Kilkuchi, J. F., & Simmons, H. (Eds.), *Developing a philosophy of nursing* (pp. 104–109). Thousand Oaks, CA: Sage.

Levine, M. E. (1995a). The rhetoric of nursing theory. *Image: Journal of Nursing Scholarship, 27*(1), 11–14.

Levine, M. E. (1995b). Myra Levine responds [letter to the editor]. *Image: Journal of Nursing Scholarship, 27,* Winter, 262.

Levine, M. E. (1996). On humanities in nursing. *Canadian Journal of Nursing Research, 27*(2), 19–23.

Martsolf, D. S., & Mickley, J. R. (1998). The concept of spirituality in nursing theories: Differing world-views and extent focus. *Journal of Advanced Nursing, 27,* 294–303.

Mefford, L. C. (1999). The relationship of nursing care to health outcomes of preterm infants: Testing a theory of health promotion for preterm infants based on Levine's Conservation Model of Nursing. (Doctoral dissertation, the University of Tennessee, 1999). Dissertation Abstracts International, 60–098, 4522.

Meleis, A. I. (1985). Myra Levine. In Meleis, A. I. (Ed.), *Theoretical nursing: Development and progress* (pp. 275–283). Philadelphia: F. A. Davis.

Newman, M. A. (1995). Margaret Newman and the rhetoric of nursing theory [letter to the editor]. *Image: Journal of Nursing Scholarship, 27,* 262–263.

The nursing theorists: Portraits of excellence: Myra Levine. (1988). Oakland: Studio III [videotape]. (Available from Fuld Video Project, 370 Hawthorne Avenue, Oakland, CA 94609.)

Peiper, B. A. (1983). Levine's nursing model. In Fitzpatrick, J. J., & Whall, A. L. (Eds.), *Conceptual models of nursing: Analysis and application* (pp. 101–115). New York: National League for Nursing.

Pond, J. B. (1990). Application of Levine's Conservation Model to nursing the homeless. In Parker, M. E. (Ed.), *Nursing theories in practice* (pp. 203–215). New York: National League for Nursing.

Pond, J. B. (1996). Nursing mourns the loss of two great leaders. *The Nursing Spectrum,* Greater Philadelphia/Tri-State edition, 5(8), May, 10–11.

Schaefer, K. M. (1991). Developing a graduate program in nursing: Integrating Levine's philosophy. In Schaefer, K. M., & Pond, J. B. (Eds.), *The conservation model: A framework for nursing practice* (pp. 209–218). Philadelphia: F. A. Davis.

Schaefer, K. M. (1996). Levine's Conservation Model: Caring for women with chronic illness. In Hinton, P. H., & Neuman, B. (Eds.), *Blueprint for use of nursing models: Education, research, practice, and administration* (pp. 187–227). New York: National League for Nursing.

Schaefer, K. M. (2002). Myra Estrin Levine: The conservation model. In Tomey, A. M., & Alligood, M. R. (Eds.), *Nursing theories and their work* (5th ed.) (pp. 212–225). St. Louis: Mosby.

Schaefer, K. M., & Pond, J. B. (1990). Effects of waterbed flotation on indicators of energy expenditure in preterm infants [letter to the editor]. *Nursing Research, 39*(5), 293.

Schaefer, K. M., & Pond, J. B. (Eds.). (1991). *The conservation model: A framework for nursing practice.* Philadelphia: F. A. Davis.

Servellen, G. M. V. (1982). The concept of individualized nursing practice. *Nursing & Health Care, 3,* 482–485.

Tompkins, E. S. (1980). Effect of restricted mobility and dominance on perceived duration. *Nursing Research, 29*(6), 333–338.

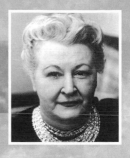

CHAPTER 10

Lydia Hall

Lydia Hall: The Care, Core, and Cure Model and Its Applications

Theris A. Touhy & Nettie Birnbach

Introducing the Theorist

In this chapter, we describe Lydia Hall and her conceptual model of nursing, her work at the Loeb Center for Nursing and Rehabilitation, the implications of her work for practice and research, and, finally, our views about how Hall might reflect on the future of nursing in the twenty-first century. The purpose of this chapter is to share the story of Lydia Hall's life and her contribution to professional nursing rather than to critique a nursing theory.

Visionary, risk taker, and consummate professional, Lydia Hall touched all who knew her in a special way. She inspired commitment and dedication through her unique conceptual framework for nursing practice that viewed professional nursing as the key to the care and rehabilitation of patients.

A 1927 graduate of the York Hospital School of Nursing in Pennsylvania, Hall held various nursing positions during the early years of her career. In the mid-1930s, she enrolled at Teachers College, Columbia University, where she earned a bachelor of science degree in 1937, and a master of arts degree in 1942. She worked with the Visiting Nurse Service of New York from 1941 to 1947 and was a member of the nursing faculty at Fordham Hospital School of Nursing from 1947 to 1950. Hall was subsequently appointed to a faculty position at Teachers College, where she developed and implemented a program in nursing consultation and joined a community of nurse leaders. At the same time, she was involved in research activities for the U.S. Health Service. Active in nursing's professional organizations, Hall also provided volunteer service to the New York City Board of Education, Youth Aid, and other community associations (Birnbach, 1988).

Hall's model, which she designed and put into place in the Loeb Center for Nursing and Rehabilitation at Montefiore Medical Center in New York, was her most significant contribution to nursing practice. Opened in 1963, the Loeb Center was the culmination of five years of planning and construction under Hall's direction. The circumstances that brought Hall and the Loeb Center together date back to 1947, when Dr. Martin Cherkasky was named director of the new hospital-based home care division of Montefiore Medical Center in Bronx, New York. At that time, Hall was employed by the Visiting Nurse Service at its Bronx office and had frequent contact with the Montefiore home care program. Hall and Cherkasky shared congruent philosophies regarding health care and the delivery of quality service, which served as the foundation for a long-standing professional relationship (Birnbach, 1988).

In 1950, Cherkasky was appointed director of the Montefiore Medical Center. During the early years of his tenure, existing traditional convalescent homes fell into disfavor. Convalescent treatment was undergoing rapid change due largely to medical advances, new pharmaceuticals, and technological discoveries. One of the homes that closed as a result of the emerging trends was the Solomon and Betty Loeb Memorial Home in Westchester County, New York. Cherkasky and Hall collaborated in convincing the board of the Loeb Home to join with Montefiore in founding the Loeb Center for Nursing and Rehabilitation. Using the proceeds from the sale of the Loeb Home, plans for the Loeb Center construction proceeded over a five-year period, from 1957 to 1962. Although the Loeb Center was, and still is, an integral part of the Montefiore physical complex, it was separately administered, with its own board of trustees that interrelated with the Montefiore board.

Under Hall's direction, nurses selected patients for the Loeb Center based on their potential for rehabilitation. Qualified professional nurses provided direct care to patients and coordinated needed services. Hall frequently described the center as "a halfway house on the road home" (Hall, 1963a, p. 2), where the nurse worked with the patients as active participants in achieving desired outcomes. Over time, the effectiveness of Hall's practice model was validated by the significant decline in the number of readmissions among former Loeb patients as compared with those who received other types of posthospital care ("Montefiore cuts," 1966).

In 1967, Hall received the Teachers College Nursing Alumni Award for distinguished achievement in nursing practice. She shared her innovative ideas about the nursing practice with numerous audiences around the country and contributed articles to nursing journals. In those articles, she referred to nurses using feminine pronouns. Because gender-neutral language was not yet an accepted style, and women comprised 96 percent of the nursing workforce, the feminine pronoun was used almost exclusively.

Hall died of heart disease on February 27, 1969, at Queens Hospital in New York. In 1984, she was inducted into the American Nurses' Association Hall of Fame. Following Hall's death, her legacy was kept alive at the Loeb Center until 1984, under the capable leadership of her friend and colleague Genrose Alfano.

Remembered by her colleagues for her passion for nursing, her flamboyant personality, and the excitement she generated, Hall was indeed a force for change. At a time when task-oriented team nursing was the preferred practice model in most institutions, she implemented a professional patient-centered framework whereby patients received a standard of care unequaled anywhere else. At the Loeb Center, Lydia Hall created an environment in which nurses were empowered, in which patients' needs were met through a continuum of care, and in which, according to Genrose Alfano, "nursing was raised to a high therapeutic level" (personal communication, January 27, 1999).

Historical Background

During the 1950s and 1960s, the health-care milieu in which Lydia Hall functioned was undergoing tremendous change. As previously stated, the type of nursing home model then in use failed to meet expectations, and care of the elderly was a growing problem. Increasing recognition that the elder population was in the greatest need of health-care insurance generated years of debate among legislators, the medical profession, and the public. Finally, in 1965, Medicare legislation was enacted that provided hospital, nursing home, and home care for those citizens age 65 and over. Medicaid was established to provide health-care services for the medically indigent, regardless of age. These programs provided a source of revenue for the nation's hospitals and, as public confidence in hospitals grew, there was concomitant growth in the need for more hospitals. Subsequent congressional legislation provided for construction of new facilities, which, in turn, created more opportunities for the employment of nurses. Undoubtedly, all of these factors were relevant to Hall as she proceeded to implement her vision.

With respect to nursing, the 1960s witnessed the growth of specialization, the movement toward preparation of nurse practitioners and clinical nurse specialists, and the emergence of new practice fields such as industrial nursing. Although most nurses worked in hospitals at that time, a beginning trend to community-based practice was evolving. In regard to nursing education, the advent of degree-granting, two-year programs in community colleges proved to be an attractive alternative to the apprenticeship model—hospital-based, diploma school education—through which most nurses had previously been prepared. And, with publication of the American Nurses' Association's position statement on educational preparation in 1965, baccalaureate education was receiving renewed recognition as the preferred method for preparing professional nurses. The correlation between higher education and professional practice seems to agree with Hall's ideas and probably elicited her support. Her model of nursing at the Loeb Center clearly required nurses to be educated, professional, and caring. Its success depended upon the ability of the nurses to relate to each patient with sensitivity and understanding. Hall was clear in her vision of the registered professional nurse as the appropriate person to fulfill that role.

Scholars and practitioners today continue to grapple with questions about how to define nursing and to demonstrate the unique contribution of professional nursing to the health and well-being of people. Lydia Hall's belief that the public deserves and can benefit from professional nursing care was articulated in her theory of nursing and was demonstrated in practice at the Loeb Center under her guidance. Hall stated:

> The program at the Loeb Center was designed to alleviate some of the growing problems which face our health-conscious public today: the complex and long-term nature of illnesses besetting all age groups; the high cost of services utilized in overcoming these illnesses; the negative reactions of the public and the health professions to patient care offered by institutions; and the confusion among all groups about the definition of nursing, its organization for service, and the kind of educational preparation it requires. (1963c, p. 805)

These questions and concerns are as relevant today as they were when Hall articulated her ideas over 30 years ago. Perhaps they are even more relevant now, as we face a rapidly increasing older population with needs for long-term care and an era of cost containment that often limits access to professional care and services.

Vision of Nursing

Lydia Hall would not have considered herself a nurse-theorist. She did not set out to develop a theory of nursing but rather to offer a view of professional nursing. Wiggins (1980, p. 10) reflected on the status of nursing theory during this time and stated: "[T]he excitement of the possibility of development by nurses of nursing theories was in its barest beginnings." Hall's observations of hospital care at the time led her to articulate her beliefs about the value of professional nursing to patient welfare. She observed that care was fragmented; patients often felt depersonalized; and patients, physicians, and nurses were voicing concern about the lack and/or poor quality of nursing care. She reflected that in the early part of the twentieth century, a person came to the hospital for care. In the 1950s and 1960s, the focus changed, and a person came to the hospital for cure. However, the health problems of the time were long-term in nature and often not subject to cure. It was Hall's belief that in

> It was Hall's belief that in spite of successes in keeping people alive, there was a failure in helping patients live fully with chronic pathology.

spite of successes in keeping people alive, there was a failure in helping patients live fully with chronic pathology. After the patient's biological crisis was stabilized, Hall believed that care should be the primary focus and that nurses were the most qualified to provide the type of care that would enable patients to achieve their maximum potential. In fact, she questioned why medicine would want the leadership and suggested that the patient with a long-term illness would come to nursing (Hall, 1965).

Hall described the two phases of medical care that she saw existing in hospitals at the time. Phase 1 is when the patient is in biological crisis with a need for intensive medicine. Phase 2 begins when the acute crisis is stabilized and the patient is in

need of a different form of medicine. Hall labeled this as "follow-up"—evaluative medicine—and felt that it is at this point that professional nursing is most important. She criticized the practice of turning over the patient's care to practical nurses and aides at this point while the professional nurse attended to new admissions in the biological crisis phase. Hall stated:

> Now when the patient reaches the point where we know he is going to live, he might be interested in learning how to live better before he leaves the hospital. But the one nurse who could teach him, the one nurse who has the background to make this a true learning situation, is now busy with the new patients in a state of biological crisis. She rarely sees those other patients who have survived this period, unless there is something investigative or potentially paining to do! The patients in the second stage of hospitalization are given over to straight comforters, the practical nurses and aides. No teaching is available and the patient doesn't change a bit. No wonder so many people keep coming back for readmission. They've never had the invitation nor the opportunity to learn from this experience. So I say, if that's the way it is, take [the patient] from the medical center at this point in his follow-up evaluative medical care period and transfer him to the Loeb Center, where nurturing will be his chief therapy and medicine will become an ancillary one. (1969, p. 87)

Hall also opposed the concept of team nursing, which was being implemented in many acute care settings at the time. According to Hall (1958), team nursing viewed nursing as a set of functions, ranging from simple to complex. Simple functions were considered those in which few factors were taken into consideration before making a nursing judgment. The tasks or activities of nursing were divided among nursing personnel, who were simply or complexly educated, with the highest educated leading the nursing team. Hall believed that the concept of team nursing was detrimental to nursing and reduced nursing to a vocation or trade. Hall (1958) stated: "There is nothing simple about patients who are complex human beings, or a nurse who is also complex and who finds herself involved in the complexities of disease and health processes in a complex helping relationship" (p. 1). Hall was convinced that patient outcomes are improved when direct care is provided by the professional nurse.

Care, Core, and Cure

Hall enumerated three aspects of the person as patient: the person, the body, and the disease. These aspects were envisioned as overlapping circles of care, core, and cure that influence each other. Hall stated:

> Everyone in the health professions either neglects or takes into consideration any or all of these, but each profession, to be a profession, must have an exclusive area of expertness with which it practices, creates new practices, new theories and introduces newcomers to its practice. (1965, p. 4)

She believed that medicine's responsibility was the area of pathology and treatment. The area of person, which, according to Hall, has been sadly neglected, belongs to a number of professions, including psychiatry, social work, and the ministry, among others. She saw nursing's expertise as the area of body as body, and also as influenced by the other two areas. Hall clearly stated that the focus of nursing is the provision of intimate bodily care. She reflected that the public has long recognized this as belonging exclusively to nursing (Hall, 1958, 1964, 1965). Being expert in the area of body involved more than simply knowing how to provide intimate bodily care. To be expert, the nurse must know how to modify the care depending on the pathology and treatment while considering the patient's unique needs and personality.

Based on her view of the person as patient, Hall conceptualized nursing as having three aspects, and she delineated the area that is the specific domain of nursing and those areas that are shared with other professions (Hall, 1955, 1958, 1964, 1965) (see Figure 10–1). Hall believed that this model reflected the nature of nursing as a professional interpersonal process. She visualized each of the three overlapping circles as an "aspect of the nursing process related to the patient, to the supporting sciences and to the underlying philosophical dynamics" (Hall, 1958, p. 1). The circles overlap and change in size as the patient progresses through a medical crisis to the rehabilitative phase of the illness. In the acute care phase, the cure circle is the largest. During the evaluation and follow-up phase, the care circle is predominant. Hall's framework for nursing has been described as the Care, Core, and Cure Model (Chinn & Jacobs, 1987; Marriner-

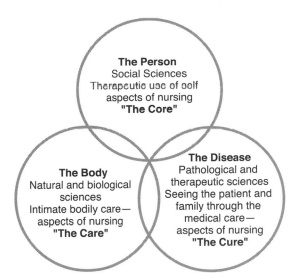

FIGURE 10–1 Care, core, and cure model. *From Hall, L. (1964, February). Nursing: What is it? The Canadian Nurse, 60(2), p. 151. Reproduced with permission from The Canadian Nurse.*

Tomey, Peskoe, & Gumm, 1989; Stevens-Barnum, 1990).

CARE

Hall suggested that the part of nursing that is concerned with intimate bodily care (e.g., bathing,

> *The part of nursing that is concerned with intimate bodily care (e.g., bathing, feeding, toileting, positioning, moving, dressing, undressing, and maintaining a healthful environment) belongs exclusively to nursing. Nursing is required when people are not able to undertake these activities for themselves.*

feeding, toileting, positioning, moving, dressing, undressing, and maintaining a healthful environment) belongs exclusively to nursing. Nursing is required when people are not able to undertake these activities for themselves. This aspect provided the opportunity for closeness and required seeing the process as an interpersonal relationship (Hall, 1958). Hall labeled this aspect "care," and she identified knowledge in the natural and biological sciences as foundational to practice. The intent of bodily care is to comfort the patient. Through this comforting, the person of the patient, as well as his or her body, responds to the physical care. Hall cautioned against viewing intimate bodily care as a task that can be performed by anyone:

> To make the distinction between a trade and a profession, let me say that the laying on of hands to wash around a body is an activity, it is a trade; but if you look behind the activity for the rationale and intent, look beyond it for the opportunities that the activity opens up for something more enriching in growth, learning and healing production on the part of the patient—you have got a profession. Our intent when we lay hands on the patient in bodily care is to comfort. While the patient is being comforted, he feels close to the comforting one. At this time his person talks out and acts out those things that concern him—good, bad and indifferent. If nothing more is done with these, what the patient gets is ventilation or catharsis, if you will. This may bring relief of anxiety and tension but not necessarily learning. If the individual who is in the comforting role has in her preparation all of the sciences whose principles she can offer a teaching-learning experience around his concerns, the ones that are most effective in teaching and learning, then the comforter proceeds to something beyond—to what I call "nurturer"—someone who fosters learning, someone who fosters growing up emotionally, someone who even fosters healing. (Hall, 1969, p. 86)

CURE

The second aspect of the nursing process is shared with medicine and is labeled the "cure." During this aspect, the nurturing process may be modified as this aspect overlaps it. Hall (1958) comments on the two ways that this medical aspect of nursing may be viewed. It may be viewed as the nurse assisting the doctor by assuming medical tasks or

> *The other view of this aspect of nursing is to see the nurse helping the patient through his or her medical, surgical, and rehabilitative care in the role of comforter and nurturer.*

functions. The other view of this aspect of nursing is to see the nurse helping the patient through his or her medical, surgical, and rehabilitative care in the role of comforter and nurturer. Hall felt that the nursing profession was assuming more and more of the medical aspects of care while at the same time giving away the nurturing process of nursing to less well-prepared persons. Hall stated:

> Interestingly enough, physicians do not have practical doctors. They don't need them . . . they have nurses. Interesting, too, is the fact that most nurses show by their delegation of nurturing to others, that they prefer being second class doctors to being first class nurses. This is the prerogative of any nurse. If she feels better in this role, why not? One good reason why not for more and more nurses is that with this increasing trend, patients receive from professional nurses second class doctoring; and from practical nurses, second class nursing. Some nurses would like the public to get first class nursing. Seeing the patient through [his or her] medical care without giving up the nurturing will keep the unique opportunity that personal closeness provides to further [the] patient's growth and rehabilitation. (1958, p. 3)

CORE

The third area that nursing shares with all of the helping professions is that of using relationships for therapeutic effect—the core. This area emphasizes the social, emotional, spiritual, and intellectual needs of the patient in relation to family, institution, community, and the world (Hall, 1955, 1958, 1965). Knowledges that are foundational to the core were based on the social sciences and on therapeutic use of self. Through the closeness offered by the provision of intimate bodily care, the patient will feel comfortable enough to explore with the nurse "who he is, where he is, where he wants to go and will take or refuse help in getting there—the patient will make amazingly more rapid progress toward recovery and rehabilitation" (Hall, 1958, p. 3). Hall believed that through this process, the patient would emerge as a whole person.

Knowledge and skills the nurse needs in order to use self therapeutically include knowing self and learning interpersonal skills. The goals of the interpersonal process are to help patients to understand themselves as they participate in problem focusing and problem solving. Hall discussed the importance of nursing with the patient as opposed to nursing at, to, or for the patient. Hall reflected on the value of the therapeutic use of self by the professional nurse when she stated:

The nurse who knows self by the same token can love and trust the patient enough to work *with* him

> *The nurse who knows self by the same token can love and trust the patient enough to work with him professionally, rather than for him technically, or at him vocationally.*

professionally, rather than *for* him technically, or *at* him vocationally. Her goals cease being tied up with "where can I throw my nursing stuff around," or "how can I explain my nursing stuff to get the patient to do what we want him to do," or "how can I understand my patient so that I can handle him better." Instead her goals are linked up with "what is the problem?" and "how can I help the patient understand himself?" as he participates in problem facing and solving. In this way, the nurse recognizes that the power to heal lies in the patient and not in the nurse unless she is healing herself. She takes satisfaction and pride in her ability to help the patient tap this source of power in his continuous growth and development. She becomes comfortable working cooperatively and consistently with members of other professions, as she meshes her contributions with theirs in a concerted program of care and rehabilitation. (1958, p. 5)

Hall believed that the role of professional nursing was enacted through the provision of *care* that facilitates the interpersonal process and invited the patient to learn to reach the *core* of his difficulties while seeing him through the *cure* that is possible. Through the professional nursing process, the patient has the opportunity of making the illness a learning experience from which he may emerge even healthier than before his illness (Hall, 1965).

The Loeb Center for Nursing and Rehabilitation

Lydia Hall was able to actualize her vision of nursing through the creation of the Loeb Center for Nursing and Rehabilitation at Montefiore Medical Center. The center's major orientation was rehabilitation and subsequent discharge to home or to a long-term care institution if further care was needed. Doctors referred patients to the center, and a professional nurse made admission decisions. Criteria for admission were based on the patient's

need for rehabilitation nursing. What made the Loeb Center uniquely different was the model of professional nursing that was implemented under Lydia Hall's guidance. The center's guiding philosophy was Hall's belief that during the rehabilitation phase of an illness experience, professional nurses were the best prepared to foster the rehabilitation process, decrease complications and recurrences, and promote health and prevent new illnesses.

> *She saw this being accomplished by the special and unique way nurses work with patients in a close interpersonal process with the goal of fostering learning, growth, and healing.*

She saw this being accomplished by the special and unique way nurses work with patients in a close interpersonal process with the goal of fostering learning, growth, and healing. At the Loeb Center, nursing was the chief therapy, with medicine and the other disciplines ancillary to nursing. A new model of organization of nursing services was implemented and studied at the center. Hall stated:

> Within this proposed organization of services, the chief therapeutic agent for the patient's rehabilitation and progress will be the special and unique way the nurse will work with the individual patient. She will be involved not only in direct bedside care but she will also be the instrument to bring the rehabilitation service of the Center to the patient. Specialists in related therapies will be available on staff as resource persons and as consultants. (1963b, p. 4)

Nursing was in charge of the total health program for the patient and was responsible for integrating all aspects of care. Only registered professional nurses were hired. The 80-bed unit was staffed with 44 professional nurses employed around the clock. Professional nurses gave direct patient care and teaching and were responsible for eight patients and their families. Senior staff nurses were available on each ward as resources and mentors for staff nurses. For every two professional nurses there was one nonprofessional worker called a "messenger-attendant." The messenger-attendants did not provide hands-on care to the patients. Instead, they performed such tasks as getting linen and supplies, thus freeing the nurse to nurse the patient (Hall, 1969). Additionally, there were four ward secretaries. Morning and evening shifts were staffed at the same ratio. Night-shift staffing was less; however, Hall (1965) noted that there were "enough nurses at night to make rounds every hour and to nurse those patients who are awake around the concerns that may be keeping them awake" (p. 2). In most institutions of that time, the number of nurses was decreased during the evening and night shifts because it was felt that larger numbers of nurses were needed during the day to get the work done. Hall took exception to the idea that nursing service was organized around work to be done rather than the needs of the patients.

The patient was the center of care at Loeb and participated actively in all care decisions. Families were free to visit at any hour of the day or night. Rather than strict adherence to institutional routines and schedules, patients at the Loeb Center were encouraged to maintain their own usual patterns of daily activities, thus promoting independence and an easier transition to home. There was no chart section labeled "Doctor's Orders." Hall believed that to order a patient to do something violated the right of the patient to participate in his or her treatment plan. Instead, nurses shared the treatment plan with the patient and helped him or her to discuss his or her concerns and become an active learner in the rehabilitation process. Additionally, there were no doctor's progress notes or nursing notes. Instead, all charting was done on a form entitled "Patient's Progress Notes." These notes included the patient's reaction to care, his concerns and feelings, his understanding of the problems, the goals he has identified, and how he sees his progress toward those goals. Hall believed that what was important to record was the patient's progress, not the duties of the nurse or the progress of the physician. Patients were also encouraged to keep their own notes to share with their caregivers.

Referring back to Hall's care, core, and cure model, the care circle enlarges at Loeb. The cure circle becomes smaller, and the core circle becomes very large. It was Hall's belief that the nurse reached the patient's person through the closeness of intimate bodily care and comfort. The interpersonal process established by the professional nurse during the provision of care was the basis for rehabilitation and learning on the part of the patient. Alfano (1982) noted that "Hall's process for nursing care was based upon a theory that incorporated

the teachings of Harry Stack Sullivan, Carl Rogers, and John Dewey" (p. 213). Nurses were taught to use a nondirective counseling approach that emphasized the use of a reflective process. Within this process, it was important for nurses to learn to know and care for self so that they could use the self therapeutically in relationship with the patient (Hall, 1965, 1969). Hall reflected:

> If the nurse is a teacher, she will concern herself with the facilitation of the patient's verbal expressions and will reflect these so that the patient can hear what he says. Through this process, he will come to grips with himself and his problems, in which case, he will learn rapidly, i.e., he will change his behavior from sickness to "wellness." (1958, p. 4)

Lydia Hall directed the Loeb Center from 1963 until her death in 1969. Genrose Alfano succeeded her in the position of director until 1984. At this time, the Loeb Center became licensed to operate as a nursing home, providing both subacute and long-term care (Griffiths, 1997b). The philosophy, structure, and organization of services established under Hall, and continued under the direction of Genrose Alfano, changed considerably in response to changes in health-care regulation and financing. Hall and others have provided detailed desciptions of the planning and design of the original Loeb Center, its daily operations, and the nursing work that was done from 1963 to 1984 (Alfano, 1964, 1969, 1982; Bowar, 1971; Bowar-Ferres, 1975; Englert, 1971; Hall, 1963a, 1963b; Henderson, 1964; Isler, 1964; Pearson, 1984).

Implications for Nursing Practice

The stories and case studies written by nurses who worked at Loeb provide the best testimony of the implications for nursing practice at the time (Alfano, 1971; Bowar, 1971; Bowar-Ferres, 1975; Englert, 1971). Griffiths and Wilson-Barnett (1998) noted: "The series of case studies from staff at the Loeb illustrate their understanding of this practice and describe a shift in the culture of care both between nurses and patient and within the nursing management structure" (p. 1185). Alfano (1964) discussed the nursing milieu, including the orientation, education, mentoring, and expectations of the nurses at the Loeb Center. Before hiring, the philosophy of nursing and the concept of professional practice were discussed with the applicant. Alfano stated: "If she agrees to try the nondirective approach and the reflective method of communication, and if she's willing to exercise all her nursing skills and to reach for a high level of clinical practice, then we're ready to join forces" (1964, p. 84). Nurses were given support in learning and developing their professional practice. Administration worked with nurses in the same manner in which they expected nurses to work with patients, emphasizing growth of self. Bowar (1971) described the role of senior resource nurse as enabling growth through a teaching-learning process grounded in caring and respect for the "integrity of each nurse as a person" (p. 301).

Staff conferences were held at least twice weekly as forums to discuss concerns, problems, or questions. A collaborative practice model between physicians and nurses evolved, and the shared knowlege of the two professions led to more effective team planning (Isler, 1964). The nursing stories published by nurses who worked at Loeb describe nursing situations that demonstrate the effect of professional nursing on patient outcomes. Additionally, they reflect the satisfaction derived from practicing in a truly professional role (Alfano, 1971; Bowar, 1971; Bowar-Ferres, 1975; Englert, 1971). Alfano stated: "The successful implementation of the professional nursing role at Loeb was associated with an institutional philosophy of nursing autonomy and with considerable authority afforded clinical nurses in their practice" (1982, p. 226). The model of professional nursing practice developed at Loeb has been compared to primary nursing (Griffiths & Wilson-Barnett, 1998).

Questions arise about why the concept of the Loeb Center was not replicated in other facilities. Alfano (1982) identified several deterrents to replication of the model. Foremost among these was her belief that many people were not convinced that it was essential for professional nurses to provide direct patient care. Additionally, she postulated that others did not share the definition of the term "professional nursing practice" that was espoused by Hall. She noted that "those who have tried to replicate the program, but have employed nonprofessional or less-skilled persons, have not produced the same results" (Alfano, 1982, p. 226). Other factors included economic incentives that favored keeping the patient in an acute care bed, and the difficulties encountered in maintaining a population of short-term rehabilitation patients in the extended care unit. Pearson (1984) suggested that the philosophy of the center may have been "threatening to established hierarchies and power relationships" (p. 54). Alfano (1982, p. 226) speculated that the Loeb Center may have been an "idea ahead of its time" and that dissatisfaction with nursing homes, the nation's excess hospital bed capacities, and an increasing emphasis on rehabilitation might contribute to replication of the Loeb model in the future.

Interestingly, the Loeb model was the prototype for the development of several nursing-led in-patient units (NLIUs) in the United Kingdom. Two British nurses, Peter Griffiths and Alan Pearson, both traveled to the Loeb Center in preparation for the development of NLIUs in the United Kingdom. Both have done extensive writing in the literature describing the units and are involved in active outcome research. In a comprehensive review of the literature, Griffiths and Wilson-Barnett (1998) identify several nursing-led in-patient units, including Loeb; they describe their structure and discuss the research that was conducted to evaluate the centers. The operational definition of nursing-led in-patient units derived from this study includes the following characteristics:

1. In-patient environment offering active treatment
2. Case mix based on nursing need
3. Nurse leadership of the multidisciplinary clinical team
4. Nursing is conceptualized as the predominant active therapy
5. Nurses have authority to admit and discharge patients (Griffiths & Wilson-Barnett, 1998, p. 1185)

Unencumbered at the present time by the financial constraints of the American health-care system, the potential for the further development of nursing-led in-patient centers in the United Kingdom seems promising. However, Griffiths (1997b) suggested that future development of NLIUs in the United Kingdom may soon be influenced by financial constraints similar to those in the United States.

Implications for Nursing Research

In addition to case study research by nurses who worked at Loeb, an 18-month follow-up study of the outcomes of care was funded by the Department of Health, Education and Welfare. Alfano (1982) presents a detailed description of the study. The purpose of the longitudinal study was to compare selected outcomes of two groups of patients exposed to different nursing environments (the Loeb program and a control group). Outcomes examined were cost of hospital stay, hospital readmissions, nursing home admissions, mortality, and return to work and social activities. Overall, findings suggested that the Loeb group achieved better outcomes at less overall cost.

> *Overall, findings suggested that the Loeb group achieved better outcomes at less overall cost.*

The findings of several other studies in nurse-led units lend further support to the benefit of the structure to patient outcomes, including prevention of complications (Daly, Phelps, & Rudy, 1991; Griffiths, 1996; Griffiths & Wilson-Barnett, 1998; Rudy, Daly, Douglas, Montenegro, Song, & Dyer, 1995). There is a critical need for research examining the effect of professional nursing care on patient outcomes in all settings. In a recent study involving 506 hospitals in 10 states, Kovner and Gergen (1998) reported that patients who have surgery done in hospitals with fewer registered nurses per patient run a higher risk of developing avoidable complications following their operation. There was a strong inverse relationship between registered nurse staffing and adverse patient events. Patients in hospitals with fewer full-time registered nurses per in-patient day had a greater incidence of urinary tract infections, pneumonia, thrombosis, pulmonary congestion, and other lung-related problems following major surgery. The authors suggested that these complications can be prevented by hands-on nursing practices and that this should be considered when developing strategies to reduce costs. Griffiths (1996) suggested the need for further research and cautioned that although clinical outcomes are important, it is equally important to study the processes of care in these units. In doing so, we will begin to understand the resources and methods of nursing care necessary to ensure positive patient outcomes.

SUMMARY

Currently, nurses practice in a health-care environment driven by financial gain, where quality is sacrificed and the patient is lost in a world of mismanaged care. More than ever, these alarming trends indicate a need to return to the basic premise of Hall's philosophy—patient-centered, therapeutic care. According to Griffiths (1997a), however, the Loeb Center presently reflects little resemblance to its former image. It now provides part subacute and part long-term care and, in fact, appears remarkably like the kind of system that Hall was trying to alter. Nursing is bogged down in a morass of paperwork, and the enthusiasm generated by the Hall model is no longer evident.

How would Lydia Hall react to these conditions, and what response might we expect if she spoke with us today? We believe she would be appalled by the diminished presence of professional nurses in health-care facilities and the impediments confronting those who remain. She would encourage us to explore new ways to provide needed nursing care within an existing chaotic climate. She would lead us in challenging the status quo and speak of the necessity for nursing leaders to have a clear vision of nursing practice and a willingness to advocate for nursing regardless of external forces seeking to undermine the profession.

She would foster scientific inquiry that addresses outcomes of care and validates the impact of professional nursing, particularly in long-term care settings. She would agree that the improvement of care to elders in nursing homes is a significant ethical issue for society and that nurses, the largest group of care providers to elders in nursing homes, play a vital role in the improvement of care. She would call upon us to develop professional models of care and demonstrate the positive outcomes for the health and well-being of elders. She would challenge the widely held belief that provision of care to this population consists only of bed and body care that can be effectively delivered by non-professional staff.

She would applaud the movement toward advanced nursing practice but would probably envision it as a means for highly educated nurses to use their expertise more effectively in providing direct patient care outside the hospital. She would encourage advanced practice nurses to continue to develop knowledge related to the nursing discipline and the unique contribution of nursing to the health of people. And she would identify community nursing organizations as an opportunity for nurses to coordinate and deliver continuity of care in the ambulatory setting and in the home.

Finally, she would urge nurses to recapture the aspects of nursing practice that have been relinquished to others—those nurturing aspects that, according to Hall (1963a), provide the opportunity for nurses to establish therapeutic, humanistic relationships with patients and make it possible for them to work together toward recovery.

References

Alfano, G. (1964). Administration means working with nurses. *American Journal of Nursing, 64,* 83–86.

Alfano, G. (1969). The Loeb Center for Nursing and Rehabilitation. *Nursing Clinics of North America, 4,* 487–493.

Alfano, G. (1971). Healing or caretaking—which will it be? *Nursing Clinics of North America, 6,* 273–280.

Alfano, G. (1982). In Aiken, L. (Ed.), *Nursing in the 1980s* (pp. 211–228). Philadelphia: J. B. Lippincott.

Birnbach, N. (1988). Lydia Eloise Hall, 1906–1969. In Bullough, V. L., Church, O. M., & Stein, A. P. (Eds.), *American nursing: A biographical dictionary* (pp. 161–163). New York: Garland Publishing.

Bowar, S. (1971). Enabling professional practice through leadership skills. *Nursing Clinics of North America, 6,* 293–301.

Bowar-Ferres, S. (1975). Loeb Center and its philosophy of nursing. *American Journal of Nursing, 75,* 810–815.

Bullough, V. L., Church, O. M., & Stein, A. P. (Eds.). (1988). *American nursing: A biographical dictionary.* New York: Garland Publishing.

Chinn, P. L., & Jacobs, M. K. (1987). *Theory and nursing.* St. Louis: Mosby.

Daly, B. J., Phelps, C., & Rudy, E. B. (1991). A nurse-managed special care unit. *Journal of Nursing Administration, 21,* 31–38.

Englert, B. (1971). How a staff nurse perceives her role at Loeb Center. *Nursing Clinics of North America, 6*(2), 281–292.

Griffiths, P. (1996). Clinical outcomes for nurse-led in-patient care. *Nursing Times, 92,* 40–43.

Griffiths, P. (1997a). In search of the pioneers of nurse-led care. *Nursing Times, 93,* 16–18.

Griffiths, P. (1997b). In search of therapeutic nursing: Subacute care. *Nursing Times, 93,* 54–55.

Griffiths, P., & Wilson-Barnett, J. (1998). The effectiveness of "nursing beds": A review of the literature. *Journal of Advanced Nursing, 27,* 1184–1192.

Hall, L. E. (1955). *Quality of nursing care.* Manuscript of an address before a meeting of the Department of Baccalaureate and Higher Degree Programs of the New Jersey League for Nursing, February 7, 1955, at Seton Hall University, Newark, New Jersey. Montefiore Medical Center Archives, Bronx, New York.

Hall, L. E. (1958). *Nursing: What is it?* Manuscript. Montefiore Medical Center Archives, Bronx, New York.

Hall, L. E. (1963a, March). *Summary of project report: Loeb Center for Nursing and Rehabilitation.* Unpublished report. Montefiore Medical Center Archives, Bronx, New York.

Hall, L. E. (1963b, June). *Summary of project report: Loeb Center for Nursing and Rehabilitation.* Unpublished report. Montefiore Medical Center Archives, Bronx, New York.

Hall, L. E. (1963c). A center for nursing. *Nursing Outlook, 11,* 805–806.

Hall, L. E. (1964). Nursing—what is it? *Canadian Nurse, 60,* 150–154.

Hall, L. E. (1965). *Another view of nursing care and quality.* Address delivered at Catholic University, Washington, DC. Unpublished report. Montefiore Medical Center Archives, Bronx, New York.

Hall, L. E. (1969). The Loeb Center for Nursing and Rehabilitation, Montefiore Hospital and Medical Center, Bronx, New York. *International Journal of Nursing Studies, 6,* 81–97.

Henderson, C. (1964). Can nursing care hasten recovery? *American Journal of Nursing, 64,* 80–83.

Isler, C. (June, 1964). New concept in nursing therapy: Care as the patient improves. *RN,* 58–70.

Kovner, C., & Gergen, P. (1998). The relationship between nurse staffing level and adverse events following surgery in acute care hospitals. *Image: Journal of Nursing Scholarship, 30,* 315–321.

Marriner-Tomey, A., Peskoe, K., & Gumm, S. (1989). Lydia E. Hall core, care, and cure model. In Marriner-Tomey, A. M. (Ed.), *Nursing theorists and their work* (pp. 109–117). St. Louis: Mosby.

Montefiore cuts readmissions 80%. (1966, February 23). *The New York Times.*

Obituaries—Lydia E. Hall. (1969). *American Journal of Nursing, 69,* 830.

Pearson, A. (1984, July 18). A centre for nursing. *Nursing Times,* 53–54.

Rudy, E. B., Daly, B. J., Douglas, S., Montenegro, H. D., Song, R., & Dyer, M. A. (1995). Patient outcomes for the chronically critically ill: Special care unit versus intensive care unit. *Nursing Research, 44,* 324–331.

Stevens-Barnum, B. J. (1990). *Nursing theory analysis, application, evaluation* (3rd ed.). Glenview, IL: Scott, Foresman/Little Brown.

Wiggins, L. R. (1980). Lydia Hall's place in the development of nursing theory. *Image, 12,* 10–12.

Bibliography

Hall, L. E. (1955). Quality of nursing care. *Public Health News (New Jersey State Department of Health), 36,* 212–215.

Hall, L. E. (1960). *Report of a work conference on nursing in long-term chronic disease and aging.* National League for Nursing as a League Exchange #50. New York: National League for Nursing.

Hall, L. E. (1963, June). *Report of Loeb Center for Nursing and Rehabilitation project report* (pp. 1515–1562). Congressional Record Hearings before the Special Subcommittee on Intermediate Care of the Committee on Veterans' Affairs. Washington, DC.

Hall, L. E. (1965). Nursing—what is it? In Baumgarten (Ed.), *Concepts of nursing home administration.* New York: Macmillan.

Hall, L. E. (1966). Another view of nursing care and quality. In Straub, M. K. (Ed.), *Continuity of patient care: The role of nursing.* Washington, DC: Catholic University of America Press.

Levenson, D. (1984). *Montefiore—the hospital as social instrument.* New York: Farrar, Straus & Giroux.

CHAPTER 11

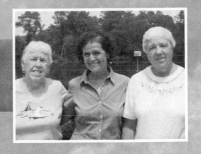

Josephine Paterson
Loretta Zderad

PART ONE: Josephine Paterson and Loretta Zderad's Humanistic Nursing Theory and Its Applications

Susan Kleiman

Introducing the Theorists

Dr. Josephine Paterson is originally from the East Coast where she attended a diploma school of nursing in New York City. She subsequently earned her bachelor's degree in nursing education from St. John's University. In her graduate work at Johns Hopkins University, she focused on public health nursing and then earned her doctor of nursing science degree from Boston University. Her doctoral dissertation was on comfort.

Dr. Loretta Zderad is from the Midwest where she attended a diploma school of nursing. She later earned her bachelor's degree in nursing education from Loyola University of Chicago. In her graduate work she majored in psychiatric nursing at the Catholic University of America. She subsequently earned her doctor of philosophy from Georgetown University. Her dissertation was on empathy.

Josephine Paterson and Loretta Zderad met in the mid-1950s while working at Catholic University. Their joint project was to create a new program that would encompass the community health component and the psychiatric component of the graduate program. This started a collaboration, dialogue, and friendship that has lasted for over 45 years. They shared and developed their concepts, approaches, and experiences of "existential phenomenology," which evolved into the formal Theory of Humanistic Nursing. They incorporated these concepts into their work as educators and shared them across the country in seminars and workshops on Humanistic Nursing Theory.

In 1971, after their work in academia, Dr. Paterson and Dr. Zderad went to the Veterans Administration (VA) hospital in Northport, MA. They were hired as "nursologists" by a forward-thinking administrator who recognized the need for staff support during a period of change in the VA system. The position of nursologist involved a three-pronged approach to the improvement of patient care through clinical practice, education, and research. These functions were integrated within the framework of Humanistic Nursing Theory. They worked with the nurses at Northport from 1971 until 1978 on this project, running workshops that incorporated their theory. In 1978 there was a change in hospital administration that entailed a reorganization of services. Dr. Paterson was assigned to the Mental Hygiene Clinic to work as a psychotherapist while Dr. Zderad became the associate chief of Nursing Service for Education. These were the positions they held when I met them as a graduate student in psychiatric mental health nursing. Dr. Paterson agreed to work with me as my clinical supervisor.

The following two years brought me a world of enrichment. For Dr. Paterson and Dr. Zderad, those years culminated in their retirement and relocation to the South. I, on the other hand, continue the work that they started—as a fellow theorist and as a friend and colleague in nursing. They have inspired me to carry on their work, using it in my nursing situations, whether in clinical, administrative, or most recently, with nursing students, and to share what I have come to know.

The Humanistic Nursing Theory was originally formulated as a way for nurses to define nursing. That is, a way to illuminate the values and meanings central to nursing experiences. Paterson and Zderad were nursing visionaries who emphasized synthesis and wholeness rather than reduction and logical/mathematical analysis. They challenged the notion that the reductionistic approach is the touchstone of explanatory power, and they postulated an "all-at-once" character of existence in nurses' experiences of being in the world. They led the way to many of the contemporary nursing theories that emphasize the caring aspects of nursing (Benner, 1984; Parse, 1981; Watson, 1988).

Introducing the Theory

Humanistic Nursing Theory is multidimensional. It speaks to the essences of nursing and embraces the dynamics of being, becoming, and change. It is an interactive nursing theory that provides a methodology for reflection and articulation of nursing essences. It is also a theory that provides a methodological bridge between theory and practice by providing a broad guide for nursing "dialogue" in a myriad of settings.

Nursing, as seen through Humanistic Nursing Theory, is the ability to struggle with another through "peak experiences related to health and suffering in which the participants are and become in accordance with their human potential" (Paterson & Zderad, 1976, p. 7). The struggle evolves within a dialogue between the participants, illuminating the possibility for each to "become" in concert with the other. According to Josephine Paterson and Loretta Zderad, in nursing, the purpose of this dialogue, or intersubjective relating, is, "nurturing the well-being and more-being of persons in need"

> *There is a call from a person, a family, a community, or from humanity for help with some health-related issue. A nurse, a group of nurses, or the community of nurses hearing and recognizing that call respond In a manner that is intended to help the caller with the health-related need. What happens during this dialogue, the "and" in the "call and response," the "between," is nursing.*

> *In nursing, the purpose of this dialogue, or intersubjective relating, is, "nurturing the well-being and more-being of persons in need."*

(1976, p. 4). Humanistic Nursing Theory is grounded in existentialism and emphasizes the lived experience of nursing. One of the existential themes that it builds on is the affirmation of being and becoming of both the patient and the nurse, who are actualized through the choices they make and the intersubjective relationships they engage in.

The new adventurer in Humanistic Nursing Theory may at first find some of these terms and phrases awkward. When I spoke to a colleague of the "moreness" and of "relating all at once," she remarked, "Oh, oh, you're beginning to sound just like them," meaning Dr. Paterson and Dr. Zderad. But this vocabulary reflects a grasp of nursing as an ever-changing process. Just as nursing in actual practice is never inert, so Humanistic Nursing Theory is dynamic. Consider Josephine Paterson's own description of humanistic nursing: "Our 'here and now' stage of Humanistic Nursing Theory development at times is experienced as an all-at-once octopus at a discotheque, stimulation personified, gyrating in many colors" (1977, p. 4).

If asked to conceptualize Humanistic Nursing Theory succinctly, I would have to say, "call and response." These three words encapsulate the core themes of this quite elegant and very profound theory. Through this paradigm, Josephine Paterson and Loretta Zderad have presented a vision of nursing that is amenable to variation in practice settings and to the changing patterns of nursing over time.

According to Humanistic Nursing Theory, there is a call from a person, a family, a community, or from humanity for help with some health-related issue. A nurse, a group of nurses, or the community of nurses hearing and recognizing that call respond in a manner that is intended to help the caller with the health-related need. What happens during this

dialogue, the "and" in the "call and response," the "between," is nursing.

In their book *Humanistic Nursing* (1976), Drs. Paterson and Zderad share with other nurses their method for exploring the "between," again emphasizing that it is the "between" that they conceive of as nursing. The method is phenomenological inquiry (Paterson & Zderad, 1976 p. 72). Engaging in the phenomenological process sensitizes the inquiring nurse to the excitement, anticipation, and uncertainty of approaching the nursing situation openly. Through a spirit of receptivity, a readiness for surprise, and the courage to experience the unknown, there is an opportunity for authentic relating and intersubjectivity. "The process leads one naturally to repeated experiencing of and reflective immersion in the lived phenomena" (Zderad, 1978, p. 8).

This immersion into the intersubjective experience and the phenomenological process helps to guide the nurse in the responsive interchange. During this interchange, the nurse calls forth all that she is (education, skills, life experiences, intuition, etc.) and integrates it into her response. A common misconception that students of Humanistic Nursing Theory may have is that it asserts that the nurse must provide what it is that the patient is calling for. Remember the response of the nurse is guided by all that she is. This includes his or her professional role, ethics, and competencies. A particular nurse may not actually be able or willing to provide what is being called for, but the process of being heard, according to this theory, is in itself a humanizing experience.

Look at the conceptual framework of Humanistic Nursing Theory in Figure 11–1 to help explain and illustrate some of its basic concepts and assumptions. Humanistic nursing is a moving process

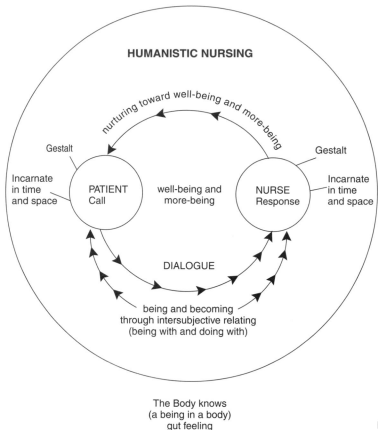

The Body knows
(a being in a body)
gut feeling

FIGURE 11–1 World of others and things.

that occurs in the living context of human beings, human beings who interface and interact with others and other things in the world. In the world of Humanistic Nursing Theory, when we speak of human beings, we mean patients (e.g., individuals, members of families, members of communities, or members of the human race) and nurses (see Figure 11–2). A person becomes a patient when he or she sends a call for help with some health-related problem. The person hearing and recognizing the call is a nurse. A nurse, by intentionally choosing to become a nurse, has made a commitment to help others with health-related needs.

It is important to emphasize that in humanistic nursing theory, each nurse and each patient is taken to be a unique human being with his or her own particular gestalt (see Figure 11–3). Gestalt, representing all that particular human beings are, which includes all past experiences, all current being, and all hopes, dreams, and fears of the future that are experienced in one's own space-time dimension. As illustrated, this gestalt includes past and current

social relationships, as well as gender, race, religion, education, work, and whatever individualized patterns for coping a person has developed. It also includes past experiences with persons in the health-care system and a patient's images and expectations of those persons.

Our gestalt is the unique expression of our individuality as incarnate human beings who exist in this particular space at this particular time, with circumscribed resources and in a physical body that senses, filters, and processes our experiences to which we assign subjective meanings. Accordingly, a nurse and a patient perceive and respond to each other as a gestalt, not just as the presentation of a sum of attributes. In humanistic nursing we say that each person is perceived as existing "all at once." In the process of interacting with patients, nurses interweave professional identity, education, intuition, and experience with all their other life experiences, creating their own tapestry, which unfolds during their responses.

One has only to observe nurses going about

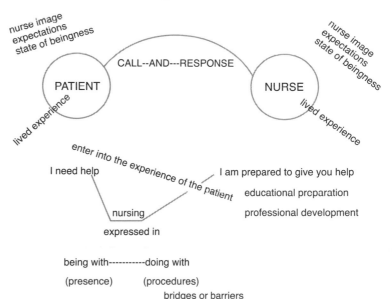

FIGURE 11–2   Shared human experience.

their nursing to see this process of interrelating as subjective human beings. Take, for example, performing the task of suctioning a patient. This task can be done with tenderness, dignity, and with masterful technical skills that make the procedure almost unnoticeable. I once watched as a nurse positioned and suctioned a patient; as she performed the task, she made sure that she also repositioned the little basket of flowers that she had placed by the patient's bedside. The repositioning of the flowers really had nothing to do with the technique of suctioning. It showed that the nurse recognized the patient as a unique human being, and she did something special to make the experience less stressful and as comfortable as possible for the patient. Comfort in this instance refers to the idea that through the relationship engendered and nurtured in intersubjective dialogue, there arises the possibility for persons to become all that they can be in particular lived situations.

PHILOSOPHICAL AND METHODOLOGICAL BACKGROUND

The phenomenological movement of the nineteenth century was in response to what its proponents called the dehumanization and objectification of the world by the logical positivists. Phenomenol-ogists proposed that human beings, the world, and their experiences of their world are inseparable. You can easily see that a nursing theory that is based in the human context lends itself to phenomenological inquiry rather than reductionism, which attempts to remove subjective humanness and strives to achieve detached objectivity. The early phenomenologists saw their goal as the examination and description of all things, including the human experience of those things, in the particular way that they reveal themselves.

Phenomenology is not only a philosophy, but it is also a method—a method that can be integrated into a general approach or way of viewing the world. Nurses who can relate to this method are inclined to cultivate it and make it a part of their everyday approach to nursing. This method is no less rigorous in its application than methods used in experimental research to build theories. The phenomenological approach is based on description, intuition, analysis, and synthesis. Of importance are training and conscientious self-criticism on the part of the unbiased inquirer as he or she investigates the phenomenon as it reveals itself. In phenomenology, a statement's validity is based on whether or not it describes the phenomenon accurately. The truth of all the statements resulting from the critical analysis of each phenomenon described

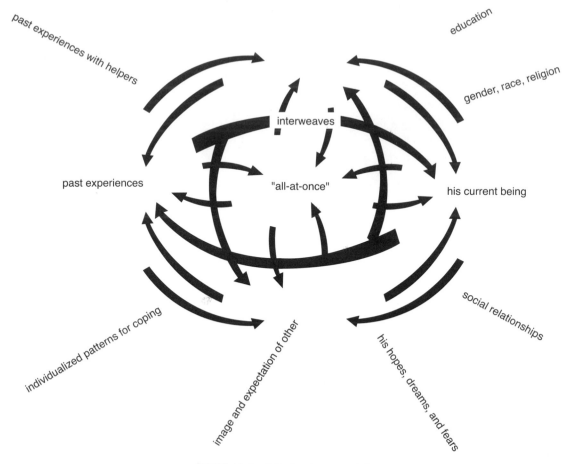

FIGURE 11–3 Patient and nurse gestalts.

can be verified by examining the phenomenon itself.

Dr. Paterson and Dr. Zderad describe five phases to their phenomenological study of nursing. These phases are presented sequentially but are actually interwoven, because as with all of Humanistic Nursing Theory, there is a constant flow between, in all directions, and all at once emanating toward a center that is nursing. The phases of humanistic nursing inquiry are:

- Preparation of the nurse knower for coming to know
- Nurse knowing the other intuitively
- Nurse knowing the other scientifically
- Nurse complementarily synthesizing known others
- Succession within the nurse from the many to the paradoxical one

Enfolded in these five phases are three concepts that are very basic to Humanistic Nursing Theory: bracketing, angular view, and noetic loci. These will be taken up as we discuss the phases of inquiry.

Preparation of the Nurse Knower for Coming to Know

In the first phase, the inquirer tries to open herself up to the unknown and to the possibly different. She consciously and conscientiously struggles with understanding and identifying her own "angular view." Angular view involves the gestalt of the unique person mentioned earlier. It includes the conceptual and experiential framework that we bring into any situation with us, a framework that is usually unexamined and casually accepted as we negotiate our everyday world. Later in the process angular view is called upon to help make sense of and give meaning to the phenomena being studied.

By identifying our angular view we are then able to bracket it purposefully so that we do not super impose it on the experience we are trying to relate to. When we bracket, we intentionally hold our own thoughts, experiences, and beliefs in abeyance. This "holding in abeyance" does not deny our unique selves but suspends them, allowing us to experience the other in his or her own uniqueness.

By intentionally bringing into present consciousness, and acknowledging what we believe to be true, we can then attempt to hold any preconceived assumptions we may have in abeyance, so that they will not prematurely intrude upon our attempts to describe the experiences of another. A personal experience that helped me to grasp the concept of bracketing and the desired state it aims to achieve occurred when I was traveling in Europe. As I entered each new country, I experienced the excitement of the unknown. I realized at the same time how alert, open, and other directed I was in this uncharted world as compared to my own daily routine at home. In my familiar surroundings, I would often fill in the blanks left by my inattentiveness to a routine experience, sometimes anticipating and answering questions even before they were asked. Contrarily bracketing requires an alertness, openness, and other directedness. According to Husserl (1970), who is considered the father of modern phenomenology, the attitude desired is that of the perpetual beginner.

Bracketing prepares the inquirer to enter the uncharted world of the other without expectations and preconceived ideas. It helps one to be open to the authentic, to the true experience of the other. Even temporarily letting go of that which shapes our own identity as the self, however, causes anxiety, fear, and uncertainty. Labeling, diagnosing, and routine add a necessary and very valuable predictability, sense of security, and means of conserving energy to our everyday existence and practice. It may also make us less open, however, to the new and different in a situation. Being open to the new and different is a necessary stance in being able to know of the other intuitively.

Nurse Knowing the Other Intuitively

Knowing the other intuitively is described by Dr. Paterson and Dr. Zderad as "moving back and forth between the impressions the nurse becomes aware of in herself and the recollected real experience of the other" (1976, pp. 88–89), which was obtained through the unbiased being with the other. This process of bracketing versus intuiting is not contra dictory. Both are necessary and interwoven parts of the phenomenological process. The rigor and validity of phenomenology are based on the ongoing referring back to the phenomenon itself. It is conceptualized as a dialectic between the impression and the real. This shifting back and forth allows for sudden insights on the nurse's part, a new overall grasp, which manifests itself in a clearer, or perhaps a new, "understanding." These understandings generate further development of the process. At this time, the nurse's general impressions are in a dialogue with her unbracketed view (see Figure 11–4).

Nurse Knowing the Other Scientifically

In the next phase, objectivity is needed as the nurse comes to know the other scientifically. Standing outside the phenomenon, the nurse examines it through analysis. She comes to know it through its parts or elements that are symbolic and known. This phase incorporates the nurse's ability to be conscious of herself and that which she has taken in, merged with, and made part of herself. "This is

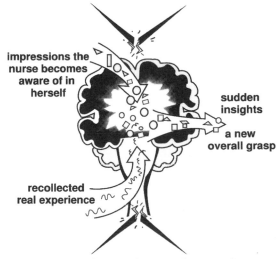

At this time the nurse's general impressions are in a dialogue with her unbracketed view

FIGURE 11–4 Nurse knowing the other intuitively. *Adapted from illustration in Briggs, J., & Peat, D. (1989). Turbulent Mirror (p. 176). New York: Harper & Row.*

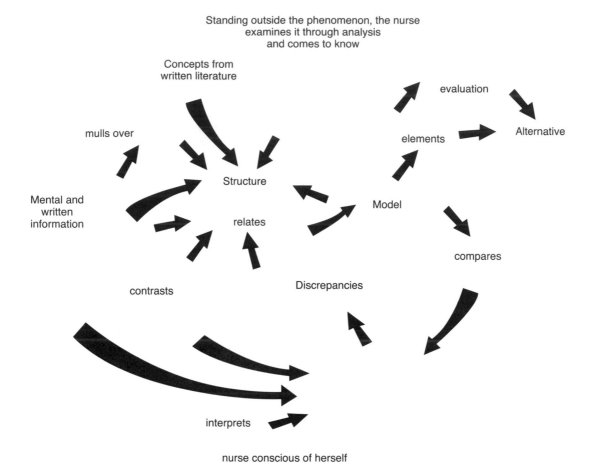

FIGURE 11–5 Nurses knowing the other scientifically. *Adapted from illustration in Briggs, J., & Peat, D. (1989). Turbulent Mirror (p. 176). New York: Harper & Row.*

the time when the nurse mulls over, analyzes, sorts out, compares, contrasts, relates, interprets, gives a name to, and categorizes" (Paterson & Zderad, 1976, p. 79). Patterns and themes are reflective of and rigorously validated by the authentic experience (Figure 11–5).

Nurse Complementarily Synthesizing Known Others

At this point the nurse personifies what has been described by Dr. Paterson and Dr. Zderad as a "noetic locus," a "knowing place" (1976, p. 43). According to this concept, the greatest gift a human being can have is the ability to relate to others, to wonder, search, and imagine about experience, and to create out of what has become known. Seeing themselves as "knowing places" inspires nurses to continue to develop and expand their community

of world thinkers through their educative and practical experiences, which then become a part of their angular view. This self-expansion, through the internalization of what others have come to know, dynamically interrelates with the nurse's human capacity to be conscious of her own lived experiences. Through this interrelationship, the subjective and objective world of nursing can be reflected upon by each nurse, who is aware of and values herself as a "knowing place" (Figure 11–6).

Succession Within the Nurse from the Many to the Paradoxical One

This is the birth of the new from the existing patterns, themes, and categories. It is in this phase that the nurse "comes up with a conception or abstraction that is inclusive of and beyond the multiplicities and contradictions" (Paterson & Zderad, 1976,

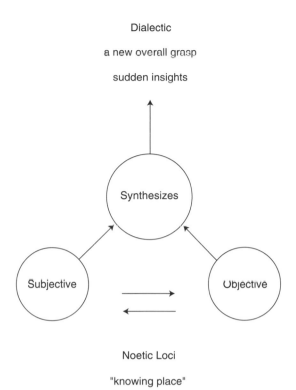

Dialectic

a new overall grasp

sudden insights

Synthesizes

Subjective

Objective

Noetic Loci

"knowing place"

FIGURE 11–6   Nurses complementarily synthesizing knowing others.

p. 81) in a process that corrects and expands her own angular view. This is the pattern of the dialectic process, which is reflected throughout Humanistic Nursing Theory. In the dialectic process there is a repetitive pattern of organizing the dissimilar into a higher level (Barnum, 1990, p. 44). At this higher level, differences are assimilated to create the new. This repetitive dialectic process of humanistic nursing is an approach that feels comfortable and natural for those who think inductively.

The pervasive theme of dialectic assimilation speaks to universal interrelatedness from the simplest to the most complex level. Human beings, by virtue of their ability to self-observe, have the unique capacity to transcend themselves and reflect on their relationship to the universe. This dialectic process has a pattern similar to that of the call-and-response paradigm of Humanistic Nursing Theory. This paradigm speaks to the interactive dialogue between two different human beings from which a unique yet universal instance of nursing emerges. The nursing interaction is limited in time and space, but the internalization of that experience adds something new to each person's angular view.

Neither is the same as before. Each is more because of that coming together. The coming together of the nurse and the patient, the between in the lived world, is nursing. Just as in the double helix of the DNA molecule (where this interweaving pattern is what structures the individual), in the fabric of Humanistic Nursing Theory this intentional interweaving between patient and nurse is what gives nursing its structure, form, and meaning.

THE CONCEPT OF COMMUNITY

The definition of community presented by Drs. Paterson and Zderad is: "Two or more persons

> *The definition of community presented by Drs. Paterson and Zderad is: "Two or more persons struggling together toward a center."*

struggling together toward a center" (1976, p. 131). In any community there is the individual and the collective known as the "community." Plato points to the microcosm and the macrocosm and proposes that the one is reflective of the many. Humanistic Nursing Theory similarly proposes that the interaction of one nurse is a reflection of the recurrent pattern of nursing and is therefore worth reflecting upon and valuing. According to Humanistic Nursing Theory, there is an inherent obligation of nurses to one another and to the community of nurses. That which enhances one of us, enhances all of us. Through openness, sharing, and caring, we each will expand our angular views, each becoming more than before. Subsequently, we take back into our nursing community these expanded selves, which in turn will touch our patients, other colleagues, and the world of health care.

PART TWO

Applications

NURSE'S REFLECTION ON NURSING

These descriptive explorations illuminate the concepts of empathy, comfort, and presence innate in applying the humanistic nursing theory to a clinical setting. Dr. Paterson (1977, p. 13) shared her experiences with a terminally ill cancer patient

"For a while I really beat on myself. I felt nothing, just a kind of indifference and numbness, as Dominic expressed his miseries, fears, and anger. I pride myself on my empathic ability. I felt so inadequate. I could not believe I could not feel with him what he was experiencing. Intellectually I knew his words, his expressions were pain-filled. My feelings of inadequacy, helplessness, and inability to control myself, came through strong. [As] I mulled reflectively about this, suddenly a light dawned amidst my puzzlement. I was experiencing what Dominic was expressing. At this time I was feeling his inadequacy, helplessness, and inability to control his cancer."

This insight brought a greater understanding between Dr. Paterson and this patient, an understanding that brought them closer so that she could endure with him in his fear-filled knowing and unknowing of dying. As his condition deteriorated, she continued to visit at his bedside. "Often after greeting me and saying what he needed he would fall asleep. First, I thought, 'It doesn't matter whether I come or not.' Then I noticed and validated that when I moved his eyes flew open. I reevaluated his sleeping during my visit. I discussed this with him. He felt safe when I sat with him. He was exhausted, staying awake, watching himself to be sure he did not die. When I was there I watched him, and he could sleep. I no longer made any move to leave before my time with him was up. I told him of this intention so that he could relax more deeply. To alleviate aloneness; this is a most expensive gift. To give this gift of time and presence in the patient's space, a person has to value the outcomes of relating."

This gift of presence is poetically described by Dr. Zderad (1978, p. 48):

Death lifts his scythe
to swipe down the young man
misdressed in hospital gown
displaced in hospital bed.
The cruel cold blade slashes
the hard mask of his nurse

silently standing there
bleeding forth her presence.

PATIENT'S REFLECTION ON NURSING

Here is an experience I was able to reflect upon after I was exposed to the process of humanistic nursing. Some time ago I attended a conference on love, intimacy, and connectedness. It was an interdisciplinary conference attended by 300 to 400 people. One of the opening speakers described the experience that had been related to him by a dear friend.

His friend had just been diagnosed with a serious form of cancer. The speaker described his friend telling him, "In the early evening the family was all around. We talked, but there was the awkwardness of not knowing what to say or what to expect. Later that night, I was in my room all alone. No longer having to be concerned about my family and what they were struggling with, I began to experience some of my own feelings. I felt so alone. Then the evening nurse who had been working with me over the last two days of testing came in. We looked at each other—neither of us said a word and she just gently touched my hand. I cried. She stayed there for . . . I don't know how long, until I placed my other hand on top of hers and gently gave it a pat. She left and I was able to go to sleep. This was one of the most intimate moments in my life. This nurse offered to be with me in the known, and unknown; somehow she also conveyed a reassurance that I did not have to go through what was coming, whatever that was, alone."

This ability to be with and endure with a patient in the process of living and dying is frequently taken for granted by us, yet it is what many times differentiates us from other professionals.

> **This ability to be with and endure with a patient in the process of living and dying is frequently taken for granted by us, yet it is what many times differentiates us from other professionals.**

PRACTICE: CLINICAL SUPERVISION

The humanistic nursing approach is useful in clinical supervision. In the process of supervision I try to understand the "call" of the nurse when she brings up a clinical issue. This usually is connected to the "call" of the patient to him or her and some issue that has arisen around the nurse's not being able to hear or respond to that call.

Consider this illustration. Ms. L. was working with a patient who had recently been told that her HIV test was positive. Although she did not have AIDS, she had been exposed to the AIDS virus, probably through her current boyfriend, who was purportedly an IV drug abuser. The original issue that came up was that the nurse was very concerned that the doctor on the interdisciplinary team, who was also the patient's therapist, was not giving the patient the support that the nurse felt the patient was calling out for. This nurse and I explored her perception that the patient did in fact seem to be reaching out. The nurse and I explored the reaching out in terms of what the patient was reaching for. It had been carefully explained to the patient that she did not have AIDS but that at some point she might come down with the illness. The patient was told that there were treatments to retard the disease but that there were no cures yet. Given this, the doctor, whose primary function is treatment and cure, was feeling ill prepared to deal with this patient; it was perhaps this sense of inadequacy that fostered avoidant behavior on his part. The nurse and I, however, came to understand that, in fact, the patient was not calling for doctoring; she was calling for nursing care. She was calling for someone to help her get through this experience in her life. With this clarified, the nurse and I began to explore the nurse's experience of hearing this call. The nurse spoke of the pain of knowing that this young woman would die prematurely. She spoke of how a friend, who reminded her of this patient, had also died and that when she associated the two she felt sad.

As we explored the nurse's angular view, we were able to identify areas that were unknown. The nurse had difficulty understanding the need or the role of the patient's relationship with her current boyfriend. We worked on helping the nurse to bracket her own thoughts and judgments, so that she could be open to the patient's experience of this relationship. Subsequently, the nurse was able to understand the patient's intense fear of being alone. As the nurse began to understand that choices are humanizing, she began to explore the need for support systems. And so to expand her own capability of being a "knowing place" and expanding her angular view, she sought out the help of the nurse practitioner in our gynecology clinic. They worked well together with this patient, who eventually was able to leave the hospital, get a part-time job, and be all that she could in her current life situation.

The nurse in the hospital grew from her experience of working with this patient. Although she is usually quite reserved and shies away from public forums, with encouragement she was able to share the experience with this patient in a large public forum. She not only shared with other professionals the role that she as a nurse played in the treatment of this patient, but she also acknowledged herself in a group of professionals as a "knowing place."

The process enfolded in Humanistic Nursing Theory is beneficial to supervisors and self-reflective practitioners in all areas of nursing. Patients call to us both verbally and nonverbally, with all sorts of health-related needs. It is important to hear the calls and know the process that lets us understand them. In hearing the calls and searching our own experiences of who we are, our personal angular view, we may progress as humanistic nurses.

RESEARCH

In an effort to better understand why some patients stayed in the day hospital and others left prematurely, the nursing staff of a psychiatric day hospital conducted a phenomenological study that investigated the experiences of patients as they entered and become engaged in treatment in a day hospital system.

The initial step in the process of preparing the nurses for this study was to expand their angular view by educating them in the phenomenological method and the unstructured interview style. In order to promote the openness of the interviewers to the experience of the patients, we used our group nursing meetings for the purpose of bracketing our angular views. In these group meetings we raised our consciousness through articulation of our own angular views. By opening ourselves to one another's experiences and points of view, we were opening ourselves to the world of other possibilities and shaking up the status quo of our own mindsets. Fifteen patients were interviewed over a period of eight months. Once the descriptions of the patients' experiences were obtained, the phenomenological method of reflecting, intuiting, analyzing, and synthesizing was used to interpret the descriptions.

We found that there were many anxiety-producing experiences on the first day in the day hospital, but very few anxiety-reducing experiences that offered the patient comfort and support. The two patients who left the study at this time found no anxiety-reducing experiences at all. Subsequently, recommendations were made to pay particular attention to reducing the anxiety of the patient on the first day. This is an example of how, through this method, corrective measures can be formulated and outcomes can be tested.

The concept of research as praxis is also illustrated in this research project. On an individual basis, the nurses related that they experienced an increased awareness of the need to be open to the patients' expressions of themselves. After reviewing the interviews of a patient who had had a particularly difficult course of treatment, one of the nurses who was on her treatment team remarked, "We weren't listening to what she was telling us—we just didn't hear the pain." Another nurse had a similar insight into a patient's experiences. She noted with some surprise that her initial impression that a patient she was working with was hostile and withholding had given way to the realization that this patient—as a result of the negative symptoms of schizophrenia—was quite empty and was really giving us all that she had to give. In future interactions with this patient, the nurse was empathic and supportive rather than judgmental and angry.

POLICY: DEVELOPING A COMMUNITY OF NURSES

Another group experience in which Humanistic Nursing Theory was utilized was the formation of a community of nurses who were mutually struggling with changes in their nursing roles. In Humanistic Nursing Theory, sharing within the community of nurses allows each nurse and the community to become more. I became aware of a common call being issued forth by nurses from my own experiences as a nurse manager.

In the report of the secretary of Health and Human Services' Commission on Nursing (December, 1988) we were told that "the perspective and expertise of nurses are a necessary adjunct to that of other health-care professionals in the policy-making, and regulatory, and standard setting process" (p. 31). The call or challenge being posed to nurses is to help create the needed changes in the health-care system today. I called to the community of nurses where I work and we joined together to struggle with this challenge. For while the importance of organized nursing power cannot be overemphasized, it is the individual nurse in her day-to-day practice who can actualize or undermine the power of the profession. As a group we strove to acknowledge and support one another as individuals of worth so that we in turn could maximize our influence as a profession.

In settings such as hospitals, the time pressure, the unending tasks, the emotional strain, and the conflicts do not allow nurses to relate, reflect, and support one another in their struggle toward a center that is nursing. This isolation and alienation does not allow for the development of either a personal or professional voice. Within our community of nurses it became clear that developing individual voices was our first task. Talking and listening to one another about our nursing worlds allowed us to become more articulate and clear about function and value as nurses. The theme of developing an articulate voice has pervaded and continues to pervade this group. There is an ever-increasing awareness of both manner and language as we interact with one another and those outside the group. The resolve for an articulate voice is even more firm as members of the group experience and share the empowering effect it can have on both personal and professional life. It has been said that "those that express themselves unfold in health, beauty, and human potential. They become unblocked channels through which creativity can flow" (Hills & Stone, 1976, p. 71).

Group members offered alternative approaches to various situations that were utilized and subsequently brought back to the group. In this way each member shared in the experience. That experience therefore became available to all members as they individually formulated their own knowledge base and expanded their angular view. As Dr. Paterson and Dr. Zderad proposed, "each person might be viewed as a community of the beings with whom she has meaningfully related" (1978, p. 45) and has a potential resource for expanding herself as a "knowing place."

Through openness and sharing we were able to differentiate our strengths. Once the members could truly appreciate the unique competence of one another, they were able to reflect that appreciation back. Through this reflection, members began to internalize and then project a competent image of themselves. They learned that this positive mirroring did not have to come from outsiders. They can reflect back to one another the image of competence and power. They, as a community of nurses, can empower one another. This reciprocity is a self-enhancing process, for "the degree to which I can create relationships which facilitate the growth of others as separate persons is a measure of the growth I have achieved in myself" (Rogers, 1976, p. 79). And so by sharing in our community of nurses we can empower one another through mutual confirmation as we help one another move toward a center that is nursing. We as nurses strive to do this with our patients. We as nurses must also strive to do this for one another and the profession of nursing.

SUMMARY

Today I perceive another call. This call is resounded in and exemplified by the following description of examining a pregnant woman: "Instead of having to approach the woman . . . to feel her breathing, you could now read the information [on her and her fetus] from across the room, from down the hall" (Rothman, 1987, p. 28).

The call I hear is for nursing. It is the call from humanity to maintain the humanness in the health-care system, which is becoming increasingly sophisticated in technology, increasingly concerned with cost containment, and increasingly less aware of and concerned with the patient as a human being. The context of Humanistic Nursing Theory is humans. The basic question it asks of nursing practice is: Is this particular intersubjective transactional nursing event humanizing or dehumanizing? Nurses as clinicians, teachers, researchers, and administrators can use the concepts and process of Humanistic Nursing Theory to gain a better understanding of the "calls" we are hearing. Through this understanding we are given direction for expanding ourselves as "knowing places" so that we can fulfill our reason for being, which, according to Humanistic Nursing Theory, is nurturing the well-being and more-being of persons in need.

References

Barnum, B. J. S. (1990). *Nursing theory: Analysis, application, evaluation.* Glenview, IL: Scott, Foresman Co.

Benner, P. (1984). *From novice to expert.* Menlo Park, CA: Addison-Wesley.

Buber, M. (1965). *The knowledge of man.* New York: Harper & Row.

Heidegger, M. (1977). *The question concerning technology.* New York: Harper & Row.

Hills, C., & Stone, R. B. (1976). *Conduct your own awareness sessions: 100 ways to enhance self-concept in the classroom.* Englewood Cliffs, NJ: Prentice-Hall.

Husserl, L. (1970). *The idea of phenomenology.* The Hague, Netherlands: Martinus Nijhoff.

May, R. (1995). *The courage to create.* New York: Norton.

Parse, R. (1981). *Man-living-health: A theory of nursing.* New York: Wiley.

Paterson, J. G. (1977). *Living until death, my perspective.* Paper presented at the Syracuse Veteran's Administration Hospital, New York.

Paterson, J. G., & Zderad, L. T. (1976). *Humanistic nursing.* New York: Wiley.

Rogers, C. R. (1976). *Perceiving, behaving, and becoming: 100 ways to enhance self-concept in the classroom.* Englewood Cliffs, NJ: Prentice-Hall.

Rothman, B. (1987). *The tentative pregnancy: Prenatal diagnosis and the future of motherhood.* New York: Penguin.

U.S. Public Health Services. (1988, December). *Secretary's commission on nursing, final report.* Washington, DC: Department of Health & Human Services.

Watson, J. (1988). *Nursing: Human science and human care.* New York: National League for Nursing.

Zderad, L. T. (1978). "From here-and-now theory: Reflections on 'how.'" In *Theory development: What? Why? How?* New York: National League for Nursing.

Nursing Theory in Nursing Practice, Education, Research, and Administration

CHAPTER 12

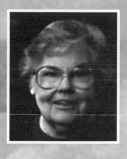

Dorothea E. Orem

PART ONE: Dorothea E. Orem's Self-Care Deficit Nursing Theory

Dorothea E. Orem

Introducing the Theorist
Views of Human Beings Specific to Nursing
Summary
References

Introducing the Theorist

Dorothea E. Orem is described as a pioneer in the development of distinctive nursing knowledge (Fawcett, 2000, p. 224). Orem contends that the term "care" describes nursing in a most general way, but does not describe nursing in a way that distinguishes it from other forms of care (Orem, 1985).

> *Nursing is distinguished from other human services and other forms of care by the way in which it focuses on human beings.*

She argues that nursing is distinguished from other human services and other forms of care by the way in which it focuses on human beings. In the 1950s, she had the foresight to recognize the need to identify the proper focus of nursing and to clarify the domain and boundaries of nursing as a field of practice in order to enhance nursing's disciplinary evolution. She began her work by seeking an answer to the question of what conditions exist in people when judgments are made about their need for nursing care. She concluded that the human condition associated with the need for nursing is the existence of a health-related limitation in the ability of persons to provide for self the amount and quality of care required (Orem, 1985). This insight provided Orem with an answer to the question, "What is nursing's phenomenon of concern?" She identified nursing's special concern as individuals' needs for self-care and their capabilities for meeting these needs.

Reprinted from *Nursing Science Quarterly* (1997), 10(1) 26–31, with permission of F. A. Davis.

Views of Human Beings Specific to Nursing

DOROTHEA E. OREM

Nursing is commonly viewed as a human health service. In this nonspecific generalization, the term "human health service" expresses what nursing is. The term implies that there are two categories of human beings: those who need the nursing service and those who produce it. The word "service" implies that nursing is a helpful activity, and the word "health" indicates that the thrust of the service is the structural and functional integrity of persons served. A nursing-specific generalization, such as a general nursing concept or theory, gives names and roles to the two categories of human beings, attributes distinct human powers and properties to each, identifies the interactions among them, and specifies the broad structural features of the processes of producing nursing. The Nursing Development Conference Group's 1971 general conceptual model

of a nursing system demonstrates the foregoing statements (Table 12–1).

In the nursing literature, views of human beings are sometimes represented as distinct from views of nursing. It is true, of course, that one can study and think about the existence of and the nature and behaviors of human beings—men, women, children—separate and apart from thoughts about nursing. But it is not true that one can study and think about nursing without incorporating into one's thought processes nursing-specific views of human beings. The integration of views of humankind within views of nursing is the focus of this discussion.

NURSING-SPECIFIC VIEWS

The powers and properties of human beings specific to nursing are named in the Nursing Development Conference Group's general concept of nursing systems presented in Table 12–1. They are further developed in Orem's 1995 work and in earlier expressions of the Self-Care Deficit Nursing Theory, with its constituent theories of self-care, self-care deficit, and nursing system. Without question it is individual human beings, through the activation of their powers for result-seeking and result-producing endeavors, who generate the processes and systems of care named "nursing."

Nursing science is knowing and seeking to extend and deepen knowing of both the structure of the nursing processes and of the internal struc-

Table 12–1	Concepts of Nursing and Nursing Systems

A *nursing system,* like other systems for the provision of personal services, is the product of a series of relations between persons who belong to different sets (classes), the set A and the set B. From a nursing perspective any member of the set A (legitimate patient) presents evidence descriptive of the complex subsets self-care agency and therapeutic self-care demand and the condition that in A demand exceeds agency due to health or health-related causes. Any member of the set B (legitimate nurse) presents evidence descriptive of the complex subset nursing agency which includes valuation of the legitimate relations between self as *nurse* and instances where, in A, certain values of the component phenomena of self-care agency and therapeutic self-care demand prevail.

B's perceptions of the conditionality of A's subset objective therapeutic self-care demand on the subset self-care agency establishes the conditionality of changes in the states of A's two subsets on the state of and changes in the state of B's subset nursing agency. The activation of the components of the subset nursing agency (change in state) by B to deliberately control or alter the state of one or both of A's subsets—therapeutic self-care demand and self-care agency— is nursing. The perceived relations among the parts of the three subsets (actual system) constitute the organization. The "mapping" of the behaviors in "mathematical or behavioral terms" provides a record of the system.

Source: From *Concept Formalization in Nursing: Process and Product* (1979). (2nd ed., p. 107), by Nursing Development Conference Group (D. E. Orem, Ed.). Boston: Little, Brown. Copyright 1979 by Dorothea E. Orem. Reprinted with permission.

ture, constitution, and nature of the powers and properties of individuals who require nursing and individuals who produce it. Harré (1970) identifies a theory as a "statement-picture" complex that supplies an account of the constitution and behavior of those entities whose interactions with each other are responsible for the manifested patterns of behaviors. The Nursing Development Conference Group's 1971 Theory of Nursing System and the general theory of nursing (the Self-Care Deficit Nursing Theory) express both the nature of the entities and the interactions of the entities responsible for the processes, the patterns of behavior, known as nursing. Both theoretical expressions had their beginning in understandings of their formulators about the reasons why individuals need and can be helped through nursing. Such understanding marks the beginning of nursing science.

It is posited that in valid general theories of nursing, the named nursing-specific conceptualizations are the human points of reference that reveal the human properties and powers—the entities investigated in nursing science. For example, in Self-Care Deficit Nursing Theory, individuals throughout their life cycles are viewed as having a continuing demand for engagement in self-care and in care of self; the constituent action components of the demand together are named the "therapeutic self-care demand." The Theory of Self-Care (Orem, 1995) offers a theoretical explanation of this continuing action demand. Individuals also are viewed as having the human power (named "self-care agency") to develop and exercise capabilities necessary for them to know and meet the components of their therapeutic self-care demands. Nursing is required when individuals' developed and operational powers and capabilities to know and meet their own therapeutic self-care demands, in whole or in part and in time-place frames of reference (that is, their self-care agency), are not adequate because of health state or health-care-related conditions.

The idea central to these nursing-specific views of individuals is that mature human beings have learned and continue to learn to meet some or all components of their own therapeutic self-care demands and the therapeutic self-care demands of their dependents. Others can know the engagement of mature and maturing human beings in self-care and dependent-care by observing their actions in time-place frames of reference and securing subjective information about what is done and what is

not done for self and dependents, including the rationales for what is done or what is not done. Both kinds of care are time-specific entities produced by individuals.

It is known that therapeutic self-care demands and self-care agency vary qualitatively and quantitatively over time for individuals. For this reason they are identified in Self-Care Deficit Nursing Theory as "patient variables" dealt with by nurses and persons in need of nursing care within the processes through which nursing is produced. As the values of each vary, the relationship between them varies. When, for health and health-care-associated reasons, individuals' self-care agency is unequal in its development or operability for meeting their existent and changing therapeutic self-care demand, a self-care deficit exists (Orem, 1995). The real or potential existence of such a health-related deficit relationship between the care demand and power of agency is the reason why individuals require nursing care.

Self-Care Deficit Nursing Theory offers the explanation that both internal and external conditions arising from or associated with health states of individuals can bring about action limitation of individuals to engage in care of self (for example, lack of knowledge or developed skills, or lack of energy) (Orem, 1995). The presence and nature of such action limitations can set up action-deficit relationships between individuals' developed and operational powers of self-care agency and the kinds and frequencies of deliberate actions to be performed to know and meet individuals' therapeutic self-care demands in time and place frames of reference.

The power of nurses to design and produce nursing care for others is the critical power that is operative in nursing. This human power with its constituent capabilities and disposition is named "nursing agency." The centrality of nursing agency as exercised by nurses in producing nursing care is made clear in the Nursing Development Conference Group's concept of nursing system (see Table 12–1). The identification and development of the power of nurses to design and produce nursing care for others are essential elements in any valid general theory of nursing. The investigation of this power and the capabilities and conditions for its exercise are critical components of nursing science.

Nurses must be knowledgeable about and skilled in investigating and calculating individuals' therapeutic self-care demands, in determining the degrees of development and operability of self-care agency, and in estimating persons' potential for regulation of the exercise or development of their powers of self-care agency. Nurses' capabilities extend to appropriately helping individuals with health-associated self-care deficits to know and meet with appropriate assistance the components of their therapeutic self-care demands and to regulate the exercise and development of their powers of self-care agency. These outcomes of nursing are contributory to the life, health, and well-being of individuals under the care of nurses. Outcomes, of course, are related to the reasons why individuals require nursing care.

Self-Care Deficit Nursing Theory, as it has been developed, builds from expressed insights about the powers and properties of persons who need nursing care and those who produce it, to the nature and constitution of those properties, to the details of the structure of the processes of providing nursing care for individuals, and to the processes for providing nursing care in multiperson situations, including family and community (Orem, 1995). These are developments of nursing's professional-technological features. In the initial and later stages of development of this general theory of nursing, developers formally recognized that nursing is a triad of interrelated action systems: a *professional-technical system,* the existence of which is dependent on the existence of an *interpersonal system,* and a *societal system* that establishes and legitimates the contractual relationship of nurses and persons who require nursing care.

Nursing students should be helped to understand and recognize in concrete nursing practice situations the tripartite features of nursing systems and the relationships among them. Theoretical nursing science differentiates content that is specifically interpersonal from professional-technological content, and it specifies content that establishes the link between interpersonal and professional-technological features of nursing and content that establishes the validity or lack of validity of a societal-contractual system.

Societal systems usually begin or are established by specifying the contracting parties and their legitimate relationships. Initial relationships may or may not endure or be legitimate throughout nursing practice situations. There may be or should be changes in both nurses and persons contracting for the care. The societal-contractual system legitimizes the interpersonal relationships of nurses and persons seeking nursing and their next of kin or their legitimate guardians. The interpersonal system is constituted from series and sequences of interaction and communication among legitimate parties necessary for the design and production of nursing in time-place frames of reference. The professional-technological nursing system is the system of action productive of nursing. It is dependent upon the initial and continuing production of an effective interpersonal system.

Comprehensive general theories of nursing address *what* nurses do, *why* they do what they do, *who* does what, and *how* they do what they do. A valid general theory of nursing thus sets forth nursing's professional-technological features specific to the production of nursing. A general theory of nursing that addresses nursing's professional-technological features provides points of articulation with interpersonal features of nursing and sets the standards for safe, effective interpersonal systems. These features also point to the legitimacy of, or need for change in, societal-contractual systems. For the initial expression of the tripartite nature of nursing systems within the frame of Self-Care Deficit Nursing Theory, see the Nursing Development Conference Group's (1979) development of a "triad of systems."

BROADER VIEWS

Nursing-specific views of individuals fit within one or more broader views of human beings. Consider, for example, the conceptual element of self-care agency in the Self-Care Deficit Nursing Theory.

Agency within this conceptual element is understood as the human power to deliberate about, make decisions about, and deliberately engage in result-producing actions or refrain from doing so. The *self-care* portion of the conceptual element specifies that agency in this context is specific to deliberating about, making decisions about, and producing the kind of care named "self-care." Thus the concept and the term "self-care agency" stand for a specialized form of agency that demands the development of specialized knowledge and action capabilities by humans. However, the power of self-care agency is necessarily attributed to human beings viewed as *persons,* for it is individuals as persons who investigate, reason, decide, and act, exercising their human powers of agency. Thus the view of human beings as self-care agents fits within the view of human beings as persons. "Agent of action" is the general term attached to persons who act deliberately to produce a foreseen result. Within the frame of reference of Self-Care Deficit Nursing Theory, persons who deliberate about and engage in self-care are referred to as "self-care agents" and their power to do so is named "self-care agency." The power of persons who are nurses and provide nursing is named "nursing agency."

The idea is that the specialized powers and characteristic properties of human beings specified in the conceptual elements of general nursing models and theories are necessarily understood within the context of broader views of human beings. Orem (1995) and the Nursing Development Conference Group (1979) suggest five broad views of human beings that are necessary for developing understanding of the conceptual constructs of Self-Care Deficit Nursing Theory and for understanding the interpersonal and societal aspects of nursing systems. The five views are summarized as follows:

The view of person. Individual human beings are viewed as embodied persons with inherent rights that become sustained public rights who live in coexistence with other persons. A mature human being "is at once a self and a person with a distinctive I and me . . . with private, publicly viable rights and able to possess changes and pluralities without endangering his [or her] constancy or unity" (Weiss, 1980, p. 128).

The view of agent. Individual human beings are viewed as persons who can bring about conditions that do not presently exist in humans or in their environmental situations by deliberately acting using valid means or technologies to bring about foreseen and desired results.

The view of user of symbols. Individual human beings are viewed as persons who use symbols to stand for things and attach meaning to them, to formulate and express ideas, and to communicate ideas and information to others through language and other means of communication.

The view of organism. Individuals are viewed as unitary living beings who grow and develop exhibiting biological characteristics of *Homo sapiens* during known stages of the human life cycle.

The view of object. Individual human beings are viewed as having the status of object subject to physical forces whenever they are unable to act to protect themselves against such forces. Inability of individuals to surmount physical forces, such as wind or forces of gravity, can arise from both the individual and prevailing environmental conditions.

The person view is central to and an integrating force for understanding and using the other four views. All other views are subsumed by the person view. The person view also is the view essential to understanding nursing as a triad of action systems. It is the view that nurses use (or should use) in all interpersonal contacts with individuals under nursing care and with their family and friends.

The person-as-agent view is the essential operational view in understanding nursing. If there is nursing, nursing agency is developed and operational. If there is self-care on the part of individuals, self-care agency is developed and operational. The agent view incorporates not only discrete deliberate actions to achieve foreseen results and the structure of processes to do so, but also the powers and capabilities of persons who are the agents or actors. The internal structure, the constitution, and the nature of the powers of nursing agency and self-care agency are content elements of nursing science. The structure of the processes of designing and producing nursing and self-care is also nursing science content.

The view of person as user of symbols is essential in understanding the nature of interpersonal systems of interaction and communication between nurses and persons who seek and receive nursing. The age and developmental state, culture, and experiences of persons receiving nursing care affect their use of symbols and the meaning they attach to events internal and external to them. The ability of nurses to be with and communicate effectively with persons receiving care and with their families incorporates the use of meaningful language and other forms of communication, knowledge of appropriate social-cultural practices, and willingness to search out the meaning of what persons receiving care are endeavoring to communicate.

The user-of-symbol view is relevant to how nurses communicate with other nurses and other health-care workers. Ideally, nurses use the language of nursing and at the same time understand and use the language of disciplines that articulate with nursing. The lack of a nursing language has been a handicap in nurses' communications about nursing to the public as well as to persons with whom they work in the health field. There can be no nursing language until the features of humankind specific to nursing are conceptualized and named and their structure uncovered.

Men, women, and children are unitary beings. They are embodied persons, and nurses must be knowing about their biological and psychobiological features. Viewing human beings as organisms brings into focus the internal structure, the constitution and nature of those human features that are the foci of the life sciences. Knowing human beings as agents or users of symbols has foundations in biology and psychology. Understanding human organic functioning, including its aberrations, requires knowledge of human physiology, environmental physiology, pathology, and other developed and developing sciences.

The object view of individual human beings is a view taken by nurses whenever they provide nursing for infants, young children, or adults unable to control their positions and movement in space and who contend with physical forces in their environment. This includes the inability to ward off physical force exerted against them by other human beings. Taking the object view carries with it a requirement for protective care of persons subject to such forces. The features of protective care are understood in terms of impending or existent environmental forces and known incapacities of individuals to manage and defend themselves in their environments, as well as in the nursing-specific views of individuals that nurses take in concrete nursing practice situations.

These five broad views of human beings subsume nursing-specific views, and they aid in understanding them and in revealing their constitution and nature. These broad views point to the sciences and disciplines of knowledge that nurses must be knowing in, and have some mastery of, in order to be effective practitioners of nursing. Establishing the linkages of nursing-specific views of human beings to the named broader views is a task of nursing scholars.

Throughout the processes of giving nursing care to individuals or multiperson units, such as families, nurses use changing combinations of the named views of human beings in accord with presenting conditions and circumstances. Nurses also may need to help individuals under nursing care to take these views about themselves. As previously stated, the person view is the guiding force.

The five described views of individual human beings also come into play when nurses think about and deal with themselves in nursing situations. They know that they have rights as persons and as nurses and that they must defend and safeguard these personal and professional rights; their powers of nursing agency must be adequate to fulfill responsibilities to meet nursing requirements of persons under their care; they must know their deficiencies, act to overcome them, or secure help to make up for them; they must be protective of their own biological well-being and act to safeguard themselves from harmful environmental forces. Nurses also have requirements for knowing nursing and articulating fields in a dynamic way. There is also a need for a nursing language that is enabling for thinking nursing within its domain and boundaries and in its articulation with other disciplines and for communicating nursing to others in nursing practice situations.

MODEL BUILDING AND THEORY DEVELOPMENT

The previously described nursing-specific views of individual human beings are necessary for understanding and identifying (1) when and why individuals need and can be helped through nursing; and (2) the structure of the processes through which the help needed is determined and produced. Nurses' continuing development of their knowing about the person, agent, symbolist, organism, and object views of individuals is essential continuing education for themselves as nurses and as nursing scholars.

Such knowing is foundational to model making and theory development in nursing. For example, Louise Hartnett-Rauckhorst (1968) developed models to make explicit what is involved physiologically and psychologically in voluntary, deliberate human action, including motor behaviors. She moved from available authoritative knowledge in the fields of physiology, psychology, and the broad field of human behavior to develop:

- A basic psychological model of action with three submodels:

  The personal frame of reference of the basic psychologic model of action.

  The veridical (coinciding with reality) frame of reference of the basic psychologic model of action.

  The sociocultural frame of reference of the basic psychologic model of action.

- A physiologic model of action.

The Hartnett-Rauckhorst theoretical models set forth structural features of the process of voluntary human action (that is, deliberate action). These models develop the agent view; however, their structure reflects the person, the user of symbols, and the organism views of individual human beings (Nursing Development Conference Group, 1979).

The study of these and other general theoretical models of deliberate action stimulated some members of the Nursing Development Conference Group to investigate and formalize the conceptual structure of self-care agency, conceptualizing it as the developed power to engage in a specific kind of deliberate action. The goal of these efforts was the construction of models to identify types of relevant information and to aid in the development of techniques for collection and analysis of data about self-care agency. By 1979, the following theoretical models were developed:

1. A model of self-care operations, and estimative, decision making, and productive operations and their results.
2. A model of power components operationally involved with and enabling for performance of self-care operations.
3. A model of human capabilities and dispositions foundational for:
   a. the development and operability of the power components.
   b. the performance of the self-care operations in time and place frames of reference.

(Refer to Orem, 1995, for descriptions of these models and highlights of their development.)

When considered together in their articulations, the three theoretical models that are descriptive and explanatory of self-care agency constitute the elements for process models of the operation of self-care agency, a process with a specified structure. The first model, self-care operations, is modeled on deliberate action. The power component model names specific enabling capabilities necessary for performing each of the named operations. (*Capabilities* are powers that can be developed or lost without a substantial change in the possessor of the power.) The foundational capabilities and dispositions model expresses physiologically or psychologically described capabilities and dispositions that permit for or facilitate or hinder persons' performance of self-care operations or the development or adequacy of the power components.

The nursing-specific view that every individual human being has a therapeutic self-care demand to be continuously met over time was conceptually developed through the construction of theoretical models using the broad views of human beings. Models of categories of constituent care requisites within the demand (universal, developmental, and health deviation types) were developed as well as a model to show the constituent content elements of a therapeutic self-care demand and their derivation (Orem, 1995). A process model of the structural elements of an action system to meet a specific self-care requisite particularized for an individual was developed as an example of what actions must be performed to meet each of the self-care requisites of individuals.

These models express the content elements of the conceptual entity therapeutic self-care demand. The models also express the derivation of the content elements, the relationships among them, and the regulatory results sought. The therapeutic self-care demand models represent what is to be known and met by individuals through their exercise of self-care agency or met for them when required by reason of self-care agency limitations.

These examples of models demonstrate that nursing theorists and scholars involved in development of Self-Care Deficit Nursing Theory used both nursing-specific and more general views of individual human beings in the process of model building. The examples also demonstrate that in model development, theorists used knowledge from more than one science or discipline of knowledge. The subjects of the models (namely, nursing systems, deliberate action, self-care agency, and therapeutic self-care demand) also differed from the sources and content elements of the respective models.

The models are offered as a means toward understanding the reality of the named entities in concrete nursing practice situations. Despite the diversity of these models, they are all directed toward knowing the structure of the processes that are operational or become operational in the production of nursing systems, systems of care for individuals or for dependent-care units or multiperson units served by nurses.

For information about models and scientific growth involving development of knowledge in individual scientists, see Wallace (1983) and Harré (1970). Black's *Models and Metaphors* (1962) was the source first used by the writer.

SUMMARY

The use of specific views of human beings by nurses or persons in other disciplines does not negate their acceptance of the unity, the oneness of each individual man, woman, or child. In human sciences, specific views of human beings identify the domain and boundaries of the science within the broad frames of humanity and society. In nursing, for example, the views of human beings expressed in Self-Care Deficit Nursing Theory identified the proper object of nursing and were enabling for the development and structuring of nursing knowledge.

Science, including models and theories, is about existent entities. A valid comprehensive theory of nursing has as its reality base individuals who need and receive nursing care and those who produce it, as well as the events of its production. Nursing exists in human societies and is something produced by human beings for other human beings when known conditions and relationships prevail. It is posited that the life experiences of nursing theorists, their observations and judgments about the world of nurses, can and do result in insights about nursing that can lead to descriptions and explanations of the human health-care service of nursing.

Nurses and nursing students who are confronted with tasks of reviewing, studying, mastering, or taking positions about extant general models or nursing theories should look for and identify the view(s) of human beings being expressed or implicit in them. The adequacy of the theories should be explored. Models and theories that purport to be general models of nursing can be adequate or deficient in their scope as related to expressing why people need and can be helped through nursing or in describing and explaining the structure of nursing processes.

In any practice field, a general model or theory incorporates not only the what and the why, but also the who and the how. The adequacy of a general theory comes into question when there is omission of any one of the named elements. The validity and specificity of theories referred to as nursing theories are in question when there is no reference to the human condition that gives rise to needs for nursing on the part of individuals, to the presence and the powers of persons qualified as nurses, to the structure of processes of production of nursing, and to the results sought.

What comes first, the view of humankind or the view of nursing in the cognitional processes of theorists, is a moot question. The writer's position is that a theorist's life experiences in and accumulated knowledge of nursing practice situations support the recognition and naming of nursing-specific views of human beings. Nursing-specific views of individual human beings are differentiated from those general views that are relevant to all the health services or even to human existence. Such general views include the view of human beings as energy fields, as living health, as culture-oriented, or as caring beings. Such general views, however helpful in understanding humankind or in identifying approaches to data collection, do not and cannot support viable nursing science, theoretical and practical.

References

Black, M. (1962). *Models and metaphors.* Ithaca, NY: Cornell University Press.

Harré, R. (1970). *The principles of scientific thinking.* Chicago: University of Chicago Press.

Fawcett, J. (2000). *Contemporary Nursing Knowledge: Analysis and evaluation of nursing models and theories.* 2nd ed. Philadelphia: F. A. Davis.

Hartnett-Rauckhorst, L. (1968). *Development of a theoretical model for the identification of nursing requirements in a selected aspect of self-care.* Unpublished master's thesis, Catholic University of America, Washington, DC.

Nursing Development Conference Group. (1979). *Concept formalization in nursing: Process and product* (2nd ed., Orem, D. E., Ed.). Boston: Little, Brown.

Orem, D. E. (1995). *Nursing: Concepts of practice.* St. Louis: Mosby-Year Book.

Orem, D. E. (1985).

Wallace, W. A. (1983). *From a realist point of view: Essays on the philosophy of science.* Washington, DC: University Press of America.

Weiss, P. (1980). *You, I, and the others.* Carbondale, IL: Southern Illinois University Press.

PART TWO:
Applications of Dorothea Orem's Self-Care Deficit Nursing Theory

Marjorie A. Isenberg

Research

Practice

Summary

References

*A*ccording to Orem (2001), it is the special focus on human beings that distinguishes or differentiates nursing from other human services. From this point of view, the role of nursing in society is to enable individuals to develop and exercise their self-care abilities to the extent that they can provide for themselves the amount and quality of care required. According to the theory, individuals whose requirements for self-care exceed their capabilities for engaging in self-care are said to be experiencing a self-care deficit. Moreover, it is the presence of an existing or potential self-care deficit that identifies those persons in need of nursing. Thus, Orem's Self-Care Deficit Nursing Theory explains when and why nursing is required.

Orem (2001) describes the Self-Care Deficit Nursing Theory as a general theory of nursing. General theories of nursing are applicable across all practice situations in which persons need nursing care. As such, the Self-Care Deficit Nursing Theory describes and explains the key concepts common to all nursing practice situations (Orem, 1995). The theory consists of four concepts about persons under the care of nurses, two nurse-related concepts, and three interrelated theories (the Theory of Nursing Systems, the Theory of Self-Care Deficit, and the Theory of Self-Care). Concepts in the general theory include, self-care, self-care agency, therapeutic self-care demand, self-care deficit, nursing agency, and nursing systems. The theory describes and explains the relationship between the capabilities of individuals to engage in self-care (self-care agency) and their requirements for self-care (therapeutic self-care demand). The term "deficit" refers to a particular relationship between self-care agency and self-care demand that is said to exist when capabilities for engaging in self-care are *less than* the demand for self-care.

The comprehensive development of the self-care concepts enhances the usefulness of the Self-Care Deficit Nursing Theory as a guide to nursing practice situations involving individuals across the life span who are experiencing health or illness, and to nurse-client situations aimed at health promotion, health restoration, or health maintenance.

According to this theory, nurses use their specialized capabilities to create a helping system in

> *Nurses use their specialized capabilities to create a helping system in situations where persons are deemed to have an existent or potential self-care deficit.*

situations where persons are deemed to have an existent or potential self-care deficit. Decisions about what type of nursing system is appropriate in a given nursing practice situation rests with the answer to the question, "Who can and should perform the self-care operations?" (Orem, 2001, p. 350). When the answer is the nurse, a wholly compensatory system of helping is appropriate. When it is concluded that the patient can and should perform all self-care actions, the nurse assumes a supportive-educative role and designs a nursing system accordingly. In nursing practice situations, the goal of nursing is to empower the person to meet their self-care requirements by doing for (wholly compensatory system), doing with (partly compensatory system), or developing agency (supportive-educative system).

This chapter focuses on the extent to which Orem's theory is offering direction to nurse scholars and scientists in advancing nursing science and professional practice. Dorothy Johnson (1959), in her treatise on nursing theory development, viewed this attribute of a theory as its value for the profession, its *social utility*.

Research

Dorothea Orem's theory is offering clear direction to nurses in the advancement of nursing science in this millennium. Orem describes nursing as a practical science that is comprised of both theoretical and practical knowledge, a point of view that is grounded in modern realism (2001, p. 170). There are parallels between Orem's description of nursing as a practical science and Donaldson and Crowley's discussion of nursing as a professional discipline. Recall that Donaldson and Crowley (1978) stated that the aim of professional disciplines is to know and to *use* knowledge to achieve the practical goal of the discipline. Both perspectives address the need for nurses to develop both theoretical and practical knowledge.

Orem (2001, p. 170) has identified a model comprised of five stages for nursing science development. Each stage is intended to yield different kinds of knowledge about persons with existent or potential health-related self-care deficits. Stages 1 and 2 of this developmental schema for science focus on the advancement of the theoretical component of nursing science. The theory is the result of Stage 1. Stage 2 is described as the study of con-

current variations between the concepts proposed within the Self-Care Deficit Nursing Theory for the purpose of verifying and further explicating the propositions (Orem, 2001, p. 171). The propositions of the Self-Care Deficit Nursing Theory provide direction to nursing researchers who aim to focus their inquiry in theory-based research.

Numerous examples of research illustrating scientific inquiry at the Stage 2 level of development are contained in the nursing literature. The aspect of the Self-Care Deficit Nursing Theory that has generated the most research of this type is the relationship posited between basic conditioning factors and self-care agency. The basic conditioning factors were identified initially by the Nursing Development Conference Group (1979) and were formalized later in a proposition linking them to self-care agency. The second proposition listed in the Self-Care Deficit Nursing Theory states that individuals' abilities to engage in self-care (self-care agency) are conditioned by age, developmental state, life experiences, sociocultural orientation, health, and available resources (Orem, 2001, p. 167). This proposition offers direction to nurses interested in engaging in theory-based research.

Basic conditioning factors are defined as "conditions or events in a time-place matrix that affect the value of person's abilities to care for themselves" (Orem). It is important to note that the influence of the basic conditioning factors on self-care agency is not assumed to be operative at all times. Nor are all the basic conditioning factors assumed to be operative at all times. Because the influence of these factors occurs within a time-place matrix, research is necessary to identify those nursing practice situations in which the factors are operative and to explain the nature of their influence on self-care agency. Based upon research findings, relationships between the basic conditioning factors and the substantive structure of self-care agency can then be made explicit. Programs of research designed in this way can verify the existence of linkages between these concepts and can explain the nature of the linkages. Scholarly work of this type is vital to the advancement of the theoretical knowledge of nursing science.

Over the past decade, nurse researchers have studied the influence of basic conditioning factors, singularly and in combination, on individuals' self-care abilities. Foremost among the basic conditioning factors studied is health state. Several studies designed to determine the nature of the influence of variations in health state on self-care abilities are reported in the research literature. Research suggests that this relationship is particularly salient in practice situations in which persons are experiencing chronic health problems. The work of selected investigators is presented here to exemplify this line of inquiry. The influence of change in health state on the self-care abilities of persons with coronary artery disease has been studied with both American and Dutch adult patient populations (Isenberg, 1991; Isenberg, Evers, & Brouns, 1987). Across these studies, changes in health state were found to be critical determinants of the quality of the self-care abilities of this patient population. As the health state of patients improved, so did their capabilities for self-care. Conversely, self-care capabilities tended to decline as patients experienced recurrence of pain and declining health. The findings revealed a positive relationship between health state and self-care agency in patients with cardiac disease.

In addition to the study of variation in health state due to pathophysiology, the conditioning influence of health state on self-care agency has also been explored in situations in which the variation in health state is due to psychopathology. West (1993) investigated the influence of clinical variations in the level of depression, conceptualized as a health-state factor, on the self-care abilities of young American women. West (1993) reported that of the basic conditioning factors studied, the level of depression (health state) was the dominant predictor of the quality of the self-care abilities of her sample. In a study with Dutch psychiatric patients, Brouns (1991) also reported that variations in mental health state significantly influenced patients' self-care capabilities. In both studies a positive relationship between health state and self-care agency was revealed. Higher levels of mental health were correlated with higher self-care agency scores. These findings verified the conditioning influence of health state on the self-care agency of patients' experience variations in physical and mental health. Moreover, the research findings clarified the nature of the influence of health state on self-care agency.

The conditioning influence of other basic factors on the self-care abilities of clinical and non-clinical populations has been the focus of inquiry of several nurse scholars. For example, Brugge

(1981) studied the influence of family as a social support system on the self-care agency of adults with diabetes mellitus. Vannoy (1989) explored the influence of basic conditioning factors on the self-care agency of persons enrolled in a weight-loss program. Schott-Baer (1989) studied the influence of family variables and caregiver variables on the self-care abilities of the spouses of patients with a cancer diagnosis. Baker (1991) explored the predictive effect of basic conditioning factors on the self-care agency and self-care in adolescents with cystic fibrosis. McQuiston (1993) investigated the influence of basic conditioning factors on the self-care capabilities of unmarried women at risk for sexually transmitted disease. Horsburgh (1994) conceptualized personality as a basic conditioning factor and tested the model with a healthy population and a comparative clinical population with chronic renal disease. O'Connor (1995) studied the influence of basic conditioning factors on the self-care abilities of a healthy and clinical adult population enrolled in a nurse-managed primary care clinic. Baiardi (1997) explored the influence of health state and caregiving factors on the self-care agency of the caregivers of cognitively impaired elders. Artinian, Magnan, Sloan, and Lange (2002) examined the influence of personal and environmental factors on the self-care behaviors among patients with congestive heart failure.

THEORY VERIFICATION AND SPECIFIC CLINICAL POPULATIONS

Opportunities to test elements of the Self-Care Deficit Nursing Theory have been greatly enhanced by the measurement work with self-care concepts that has transpired over the past 20 years. It is important to note that the theory-testing studies cited above were made possible by the development and psychometric testing of instruments to measure the theoretical concepts. Instruments are currently available to measure the self-care agency of adolescent populations (Denyes, 1982), adult populations (Evers, Isenberg, Philipsen, Senten, & Brouns, 1993; Geden & Taylor, 1991; Hanson & Bickel, 1985), and elderly populations (Biggs, 1990). The availability of valid and reliable measures of self-care agency has been vital to the advancement of the theoretical component of self-care nursing science.

In addition to the theory verification line of

research, the Self-Care Deficit Nursing Theory is being used to guide research programs to identify the self-care requisites and self-care behaviors of specific clinical populations. Intervention studies designed to enhance self-care performance are also under way. For example, Dodd has launched a program of research focused on the self-care of cancer patients who were receiving chemotherapy or radiation therapy. Her early descriptive studies clarified the health-deviation self-care requisites of this population and documented the therapeutic self-care demand (Dodd, 1982, 1984). More recent work described specific self-care behaviors initiated by patients receiving these therapies and led to the identification of a patient profile of self-care that can be used in practice to target specific patient groups who are in most need of nursing interventions (Dodd, 1997). Dodd's intervention studies demonstrated that with targeted information, patients can learn more about their treatment and can perform more effective self-care behaviors (Dodd, 1997). Her work has advanced to conducting randomized control trials to test a self-care intervention called PRO-SELF© to decrease chemotherapy-related morbidity (Dodd, 1997). Through her 20-year program of descriptive, predictive, and intervention studies based on self-care theory, Dodd's research has demonstrated how to enhance patients' knowledge of their treatment and how to increase effective self-care activities. Dodd clearly qualifies as a pioneer in self-care theory-based research.

Investigators have used Orem's theory to identify the self-care requisites and self-care capabilities of patients across a broad range of health deviations. Based on the theory, Utz and Ramos (1993) have conducted a sequence of studies to explore and describe the self-care needs of people with symptomatic mitral valve prolapse. The self-care capabilities and the self-care needs (requisites) of persons with rheumatoid arthritis have also been described. The most frequently reported universal self-care requisites for these clients were the maintenance of a balance between activity and rest, the promotion of normalcy, and the prevention of hazards (Ailinger & Dear, 1997). Duration of illness (health state) and educational level were found to be related to self-care agency (Ailinger & Dear, 1993). Aish (1993) tested the effect of an Orem-based nursing intervention on the nutritional self-care of myocardial infarction patients. A supportive-educative nursing system was reported to be effective in promoting healthy low-fat eating behavior (Aish, 1993). Metcalfe (1996) studied the therapeutic self-care demand, self-care agency, and the self-care actions of individuals with chronic obstructive lung disease. Health state was found to offer significant explanation of variations in the self-care actions of this population. Based on the universal, developmental, and health deviation self-care requisites, Riley (1996) developed a tool to measure the performance and frequency of the self-care actions of patients with chronic obstructive lung disease. This tool has the potential to be useful as an outcome measure in future intervention studies designed to enhance the self-care abilities of this population.

Moore (1995) has used the Self-Care Deficit Nursing Theory as the basis for her program of research with children. She has developed the Child and Adolescent Self-Care Practice questionnaire, which can be used to assess the self-care performance of children and adolescents. In a study of children with cancer, Mosher and Moore (1998) reported a significant relationship between self-concept and self-care. Children with higher self-concept scores were found to perform more self-care activities than children with low self-concept scores (Mosher & Moore, 1998).

THE CROSS-CULTURAL AND INTERNATIONAL RESEARCH APPLICATIONS

The utility of the Self-Care Deficit Nursing Theory beyond our national borders can be explained in

> *The utility of the Self-Care Deficit Nursing Theory beyond our national borders can be explained in part by the fact that Orem's intention was to develop a general theory of nursing that would be useful in describing and explaining universal nursing knowledge.*

part by the fact that Orem's intention was to develop a general theory of nursing that would be useful in describing and explaining universal nursing knowledge. The theory's applicability beyond Western civilizations may be further explained by the inclusion of culture as a primary influence on people's care beliefs and practices. According to the theory, "self-care" is described as learned behavior, and the activities of self-care are learned according to the beliefs and practices that characterize the cultural way of life of the group to which the individual belongs (Orem, 2001). The individual first learns about cultural standards within the family. Thus, the self-care practices that individuals employ should be understood and examined by nurses within the cultural context of social groups and within the health-care systems of societal groups. The theory provides a means to study the types of self-care needs identified by specific cultural groups and the acceptable cultural self-care practices to meet the needs (Meleis, Isenberg, Koerner, Lacey, & Stern, 1995).

In contrast to these studies that are focused on clinical populations experiencing health deviation self-care requisites, Hartweg's research centers on health promotion and has been extended cross-culturally. Hartweg (1990) conceptualized health promotion self-care within Orem's Self-Care Deficit Nursing Theory and went on to explore through a descriptive study the self-care actions performed by healthy middle-aged women to promote well-being. The women studied were able to identify over 8,000 diverse self-care actions, the majority of which were related to the universal self-care requisites (Hartweg, 1993). The interview guide used with this American population has recently been validated with healthy, middle-aged Mexican American women in a comparative study (Hartweg & Berbiglia, 1996). Whetstone (1987) and Whetstone and Hansson (1989) also conducted cross-cultural comparative studies using self-care concepts. They compared the meanings of self-care among Americans, German, and Swedish populations.

In addition to the cross-cultural comparative research, the Self-Care Deficit Nursing Theory is being applied in studies with specific cultural groups. In an ethnographic study based on concepts within Orem's theory, Villarruel (1995) explored the cultural meanings, expressions, self-care, and dependent care actions related to pain with a Mexican American population and commented on the theory's use with this population. Dashiff (1992) applied Orem's theory in her description of the self-care capabilities of young African American women prior to menarche.

Nurse scientists beyond our national borders are currently using the Self-Care Deficit Nursing Theory as a basis for their research. Professor Georges Evers at the Catholic University of Leuven in Belgium has developed an extensive program of research based on the theory. His program includes descriptive and explanatory studies of the self-care requisites and self-care capabilities of diverse clinical populations, the development and psychometric testing of instruments to measure self-care concepts, and the testing of interventions to enhance self-care performance (Evers, 1998).

Orem's theory is also being applied by Jaarsma and colleagues as a basis for an ongoing program of research with cardiac patients in the Netherlands. Using a questionnaire derived from the self-care requisites described in the Self-Care Deficit Nursing Theory, Jaarsma, Kastermans, Dassen, and Philipsen (1995) identified problems frequently encountered by cardiac patients in the early recovery phase from coronary artery bypass surgery or myocardial infarction. With a population of patients with advanced heart failure, Jaarsma, Halfens, Senten, Saad, and Dracup (1998) identified the therapeutic self-care demand of this population and then developed a supportive-educative program designed to enhance their self-care abilities.

The global nature of this theory is apparent. The book *Nursing: Concepts of Practice* (Orem, 1985) has been translated into Dutch, French, German, Italian, Spanish, and Japanese. Records cited in a CINAHL index search of the nursing literature included publications describing the application of the Self-Care Deficit Nursing Theory in nursing situations in Australia, Belgium, Denmark, Finland, Germany, the Netherlands, Norway, Portugal, Sweden, Switzerland, the United Kingdom, Hong Kong, Taiwan, Thailand, Turkey, Canada, Mexico, the United States, and Puerto Rico.

Moreover, over the past 15 years, the author has been privileged to be a part of an international network of nurse scholars and scientists focused on the development of disciplinary knowledge derived from the Self-Care Deficit Nursing Theory. Our collaborative work began in 1983 when the author was invited as a consultant to the faculty of health sciences at the University of Maastricht in the Netherlands to assist faculty and students in developing programs of nursing theory–based research. Initially, our work focused primarily on the teaching of nursing science seminars for nurses throughout the Netherlands. In 1986, we extended the seminars to include nurses from all parts of Europe.

Over the subsequent five years, approximately 200 nurses from 12 European countries participated in the seminars. The participants studied the Self-Care Deficit Nursing Theory, research methodology, and the interrelatedness of theory and research. Each participant developed a self-care theory-based research project that could be implemented in his or her home settings.

Our first collaborative research project involved the development of an instrument to measure Orem's theoretical concept of self-care agency. The English and Dutch versions of the Appraisal of Self-Care Agency (ASA) Scale were the products of this endeavor. To date, the ASA Scale has been translated and validated for research use with populations in the following countries: Belgium, Denmark, Finland, Canada (French-speaking), Germany, Norway, Sweden, Switzerland (German-speaking), Japan, Korea, Thailand, Turkey, and Mexico.

This collaborative project provided the team with the opportunity to identify universal nursing knowledge and, by means of transnational comparisons, identify culture-specific knowledge. The current shared programs of research focus on: (1) influences of aging on the self-care abilities of Americans (Jirovec & Kasno, 1990), Canadians (Ward-Griffin & Bramwell, 1990), Danes (Lorensen, Holter, Evers, Isenberg, & Van Achterberg, 1993), Dutch (Evers, Isenberg, Philipsen, Senten, & Brouns, 1993), Finns (Katainen, Merlainen, & Isenberg, 1993), Norwegians (Van Achterberg et al., 1991), and Swedes (Soderhamn, Evers, & Hamrin, 1996); and (2) influence of chronic health problems, such as coronary artery disease, on the self-care abilities of Americans (Isenberg, 1987, 1993), Canadians (Aish & Isenberg, 1996), and Dutch clients (Isenberg, 1993; Isenberg, Evers, & Brouns, 1987; Senten, Evers, Isenberg, & Philipsen, 1991). Using the Mexican version of the ASA Scale to measure self-care agency, Professor Esther Gallegos at the University of Nuevo Leon in Monterrey, Mexico, recently completed a study of the influence of social, family, and individual conditioning factors on the self-care abilities and practices of Mexican women. The results of her study indicated that health state was the predominant predictor of women's self-care agency and self-care performance (Gallegos, 1997). The level of poverty experienced by the Mexican women also had a significant influence on their self-care performance.

One of the challenges of international collaborative research deals with establishing sources for funding to carry out the scientific work. The research work cited above was funded in part by a variety of agencies: the Netherlands Heart Foundation, the Swiss National Fund, Fulbright Scholarship, Finnish Academy of Science, and the Kellogg Foundation. Our collaborative work was further enhanced by the generous support that each of us received from our respective institutions: Wayne State University, United States; University of Maastricht, the Netherlands; Catholic University of Leuven, Belgium; University of Oslo, Norway; University of Nuevo Leon, Mexico; St. Gallen Hospital, Switzerland; and University of Kuopio, Finland.

To this network of nurse scientists, international collaboration has provided an opportunity and a means to pursue a shared vision and address a shared challenge. By means of shared ideas, resources, research designs, and instruments, we are advancing nursing science derived from the Self-Care Deficit Nursing Theory. To date, specific propositions of the theory have been tested in nine countries. Through this theory testing program of research, data are being accrued that will provide answers to the question, "To what extent is the Self-Care Deficit Nursing Theory relevant to the global community?" The findings of the transnational comparative studies are identifying universal elements of the theory and suggest that the translated versions of the ASA Scale are cross-nationally valid.

Furthermore, the idea to organize a forum for self-care scientists and scholars originated with this group. In 1991, the International Orem Society for Nursing Science and Scholarship was founded. The society's mission is to advance nursing science and scholarship through the use of Dorothea E. Orem's nursing conceptualizations in nursing education, practice, and research. The society cosponsors a Biennial International Self-Care Conference with the University of Columbia, Missouri, and publishes a quarterly newsletter, which has recently been expanded to a journal.

Practice

In this section, we focus on the ways in which the Self-Care Deficit Nursing Theory is guiding nursing research because the theory's utility to nursing practice is well-documented in the literature. Nonetheless, it would be remiss not to comment on the extensive applications of the theory to nursing practice. Since the pioneering efforts of Crews (1972) and Backscheider (1974) in the use of the theory in structuring and organizing nursing care to patients in nurse-managed clinics, nurse scholars have been proclaiming the usefulness of the theory as a guide to practice. The theory has been used to guide practice across a wide range of nursing situations in all types of care settings, ranging from neonatal intensive care units (Tolentino, 1990) to nursing home facilities (Anna, Christensen, Hohon, Ord, & Wells, 1978). The theory's relevance to the care of patients in intensive care units has also been examined. Jacobs (1990) concluded that although most patients require wholly compensatory systems of care, patient situations do exist in which partly compensatory or supportive-educative systems of care are more appropriate.

Orem-based nursing practice has been extensively described in the care of patients of various ages with all kinds of health-deviation self-care requisites and developmental requisites. For example, the theory has been applied to the long-term care of ambulatory adolescent transplant recipients. Nursing services based on Orem's theory were found to significantly enhance the quality of life of this adolescent population (Norris, 1991). Haas (1990) also reported on the usefulness of the Self-Care Deficit Nursing Theory as a basis for nursing practice aimed at meeting the care demands of children with long-term chronic health problems. Clearly, the extent of the documentation of this work far exceeds the scope of this chapter. Selected citations appear in the bibliography.

SUMMARY

Dorothea E. Orem contended that identification of nursing's focus would enhance the productivity of nurse scholars and scientists. She set forth the premise that the Self-Care Deficit Nursing Theory was the foundation for developing nursing science, and then described her views of nursing science. The abundance of Orem-based research documented in the literature today supports the validity of her convictions and the social utility of the theory for the profession in guiding the research and scholarship of nurses worldwide.

References

Ailinger, R. L., & Dear, M. R. (1993). Self-care agency in persons with rheumatoid arthritis. *Arthritis Care and Research, 6*(3), 134–140.

Ailinger, R. L., & Dear, M. R. (1997). An examination of the self-care needs of clients with rheumatoid arthritis . . . including commentary by Popovich, J. *Rehabilitation Nursing, 22*(3), 135–140.

Aish, A. E. (1993). *An investigation of a nursing system to support nutritional self-care in post myocardial infarction patients.* Unpublished doctoral dissertation, Wayne State University, Detroit.

Aish, A. E., & Isenberg, M. A. (1996). Effects of Orem-based nursing intervention on nutritional self-care of myocardial infarction patients. *International Journal of Nursing Studies, 33*(3), 259–270.

Anna, D. J., Christensen, D. G., Hohon, S. A., Ord, L., & Wells, S. R. (1978). Implementing Orem's conceptual framework. *Journal of Nursing Administration, 8*(11), 8–11.

Artinian, N. T., Magnan, M., Sloan, M., and Lange, M. P. (2002). Self-care behaviors among patients with heart failure. *Heart Lung, 31*(3), 161–172.

Backscheider, J. E. (1974). Self-care requirements, self-care capabilities and nursing systems in the diabetic nurse management clinic. *American Journal of Public Health, 64*, 1138–1146.

Baiardi, J. (1997). *The influence of health status, burden, and degree of cognitive impairment on the self-care agency and dependent-care agency of caregivers of elders.* Unpublished doctoral dissertation, Wayne State University, Detroit.

Baker, L. K. (1991). *Predictors of self-care in adolescents with cystic fibrosis: A test and explication of Orem's theories of self-care and self-care deficit.* Unpublished doctoral dissertation, Wayne State University, Detroit.

Biggs, A. J. (1990). Family caregiver versus nursing assessments of elderly self-care abilities. *Journal of Gerontological Nursing, 16*(8), 11–16.

Black, M. (1962). *Models and metaphors.* Ithaca, NY: Cornell University Press.

Brouns, G. (1991). *Self-care agency of psychiatric patients: A validity and reliability study of the ASA-Scale.* Unpublished master's thesis, University of Limburg, Maastricht, the Netherlands.

Brugge, P. (1981). *The relationship between family as a social support system, health status, and exercise of self-care agency in the adult with a chronic illness.* Unpublished doctoral dissertation, Wayne State University, Detroit.

Crews, J. (1972). Nurse-managed cardiac clinics. *Cardio-Vascular Nursing, 8*, 15–18.

Dashiff, C. J. (1992). Self-care capabilities in black girls in anticipation of menarche. *Health Care for Women International, 13*(1), 67–76.

Denyes, M. J. (1982). Measurement of self-care agency in adolescents. *Nursing Research, 31*, 63.

Dodd, M. J. (1982). Assessing patient self-care for side effects of cancer chemotherapy—part 1. *Cancer Nursing, 5*, 447–451.

Dodd, M. J. (1984). Patterns of self-care in cancer patients receiving radiation therapy. *Oncology Nursing Forum, 11*, 23–27.

Dodd, M. J. (1997). Self-care: Ready or not! *Oncology Nursing Forum, 24*(6), 983–990.

Donaldson, S. K., & Crowley, D. M. (1978). The discipline of nursing. *Nursing Outlook, 26*(2), 113–120.

Evers, G. (1998). *Meten van zelfzorg: Verpleegkundige instrumenten voor onderzoek en klinische praktijk.* [Measurement of Self-Care: Nursing instruments for research in clinical practice.] Belgium: Universitaire Pers Leuven.

Evers, G. C. M., Isenberg, M. A., Philipsen, H., Senten, M., & Brouns, G. (1993). Validity testing of the Dutch translation of the appraisal of the self-care agency ASA-scale. *International Journal of Nursing Studies, 30*(4), 331–342.

Fawcett, J. (1995). *Analysis and evaluation of conceptual models of nursing.* Philadelphia: F. A. Davis.

Gallegos, E. (1997). *The effect of social, family and individual conditioning factors on self-care agency and universal self-care of adult Mexican women.* Unpublished doctoral dissertation, Wayne State University, Detroit.

Geden, E., & Taylor, S. (1991). Construct and empirical validity of the self-as-carer inventory. *Nursing Research, 40*(1), 47–50.

Haas, D. L. (1990). Application of Orem's self-care deficit theory to the pediatric chronically ill population. *Issues in Comprehensive Pediatric Nursing, 13,* 253–264.

Hanson, B. R., & Bickel, L. (1985). Development and testing of the questionnaire on perception of self-care agency. In Riehl-Sisca, J. (Ed.), *The science and art of self-care* (pp. 271–278). Norwalk, CT: Appleton-Century-Crofts.

Hanucharurnkul, S. (1989). Predictors of self-care in cancer patients receiving radiotherapy. *Cancer Nursing, 12*(1), 21–27.

Harré, R. (1970). *The principles of scientific thinking.* Chicago: University of Chicago Press.

Hartnett-Rauckhorst, L. (1968). *Development of a theoretical model for the identification of nursing requirements in a selected aspect of self-care.* Unpublished master's thesis, Catholic University of America, Washington, DC.

Hartweg, D. L. (1990). Health promotion self-care within Orem's general theory of nursing. *Journal of Advanced Nursing, 15*(1), 35–41.

Hartweg, D. L. (1993). Self-care actions of healthy, middle-aged women to promote well-being. *Nursing Research, 42*(4), 221–227.

Hartweg, D. L., & Berbiglia, V. A. (1996). Determining the adequacy of a health promotion self-care interview guide with healthy, middle-aged, Mexican-American women: A pilot study. *Health Care for Women, 17*(1), 57–68.

Horsburgh, M. E. (1994). *The contribution of personality to adult well-being: Test and explication of Orem's theory of self-care.* Unpublished doctoral dissertation, Wayne State University, Detroit.

Isenberg, M. (1987). International research project to test Orem's Self-Care Deficit Theory of Nursing. *Proceedings of scientific session of the 29th Biennial Convention of Sigma Theta Tau International.* Sigma Theta Tau, San Francisco, California.

Isenberg, M. A. (1991). Insights from Orem's nursing theory on differentiating nursing practice. In Goertzen, E. E. (Ed.), *Differentiating nursing practice: Into the twenty-first century* (pp. 45–49). Kansas City, MO: American Academy of Nursing.

Isenberg, M. (1993). The influence of health state on the self-care agency of persons with coronary artery disease. *Proceedings of Sigma Theta Tau International Research Congress* (Madrid, Spain). Indianapolis: Sigma Theta Tau.

Isenberg, M., Evers, G. C. M., & Brouns, G. (1987). An international research project to test Orem's self-care deficit theory.

Proceedings of the International Research Congress. Edinburgh, United Kingdom: University of Edinburgh.

Jaarsma, T., Halfens, R., Senten, M., Saad, H., & Dracup, K. (1998). Developing a supportive-educative program for patients with advanced heart failure within Orem's general theory of nursing. *Nursing Science Quarterly, 11*(2), 79–85.

Jaarsma, T., Kastermans, M., Dassen, T., & Philipsen, H. (1995). Problems of cardiac patients in early recovery. *Journal of Advanced Nursing, 21*(1), 21–27.

Jacobs, C. J. (1990). Orem's self-care model: Is it relevant to patients in intensive care? *Intensive Care Nursing, 6*(2), 100–103.

Jirovec, M. M., & Kasno, J. (1990). Self-care agency as a function of patient-environmental factors among nursing home residents. *Research in Nursing and Health, 13,* 303–309.

Johnson, D. E. (1959). The nature of a science of nursing. *Nursing Outlook, 7*(5), 291–294.

Katainen, A. L., Merlainen, P., & Isenberg, M. (1993). Reliability and validity testing of Finnish version of the appraisal of self-care agency (ASA) scale. *Proceedings of the Sigma Theta Tau International Research Congress* (Madrid, Spain). Indianapolis: Sigma Theta Tau.

Lorensen, M., Holter, I. M., Evers, G. C. M., Isenberg, M. A., & Van Achterberg, T. (1993). Cross-cultural testing of the "Appraisal of Self-Care Agency: ASA Scale" in Norway. *International Journal of Nursing Studies, 30*(1), 15–23.

McQuiston, C. M. (1993). *Basic conditioning factors and self-care agency of unmarried women at risk for sexually transmitted disease.* Unpublished doctoral dissertation, Wayne State University, Detroit.

Meleis, A. I., Isenberg, M. A., Koerner, J. E., Lacey, B., & Stern, P. (1995). *Diversity, marginalization, and culturally competent health care issues in knowledge development.* Washington, DC: American Academy of Nursing.

Metcalfe, S. A. (1996). *Self-care actions as a function of therapeutic self-care demand and self-care agency in individuals with chronic obstructive pulmonary disease.* Unpublished doctoral dissertation, Wayne State University, Detroit.

Moore, J. B. (1995). Measuring the self-care practice of children and adolescents: Instrument development. *Maternal Child Nursing Journal, 23*(3), 101–108.

Mosher, R. B., & Moore, J. B. (1998). The relationship of self-concept and self-care in children with cancer. *Nursing Science Quarterly, 11*(3), 116–122.

Norris, M. K. G. (1991). Applying Orem's theory to the long-term care of adolescent transplant recipients. *American Nephrology Nurses Association Journal, 18,* 45–47, 53.

Nursing Development Conference Group. (1979). *Concept formalization in nursing: Process and product* (2nd ed.). Boston: Little, Brown.

O'Connor, N. A. (1995). *Maieutic dimensions of self-care agency: Instrument development.* Unpublished doctoral dissertation, Wayne State University, Detroit.

Orem, D. E. (1971). *Nursing: Concepts of practice.* New York: McGraw-Hill.

Orem, D. E. (1985). *Nursing: Concepts of practice* (3rd ed.). New York: McGraw-Hill.

Orem, D. E. (1995). *Nursing: Concepts of practice* (5th ed.). New York: McGraw-Hill.

Orem, D. E. (2001). *Nursing: Concepts of practice* (6th ed.). St. Louis: Mosby.

Richardson, A., & Ream, E. K. (1997). Self-care behaviours initiated by chemotherapy patients in response to fatigue. *International Journal of Nursing Studies, 34*(1), 35–43.

Riley, P. (1996). Development of a COPD self-care action scale. *Rehabilitation Nursing Research, 5*(1), 3–8.

Schott-Baer, D. (1989). *Family culture, family resources, dependent care, caregiver burden and self-care agency of spouses of cancer patients.* Unpublished doctoral dissertation, Wayne State University, Detroit.

Senten, M. C., Evers, G. C. M., Isenberg, M., & Philipsen, H. (1991). Veranderingen in selfsorg na coronair bypass operatie, een prospectieve stude [Changes in self-care following coronary artery bypass surgery, a prospective study.] *Verplegkuude, 5*(1), 34–43.

Soderhamn, O., Evers, G., & Hamrin, E. (1996). A Swedish version of the Appraisal of Self-Care Agency (ASA) scale. *Scandinavian Journal of Caring, 10*(1), 3–9.

Tolentino, M. B. (1990). The use of Orem's self-care model in the neonatal intensive care unit. *Journal of Obstetric, Gynecologic, and Neonatal Nursing, 19,* 496–500.

Utz, S. W., & Ramos, M. C. (1993). Mitral valve prolapse and its effects: A programme of inquiry within Orem's self-care deficit theory of nursing. *Journal of Advanced Nursing, 18,* 742–751.

Van Achterberg, T., Lorensen, M., Isenberg, M., Evers, G. C. M., Levin, E., & Philipsen, H. (1991). The Norwegian, Danish and Dutch version of the appraisal of self-care agency scale: Comparing reliability aspects. *Scandinavian Journal of Caring Science, 5*(1), 1–8.

Vannoy, B. (1989). *The relationship among motivational dispositions, basic conditioning factors, and the power element of self-care agency in people beginning a weight loss program.* Unpublished doctoral dissertation, Wayne State University, Detroit.

Villarruel, A. M. (1995). Mexican-American cultural meanings, expressions, self-care and dependent care actions associated with experiences of pain. *Research in Nursing & Health, 18*(5), 427–436.

Wallace, W. A. (1983). *From a realist point of view: Essays on the philosophy of science.* Washington, DC: University Press of America.

Ward-Griffin, C., & Bramwell, L. (1990). The congruence of elderly client and nurse perceptions of the clients' self-care agency. *Journal of Advanced Nursing, 15*(9), 1070–1077.

Weiss, P. (1980). *You, I, and the others.* Carbondale, IL: Southern Illinois University Press.

West, P. (1993). *The relationship between depression and self-care agency in young adult women.* Unpublished doctoral dissertation, Wayne State University, Detroit.

Whetstone, W. R. (1987). Perceptions of self-care in East Germany: A cross-cultural empirical investigation. *Journal of Advanced Nursing, 12,* 167–176.

Whetstone, W. R., & Hansson, A. M. O. (1989). Perceptions of self-care in Sweden: A cross-cultural replication. *Journal of Advanced Nursing, 14*(11), 962–969.

Bibliography

Ailinger, R. L. (1993). Patient's explanations of rheumatoid arthritis. *Western Journal of Nursing Research, 15*(3), 340–351.

Allison, S. E. (1985). *Structuring nursing practice based on Orem's theory of nursing: A nurse administrator's perspective.* Norwalk, CT: Appleton-Century-Crofts.

Allison, S. E., McLaughlin, K., & Walker, D. (1991). Nursing theory: A tool to put nursing back into nursing administration. *Nursing Administration Quarterly, 15*(3), 72–78.

Anderson, J. A. (2001). Understanding homeless adults by testing the theory of self-care. *Nursing Science Quarterly, 14*(1), 59–67.

Angeles, D. M. (1991). An Orem-based NICU orientation checklist. *Neonatal-Nater, 9*(7), 43–48.

Berbiglia, V. A. (1991). A case study: Perspectives on a self-care deficit nursing theory-based curriculum. *Journal of Advanced Nursing, 16,* 1158–1163.

Bidigare, S. A., & Oermann, M. H. (1991). Attitudes and knowledge of nurses regarding organ procurement. *Heart and Lung, 20,* 20–24.

Biley, F., & Dennerley, M. (1990). Orem's model: A critical analysis . . . part 2. *Nursing (London): The Journal of Clinical Practice, Education and Management, 4*(13), 21–22.

Bliss-Holtz, V. J. (1988). Primiparas' prenatal concern for learning infant care. *Nursing Research, 37,* 20–24.

Bliss-Holtz, V. J. (1991). Developmental tasks of pregnancy and prenatal education. *International Journal of Childbirth Education, 6*(1), 29–31.

Campbell, J. C. (1986). Nursing assessment for risk of homicide with battered women. *Advances in Nursing Science, 8*(4), 36–51.

Campbell, J. C. (1989). A test of two explanatory models of women's responses to battering. *Nursing Research, 38,* 18–24.

Conn, V. (1991). Self-care actions taken by older adults for influenza and colds. *Nursing Research, 40,* 176–181.

Conn, V. S., Taylor, S. G., & Kelley, S. (1991). Medication regimen complexity and adherence among older adults. *Image: Journal of Nursing Scholarship, 23,* 231–235.

Dellasega, C. (1995). SCOPE: A practical method for assessing the self-care status of elderly persons. *Rehabilitation Nursing Research, 4*(4), 128–135.

Denyes, M. J. (1988). Orem's model used for health promotion: Directions from research. *Advances in Nursing Science Research, 11*(1), 13–21.

Denyes, M. J. (1993). Response to "Predictors of children's self-care performance: Testing the theory of self-care deficit." *Scholarly Inquiry for Nursing Practice, 7,* 213–217.

Denyes, M. J., Neuman, B. M., & Villarruel, A. M. (1991). Nursing actions to prevent and alleviate pain in hospitalized children. *Issues in Comprehensive Pediatric Nursing, 14,* 31–48.

Denyes, M. J., O'Connor, N. A., Oakley, D., & Ferguson, S. (1989). Integrating nursing theory, practice and research through collaborative practice. *Journal of Advanced Nursing, 14,* 141–145.

Dodd, M. J. (1983). Self-care for side effects in cancer chemotherapy: An assessment of nursing interventions—part 2. *Cancer Nursing, 6,* 63–67.

Dodd, M. J. (1984). Measuring informational intervention for chemotherapy knowledge and self-care behavior. *Research in Nursing and Health, 7,* 43–50.

Dodd, M. J. (1987). Efficacy of proactive information on self-care in radiation therapy patients. *Heart and Lung, 16,* 538–544.

Dodd, M. J. (1988a). Efficacy of proactive information on self-care in chemotherapy patients. *Patient Education and Counseling, 11,* 215–225.

Dodd, M. J. (1988b). Patterns of self-care in patients with breast cancer. *Western Journal of Nursing Research, 10,* 7–24.

Dodd, M. J. (1997). Self-Care: Ready or not! *Oncology Nursing Forum, 24*(6), 983–990.

Dowd, T. T. (1991). Discovering older women's experience of urinary incontinence. *Research in Nursing and Health, 14,* 179–186.

Dowd, T. (1993). *Relationships among health state factors, foundational capabilities, and urinary incontinence self-care in women.* Unpublished doctoral dissertation, Wayne State University, Detroit.

Evers, G. (1989). *Appraisal of self-care agency scale: Validity and reliability testing with Dutch populations.* Van Gorcum: Assen/Maastricht.

Ewing, G. (1989). The nursing preparation of stoma patients for self-care. *Journal of Advanced Nursing, 14,* 411–420.

Fawcett, J., Ellis, V., Underwood, P., Naqvi, A., & Wilson, D. (1990). The effect of Orem's self-care model on nursing care in a nursing home setting. *Journal of Advanced Nursing, 15,* 659–666.

Frey, M. A., & Denyes, M. J. (1989). Health and illness self-care in adolescents with IDDM: A test of Orem's theory. *Advances in Nursing Sciences, 12*(1), 67–75.

Frey, M. A., & Fox, M. A. (1990). Assessing and teaching self-care to youths with diabetes mellitus. *Pediatric Nursing, 16,* 597–800.

Furlong, S. (1996). Self-care: The application of a ward philosophy. *Journal of Clinical Nursing, 5*(2), 85–90.

Gast, H. L., Denyes, M. J., Campbell, J. C., Hartweg, D. L., Schott-Baer, D., & Isenberg, M. (1989). Self-care agency: Conceptualizations and operationalizations. *Advances in Nursing Science, 12*(1), 26–38.

Gaut, D. A., & Kieckhefer, G. M. (1988). Assessment of self-care agency in chronically ill adolescents. *Journal of Adolescent Health Care, 9,* 55–60.

Hanucharurnkul, S. (1989). Comparative analysis of Orem's and King's theories. *Journal of Advanced Nursing, 15,* 35–41.

Hanucharurnkul, S., & Vinya-nguag, P. (1991). Effects of promoting patients' participation in self-care on postoperative recovery and satisfaction with care. *Nursing Science Quarterly, 4*(1), 14–20.

Harris, J. L., & Williams, L. K. (1991). Universal self-care requisites as identified by homeless elderly men. *Journal of Gerontological Nursing, 17*(6), 39–43.

Hartweg, D. L. (1991). *Dorothea Orem: Self-care deficit theory.* Newbury Park, CA: Sage.

Hartweg, D. L., & Metcalfe, S. (1986). Self-care attitude changes of nursing students enrolled in a self-care curriculum—a longitudinal study. *Research in Nursing and Health, 9,* 347–353.

Hiromoto, B. M., & Dungan, J. (1991). Contract learning for self-care activities: A protocol study among chemotherapy outpatients. *Cancer Nursing, 14,* 148–154.

Horsburgh, M. E. (1994). *The contribution of personality to adult well-being: Test and explication of Orem's theory of self-care.* Unpublished doctoral dissertation, Wayne State University, Detroit.

Humphreys, J. (1991). Children of battered women: Worries about their mothers. *Pediatric Nursing, 17,* 342–345, 354.

Ip, W., Chau, J., Leung, M., Leung, Y., Foo, Y., & Chang, A. M. (1996). Research forum: Relationship between self-concept and perception of self-care ability of elderly in a Hong Kong hostel. *Hong Kong Nursing Journal, 72,* 6–12.

Jenny, J. (1991). Self-care deficit theory and nursing diagnosis: A test of conceptual fit. *Journal of Nursing Education, 30*(5), 227–232.

Jirovec, M. M., & Kasno, J. (1993). Predictors of self-care abilities among the institutionalized elderly. *Western Journal of Nursing Research, 15,* 314–326.

Jopp, M., Carroll, M. C., & Waters, L. (1993). Using self-care theory to guide nursing management of the older adult after hospitalization. *Rehabilitation Nursing, 18,* 91–94.

Kearney, B. Y., & Fleischer, B. J. (1979). Development of an instrument to measure exercise of self-care agency. *Research in Nursing and Health, 2,* 25–34.

Kerkstra, A., Castelein, E., & Philipsen, H. (1991). Preventive home visits to elderly people by community nurses in the Netherlands. *Journal of Advanced Nursing, 16,* 631–637.

Kirkpatrick, M. K., Brewer, J. A., & Stocks, B. (1990). Efficacy of self-care measures for perimenstrual syndrome (PMS). *Journal of Advanced Nursing, 15,* 281–285.

Leininger, M. (1992). Self-care ideology and cultural incongruities: Some critical issues. *Journal of Transcultural Nursing, 4*(1), 2–4.

Magnan, M. A. (2001). *Self-care and health in persons with cancer-related fatigue: Refinement and evaluation of Orem's self-care framework.* Unpublished doctoral dissertation, Wayne State University, Detroit.

Malik, U. (1992). Women's knowledge, beliefs, and health practices about breast cancer, and breast self-examination. *Nursing Journal of India, 83,* 186–190.

McBride, S. (1987). Validation of an instrument to measure exercise of self-care agency. *Research in Nursing and Health, 10,* 311–316.

McDermott, M. A. N. (1993). Learned helplessness as an interacting variable with self-care agency: Testing a theoretical model. *Nursing Science Quarterly, 6,* 28–38.

McQuiston, C. M., & Campbell, J. C. (1997). Theoretical substruction: A guide for theory testing research. *Nursing Science Quarterly, 10*(3), 117–123.

Moore, J. B. (1993). Predictors of children's self-care performance: Testing the theory of self-care deficit. *Scholarly Inquiry for Nursing Practice, 7,* 199–212.

Moore, J. B., & Gaffney, K. F. (1989). Development of an instrument to measure mothers' performance of self-care activities for children. *Advances in Nursing Science, 12*(1), 76–83.

Moore, J. B., & Pichler, V. H. (2002). Measurement of Orem's basic conditioning factors: a review of published research. *Nursing Science Quarterly, 13*(2), 137–142.

Morales-Mann, E. T., & Jiang, S. L. (1993). Applicability of Orem's conceptual framework: A cross-cultural point of view. *Journal of Advanced Nursing, 18,* 737–741.

Nursing Development Conference Group. (1973). *Concept formalization in nursing: Process and product.* Boston: Little, Brown.

Orem, D. E. (1980). *Nursing: Concepts of practice* (2nd ed.). New York: McGraw-Hill.

Orem, D. E. (1983a). *The family coping with a medical illness: Analysis and application of Orem's theory.* New York: Wiley.

Orem, D. E. (1983b). *The family experiencing emotional crisis:*

Analysis and application of Orem's self-care deficit theory. New York: Wiley.

Orem, D. E. (1983c). *The self-care deficit theory of nursing: A general theory.* New York: Wiley.

Orem, D. E. (1987). *Orem's general theory of nursing.* Philadelphia: W. B. Saunders.

Orem, D. E. (1990). A nursing practice theory in three parts, 1956–1989. In Parker, M. (Ed.), *Nursing theories in practice.* New York: National League for Nursing.

Orem, D. E. (1991). *Nursing: Concepts of practice* (4th ed.). New York: McGraw-Hill.

Orem, D. E., Taylor, S. G., & Renpenning, K. M. (2001). *Nursing: Concepts of Practice* (6th ed.). Elsevier Science.

Rhodes, V. A., Watson, P. M., & Hanson, B. M. (1988). Patients' descriptions of the influence of tiredness and weakness on self-care abilities. *Cancer Nursing, 11,* 186–194.

Richardson, A. (1992). Studies exploring self-care for the person coping with cancer treatment: A review. *International Journal of Nursing Studies, 29,* 191–204.

Richardson, A., & Ream, E. K. (1997). Self-care behaviours initiated by chemotherapy patients in response to fatigue. *International Journal of Nursing Studies, 34*(1), 35–43.

Riesch, S. K. (1988). Changes in the exercise of self-care agency. *Western Journal of Nursing Research, 10,* 257–273.

Riesch, S. K., & Hauck, M. R. (1988). The exercise of self-care agency: An analysis of construct and discriminant validity. *Research in Nursing and Health, 11,* 245–255.

Roberson, M. R., & Kelley, J. H. (1996). Using Orem's theory in transcultural settings: A critique. *Nursing Forum, 31*(3), 22–28.

Schott-Baer, D. (1993). Dependent care, caregiver burden, and self-care agency of spouse caregivers. *Cancer Nursing, 16,* 230–236.

Simmons, S. J. (1990a). The health-promoting self-care system model: Directions for nursing research and practice. *Journal of Advanced Nursing, 15*(10), 1162–1166.

Simmons, S. J. (1990b). The health-promoting self-care system model: Directions for nursing research and practice. *Journal of Advanced Nursing, 15*(10), 1162–1166.

Smith, M. C. (1979). Proposed metaparadigm for nursing research and theory development: An analysis of Orem's self-care theory. *Image, 11,* 75–79.

Smits, J., & Kee, C. C. (1992). Correlates of self-care among the independent elderly: Self-concept affects well-being. *Journal of Gerontological Nursing, 18*(9), 13–18.

Spearman, S. A., Duldt, B. W., & Brown, S. (1993). Research testing theory: Selective review of Orem's self-care theory. *Journal of Advanced Nursing, 18*(10), 1626–1631.

Spitzer, A., Bar-Tal, Y., & Ziv, L. (1996). The moderating effect of age on self-care. *Western Journal of Nursing Research, 18*(2), 136–148.

Urbancic, J. C. (1992a). Empowerment support with adult female survivors of childhood incest: Part I—Theories and research. *Archives of Psychiatric Nursing, 6,* 275–281.

Urbancic, J. C. (1992b). Empowerment support with adult female survivors of childhood incest: Part II—Application of Orem's method helping. *Archives of Psychiatric Nursing, 6,* 282–286.

Utz, S. W. (1990). Motivating self-care: A nursing approach. *Holistic Nursing Practice, 4*(2), 13–21.

Villarruel, A. M., & Denyes, M. J. (1991). Pain assessment in children: Theoretical and empirical validity. *Advances in Nursing Science, 14*(2), 32–41.

Villarruel, A. M., & Denyes, M. J. (1997). International scholarship: Testing Orem's theory with Mexican Americans. *Image: Journal of Nursing, 29*(3), 283–288.

Weaver, M. T. (1987). Perceived self-care agency: A LISREL factor analysis of Bickel and Hanson's questionnaire. *Nursing Research, 36,* 381–387.

Weber, N. A. (2000). *Explication of the structure of the secondary concept of women's self-care developed within Orem's self-care deficit theory: Instrumentation, psychometric evaluation and theory-testing.* Unpublished dissertation, Wayne State University, Detroit.

CHAPTER 13

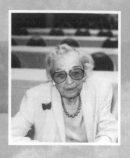

Martha E. Rogers

PART ONE: Martha E. Rogers' Science of Unitary Human Beings

Violet M. Malinski

Introducing the Theorist
Introducing the Theory
Separate Theories Implicit in Science of Unitary Human Beings
Summary
Bibliography

Introducing the Theorist

Martha E. Rogers, one of nursing's foremost scientists, was a staunch advocate for nursing as a basic science. She believed that the art of practice could be developed only as the science of nursing evolved. A common refrain throughout her career was the need to differentiate skills, techniques, and ways of using knowledge from the body of knowledge that guides practice to promote health and well-being for humankind. "The practice of nursing is not nursing. Rather, it is the use of nursing knowledge for human betterment" (Rogers, 1994a, p. 34). Rogers identified the unitary human being and the environment as the central concern of nursing, rather than health and illness. She repeatedly emphasized the need for nursing science to encompass beings in space as well as on Earth. Who was this visionary who introduced a new worldview to nursing?

Martha Elizabeth Rogers was born in Dallas, Texas, on May 12, 1914, a birthday she shared with Florence Nightingale. Her parents soon returned home to Knoxville, Tennessee, where Martha and her three siblings grew up.

Rogers spent two years at the University of Tennessee in Knoxville before entering the nursing program at Knoxville General Hospital. Next, she attended George Peabody College in Nashville, Tennessee, where she earned her bachelor of science degree in public health nursing, choosing that field as her professional focus.

Rogers spent the next 13 years in rural public health nursing in Michigan, Connecticut, and Arizona, where she established the first Visiting Nurse Service in Phoenix, serving as its executive director (Hektor, 1989, 1994). Recognizing the need for advanced education, she took a break during this period and returned to academia, earning her master's degree in nursing from Teachers College, Columbia University, in the program developed by another nurse theorist, Hildegard Peplau. In 1951, she returned to academia, this time earning a master's of public health and a doctor of science degree from Johns Hopkins University in Baltimore, Maryland.

In 1954 Rogers was appointed head of the Division of Nursing at New York University (NYU), beginning the second phase of her career overseeing baccalaureate, master's, and doctoral programs in nursing and developing the nursing science she knew was integral to the knowledge base nurses needed. She articulated the need for a "valid baccalaureate education" that would serve as the base for graduate and doctoral studies in nursing. Such a program, she believed, required five years of study in theoretical content in nursing as well as liberal arts and the biological, physical, and social sciences. Under her leadership, NYU established such a program. At the doctoral level, Rogers opposed the federally funded nurse-scientist doctoral programs that prepared nurses in other disciplines rather than in the science of nursing. During the 1960s she successfully shifted the focus of doctoral research from nurses and their functions to human beings in mutual process with the environment. She wrote three books that explicated her ideas: *Educational Revolution in Nursing* (1961), *Reveille in Nursing*

(1964), and the landmark *An Introduction to the Theoretical Basis of Nursing* (1970). From 1963 to 1965 she edited *Nursing Science,* a journal that was far ahead of its time; this journal offered content on theory development and the emerging science of nursing plus research and issues in education and practice.

Along with a number of nursing colleagues, Rogers established the Society for Advancement in Nursing in 1974. Among other issues, this group supported differentiation in education and practice for professional and technical careers in nursing. They drafted legislation to amend the Education Law in New York State proposing licensure as an independent nurse (IN) for those who had a minimum of a baccalaureate degree. It also introduced a new exam and licensure as a registered nurse (RN) for those with either a diploma or an associate degree in nursing who passed the traditional boards (Governing Council of the Society for Advancement in Nursing, 1977, 1994).

Rogers is best remembered for the paradigm she introduced to nursing, the science of unitary human beings, which displays her visionary, future-oriented perspective. Her theoretical ideas appeared in embryonic form in her two earlier books and were fleshed out in the 1970a book, then revised and refined in a number of articles and book chapters written between 1980 and 1994. She helped create the Society of Rogerian Scholars, Inc., chartered in New York in 1988, as one avenue for furthering the development of this nursing science.

Rogers died in 1994, leaving a rich legacy in her writings on nursing science, the space age, research, education, and professional and political issues in nursing.

Introducing the Theory

The historical evolution of the Science of Unitary Human Beings has been described by Malinski and Barrett (1994). This chapter presents the science in its current form and identifies work in progress to expand it further.

ROGERS' WORLDVIEW

Rogers (1994a) identified the unique focus of nursing as "the irreducible human being and its

> *The unique focus of nursing as "the irreducible human being and its environment, both identified as energy fields."*

environment, both identified as energy fields" (p. 33). "Human" encompasses both *Homo sapiens* and *Homo spatialis,* the evolutionary transcendence of humankind as we voyage into space, and environment encompasses outer space. This perspective necessitates a new worldview, out of which emerges the Science of Unitary Human Beings, "a pandimensional view of people and their world" (Rogers, 1992, 1994, p. 257).

Rogers described the new worldview underpinning her conceptual system to students and colleagues beginning in 1968. It has been available in print with some revisions in language since 1986 (Madrid & Winstead-Fry, 1986; Malinski, 1986; Rogers, 1990a, 1990b, 1992, 1994a, 1994b). Rogers (1992) described the evolution from older to newer worldviews in such shifting perspectives as cell theory to field theory, entropic to negentropic universe, three dimensional to pandimensional, person-environment as dichotomous to person-environment as integral, causation and adaptation to mutual process, dynamic equilibrium to innovative growing diversity, homeostasis to homeodynamics, waking as a basic state to waking as an evolutionary emergent, and closed to open systems. She pointed

> *In a universe of open systems, energy fields are continuously open, infinite, and integral with one another.*

out that in a universe of open systems, energy fields are continuously open, infinite, and integral with one another. Change that is predictable, brought about by a linear, causal chain of events, gives way to change that is diverse, creative, innovative, and unpredictable.

Rogers was aware that the world looks very different from the vantage point of the newer view as contrasted with the older, traditional worldview. She pointed out that we are already living in a new reality, one that is "a synthesis of rapidly evolving, accelerating ways of using knowledge" (Rogers, 1994a, p. 33), even if people are not always fully aware that these shifts have occurred or are in process. She urged that nurses be visionary, looking

forward and not backward, and not allowing themselves to become stuck in the present, in the details of how things are now, but envision how they might be in a universe where continuous change is the only given. Rogers (1994b) cautioned that, although traditional modalities of practice and methods of research serve a purpose, they are inadequate for the newer worldview, which urges nurses to use the knowledge base of Rogerian nursing science creatively in order to develop innovative new modalities and research approaches that would promote the betterment of humankind.

POSTULATES OF ROGERIAN NURSING SCIENCE

Rogers (1992) identified four fundamental postulates:

- energy fields,
- openness,
- pattern, and
- pandimensionality, formerly called both four-dimensionality and multidimensionality.

> *Rogers identified four fundamental postulates: energy fields, openness, pattern, and pandimensionality.*

In their irreducible unity, they form reality as experienced in this worldview. Rogers (1990a, 1994a, 1994b) defined the energy field as "the fundamental unit of the living and the non-living," noting that the energy field is infinite and dynamic, meaning that it is continuously moving and flowing (1990a, p. 7). She identified two energy fields of concern to nurses, which are distinct but not separate: the human field, or unitary human being, and the environmental field. The human field can be conceptualized as one person or a group, family, or community. The human and environmental fields are irreducible; they cannot be broken down into component parts or subsystems. Parts have no meaning in unitary science. For example, the unitary human is not described as a bio-psycho-sociocultural or body-mind-spirit entity. Rogers interpreted such designations as representative of current uses of "holistic," meaning a summation of parts to arrive at the whole, where a nurse would assess the domains, subsystems, or components identified, then synthesize the accumulated data to arrive at a picture of the total person. Instead, Rogers maintained that each field, human and environmental, is identified by pattern, defined as "the distinguishing characteristic of an energy field perceived as a single wave" (Rogers, 1990a, p. 7). Pattern manifestations and characteristics are specific to the whole.

Because human and environmental fields are integral with each other, they cannot be separated. They are always in mutual process. A concept like adaptation, a change in one preceding a change in another, loses meaning in this nursing science. Change occurs simultaneously for human and environment.

The fields are pandimensional, defined as "a non-linear domain without spatial or temporal attributes" (Rogers, 1992, p. 28). Pandimensional reality transcends traditional notions of space and time, which can be understood as perceived boundaries only. Examples of pandimensionality include phenomena commonly labeled "paranormal" that are, in Rogerian nursing science, manifestations of the changing diversity of field patterning and examples of pandimensional awareness.

The postulate of openness resonates throughout the previous discussion. In an open universe, there are no boundaries other than perceptual ones. Therefore, human and environment are not separated by boundaries. The energy of each flows continuously through the other in an unbroken wave. Rogers repeatedly emphasized that person and environment are energy fields—but they do not have energy fields, such as auras, surrounding them. In an open universe, there are multiple potentials and possibilities. Nothing is predetermined or foreordained. Causality breaks down, paving the way for a creative, unpredictable future. People experience their world in multiple ways, evidenced by the diverse manifestations of field patterning that continuously emerge.

Rogers (1992, 1994a) described pattern as changing continuously while giving identity to each unique human-environmental field process. Although pattern is an abstraction, not something that can be observed directly, "it reveals itself through its manifestations" (Rogers, 1992, p. 29). Individual characteristics of a particular person are not characteristics of field patterning. Pattern manifestations reflect the human-environmental field mutual process as a unitary, irreducible whole.

Person and environment cannot be examined or understood as separate entities. Pattern manifestations reveal the relative diversity, lower frequency, and higher frequency patterning of this human-environmental mutual field process. Rogers identified some of these manifestations as lesser and greater diversity; longer, shorter, and seemingly continuous rhythms; slower, faster, and seemingly continuous motion; time experienced as slower, faster, and timeless; pragmatic, imaginative, and visionary; and longer sleeping, longer waking, and beyond waking. She explained "seems continuous" as "a wave frequency so rapid that the observer perceives it as a single, unbroken event" (Rogers, 1990a, p. 10). This view of the ongoing process of change is captured in Rogers' principles of homeodynamics.

PRINCIPLES OF HOMEODYNAMICS

Like adaptation, homeostasis—maintaining balance or equilibrium—is an outdated concept in the worldview represented in Rogerian nursing science. Rogers chose "homeodynamics" to convey the dynamic, ever-changing nature of life and the world. Her three principles of homeodynamics—resonancy, helicy, and integrality—describe the nature of change in the human-environmental field process. *Resonancy* specifies the "continuous change from lower to higher frequency wave patterns in human and environmental fields" (Rogers, 1990a, p. 9). Resonancy presents the way change occurs. Although Rogers stated that this process is nonlinear, she was unable to move away from the language of "from lower to higher" in the principle itself, which seems to indicate a linear progression. Rogers (1990b) elaborated: "[I]ndividuals experience lesser diversity and greater diversity . . . time as slower, faster, or unmoving. Individuals are sometimes pragmatic, sometimes imaginative, and sometimes visionary. Individuals experience periods of longer sleeping, longer waking, and periods of beyond waking" (p. 10).

Resonancy, then, specifies change flowing in lower and higher frequencies that continually fluctuate, rather than flow from lower to higher frequencies. Both lower and higher frequency awareness and experiencing are essential to the wholeness of rhythmical patterning. As Phillips (1994, p. 15) described it, "[W]e may find that growing diversity of pattern is related to a dialectic of low frequency–high frequency, similar to that of order-disorder in chaos theory. When the rhythmicities of lower-higher frequencies work together, they yield innovative, diverse patterns."

Helicy is the "continuous innovative, unpredictable, increasing diversity of human and environmental field patterns" (Rogers, 1990a, p. 8). This principle describes the nature of change. *Integrality* is "continuous mutual human field and environmental field process" (Rogers, 1990a, p. 8). It specifies the context of change as the integral human-environmental field process where person and environment are inseparable.

Together the principles suggest that the mutual patterning process of human and environmental fields changes continuously, innovatively, and unpredictably, flowing in lower and higher frequencies. Rogers (1990a, p. 9) believed that they serve as guides both to the practice of nursing and to research in the science of nursing.

Separate Theories Implicit in Science of Unitary Human Beings

Rogers clearly stated her belief that multiple theories can be derived from the Science of Unitary

> *Rogers clearly stated her belief that multiple theories can be derived from the Science of Unitary Human Beings.*

Human Beings. They are specific to nursing and reflect not what nurses do, but an understanding of people and our world (Rogers, 1992). Nursing education is identified by transmission of this theoretical knowledge, and nursing practice is the creative use of this knowledge. Nursing research uses it to illuminate the nature of the human-environmental field change process and its many unpredictable potentials.

THEORY OF ACCELERATING EVOLUTION

The theory of accelerating evolution suggests that the only "norm" is accelerating change. Higher frequency field patterns that manifest growing diversity open the door to wider ranges of experiences and behaviors, calling into question the very idea of

"norms" as guidelines. Human and environmental field rhythms are speeding up. We experience faster environmental motion now than ever before, in cars and high-speed trains and planes, for example. It is common for people to experience time as rapidly speeding by. People are living longer. Rather than viewing aging as a process of decline or as "running down," as in an entropic worldview, this theory views aging as a creative process whereby field patterns show increasing diversity in such manifestations as sleeping, waking, and dreaming.

Rogers hypothesized that hyperactive children provide a good example of speeded-up rhythms relative to other children. They would be expected to show indications of faster rhythms, increased motion, and other behaviors indicative of this shift. She expected that relative diversity would manifest in different patterns for individuals within any age cohort, concluding that chronological age is not a valid indicator of change in this system: "[I]n fact, as evolutionary diversity continues to accelerate, the range and variety of differences between individuals also increase; the more diverse field patterns evolve more rapidly than the less diverse ones" (Rogers, 1992, p. 30).

THEORY OF EMERGENCE OF PARANORMAL PHENOMENA

The theory of the emergence of paranormal phenomena suggests that experiences commonly labeled "paranormal" are actually manifestations of the changing diversity and innovation of field patterning. They are pandimensional forms of awareness, examples of pandimensional reality that manifest visionary, beyond waking potentials. Meditation, for example, transcends traditionally perceived limitations of time and space, opening the door to new and creative potentials. Therapeutic touch provides another example of such pandimensional awareness. Both participants often share similar experiences during therapeutic touch, such as a visualization sharing common features that evolves spontaneously for both, a shared experience arising within the mutual process both are experiencing, with neither able to lay claim to it as a personal, private experience. Precognition, déjà vu, and clairvoyance become normal rather than paranormal experiences.

McEvoy (1990) hypothesized that the process of dying exemplifies four-dimensional awareness and thus encompasses paranormal events such as out-of-body and apparitional experiences. She cited Margeneau's discussion in "Science, Creativity, and Psi," identifying paranormal experiences as the ability to perceive within a four-dimensional world: "It is our human lot to look at the four-dimensional world through a slit-like opening.... Whenever the slit opens, and for some people the slit only opens at the time of death, you see more than a segmented three-dimensional slice of the four-dimensional universe" (cited in McEvoy, 1990, p. 211). Death itself is a transition, not an end, a manifestation of increasing diversity as energy fields transform.

RHYTHMICAL CORRELATES OF CHANGE

Rogers' third theory, Rhythmical Correlates of Change, was changed to "Manifestations of Field Patterning in Unitary Human Beings," discussed earlier. Here Rogers suggested that evolution is an irreducible, nonlinear process characterized by increasing diversity of field patterning. She offered some manifestations of this relative diversity, including the rhythms of motion, time experience, and sleeping-waking, encouraging others to suggest further examples. The next part of this chapter covers Rogerian science-based practice and research in more detail.

PRACTICE

Rogers identified noninvasive modalities as the basis for nursing practice now and in the future.

> Nurses must use "nursing knowledge in non-invasive ways in a direct effort to promote well-being."

She said that nurses must use "nursing knowledge in non-invasive ways in a direct effort to promote well-being" (Rogers, 1994a, p. 34). This focus gives nurses a central role in health care rather than medical care. She also noted that health services should be community-based, not hospital-based. Hospitals are properly used to provide satellite services in specific instances of illness and trauma; they do not provide health services. Rogers urged nurses to develop autonomous, community-based nursing centers.

In a 1990 panel discussion among Rogers and five other theorists, Rogers maintained that "[o]ur primary concern ... is to focus on people wherever they are and to help them get better, whatever that means.... Our job is better health, and people do better making their own choices. The best prognosis is for the individual who is non-compliant" (Randell, 1992, p. 181). She was an advocate for people's rights to make their own informed choices in the belief that this would improve well-being. In yet another panel discussion in 1991, Rogers explained that greater diversity necessitates "services that are far more individualized than we have ever provided" (Takahashi, 1992, p. 89), and went on to reiterate her lack of support for nursing diagnosis. Individualizing health care also negates the need for care plans, care mapping, and so on.

Rogers consistently identified the need for individualized, community-based health services incorporating noninvasive modalities. She offered examples from those currently in use, such as therapeutic touch, meditation, imagery, humor, and laughter, while stating her belief that new ones will emerge out of the evolution toward spacekind (Rogers, 1994b). The principles of homeodynamics provide a way to understand the process of human-environmental change, paving the way for Rogerian theory-based practice.

RESEARCH

Rogers maintained that both qualitative and quantitative research methods were appropriate for

> Rogers maintained that both qualitative and quantitative research methods were appropriate for Rogerian science–based research, with the nature of the question and the phenomena under investigation guiding the selection.

Rogerian science–based research, with the nature of the question and the phenomena under investigation guiding the selection. However, she cautioned that neither is totally adequate for the new worldview and encouraged the development of new methods.

Pattern manifestations have provided a common research focus, highlighting the need for tools by which they can be measured. The earliest such tool, developed by Ference (1986) in her 1979 dissertation, is the Human Field Motion Tool, a semantic differential scale rating two concepts: "my motor is running" and "my field expansion."

Barrett (1986, 1990) developed the next tool in her 1983 dissertation. The power as knowing participation in change tool (PKPCT) uses the semantic differential technique to rate the four concepts of her power theory—awareness, choices, freedom to act intentionally, and involvement in creating changes.

Paletta (1990) developed the Temporal Experience Scales using metaphors to capture the experiences of time dragging, time racing, and timelessness. Johnston (1994; Watson et al., 1997) developed the Human Field Image Metaphor Scale to measure awareness of the infinite wholeness of the human field. Gueldner (cited in Watson et al., 1997) developed the Index of Field Energy, composed of 18 pairs of line drawings judged to represent low and high frequency descriptions of a concept. Respondents indicate how they feel now along a seven-point scale. Hastings-Tolsma's (Watson et al., 1997) Diversity of Human Field Pattern Scale explores diverse pattern changes and personal preferences for participation in change. Watson's (Watson et al., 1997) Assessment of Dream Experience Scale explores dreaming as a beyond-waking experience. Leddy (1995) developed the Person-Environment Participation Scale and the Leddy Healthiness Scale (1996).

Currently, researchers are using Rogerian tools such as those described, developing new Rogerian tools, and developing creative, new research methods. Innovative potentials for promoting the well-being of people and their environment emerge daily as nurses apply the knowledge gained through Rogerian nursing science. Rogers' challenge has been eagerly taken up by a community of committed scholars.

SUMMARY

The Science of Unitary Human Beings reflects Rogers' optimism and hope for the future. She envisioned humankind poised "on the threshold of a fantastic and unimagined future" (Rogers, 1992, p. 33), looking toward space while simultaneously engaging in a transformative Rogerian revolution in health care on Earth. One manifestation will surely be the establishment of autonomous Rogerian nursing centers here on Earth and ultimately in space.

Bibliography

Rogers, M. F. (1961). *Educational revolution in nursing.* New York: Macmillan.

Rogers, M. F. (1963a). Building a strong educational foundation. *American Journal of Nursing, 63*(6), 94–95.

Rogers, M. F. (1963b). Courage of their convictions. *Nursing Science, 1,* 44–47.

Rogers, M. F. (1963c). Some comments on the theoretical basis of nursing practice. *Nursing Science, 1,* April–May.

Rogers, M. F. (1964). *Reveille in nursing.* Philadelphia: F. A. Davis.

Rogers, M. F. (1965). What the public demands of nursing today. *RN, 28,* January, 80.

Rogers, M. F. (1966). Research in nursing. *Nursing Forum,* January.

Rogers, M. F. (1967). Professional commitment. *Image,* December.

Rogers, M. F. (1968a). For public safety: Higher education's responsibility for professional education in nursing. *Hartwick Review, 5*(1), 21–25.

Rogers, M. F. (1968b). Nursing science: Research and researchers. *Teachers College Record, 69,* 469–476.

Rogers, M. F. (1969a). Nursing research: Relevant to practice. *Proceedings of the fifth nursing research conference.* New York: American Nurses' Association.

Rogers, M. F. (1969b). Regional planning for graduate education in nursing. *Proceedings of the National Committee of Deans of Schools of Nursing having accredited graduate programs in nursing.* New York: National League for Nursing.

Rogers, M. F. (1970a). *An introduction to the theoretical basis of nursing.* Philadelphia: F. A. Davis.

Rogers, M. F. (1970b). Yesterday a nurse—today a manager—what now? *Journal of the New York State Nurses' Association, 1*(1), 15–21.

Rogers, M. F. (1972a). Nurses' expanding role and other euphemisms. *Journal of the New York State Nurses' Association, 3*(4), 5–10.

Rogers, M. F. (1972b). Nursing: To be or not to be? *Nursing Outlook, 20,* 42–46.

Rogers, M. F. (1975a). Euphemisms and nursing's future. *Image, 7*(2), 3–9.

Rogers, M. F. (1975b). Nursing is coming of age. *American Journal of Nursing, 75*(10), 1834–1843, 1859.

Rogers, M. F. (1977). Nursing: To be or not to be. In Bullough, B., & Bullough, V. (Eds.), *Expanding horizons for nursing.* New York: Springer.

Rogers, M. F. (1978a). A 1985 dissent. *Health/PAC Bulletin, 80,* January–February, 32–34.

Rogers, M. F. (1978b). Emerging patterns in nursing education. In *Current perspectives in nursing education* (Vol. II, pp. 1–8). St. Louis: Mosby.

Rogers, M. F. (1978c). Legislative and licensing problems in health care. *Nursing Administration Quarterly, 2*(3).

Rogers, M. F. (1980). Nursing: A science of unitary man. In Riehl, J. P., & Roy, C. (Eds.), *Conceptual models for nursing practice* (2nd ed., pp. 329–337). New York: Appleton-Century-Crofts.

Rogers, M. F. (1981). Science of unitary man: A paradigm for nursing. In Laskar, G. E. (Ed.), *Applied systems and cybernetics, Vol. 4. Systems research in health care, biocybernetics and ecology* (pp. 1719–1722). New York: Pergamon.

Rogers, M. F. (1983a). The family coping with a surgical crisis: Analysis and application of Rogers' theory of nursing. In Clements, I. W., & Roberts, F. B. (Eds.), *Family health: A theoretical approach to nursing care* (pp. 390–391). New York: Wiley.

Rogers, M. F. (1983b). Science of unitary human beings: A paradigm for nursing. In Clements, I. W., & Roberts, F. B. (Eds.), *Family health: A theoretical approach to nursing care* (pp. 219–227). New York: Wiley.

Rogers, M. F. (1985a). The nature and characteristics of professional education for nursing. *Journal of Professional Nursing, 1*, 381–383.

Rogers, M. F. (1985b). The need for legislation for licensure to practice professional nursing. *Journal of Professional Nursing, 1*, 384.

Rogers, M. F. (1985c). Nursing education: Preparation for the future. In *Patterns in education: The unfolding of nursing* (pp. 11–14). New York: National League for Nursing.

Rogers, M. F. (1985d). Science of unitary human beings: A paradigm for nursing. In Wood, R., & Kekahbah, J. (Eds.), *Examining the cultural implications of Martha E. Rogers' science of unitary human beings* (pp. 13–23). Pawhuska, OK: Wood-Kekahbah Associates.

Rogers, M. F. (1986). Science of unitary human beings. In Malinski, V. M. (Ed.), *Explorations on Martha Rogers' science of unitary human beings* (pp. 3–8). Norwalk, CT: Appleton-Century-Crofts.

Rogers, M. F. (1987a). Nursing research in the future. In Roode, J. (Ed.), *Changing patterns in nursing education* (pp. 121–123). New York: National League for Nursing.

Rogers, M. F. (1987b). Rogers' science of unitary human beings. In Parse, R. R. (Ed.), *Nursing science: Major paradigms, theories, and critiques* (pp. 139–146). Philadelphia: Saunders.

Rogers, M. F. (1988). Nursing science and art: A prospective. *Nursing Science Quarterly, 1*, 99–102.

Rogers, M. F. (1989). Nursing: A science of unitary human beings. In Riehl-Sisca, J. P. (Ed.), *Conceptual models for nursing practice* (3rd ed., pp. 181–188). Norwalk, CT: Appleton & Lange.

Rogers, M. F. (1992). Nightingale's Notes on Nursing: Prelude to the 21st century. In Nightingale, F. N. *Notes on nursing: What it is, and what it is not* (Commemorative edition, pp. 58 62). Philadelphia: Lippincott. (Originally published in 1854.)

Rogers, M. F. (1994). The science of unitary human beings: Current perspectives. *Nursing Science Quarterly, 7*, 33–35.

PART TWO:
Applications of Rogers' Science of Unitary Human Beings
Howard K. Butcher

Practice
Research
Summary
References

Rogers' (1970, 1980, 1988, 1992) Science of Unitary Human Beings is a major conceptual system unique to nursing that offers nurses a radically new way of viewing persons and their universe. It is concordant with the most contemporary emerging scientific theories describing a worldview of wholeness (Bohm, 1980; Briggs & Peat, 1984, 1989; Capra, 1996; Lovelock, 1991; Mitchell, 1996; Sheldrake, 1988; Talbot, 1991; Woodhouse, 1996).

> *New worldviews require new ways of thinking, sciencing, languaging, and practicing.*

New worldviews require new ways of thinking, sciencing, languaging, and practicing. Rogers' nursing science postulates a pandimensional universe of mutually processing human and environmental energy fields manifesting as continuously innovative, increasingly diverse, creative, and unpredictable unitary field patterns.

A hallmark of a maturing scientific practice discipline is the development of specific practice and research methods evolving from the discipline's extant conceptual systems. Rogers (1992) asserted that practice and research methods must be consistent with the Science of Unitary Human Beings in order to study irreducible human beings in mutual process with a pandimensional universe. Therefore, Rogerian practice and research methods must be congruent with Rogers' postulates and principles if they are to be consistent with Rogerian science.

Practice

The goal of nursing practice is the promotion of well-being and human betterment. Nursing is a service to people wherever they may reside. Nursing practice—the art of nursing—is the creative application of substantive scientific knowledge developed through logical analysis, synthesis, and research. Since the 1960s, the nursing process has been the dominant nursing practice method. The nursing process is an appropriate practice methodology for many nursing theories. However, there has been some confusion in the nursing literature concerning the use of the traditional nursing process within Rogers' Nursing Science.

In early writings, Rogers (1970) did make reference to nursing process and nursing diagnosis. But in later years she asserted that nursing diagnoses were not consistent with her scientific system. Rogers (quoted in Smith, 1988, p. 83) stated:

> [N]ursing diagnosis is a static term that is quite inappropriate for a dynamic system . . . it [nursing diagnosis] is an outdated part of an old worldview, and I think by the turn of the century, there is going to be new ways of organizing knowledge.

Furthermore, nursing diagnoses are particularistic and reductionistic labels describing cause and effect (i.e., "related to") relationships inconsistent with a "nonlinear domain without spatial or temporal attributes" (Rogers, 1992, p. 29). The nursing process is a stepwise sequential process inconsistent with a nonlinear or pandimensional view of reality. In addition, the term "intervention" is not consistent with Rogerian science. *Intervention* means to "come, appear, or lie between two things" (American Heritage Dictionary, 2000, p. 916). The

principle of integrality describes the human and environmental field as integral and in mutual process. Energy fields are open, infinite, dynamic, and constantly changing. The human and environmental fields are inseparable, so one cannot "come between." The nurse and the client are already inseparable and interconnected. Outcomes are also inconsistent with Rogers' principle of helicy: that expected outcomes infer predictability. The principle of helicy describes the nature of change as being unpredictable. Within an energy-field perspective, nurses in mutual process assist clients in actualizing their field potentials by enhancing their ability to participate knowingly in change (Butcher, 1997).

Given the inconsistency of the traditional nursing process with Rogers' postulates and principles, the Science of Unitary Human Beings requires the development of new and innovative practice methods derived from and consistent with the conceptual system. Over the last decade, a number of practice methods have been derived from Rogers' postulates and principles.

BARRETT'S ROGERIAN PRACTICE METHOD

Barrett's two-phase Rogerian practice methodology for health patterning is the accepted alternative to the nursing process for Rogerian practice and is currently the most widely used Rogerian practice model. Barrett's (1988) practice model was derived from the Science of Unitary Human Beings and consisted of two phases: pattern manifestation appraisal and deliberative mutual patterning. Barrett (1998) expanded and updated the methodology by refining each of the phases, now more appropriately referred to as "processes." Each of the processes have also been renamed for greater clarity and precision. *Pattern manifestation knowing* is the continuous process of apprehending the human and environmental field (Barrett, 1998). "Appraisal" means to estimate an amount or to judge the value of something, negating the egalitarian position of the nurse, whereas "knowing" means to recognize the nature, achieve an understanding, or become familiar or acquainted with something. *Voluntary mutual patterning* is the continuous process whereby the nurse assists clients in freely choosing—with awareness—ways to participate in their well-being (Barrett, 1998). The change to the term "voluntary" emphasizes freedom, spontaneity, and choice of action. The nurse does not invest in changing the client in a particular direction, but rather facilitates and mutually explores with the client options and choices and provides information and resources so the client can make informed decisions regarding his or her health and well-being. Thus, clients feel free to choose with awareness how they want to participate in their own change process.

The two processes are continuous and nonlinear and are therefore not necessarily sequential. Patterning is continuous and occurs simultaneously with knowing. Control and predictability are not consistent with Rogers' postulate of pandimensionality and principles of integrality and helicy. Rather, acausality allows for freedom of choice and means outcomes are unpredictable. The goal of voluntary mutual patterning is the actualization of *potentialities* for well-being through knowing participation in change.

COWLING'S ROGERIAN PRACTICE CONSTITUENTS

Cowling (1990) proposed a template comprising 10 constituents for the development of Rogerian practice models. Cowling (1993b, 1997) refined the template and proposed that "pattern appreciation" was a method for unitary knowing in both Rogerian nursing research and practice. Cowling preferred the term "appreciation" rather than "assessment" or "appraisal" because *appraisal* is associated with evaluation. *Appreciation* has broader meaning, which includes "being full aware or sensitive to or realizing; being thankful or grateful for; and enjoying or understanding critically or emotionally" (Cowling, 1997, p. 130). Pattern appreciation has a potential for deeper understanding.

The first constituent for unitary pattern appreciation identifies the human energy field emerging from the human/environment mutual process as the basic referent. Pattern manifestations emerging from the human-environment mutual process are the focus of nursing care. Next, the person's experiences, perceptions, and expressions are unitary manifestations of pattern and provide a focus for pattern appreciation. Third, "pattern appreciation requires an inclusive perspective of what counts as pattern information (energetic manifestations)"

(Cowling, 1993b, p. 202). Thus, any information gathered from and about the client, family, or community—including sensory information, feelings, thoughts, values, introspective insights, intuitive apprehensions, lab values, and physiological measures—are viewed as "energetic manifestations" emerging from the human/environmental mutual field process.

The fourth constituent is that the nurse uses pandimensional modes of awareness when appreciating pattern information. In other words, intuition, tacit knowing, and other forms of awareness beyond the five senses are ways of apprehending manifestations of pattern. Fifth, all pattern information has meaning only when conceptualized and interpreted within a unitary context. Synopsis and synthesis are requisites to unitary knowing. *Synopsis* is a process of deliberately viewing together all aspects of a human experience (Cowling, 1997). Interpreting pattern information within a unitary perspective means that all phenomena and events are related nonlinearly. Also, phenomena and events are not discrete or separate but rather coevolve together in mutual process. Furthermore, all pattern information is a reflection of the human/environment mutual field process. The human and environmental fields are inseparable. Thus, any information from the client is also a reflection of his or her environment. Physiological and other reductionistic measures have new meaning when interpreted within a unitary context. For example, a blood pressure measurement interpreted within a unitary context means the blood pressure is a manifestation of pattern emerging from the entire human/environmental field mutual process rather than being simply a physiological measure. Thus, any expression from the client is unitary and not particular by reflecting the unitary field from which it emanates (Cowling, 1993b).

The sixth constituent in Cowling's practice method describes the format for documenting and presenting pattern information. Rather than stating nursing diagnoses and reporting "assessment data" in a format that is particularistic and reductionistic by dividing the data into categories or parts, the nurse constructs a "pattern profile." Usually the pattern profile is in the form of a narrative summarizing the client's experiences, perceptions, and expression inferred from the pattern appreciation process. The pattern profile tells the story of the client's situation and should be expressed in as many of the client's own words as possible. Relevant particularistic data such as physiological data interpreted within a unitary context may be included in the pattern profile. Cowling (1990, 1993b) also identified additional forms of pattern profiles, including single words or phrases and listing pattern information, diagrams, pictures, photographs, or metaphors that are meaningful in conveying the themes and essence of the pattern information.

Seventh, the primary source for verifying pattern appreciation and profile is the client. Verifying can occur by sharing the pattern profile with the client for revision and confirmation. During verification, the nurse also discusses options, mutually identifies goals, and plans mutual patterning strategies. Sharing the pattern profile with the client enhances participation in the planning of care and facilitates the client's knowing participation in the change process (Cowling, 1997).

The eighth constituent identifies knowing participation in change as the foundation for health patterning. Knowing participation in change is being aware of what one is choosing to do, feeling free to do it, doing it intentionally, and being actively involved in the change process. The purpose of health patterning is to assist clients in knowing participation in change (Barrett, 1988). Ninth, pattern appreciation incorporates the concepts and principles of unitary science, and approaches for health patterning are determined by the client. Last, knowledge derived from pattern appreciation reflects the unique patterning of the client (Cowling, 1997).

THE UNITARY PATTERN-BASED PRACTICE METHOD

Butcher (1997, 1999a, 2001) synthesized Cowling's Rogerian practice constituents with Barrett's practice method to develop a more inclusive and comprehensive practice model. The *unitary pattern-based practice method* consists of two nonlinear and simultaneous processes: pattern manifestation appreciation and knowing, and voluntary mutual patterning. The focus of nursing care guided by Rogers' nursing science is on recognizing manifestations of patterning through *pattern manifestation knowing and appreciation* and by facilitating the client's ability to participate knowingly in change, harmonizing person/environment integral-

ity, and promoting healing potentialities and well-being through *voluntary mutual patterning*.

Pattern Manifestation Knowing and Appreciation

Pattern manifestation knowing and appreciation is the process of identifying manifestations of patterning emerging from the human/environmental field mutual process and involves focusing on the client's experiences, perceptions, and expressions. "Knowing" refers to apprehending pattern manifestations (Barrett, 1988), whereas "appreciation" seeks for a perception of the "full force of pattern" (Cowling, 1997).

Pattern is the distinguishing feature of the human/environmental field. Everything experienced, perceived, and expressed is a manifestation

> *Pattern is the distinguishing feature of the human/environmental field. Everything experienced, perceived, and expressed is a manifestation of patterning.*

of patterning. During the process of pattern manifestation knowing and appreciation, the nurse and client are coequal participants. In Rogerian practice, nursing situations are approached and guided by a set of Rogerian-ethical values, a scientific base for practice, and a commitment to enhance the client's desired potentialities for well-being.

Rogerian ethics are pattern manifestations emerging from the human/environmental field mutual process that reflect those ideals concordant with Rogers' most cherished values and are indicators of the quality of knowing participation in change (Butcher, 1999b). Thus, unitary pattern-based practice includes making the Rogerian values of reverence, human betterment, generosity, commitment, diversity, responsibility, compassion, wisdom, justice-creating, openness, courage, optimism, humor, unity, transformation, and celebration intentional in the human/environmental field mutual process (Butcher, 1999b, 2000).

Unitary pattern-based practice begins by creating an atmosphere of openness and freedom so clients can freely participate in the process of knowing participation in change. Approaching the nursing situation with an appreciation of the uniqueness of each person and with unconditional love, compassion, and empathy can help create an atmosphere of openness and healing patterning. Rogers (1966/1994) defined nursing as a humanistic science dedicated to compassionate concern for human beings. Compassion includes energetic acts of unconditional love and means (a) recognizing the interconnectedness of the nurse and client by being able to fully understand and know the suffering of another, (b) creating actions designed to transform injustices, and (c) not only grieving in another's sorrow and pain, but also rejoicing in another's joy (Butcher, 2002b).

Pattern manifestation knowing and appreciation involves focusing on the experiences,

> *Pattern manifestation knowing and appreciation involves focusing on the experiences, perceptions, and expressions of a health situation, revealed through a rhythmic flow of communion and dialogue.*

perceptions, and expressions of a health situation, revealed through a rhythmic flow of communion and dialogue. In most situations, the nurse can initially ask the client to describe his or her health situation and concern. The dialogue is guided toward focusing on uncovering the client's experiences, perceptions, and expressions related to the health situation as a means to reaching a deeper understanding of unitary field pattern. Humans are constantly all-at-once experiencing, perceiving, and expressing (Cowling, 1993a). Experience involves the rawness of living through sensing and being aware as a source of knowledge and includes any item or ingredient the client senses (Cowling, 1997). The client's own observations and description of his or her health situation includes his or her experiences. "Perceiving is the apprehending of experience or the ability to reflect while experiencing" (Cowling, 1993a, p. 202). Perception is making sense of the experience through awareness, apprehension, observation, and interpreting. Asking clients about their concerns, fears, and observations is a way of apprehending their perceptions. Expressions are manifestations of experiences and perceptions that reflect human field patterning. In addition, expressions are any form of information that comes forward in the encounter with the client. All expressions are energetic manifestations of field pattern. Body language, communication patterns, gait, behaviors, lab values, and vital

signs are examples of energetic manifestations of human/environmental field patterning.

Since all information about the client/environment/health situation is relevant, various health assessment tools, such as the comprehensive holistic assessment tool developed by Dossey, Guzzetta, and Keegan (2000), may also be useful in pattern knowing and appreciation. However, all information must be interpreted within a unitary context. A *unitary context* refers to conceptualizing all information as energetic/dynamic manifestations of pattern emerging from a pandimensional human/environment mutual process. All information is interconnected, is inseparable from environmental context, unfolds rhythmically and acausally, and reflects the whole. Data are not divided or understood by dividing information into physical, psychological, social, spiritual, or cultural categories. Rather, a focus on experiences, perceptions, and expressions is a synthesis more than and different from the sum of parts. From a unitary perspective, what may be labeled as abnormal processes, nursing diagnoses, illness or disease are conceptualized as episodes of discordant rhythms or nonharmonic resonancy (Bultemeier, 2002).

A unitary perspective in nursing practice leads to an appreciation of new kinds of information that may not be considered within other conceptual approaches to nursing practice. The nurse is open to using multiple forms of knowing, including pandimensional modes of awareness (intuition, meditative insights, tacit knowing) throughout the pattern manifestation knowing and appreciation process. Intuition and tacit knowing are artful ways to enable seeing the whole, revealing subtle patterns, and deepening understanding. Pattern information concerning time perception, sense of rhythm or movement, sense of connectedness with the environment, ideas of one's own personal myth, and sense of integrity are relevant indicators of human/environment/health potentialities (Madrid & Winstead-Fry, 1986). A person's hopes and dreams, communication patterns, sleep-rest rhythms, comfort-discomfort, waking–beyond waking experiences, and degree of knowing participation in change provide important information regarding each client's thoughts and feelings concerning a health situation.

The nurse can also use a number of pattern appraisal scales, as mentioned in Part 1 of this chapter, derived from Rogers' postulates and principles to enhance the collecting and understanding of relevant information specific to Rogerian science. In addition to those mentioned in Part 1, Paletta (1990) developed a tool consistent with Rogerian science that measures the subjective awareness of temporal experience.

The pattern manifestation knowing and appreciation is enhanced through the nurse's ability to *grasp meaning,* create a *meaningful connection,* and *participate knowingly* in the client's change process (Butcher, 1999a). "*Grasping meaning* entails using sensitivity, active listening, conveying unconditional acceptance, while remaining fully open to the rhythm, movement, intensity, and configuration of pattern manifestations" (Butcher, 1999a, p. 51). Through integrality, nurse and client are always connected in mutual process. However, a *meaningful connection* with the client is facilitated by creating a rhythm and flow through the intentional expression of unconditional love, compassion, and empathy. Together, in mutual process, the nurse and client explore the meanings, images, symbols, metaphors, thoughts, insights, intuitions, memories, hopes, apprehensions, feelings, and dreams associated with the health situation.

When initial pattern manifestation knowing and appreciation is complete, the nurse synthesizes all the pattern information into a meaningful pattern profile. The pattern profile is an expression of the person/environment/health situation's essence. The nurse weaves together the expressions, perceptions, and experiences in a way that tells the client's story. The pattern profile reveals the hidden meaning embedded in the client's human/environmental mutual field process. Usually the pattern profile is in a narrative form that describes the essence of the properties, features, and qualities of the human/environment/health situation. In addition to a narrative form, the pattern profile may also include diagrams, poems, listings, phrases, and/or metaphors. Interpretations of any measurement tools may also be incorporated into the pattern profile.

Voluntary Mutual Patterning

Voluntary mutual patterning is a process of transforming human/environmental field patterning. The goal of voluntary mutual patterning is to facilitate each client's ability to participate knowingly in change, harmonize person/environment integrality, and promote healing potentialities, lifestyle changes, and well-being in the client's desired direction of change without attachment to predetermined outcomes. The process is mutual in that both the nurse and the client are changed with each encounter, each patterning one another and co-evolving together. "Voluntary" signifies freedom of choice or action without external compulsion (Barrett, 1998). The nurse has no investment in changing the client in a particular way.

Whereas patterning is continuous, voluntary mutual patterning may begin by sharing the pattern profile with the client. Sharing the pattern profile with the client is a means of validating the interpretation of pattern information and may spark further dialogue, revealing new and more in-depth information. Sharing the pattern profile with the client facilitates pattern recognition and also may enhance the client's knowing participation in his or her own change process. An increased awareness of one's own pattern may offer new insight and increase one's desire to participate in the change process. In addition, the nurse and client can continue to explore goals, options, choices, and voluntary mutual patterning strategies as a means to facilitate the client's actualization of his or her human/environmental field potentials.

A wide variety of mutual patterning strategies may be used in Rogerian practice, including many "interventions" identified in the Nursing Intervention Classification (McCloskey & Bulechek, 2004). However, "interventions," within a unitary context, are not linked to nursing diagnoses and are reconceptualized as *voluntary mutual patterning strategies,* and the activities are reconceptualizied as *patterning activities.* Rather than linking voluntary mutual patterning strategies to nursing diagnoses, the strategies emerge in dialogue whenever possible out of the patterns and themes described in the pattern profile. Furthermore, Rogers (1988, 1992, 1994) placed great emphasis on modalities that are traditionally viewed as holistic and noninvasive. In particular, therapeutic touch, guided imagery, and the use of humor, sound, dialogue, affirmations, music, massage, journaling, expressive emotional writing, exercise, nutrition, reminiscence, aroma, light, color, artwork, meditation, storytelling, literature, poetry, movement, and dance are just a few of the voluntary mutually patterning strategies consistent with a unitary perspective. Sharing of knowledge through health education and providing health education literature and teaching also have the potential to enhance knowing participation in change. These and other noninvasive modalities are well described and documented in both the Rogerian literature (Barrett, 1990; Madrid, 1997; Madrid & Barrett, 1994) and in the holistic nursing practice literature (Dossey, 1997; Dossey, Guzzetta, & Keegan, 2000).

Evaluation is continuous and is integral both to pattern manifestation knowing and appreciation and to voluntary mutual patterning. The nurse is continuously evaluating changes in patterning emerging from the human/environmental field mutual process. While the concept of "outcomes" is incompatible with Rogers' notions of unpredictability, outcomes in the Nursing Outcomes Classification (Moorhead, Johnson, Maas, 2004) can be reconceptualizied as potentialities of change or "client potentials" (Butcher, 1997, p. 29), and the indicators can be used as a means to evaluate the client's desired direction of pattern change. At various points in the client's care, the nurse can also use the scales derived from Rogers' science (previously discussed) to coexamine changes in pattern. Regardless of which combination of voluntary patterning strategies and evaluation methods are used, the intention is for clients to actualize their potentials related to their desire for well-being and betterment.

The unitary pattern-based practice method identifies that aspect that is unique to nursing and expands nursing practice beyond the traditional biomedical model that dominates much of nursing. Rogerian nursing practice does not necessarily need to replace hospital-based and medically driven nursing interventions and actions for which nurses hold responsibility. Rather, unitary pattern-based practice complements medical practices and places treatments and procedures within an acausal, pandimensional, rhythmical, irreducible, and unitary context. Unitary pattern-based practice brings about a new way of thinking and being in nursing that distinguishes nursing from other health-care professionals and offers new and innovative ways for clients to reach their desired health potentials.

SELECTED ROGERIAN THEORIES

In addition to the processes of the unitary pattern-based practice method, a number of Rogerian theories have been developed that are useful in informing the pattern manifestation knowing and appreciation and voluntary mutual patterning processes.

Theory of Power as Knowing Participation in Change

Barrett's (1989) Theory of Power as Knowing Participation in Change was derived directly from Rogers' postulates and principles, and it interweaves awareness, choices, freedom to act intentionally, and involvement in creating changes. Power is a natural continuous theme in the flow of life experiences and dynamically describes how human beings participate with the environment to actualize their potential. Barrett (1983) pointed out that most theories of power are causal and define power as the ability to influence, prevent, or cause change with dominance, force, and hierarchy. Power, within a Rogerian perspective, is being aware of what one is choosing to do, feeling free to do it, doing it intentionally, and being actively involved in the change process. A person's ability to participate knowingly in change varies in given situations. Thus, the intensity, frequency, and form in which power manifests vary. Power is neither inherently good nor evil; however, the form in which power manifests may be viewed as either constructive or destructive, depending on one's value perspective (Barrett, 1989). Barrett (1989) stated that her theory does not value different forms of power, but instead recognizes differences in power manifestations.

The Power as Knowing Participation in Change Tool (PKPCT), mentioned earlier, is a measure of one's relative frequency of power. Barrett (1989) suggests that the Power Theory and the PKPCT may be useful in a wide variety of nursing situations. Barrett's Power Theory is useful with clients who are experiencing hopelessness, suicidal ideation, hypertension and obesity, drug and alcohol dependence, grief and loss, self-esteem issues, adolescent turmoil, career conflicts, marital discord, cultural relocation trauma, or the desire to make a lifestyle change. In fact, all health/illness experiences involve issues concerning knowing participation in change.

During pattern manifestation knowing and appreciation, the nurse invites the client to complete the PKPCT as a means to identify the client's power pattern. To prevent biased responses, the nurse should refrain from using the word "power." The power score is determined on each of the four sub-scales: awareness, choices, freedom to act intentionally, and involvement in creating changes. The scores are documented as part of the client's pattern profile and shared with the client during voluntary mutual patterning. Scores are considered as a tentative and relative measure of the ever-changing nature of one's field pattern in relation to power.

Instead of focusing on issues of control, the nurse helps the client identify the changes and the direction of change the client desires to make. Using open-ended questions, the nurse and the client mutually explore choices and options and identify barriers preventing change, strategies, and resources to overcome barriers; the nurse facilitates the client's active involvement in creating the changes. For example, asking the questions, "What do you want?" "What choices are open to you now?" "How free do you feel to do what you want to do?" and "How will you involve yourself in creating the changes you want?" can enhance the client's awareness, choice-making, freedom to act intentionally, and his or her involvement in creating change (Barrett, 1998).

A wide range of voluntary mutual patterning strategies may be used to enhance knowing participation in change, including meaningful dialogue, dance/movement/motion, sound, light, color, music, rest/activity, imagery, humor, therapeutic touch, bibliotherapy, journaling, drawing, and nutrition (Barrett, 1998). The PKPCT can be used at intervals to evaluate the client's relative changes in power.

Theory of Kaleidoscoping in Life's Turbulence

Butcher's (1993) Theory of Kaleidoscoping in Life's Turbulence was derived from Rogers' Science of Unitary Human Beings, chaos theory (Briggs & Peat, 1989; Peat, 1991), and Csikszentmihalyi's (1990) Theory of Flow. It focuses on facilitating well-being and harmony amid turbulent life events. Turbulence is a dissonant commotion in the human/environmental field characterized by chaotic and unpredictable change. Any crisis may be viewed as a turbulent event in the life process. Nurses often work closely with clients who are in a "crisis." The turbulent life event may be an illness, the uncertainty of a medical diagnosis, marital discord, or loss of a loved one. Turbulent life events are often chaotic in nature, unpredictable, and always transformative.

Kaleidoscoping is a way of engaging in a mutual process with clients who are in the midst of experiencing a turbulent life event by mutually *flowing with turbulent manifestations of patterning* (Butcher, 1993). *Flow* is an intense harmonious involvement in the human/environment mutual field process. The term "kaleidoscoping" was used because it evolves directly from Rogers' writings and conveys the unpredictable continuous flow of patterns, sometimes turbulent, that one experiences when looking through a kaleidoscope. Rogers (1970) explained that the "organization of the living system is maintained amidst kaleidoscopic alterations in the patterning of system" (p. 62).

The Theory of Kaleidoscoping with Turbulent Life Events is used in conjunction with the pattern manifestation knowing and appreciation and voluntary mutual patterning processes. In addition to engaging in the processes already described in pattern manifestation knowing and appreciation, the nurse identifies manifestations of patterning and mutually explores the meaning of the turbulent situation with the client. A pattern profile describing the essence of the client's experiences, perceptions, and expressions related to the turbulent life event is constructed and shared with the client.

In the theory of kaleidoscoping, voluntary mutual patterning also incorporates the processes of transforming turbulent events by *cultivating purpose, forging resolve,* and *recovering harmony* (Butcher, 1993). *Cultivating purpose* involves assisting clients in identifying goals and developing an action system. The action system is comprised of patterning strategies designed to promote harmony amid adversity and facilitate the actualization of the potential for well-being.

In moments of turbulence, clients may want to increase their awareness of the complexity of the situation. Creative suspension is a technique that may be used to facilitate comprehension of the situation's complexity (Peat, 1991). Guided imagery is a useful strategy for facilitating creative suspension because it potentially enhances the client's ability to enter a timeless suspension directed toward visualizing the whole situation and facilitating the creation of new strategies and solutions. *Forging resolve* is assisting the clients in becoming involved and immersed in their action system. Because chaotic and turbulent systems are infinitely sensitive, actions are "gentle" or subtle in nature and are distributed over the entire system involved in the change process. Entering chaotic systems with a "big splash" or trying to force a change in a particular direction will likely lead to increased turbulence (Butcher, 1993).

Forging resolve involves incorporating flow experiences into the change process. Flow experiences promote harmonious human/environmental field patterns. There are a wide range of flow experiences that can be incorporated into the daily activities: art, music, exercise, reading, gardening, meditation, dancing, sports, sailing, swimming, carpentry, sewing, yoga, or any activity that is a source of enjoyment, concentration, and deep involvement. The incorporating of flow experiences into daily patterns potentiates the recovering of harmony. *Recovering harmony* is achieving a sense of courage, balance, calm, and resilience amid turbulent and threatening life events. The art of kaleidoscoping with turbulence is a mutual creative expression of beauty and grace and is a way of enhancing perseverance through difficult times.

Personalized Nursing LIGHT Practice Model

The final Rogerian theory discussed in this overview is the successful Personalized Nursing LIGHT Practice Model (Anderson & Smereck, 1989, 1992, 1994). For more than 10 years, the model has been used by the Personalized Nursing Corporation, an independent, nurse-owned, nurse-managed company providing outreach nursing care to high-risk and active drug users in Detroit, Michigan. The goal of the LIGHT model is to assist clients in improving their sense of well-being. With a higher sense of well-being, clients are less likely to continue to engage in high-risk drug-related behaviors. Drug-addicted behaviors are postulated to be a painful means to experience an awareness of integrality. During the pattern manifestation knowing and appreciation process, clients are asked to name a painful experience, are encouraged to "be in the moment" in a safe place with the experience/feeling, are asked to identify the choices they usually make during the painful experience, and are then asked to identify pattern manifestations associated with their usual choices.

The acronym LIGHT guides the voluntary mutual patterning process. Nurses:

- Love the client,
- Intend to help,
- Give care gently,
- Help the client improve well-being, and
- Teach the healing process of the LIGHT model.

Clients make progress toward well-being as they learn to:

- Love themselves,
- Identify concerns,
- Give themselves goals,
- Have confidence and help themselves, and
- Take positive action.

In a three-year pre- and postcontrol treatment group study involving 744 participants, clients who received nursing care with the LIGHT model improved their sense of well-being associated with a decrease in high-risk drug behaviors (Anderson & Hockman, 1997).

Research

Research is the bedrock of nursing practice. The Science of Unitary Human Beings has a long

> **Research is the bedrock of nursing practice.**

history of theory-testing research. As new practice theories and health patterning modalities evolve from the Science of Unitary Human Beings, there remains a need to test the viability and usefulness of Rogerian theories and voluntary health patterning strategies. The mass of Rogerian research has been reviewed in a number of publications (Caroselli & Barrett, 1998; Dykeman & Loukissa, 1993; Fawcett, 2000; Fawcett & Alligood, 2003; Malinski, 1986; Phillips, 1989b; Watson, Barrett, Hastings-Tolsma, Johnson, & Gueldner, 1997). Rather than repeat the reviews of Rogerian research, the following section describes current methodological trends within the Science of Unitary Human Beings to assist researchers interested in Rogerian science in making methodological decisions.

Although there is some debate among Rogerian scholars and researchers concerning the choice of an appropriate methodology in Rogerian research, Rogers (1994) maintained that both quantitative and qualitative methods may be useful for advancing Rogerian science. Similarly, Barrett (1996), Barrett and Caroselli (1998), Barrett, Cowling, Carboni, and Butcher (1997), Cowling (1986), Smith & Reeder (1996), and Rawnsley (1994) have all advocated for the appropriateness of multiple methods in Rogerian research. Conversely, Butcher (cited in Barrett et al., 1997), Butcher (1994), and Carboni (1995b) have argued that the ontological and epistemological assumptions of causality, reductionism, particularism, control, prediction, and linearity of quantitative methodologies are inconsistent with Rogers' unitary ontology and participatory epistemology. Later, Fawcett (1996) also questioned the congruency between the ontology and epistemology of Rogerian science and the assumptions embedded in quantitative research designs; like Carboni (1995) and Butcher (1994), she concluded that interpretive/qualitative methods may be more congruent with Rogers' ontology and epistemology.

This chapter presents an inclusive view of methodologies. Nevertheless, the researcher needs to present an argument as to how the design of the study and interpretations of results are congruent with Rogers' postulates and principles. Furthermore, nurses interested in engaging in Rogerian research are encouraged to use, test, and refine the developed research methods and tools that are consistent with the ontology and epistemology of the science of unitary human beings.

CRITERIA FOR ROGERIAN INQUIRY

The criteria for developing Rogerian research methods presented in this chapter are a synthesis and modification of the Criteria of Rogerian Inquiry developed by Butcher (1994) and the Characteristics of Operational Rogerian Inquiry developed by Carboni (1995b). The criteria may be a useful guide in designing research investigations guided by the Science of Unitary Human Beings.

1. *A priori nursing science:* All research flows from a theoretical perspective. Every step of the inquiry, including the type of questions asked, the conceptualization of phenomena of concern, choice of research design, selection of participants, selection of instruments, and interpretation of findings is guided by the science of unitary human beings. The researcher explicitly identi-

fies the science of unitary human beings as the conceptual orientation of the study. Nursing research must be grounded in a theoretical perspective unique to nursing in order for the research to contribute to the advance of nursing science.

2. *Creation:* The Rogerian research endeavor is a creative and imaginative process for discovering new insights and knowledge concerning unitary human beings in mutual process with their environment.

3. *Irreducible human/environmental energy fields are the focus of Rogerian inquiry:* Energy fields are postulated to constitute the fundamental unit of the living and nonliving. Both human beings and the environment are understood as dynamic energy fields that cannot be reduced to parts.

4. *Pattern manifestations are indicators of change:* Pattern is the distinguishing characteristic of an energy field and gives identity to the field. Pattern manifestations are the source of information emerging from the human/environmental mutual field process and are the only valid reflections of the energy field. The phenomenon of concern in Rogerian inquiry is conceptualized and understood as manifestations of human/environmental energy mutual process.

5. *Pandimensional awareness:* Rogerian inquiry recognizes the pandimensional nature of reality. All forms of awareness are relevant in a pandimensional universe. Thus, intuition, both tacit and mystical, and all forms of sensory knowing are relevant ways of apprehending manifestations of patterning.

6. *Human instrument is used for pattern knowing and appreciation:* The researchers use themselves as the primary pattern-apprehending instrument. The human instrument is the only instrument sensitive to, and which has the ability to interpret and understand, pandimensional potentialities in human/environmental field patterning. Pattern manifestation knowing and appreciation is the process of apprehending information or manifestations of patterning emerging from the human/environmental field mutual process. The process of pattern knowing and appreciation is the same in the research endeavor as described earlier in the Rogerian practice methodology.

7. *Both quantitative and qualitative methods are*

appropriate: Quantitative methods may be used when the design, concepts, measurement tools, and results are conceptualized and interpreted in a way consistent with Rogers' nursing science. It is important to note that because of the incongruency between ontology and epistemology of Rogerian science with assumptions in quantitative designs, Carboni (1995b) argues that the researcher must select qualitative methods exclusively over quantitative methods. Barrett and Caroselli (1998), however, recognize the inconsistencies of quantitative methods with Rogerian science and argue that the "research question drives the choice of method; hence, both qualitative and quantitative methods are not only useful but necessary" (p. 21). The ontological and epistemological congruence is reflected in the nature of questions asked and their theoretical conceptualization (Barrett, 1996). However, qualitative designs, particularly those that have been derived from the postulates and principles of the science of unitary human beings, are *preferred* because the ontology and epistemology of qualitative designs are more congruent with Rogers' notions of unpredictability, irreducibility, acausality, integrality, continuous process, and pattern (Barrett et al., 1997; Butcher, 1994).

8. *Natural setting:* Rogerian inquiry is pursued in the natural settings where the phenomenon of inquiry occurs naturally, because the human field is inseparable and in mutual process with the environmental field. Any "manipulation" of "variables" is inconsistent with mutual process, unpredictability, and irreducibility.

9. *The researcher and the researcher-into are integral:* The principle of integrality implies that the researcher is inseparable and in mutual process with the environment and the participants in the study. Each evolves during the research process. The researcher's values are also inseparable from the inquiry. "Objectivity" and "bracketing" are not possible when the human and environmental field are integral to each other.

10. *Purposive sampling:* The researcher uses purposive sampling to select participants who manifest the phenomenon of interest. Recognition of the integrality of all that is tells us that information about the whole is available in individuals, groups, and settings; therefore, representative samples are not required to capture manifestations of patterning reflective of the whole.

11. *Emergent design:* The Rogerian researcher is aware of dynamic unpredictability and continuous change and is open to the idea that patterns in the inquiry process may change in the course of the study that may not have been envisioned in advance. Rather than adhere to pre-ordained rigid patterns of inquiry, the research design may change and evolve during the inquiry. It is essential that the researcher document and report any design changes.

12. *Pattern synthesis:* Rogerian science emphasizes synthesis rather than analysis. *Analysis* is the separation of the whole into its constituent parts. The separation of parts is not consistent with Rogers' notion of integrality and irreducible wholes. Patterns are manifestations of the whole emerging from the human/environmental mutual field process. Synthesis allows for creating and viewing a coherent whole. Therefore, data are not "analyzed" within Rogerian inquiry but are "synthesized." Data-processing techniques that put emphasis on information or pattern synthesis are preferred over techniques that place emphasis on data "analysis."

13. *Shared description and shared understanding:* Mutual process is enhanced by including participants in the process of inquiry where possible. For example, sharing of results with participants in the study enhances shared awareness, understanding, and knowing participation in change. Furthermore, participants are the best judges of the authenticity and validity of their own experiences, perceptions, and expressions. Participatory action designs and focus groups conceptualized within Rogerian science may be ways to enhance mutual exploration, discovery, and knowing participation in change.

14. *Evolutionary interpretation:* The researcher interprets all the findings within the perspective of the Science of Unitary Human Beings. Thus, the findings are understood and presented within the context of Rogers' postulates of energy fields, pandimensionality, openness, pattern, and the principles of integrality, resonancy, and helicy. Evolutionary interpretation provides *meaning* to the findings within a

Rogerian science perspective. Interpreting the findings within a Rogerian perspective advances Rogerian science, practice, and research.

POTENTIAL ROGERIAN RESEARCH DESIGNS

Cowling (1986) was among the first to suggest a number of research designs that may be appropriate for Rogerian research, including philosophical, historical, and phenomenological ones. There is strong support for the appropriateness of phenomenological methods in Rogerian science. Reeder (1986) provided a convincing argument demonstrating the congruence between Husserlian phenomenology and the Rogerian science of unitary human beings:

> [G]iven the congruency between Husserlian phenomenology and the Rogerian conceptual system, a sound, convincing rationale is established for the use of this philosophy of science as an alternative for basic theoretical studies in Rogerian nursing science.... Nursing research in general requires a broader range of human experience than sensory experience (whether intuitive or perceptive) in the development and testing of conceptual systems for gaining better access to multifaceted phenomena.... Husserlian phenomenology as a rigorous science provides just such an experience. (p. 62)

Experimental and quasi-experimental designs are problematic because of assumptions concerning causality; however, these designs may be appropriate for testing propositions concerning differences in the change process in relation to "introduced environmental change" (Cowling, 1986, p. 73). The researcher must be careful to interpret the findings in a way that is consistent with Rogers' notions of unpredictability, integrality, and nonlinearity. Emerging interpretive evaluation methods, such as Guba and Lincoln's (1989) Fourth Generation Evaluation, offer an alternative means for testing for differences in the change process within and/or between groups more consistent with the Science of Unitary Human Beings.

Cowling (1986) contended that in the early stages of theory development, designs that generate descriptive and explanatory knowledge are relevant to the Science of Unitary Human Beings. For example, correlational designs may provide evidence of patterned changes among indices of the human field. Advanced and complex designs with multiple indicators of change that may be tested using linear structural relations (LISREL) statistical analysis may also be a means to uncover knowledge about the pattern of change rather than just knowledge of parts of a change process (Phillips, 1990a). Barrett (1996) suggests that canonical correlation may be useful in examining relationships and patterns across domains and may also be useful for testing theories pertaining to the nature and direction of change. Another potentially promising area yet to be explored is participatory action and cooperative inquiry (Reason, 1994), because of their congruence with Rogers' notions of knowing participation in change, continuous mutual process, and integrality. Cowling (1998) proposed that a case-oriented approach is useful in Rogerian research, because case inquiry allows the researcher to attend to the whole and strives to comprehend his or her essence.

SELECTING A FOCUS OF ROGERIAN INQUIRY

In selecting a focus of inquiry, concepts that are congruent with the Science of Unitary Human Beings are most relevant. The focus of inquiry flows from the postulates, principles, and concepts relevant to the conceptual system. Noninvasive voluntary patterning modalities, such as guided imagery, therapeutic touch, humor, sound, dialogue, affirmations, music, massage, journaling, written emotional expression, exercise, nutrition, reminiscence, aroma, light, color, artwork, meditation, storytelling, literature, poetry, movement, and dance, provide a rich source for Rogerian science-based research. Creativity, mystical experiences, transcendence, sleeping-beyond-waking experiences, time experience, and paranormal experiences as they relate to human health and well-being are also of interest in this science. Feelings and experiences are a manifestation of human/environmental field patterning and are a manifestation of the whole (Rogers, 1970); thus, feelings and experiences relevant to health and well-being are an unlimited source for potential Rogerian research. Discrete particularistic biophysical phenomena are usually not an appropriate focus for inquiry because Rogerian science focuses on irreducible wholes.

Diseases or medical diagnoses are not the focus of Rogerian inquiry. Disease conditions are conceptualized as labels and as manifestations of patterning emerging acausally from the human/environmental mutual process. New concepts that describe unitary phenomena may be developed through research. Dispiritedness (Butcher, 1996), power (Barrett, 1983), perceived dissonance (Bultemeier, 2002), and human field image (Johnson, 1994; Phillips, 1990b) are examples of concepts developed through research within Rogers' nursing science, while spirituality (Malinski, 1991, 1994; Woods, 1994), compassion (Butcher, 2002b), caring (Smith, 1999), and energy (Leddy, 2003; Todaro-Franceschi, 1999) are examples of concepts that have been reconceptualizied in

> *Researchers need to ensure that concepts and measurement tools used in the inquiry are defined and conceptualized within a unitary perspective.*

a way congruent with Rogers' principles and postulates. Researchers need to ensure that concepts and measurement tools used in the inquiry are defined and conceptualized within a unitary perspective.

MEASUREMENT OF ROGERIAN CONCEPTS

The Human Field Motion Test (HFMT) is an indicator of the continuously moving position and flow of the human energy field. Two major concepts—"my motor is running" and "my field expansion"—are rated using a semantic differential technique (Ference, 1979). Examples of indicators of higher human field motion include feeling imaginative, visionary, transcendent, strong, sharp, bright, and active. Indicators of relative low human field motion include feeling dull, weak, dragging, dark, pragmatic, and passive. The tool has been widely used in numerous Rogerian studies.

The Power as Knowing Participation in Change Tool (PKPCT) has been used in over 26 major research studies (Caroselli & Barrett, 1998) and is a measure of one's capacity to participate knowingly in change as manifested by awareness, choices, freedom to act intentionally, and involvement in creating changes using semantic differential scales. Statistically significant correlations have been found between power as measured by the PKPCT and the following: human field motion, life satisfaction, spirituality, purpose in life, empathy, transformational leadership style, feminism, imagi-

nation, and socioeconomic status. Inverse relations with power have been found with anxiety, chronic pain, personal distress, and hopelessness (Caroselli & Barrett, 1998).

A number of new tools have been developed that are rich sources of measures of concepts congruent with unitary science. The Human Field Image Metaphor Scale (HFMIS) used 25 metaphors that capture feelings of potentiality and integrality rated on a Likert-type scale. For example, the metaphor "I feel at one with the universe" reflects a high degree of awareness of integrality; "I feel like a worn-out shoe" reflects a more restricted perception of one's potential (Johnston, 1994; Watson et al., 1997). Future research may focus on developing an understanding of how human field image changes in a variety of health-related situations or how human field image changes in mutual process with selected patterning strategies.

Diversity is inherent in the evolution of the human/environmental mutual field process. The evolution of the human energy field is characterized by the creation of more diverse patterns reflecting the nature of change. The Diversity of Human Field Pattern Scale (DHFPS) measures the process of diversifying human field pattern and may also be a useful tool to test theoretical propositions derived from the postulates and principles of Rogerian science to examine the extent of selected patterning modalities designed to foster harmony and well-being (Hastings-Tolsma, 1992; Watson et al., 1997). Other measurement tools developed within and unitary science perspective that may be used in a wide variety of research studies and in combination with other Rogerian measurements include:

- Assessment of Dream Experience Scale, which measures the diversity of dream experience as a beyond-waking manifestation using a 20-item Likert scale (Watson, 1993; Watson et al., 1997);
- Temporal Experience Scale (TES), which measures the subjective experience of temporal awareness (Paletta, 1990);
- Leddy's (1995) Person-Environment Participation Scale, which measures expansiveness and ease of participation in the continuous human/environmental mutual field process using semantic differential scales; and
- Mutual Exploration of the Healing Human Field–Environmental Field Relationship Crea-

tive Measurement Instrument developed by Carboni (1992), which is a creative qualitative measure designed to capture the changing configurations of energy field pattern of the healing human/environmental field relationship.

MEASURES SPECIFIC TO SCIENCE OF UNITARY HUMAN BEINGS

Although the quantitative measures provide a rich source for future research, Rogerian researchers are encouraged to use methods developed specific to the Science of Unitary Human Beings. Three methods have been developed: Rogerian Process of Inquiry, the Unitary Field Pattern Portrait Research Method, and Unitary Case Inquiry. Each method was derived from Rogers' unitary ontology and participatory epistemology and is congruent with the criteria for Rogerian inquiry presented earlier in this chapter.

Rogerian Process of Inquiry

Carboni (1995b) developed the Rogerian Process of Inquiry from her characteristics of Rogerian inquiry. The method's purpose is to investigate the dynamic enfolding-unfolding of the human field–environmental field energy patterns and the evolutionary change of configurations in field patterning of the nurse and participant. Rogerian Process of Inquiry transcends both matter-centered methodologies espoused by empiricists and thought-bound methodologies espoused by phenomenologists and critical theorists (Carboni, 1995b). Rather, this process of inquiry is evolution-centered and focuses on changing configurations of human and environmental field patterning.

The flow of the inquiry starts with a summation of the researcher's purpose, aims, and visionary insights. Visionary insights emerge from the study's purpose and researcher's understanding of Rogerian science. Next, the researcher focuses on becoming familiar with the participants and the setting of the inquiry. Shared descriptions of energy field perspectives are identified through observations and discussions with participants and processed through mutual exploration and discovery. The researcher uses the Mutual Exploration of the Healing Human Field–Environmental Field Relationship Creative Measurement Instrument (Carboni, 1992) as a way to identify, understand, and creatively measure human and environmental

energy field patterns. Together, the researcher and the participants develop a shared understanding and awareness of the human/environmental field patterns manifested in diverse multiple configurations of patterning. All the data are synthesized using inductive and deductive data synthesis. Through the mutual sharing and synthesis of data, unitary constructs are identified. The constructs are interpreted within the perspective of unitary science, and a new unitary theory may emerge from the synthesis of unitary constructs. Carboni (1995b) also developed special criteria of trustworthiness to ensure the scientific rigor of the findings conveyed in the form of a Pandimensional Unitary Process Report. Carboni's research method affords a way of creatively measuring manifestations of field patterning emerging during coparticipation of the researcher and participant's process of change.

The Unitary Field Pattern Portrait Research Method

The Unitary Field Pattern Portrait (UFPP) research method (Butcher, 1994, 1996, 1998) was developed at the same time Carboni was developing the Unitary Process of Inquiry and was derived directly from the criteria of Rogerian inquiry. The purpose of the UFPP research method is to create a unitary understanding of the dynamic kaleidoscopic and symphonic pattern manifestations emerging from the pandimensional human/environmental field mutual process as a means to enhance the understanding of a significant phenomenon associated with human betterment and well-being. There are eight essential aspects in the method, as described here. The UFPP (see Figure 13–1) also includes three essential processes. Each aspect is described here in relation to the essential processses.

1. *Initial engagement* is a passionate search for a research question of central interest to understanding unitary phenomena associated with human betterment and well-being.
2. *A priori nursing science* identifies the Science of Unitary Human Beings as the researcher's perspective. It guides all processes of the research method, including the interpretation of findings.
3. *Immersion* involves becoming steeped in the research topic. The researcher may immerse himself or herself in any activity that enhances the integrality of the researcher and the research topic.

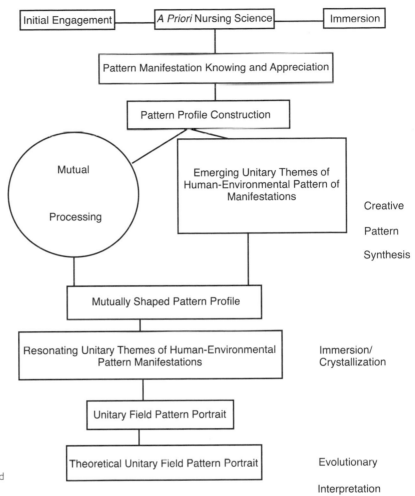

FIGURE 13–1 The Unitary Field
Pattern Portrait Research Method.

4. *Pattern manifestation knowing and appreciation* includes participant selection, in-depth dialoguing, and recording pattern manifestations. Participant selection is made using intensive purposive sampling. Patterning manifestation knowing and appreciation occurs in a natural setting and involves using pandimensional modes of awareness during in-depth dialoguing. The activities described earlier in the pattern manifestation knowing and appreciation process section of the practice method are used in this research method. However, in the UFPP research method, the focus of pattern appreciation and knowing is on experiences, perceptions, and expressions associated with the phenomenon of concern. The researcher also maintains an informal conversational style while focusing on revealing the rhythm, flow, and con-

figurations of the pattern manifestations emerging from the human/environmental mutual field process associated with the research topic. The dialogue is taped and transcribed. The researcher maintains observational, methodological, and theoretical field notes, and a reflexive journal. Any artifacts the participant wishes to share that illuminate the meaning of the phenomenon may also be included.

a. *Unitary field pattern profile* is a rich description of the participants' experiences, perceptions, and expressions created through a process of *creative pattern synthesis*. All the information collected for each participant is synthesized into a narrative statement revealing the essence of the participant's description of the phenomenon of concern. The field pattern profile is in the language of the participant and is then shared with the participant for verification and revision.

b. *Mutual processing* involves constructing the mutual unitary field pattern profile by mutually sharing an emerging joint or shared profile with each successive participant at the end of each participant's pattern manifestation knowing and appreciation process. For example, at the end of the fourth participant's interview, a joint construction of the phenomenon is shared with the participant for comment. The joint construction (mutual unitary field pattern profile) at this phase would consist of a synthesis of the profiles of the first three participants. After verification of the fourth participant's pattern profile, the profile is folded into the emerging mutual unitary field pattern profile. Pattern manifestation knowing and appreciation continues until there are no new pattern manifestations to add to the mutual unitary field pattern profile. If it is not possible to either share the pattern profile with each participant or create a *mutually constructed unitary field pattern profile*, the research may choose to bypass the mutual processing phase.

c. The *unitary field pattern portrait* is created by identifying emerging unitary themes from each participant's field pattern profile, sorting the unitary themes into common categories and creating the resonating unitary themes of human/environmental pattern manifestations through *immersion and crystallization*, which involves synthesizing the resonating themes into a descriptive portrait of the phenomenon. The unitary field pattern portrait is expressed in the form of a vivid, rich, thick, and accurate aesthetic rendition of the universal patterns, qualities, features, and themes exemplifying the essence of the dynamic kaleidoscopic and symphonic nature of the phenomenon of concern.

d. The unitary field pattern portrait is interpreted from the perspective of the Science of Unitary Human Beings using the process of *evolutionary interpretation* to create a *theoretical unitary field pattern portrait* of the phenomenon. The purpose of theoretical unitary field pattern portrait is to explicate the theoretical structure of the phenomenon from the perspective of Rogers' nursing science. The

theoretical unitary field pattern portrait is expressed in the language of Rogerian science, thereby lifting the unitary field pattern portrait from the level of description to the level of unitary science. Scientific rigor is maintained throughout processes by using the criteria of trustworthiness and authenticity. The findings of the study are conveyed in a Unitary Field Pattern Report.

Unitary Appreciative Inquiry

Cowling (2001) recently explicated the processes of Unitary Appreciative Inquiry as a method grounded in Rogerian science for "uncovering the wholeness and essence of human existence to inform the development of nursing science and guide the practice of nursing" (p. 32). Cowling's method may be used with individuals, groups, or communities and includes appreciative knowing, participatory, synoptic, and transformative processes. Human life is viewed as a miracle of a variety of ordinary and extraordinary forces characterized by unknowable mystery. The researcher and participant are equals in a participatory mutual process where outcomes are not imposed and change unfolds acausally and unpredictably. The inquirer examines all pattern information synoptically by viewing all experiences, perceptions, and expressions as interrelated in a way that reflects the inherent wholeness of a phenomenon or situation. The elements of the approach in unitary appreciative inquiry (Cowling, 2001) include:

1. The scientist/practitioner seeks out to explore a life situation, phenomenon, or concern from a unitary perspective.
2. Describe the endeavor with the aim of appreciating the wholeness, uniqueness, and essence of the particular situation, phenomenon, or concern.
3. Gain human subject's approval and informed consent.
4. Approach participants as partners in a coequal participative appreciative endeavor.
5. Information is collected in the form of dialogue, discussion, interview, observation, or any practice that illuminates the underlying human life pattern.
6. Documentation of the experience, perceptions, and expressions can be accomplished through journaling, audiotaping, videotaping, photo

graphing, recording music, or creating meaningful products.

7. Maintain theoretic, methodologic, reflective, and peer review notes.

8. Engagement with participants is negotiated and may last from several weeks to more than a year.

9. Construct a pattern profile using synopsis that meaningfully represents the person's experiences, perceptions, and expressions of participants and captures the wholeness, uniqueness, and essence of life. The profile may be created by the scientist/practitioner, the participants, or as a joint venture. The profile is often in the form of a story and may be shared with the participant.

10. The pattern profile may be used in unitary theory by seeking universals that may exist across cases while acknowledging the individual differences.

SUMMARY

"Nursing is the study of caring for persons experiencing human-environment-health transitions" (Butcher, 2004, p. 76). If nursing's content and contribution to the betterment of the health and well-being of a society is not distinguishable from other disciplines and has nothing unique or valuable to offer, then nursing's continued existence may be questioned. Thus, nursing's survival rests on its ability to make a *difference* in promoting the health and well-being of people. Making a difference refers to nursing's contribution to the client's desired health goals, and offering care is *distinguishable* from the services of other disciplines.

Every discipline's uniqueness evolves from its philosophical and theoretical perspective. The Science of Unitary Human Beings offers nursing a *distinguishable* and new way of conceptualizing health events concerning human well-being that is congruent with the most contemporary scientific theories. As with all major theories embedded in a new worldview, new terminology is needed to create clarity and precision of understanding and meaning. Rogers' nursing science leads to a new understanding of the experiences, perceptions, and expressions of health events and leads to innovative ways of practicing nursing. There is an ever-growing body of literature demonstrating the application of Rogerian science to practice and research. Rogers' nursing science is applicable in all nursing situations. Rather than focusing on disease and cellular biological processes, the Science of Unitary Human Beings focuses on human beings as irreducible wholes inseparable from their environment.

For 30 years, Rogers advocated that nurses should become the experts and providers of noninvasive modalities that promote health. Now, the growth of "alternative medicine" and noninvasive practices is outpacing the growth of traditional medicine. If nursing continues to be dominated by biomedical frameworks that are indistinguishable from medical care, nursing will lose an opportunity to become expert in holistic health-care modalities.

The Science of Unitary Human Beings offers nursing a distinguishable and new way of conceptualizing health events concerning human well-being that is congruent with the most contemporary scientific theories.

References

American Heritage Dictionary. (2000). (4th edition). New York: Houghton Mifflin.

Anderson, M. D., & Hockman, E. M. (1997). Well-being and high-risk drug use among active drug users. In Madrid, M. (Ed.), *Patterns of Rogerian knowing* (pp. 152–166). New York: National League for Nursing.

Anderson, M. D., & Smereck, G. A. D. (1989). Personalized LIGHT model. *Nursing Science Quarterly, 2,* 120–130.

Anderson, M. D., & Smereck, G. A. D. (1992). The consciousness rainbow: An explication of Rogerian field pattern manifestation. *Nursing Science Quarterly, 5,* 72–79.

Anderson, M. D., & Smereck, G. A. D. (1994). Personalized nursing: A science-based model of the art of nursing. In Madrid, M., & Barrett, E. A. M. (Eds.), *Rogers' scientific art of nursing practice* (pp. 261–283). New York: National League for Nursing.

Barrett, E. A. M. (1983). *An empirical investigation of Martha E. Rogers' principle of helicy: The relationship of human field motion and power.* Unpublished dissertation, New York University, New York.

Barrett, E. A. M. (1986). Investigation of the principle of helicy: The relationship of human field motion and power. In Malinski, V. M. (Ed.), *Explorations on Martha Rogers' science of unitary human beings* (pp. 173–184). Norwalk, CT: Appleton-Century-Crofts.

Barrett, E. A. M. (1988). Using Rogers' science of unitary human beings in nursing practice. *Nursing Science Quarterly, 1,* 50–51.

Barrett, E. A. M. (1989). A nursing theory of power for nursing practice: Derivation from Rogers' paradigm. In Riehl-Sisca, J. (Ed.), *Conceptual models for nursing practice* (3rd ed., pp. 207–217). Norwalk, CT: Appleton & Lange.

Barrett, E. A. M. (1990). Health patterning with clients in a private practice environment. In Barrett, E. A. M. (Ed.), *Visions of Rogers' science-based practice* (pp. 105–115). New York: National League for Nursing.

Barrett, E. A. M. (1990). Rogers' science-based nursing practice. In Barrett, E. A. M. (Ed.), *Visions of Rogers' science-based nursing.* New York: National League for Nursing.

Barrett, E. A. M. (1992). Innovative imagery: A health patterning modality for nursing practice. *Journal of Holistic Nursing, 10,* 154–166.

Barrett, E. A. M. (1996). Canonical correlation analysis and its use in Rogerian research. *Nursing Science Quarterly, 9,* 50–52.

Barrett, E. A. M. (1998). A Rogerian practice methodology for health patterning. *Nursing Science Quarterly, 11,* 136–138.

Barrett, E. A. M., & Caroselli, C. (1998). Methodological ponderings related to the power as knowing participation in change tool. *Nursing Science Quarterly, 11,* 17–22.

Barrett, E. A. M., Cowling, W. R. I., Carboni, J. T., & Butcher, H. K. (1997). Unitary perspectives on methodological practices. In Madrid, M. (Ed.), *Patterns of Rogerian knowing* (pp. 47–62). New York: National League for Nursing.

Bohm, D. (1980). *Wholeness and the implicate order.* London: Ark Paperbacks.

Briggs, J. P., & Peat, F. D. (1984). *Looking glass universe: The emerging science of wholeness.* New York: Simon & Schuster.

Briggs, J., & Peat, F. D. (1989). *Turbulent mirror: An illustrated guide to chaos theory and the science of wholeness.* New York: Harper & Row.

Bultemeier, K. (2002). Rogers' Science of Unitary Human Beings in nursing practice. In Alligood, M. R., & Marriner-Tomey, A. (Eds.), *Nursing theory: Utilization and application* (pp. 267–288). St. Louis: Mosby.

Butcher, H. K. (1993). Kaleidoscoping in life's turbulence: From Seurat's art to Rogers' nursing science. In Parker, M. E. (Ed.), *Patterns of nursing theories in practice* (pp. 183–198). New York: National League for Nursing.

Butcher, H. K. (1994). The unitary field pattern portrait method: Development of research method within Rogers' science of unitary human beings. In Madrid, M., & Barrett, E. A. M. (Eds.), *Rogers' scientific art of nursing practice* (pp. 397–425). New York: National League for Nursing.

Butcher, H. K. (1996). A unitary field pattern portrait of dispiritedness in later life. *Visions: The Journal of Rogerian Nursing Science, 4,* 41–58.

Butcher, H. K. (1997). Energy field disturbance. In McFarland, G. K., & McFarlane, E. A. (Eds.), *Nursing diagnosis and intervention* (3rd ed., pp. 22–33). St. Louis: Mosby.

Butcher, H. K. (1998). Crystallizing the processes of the unitary field pattern portrait research method. *Visions: The Journal of Rogerian Nursing Science, 6,* 13–26.

Butcher, H. K. (1999a). The artistry of Rogerian practice. *Visions: The Journal of Rogerian Nursing Science, 7,* 49–54.

Butcher, H. K. (1999b). Rogerian-ethics: An ethical inquiry into Rogers' life and science. *Nursing Science Quarterly, 12,* 111–117.

Butcher, H. K. (2000). Critical theory and Rogerian science: Incommensurable or reconcilable. *Visions: The Journal of Rogerian Nursing Science, 8,* 50–57.

Butcher, H. K. (2001). Nursing science in the new millennium: Practice and research within Rogers' science of unitary human beings. In Parker, M. (Ed.), *Nursing theories and nursing practice* (pp. 205–226). Philadelphia: F. A. Davis.

Butcher, H. K. (2002a). On fire flies and stars: Envisioning luminescent beacons for advancing nursing and Rogerian science. *Visions: The Journal of Rogerian Nursing Science, 10,* 57–67.

Butcher, H. K. (2002b). Living in the heart of helicy: An inquiry into the meaning of compassion and unpredictability in Rogers' nursing science. *Visions: The Journal of Rogerian Nursing Science, 10,* 6–22.

Butcher, H. K. (2004). Nursing's distinctive knowledge. In Haynes, L., Butcher, H., & Boese, T. (Eds.), *Nursing in contemporary society: Issues, trends, and transition to practice* (pp. 71–103). Upper Saddle River, NJ: Prentice Hall.

Capra, F. (1996). *The web of life: A new understanding of living systems.* New York: Anchor Books.

Carboni, J. T. (1992). Instrument development and the measurement of unitary constructs. *Nursing Science Quarterly, 5,* 134–142.

Carboni, J. T. (1995a). Enfolding health-as-wholeness-and-harmony: A theory of Rogerian nursing practice. *Nursing Science Quarterly, 8,* 71–78.

Carboni, J. T. (1995b). A Rogerian process of inquiry. *Nursing Science Quarterly, 8,* 22–37.

Caroselli, C., & Barrett, E. A. M. (1998). A review of the power as knowing participation in change literature. *Nursing Science Quarterly, 11,* 9–16.

Cowling, W. R. I. (1986). The science of unitary human beings: Theoretical issues, methodological challenges, and research realities. In Malinski, V. M. (Ed.), *Explorations on Martha Rogers' science of unitary human beings* (pp. 65–78). Norwalk, CT: Appleton-Century-Crofts.

Cowling, W. R. I. (1990). A template for unitary pattern-based nursing practice. In Barrett, E. A. M. (Ed.), *Visions of Rogers' science-based nursing* (pp. 45–65). New York: National League for Nursing.

Cowling, W. R. I. (1993a). Unitary knowing in nursing practice. *Nursing Science Quarterly, 6,* 201–207.

Cowling, W. R. I. (1993b). Unitary practice: Revisionary assumptions. In Parker, M. E. (Ed.), *Patterns of nursing theories in practice* (pp. 199–212). New York: National League for Nursing.

Cowling, W. R. I. (1997). Pattern appreciation: The unitary science/practice of reaching essence. In Madrid, M. (Ed.), *Patterns of Rogerian knowing* (pp. 129–142). New York: National League for Nursing.

Cowling, W. R. I. (1998). Unitary case inquiry. *Nursing Science Quarterly, 11,* 139–141.

Cowling, W. R. I. (2001). Unitary appreciative inquiry. *Advances in Nursing Science, 23*(4), 32–48.

Csikszentmihalyi, M. (1990). *Flow: The psychology of optimal experience*. New York: Harper & Row.

Dochteman, J. M., & Bulechek, G. M. (Eds.). (2004). *Nursing interventions classification (NIC)* (4th ed). St. Louis: Mosby.

Dossey, B. (1997). *Core curriculum for holistic nursing*. Gaithersburg, MD: Aspen.

Dossey, B., Guzzetta, C., & Keegan, L. (2000). *Holistic nursing: A handbook for practice*. Gaithersburg, MD: Aspen.

Dykeman, M. C., & Loukissa, D. (1993). The science of unitary human beings: An integrative review. *Nursing Science Quarterly, 6*, 179–188.

Fawcett, J. (1996). Issues of (in) compatibility between the worldview and research views of the science of unitary human beings: An invitation to dialogue. *Visions: The Journal of Rogerian Nursing Science, 4*, 5–11.

Fawcett, J. (2000). *Analysis and evaluation of contemporary nursing knowledge: Nursing models and theories*. Philadelphia: F. A. Davis.

Fawcett, J., & Alligood, M. R. (2003). The science of unitary human beings: Analysis of qualitative research approaches. *Visions: The Journal of Rogerian Nursing Science, 11*, 7–20.

Ference, H. (1979). *The relationship of time experience, creativity traits, differentiation, and human field motion*. Unpublished doctoral dissertation, New York University, New York.

Ference, H. M. (1986). The relationship of time experience, creativity traits, differentiation, and human field motion. In Malinski, V. M. (Ed.), *Explorations on Rogers' science of unitary human beings* (pp. 95–105). Norwalk, CT: Appleton-Century-Crofts.

Governing Council of the Society for the Advancement of Nursing (SAIN). (1977/1994). SAIN Perspective. In Malinski, V. M., & Barrett, E. A. M. (Eds.), *Martha E. Rogers: Her life and her work* (pp. 182–191). Philadelphia: F. A. Davis. (Reprinted from *SAIN Newsletter*, pp. 4–6, 1977, January.)

Guba, E. G., & Lincoln, Y. S. (1989). *Fourth generation evaluation*. Newbury Park, CA: Sage.

Guzzetta, C. E. (Ed.). (1998). *Essential readings in holistic nursing*. Gaithersburg, MD: Aspen.

Hastings-Tolsma, M. T. (1992). *The relationship among diversity and human field pattern, risk taking, and time experience: An investigation of Rogers' principles of homeodynamics*. Unpublished doctoral dissertation, New York University, New York.

Heggie, J., Garon, M., Kodiath, M., & Kelly, A. (1994). Implementing the science of unitary human beings at the San Diego Veterans Affairs Medical Center. In Madrid, M., & Barrett, E. A. M. (Eds.), *Rogers' scientific art of nursing practice* (pp. 285–304). New York: National League for Nursing.

Hektor, L. M. (1989/1994). Martha E. Rogers: A life history. In Malinski, V. M. & Barrett, E. A. M. (Eds.), *Martha E. Rogers: Her life and her work* (pp. 10–27). Philadelphia: F. A. Davis. (Reprinted from *Nursing Science Quarterly, 2*, 63–73.)

Johnston, L. W. (1994). Psychometric analysis of Johnson's Human Field Metaphor Scale. *Visions: The Journal of Rogerian Nursing Science, 2*, 7–11.

Leddy, S. K. (1995). Measuring mutual process: Development and psychometric testing of the person-environment participation scale. *Visions: The Journal of Rogerian Nursing Science, 3*, 20–31.

Leddy, S. K. (1996). Development and psychometric testing of the Leddy Healthiness Scale. *Research in Nursing and Health, 19*, 431–440.

Leddy, S. K. (2003). A unitary energy-based nursing practice theory: Theory and application. *Visions: The Journal of Rogerian Nursing Science, 11*, 21–28.

Leddy, S. K., & Fawcett, J. (1997). Testing the theory of healthiness: Conceptual and methodological issues. In Madrid, M. (Ed.), *Patterns of Rogerian knowing* (pp. 75–86). New York: National League for Nursing.

Lovelock, J. E. (1991). *Gaia*. Oxford: Oxford University Press.

Madrid, M. (Ed.). (1997). *Patterns of Rogerian knowing*. New York: National League for Nursing.

Madrid, M., & Barrett, E. A. M. (Eds.). (1994). *Rogers' scientific art of nursing practice*. New York: National League for Nursing.

Madrid, M., & Winstead-Fry, P. (1986). Rogers' conceptual model. In Winstead-Fry, P. (Ed.), *Case studies in nursing theory* (pp. 73–102). New York: National League for Nursing.

Malinski, V. M. (1986). Further ideas from Martha Rogers. In Malinski, V. M. (Ed.), *Explorations on Martha Rogers' Science of Unitary Human Beings* (pp. 9–14). Norwalk, CT: Appleton-Century-Crofts.

Malinski, V. M. (1991). Spirituality as integrality: A Rogerian perspective on the path of healing. *Journal of Holistic Nursing, 9*, 54–64.

Malinski, V. M. (1994). Spirituality: A pattern manifestation of the human/environmental mutual process. *Visions: The Journal of Rogerian Nursing Science, 2*, 12–18.

Malinski, V. M. (1994). A family of strong-willed women. In Malinski, V. M., & Barrett, E. A. M. (Eds.), *Martha E. Rogers: Her life and her work* (pp. 3–9). Philadelphia: F. A. Davis.

Malinski, V. M., & Barrett, E. A. M. (Eds.) (1994). *Martha E. Rogers: Her life and her work*. Philadelphia: F. A. Davis.

McEvoy, M. D. (1990). The relationships among the experience of dying, the experience of paranormal events, and creativity in adults. In Barrett, E. A. M. (Ed.), *Visions of Rogers' science-based nursing* (pp. 209–228). New York: National League for Nursing.

Mitchell, E. (1996). *The way of the explorer*. New York: Putnam.

Moorhead, S., Johnson, M., & Maas, M. (2004). *Nursing outcomes classification (NOC)*. St Louis: Mosby.

Morwessel, N. J. (1994). Developing an effective pattern appraisal to guide nursing care of children with heart variations and their families. In Madrid, M., & Barrett, E. A. M. (Eds.), *Rogers' scientific art of nursing practice* (pp. 147–161). New York: National League for Nursing.

Paletta, J. L. (1990). The relationship of temporal experience to human time. In Barrett, E. A. M. (Ed.), *Visions of Rogers' science-based nursing* (pp. 239–253). New York: National League for Nursing.

Parker, K. P. (1989). The theory of sentience evolution: A practice-level theory of sleeping, waking, and beyond waking patterns based on the science of unitary human beings. *Rogerian Nursing Science News, 2*(1), 4–6.

Peat, F. D. (1991). *The philosopher's stone: Chaos, synchronicity, and the hidden world of order*. New York: Bantam.

Phillips, J. (1988). The looking glass of nursing research. *Nursing Science Quarterly, 1*, 96.

Phillips, J. (1989a). Qualitative research: A process of discovery. *Nursing Science Quarterly, 2*, 5–6.

Phillips, J. (1989b). Science of unitary human beings: Changing research perspectives. *Nursing Science Quarterly, 2*, 57–60.

Phillips, J. R. (1990a). Research and the riddle of change. *Nursing Science Quarterly, 3*, 55–56.

Phillips, J. R. (1990b). Changing human potentials and future visions of nursing. In Barrett, E. A. M. (Ed.), *Visions of Rogers' science-based nursing* (pp. 13–25). New York: National League for Nursing.

Phillips, J. R. (1994). The open-ended nature of the science of unitary human beings. In Madrid, M., & Barrett, E. A. M. (Eds.), *Rogers' scientific art of nursing practice* (pp. 11–25). New York: National League for Nursing.

Randell, B. P. (1992). Nursing theory: The 21st century. *Nursing Science Quarterly, 5,* 176–184.

Rawnsley, M. M. (1994). Multiple field methods in unitary human field science. In Madrid, M., & Barrett, E. A. M. (Eds.), *Rogerian scientific art of nursing practice* (pp. 381–395). New York: National League for Nursing.

Reason, P. (1994). Three approaches to participative inquiry. In Denzin, N. K., & Lincoln, Y. S. (Eds.), *Handbook of qualitative research* (pp. 324–339). Thousand Oaks, CA: Sage.

Reeder, F. (1986). Basic theoretical research in the conceptual system of unitary human beings. In Malinski, V. M. (Ed.), *Explorations on Martha E. Rogers' science of unitary human beings* (pp. 45–64). Norwalk, CT: Appleton-Century-Crofts.

Rogers, M. E. (1970). *An introduction to the theoretical basis of nursing.* Philadelphia: F. A. Davis.

Rogers, M. E. (1980). Nursing: A science of unitary man. In Riehl, J. P., & Roy, C. (Eds.), *Conceptual models for nursing practice* (2nd ed., pp. 329–337). New York: Appleton-Century-Crofts.

Rogers, M. E. (1966/1994). Epilogue. In Malinski, V. M., & Barrett, E. A. M. (Eds.), *Martha E. Rogers and her work* (pp. 337–338). Philadelphia: F. A. Davis. (Reprinted from the *Education Violet,* the New York University newspaper, 1966.)

Rogers, M. E. (1988). Nursing science and art: A prospective. *Nursing Science Quarterly, 1,* 99–102.

Rogers, M. E. (1990a). Nursing: Science of unitary, irreducible human beings: Update 1990. In Barrett, E. A. M. (Ed.), *Visions of Rogers' science-based nursing* (pp. 5–11). New York: National League for Nursing.

Rogers, M. E. (1990b). Space-age paradigm for new frontiers in nursing. In Parker, M. E. (Ed.), *Nursing theories in practice* (pp. 105–113). New York: National League for Nursing.

Rogers, M. E. (1992). Nursing and the space age. *Nursing Science Quarterly, 5,* 27–34.

Rogers, M. E. (1994). Nursing science evolves. In Madrid, M., & Barrett, E. A. M. (Eds.), *Rogers' scientific art of nursing practice* (pp. 3–9). New York: National League for Nursing.

Rogers, M. E. (1994a). The science of unitary human beings: Current perspectives. *Nursing Science Quarterly, 7,* 33–35.

Sheldrake, R. (1988). *The presence of the past: Morphic resonance and the habits of nature.* New York: Times Books.

Smith, D. W. (1994). Toward developing a theory of spirituality. *Visions: The Journal of Rogerian Nursing Science, 2,* 35–43.

Smith, M. C. (1999). Caring and the science of unitary human beings. *Advances in Nursing Science, 21*(4), 14–28.

Smith, M. C., & Reeder, F. (1996). Clinical outcomes research and Rogerian science: Strange or emergent bedfellows. *Visions: The Journal of Rogerian Nursing Science, 6,* 27–38.

Smith, M. J. (1988). Perspectives on nursing science. *Nursing Science Quarterly, 1,* 80–85.

Takahashi, T. (1992). Perspectives on nursing knowledge. *Nursing Science Quarterly, 5,* 86–91.

Talbot, M. (1991). *The holographic universe.* New York: HarperCollins.

Todaro-Franceschi, V. (1999). *The enigma of energy: Where science and religion converge.* New York: Crossroad Publishing.

Tudor, C. A., Keegan-Jones, L., & Bens, E. M. (1994). Implementing Rogers' science-based nursing practice in a pediatric nursing service setting. In Madrid, M., & Barrett, E. A. M. (Eds.), *Rogers' scientific art of nursing practice* (pp. 305–322). New York: National League for Nursing.

Watson, J. (1993). *The relationships of sleep-wake rhythm, dream experience, human field motion, and time experience in older women.* Unpublished doctoral dissertation, New York University, New York.

Watson, J., Barrett, E. A. M., Hastings-Tolsma, M., Johnston, L., & Gueldner, S. (1997). Measurement in Rogerian Science: A review of selected instruments. In Madrid, M. (Ed.), *Patterns of Rogerian knowing* (pp. 87–99). New York: National League for Nursing.

Woodhouse, M. B. (1996). *Paradigm wars: Worldviews for a new age.* Berkeley, CA: Frog, Ltd.

Woodward, T. A., & Heggie, J. (1997). Rogers in reality: Staff nurse application of the science of unitary human beings in the clinical setting following changes in an orientation program. In Madrid, M. (Ed.), *Patterns of Rogerian knowing* (pp. 239–248). New York: National League for Nursing.

CHAPTER 14

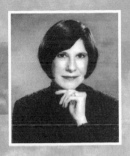

Rosemarie Rizzo Parse

PART ONE: Rosemarie Rizzo Parse's Human Becoming School of Thought

Rosemarie Rizzo Parse

| Introducing the Theorist |
| Introducing the Theory: The Human Becoming School of Thought |
| Summary |

Introducing the Theorist

Rosemarie Rizzo Parse is professor and Niehoff chair at Loyola University in Chicago. She is founder and editor of *Nursing Science Quarterly*; president of Discovery International, Inc., which sponsors international nursing theory conferences; and founder of the Institute of Human Becoming, where she teaches the ontological, epistemological, and methodological aspects of the human becoming school of thought. Her most recent work is *Community: A Human Becoming Perspective*

(2003a). Previous works include *Nursing Fundamentals* (1974); *Man-Living-Health: A Theory of Nursing* (1981); *Nursing Research: Qualitative Methods* (1985); *Nursing Science: Major Paradigms, Theories, and Critiques* (1987); *Illuminations: The Human Becoming Theory in Practice and Research* (1995); *The Human Becoming School of Thought* (1998); *Hope: An International Human Becoming Perspective* (1999); and *Qualitative Inquiry: The Path of Sciencing* (2001b). Her theory is a guide for practice in health-care settings in the United States, Canada, Finland,

Sweden, and many other countries; her research methodology is used as a method of inquiry by nurse scholars in Australia, Canada, Denmark, Finland, Greece, Italy, Japan, South Korea, Sweden, the United Kingdom, the United States, and other countries on five continents.

Dr. Parse is a graduate of Duquesne University in Pittsburgh, and she received her master's and doctorate from the University of Pittsburgh. She was on the faculty of the University of Pittsburgh, was dean of the Nursing School at Duquesne University, and from 1983 to 1993 was professor and coordinator of the Center for Nursing Research at Hunter College of the City University of New York.

Introducing the Theory: The Human Becoming School of Thought

Presently, nurse leaders in research, administration, education, and practice are focusing attention on expanding the knowledge base of nursing through enhancement of the discipline's frameworks and theories. Nursing is a discipline and a profession. The goal of the *discipline* is to expand knowledge about human experiences through creative conceptualization and research. This knowledge is the

> *Knowledge of the discipline is the scientific guide to living the art of nursing.*

scientific guide to living the art of nursing. The discipline-specific knowledge is given birth and fostered in academic settings where research and education move the knowledge to new realms of understanding. The goal of the *profession* is to provide service to humankind through living the art of the science. Members of the nursing profession are responsible for regulating the standards of practice and education based on disciplinary knowledge that reflects safe health service to society in all settings.

THE DISCIPLINE OF NURSING

The discipline of nursing encompasses at least two paradigmatic perspectives related to the human-universe-health process. One view is of the human as body-mind-spirit (totality paradigm) and the

other is of the human as unitary (simultaneity paradigm) (Parse, 1987). The body-mind-spirit perspective is particulate—focusing on the bio-psycho-social-spiritual parts of the whole human as the human interacts with and adapts to the environment. Health is considered a state of biological, psychological, social, and spiritual well-being. This ontology leads to research and practice on phenomena related to preventing disease and maintaining and promoting health according to societal norms. In contrast, the unitary perspective is a view of the human-universe process as irreducible, unpredictable, and ever-changing. Health is considered a process of changing value priorities. It is not a static state but, rather, is ever-changing as the human chooses ways of living. This ontology leads to research and practice on patterns (Rogers, 1992), lived experiences, and quality of life (Parse, 1981, 1992, 1997a, 1998a). Because the ontologies of these paradigmatic perspectives lead to different research and practice modalities, they lead to different professional services to humankind.

THE PROFESSION OF NURSING

The profession of nursing consists of people educated according to nationally regulated, defined, and monitored standards. The standards and regulations are to preserve the safety of health care for members of society. The nursing regulations and standards are specified predominantly in medical/scientific terms. This is according to tradition and is largely related to nursing's early subservience to medicine. Recently, the nurse leaders in health-care systems and in regulating organizations have been developing standards (Mitchell, 1998) and regulations (Damgaard & Bunkers, 1998) consistent with discipline-specific knowledge as articulated in the theories and frameworks of nursing. This is a very significant development that will fortify the identity of nursing as a discipline with its own body of knowledge—one that specifies the service that society can expect from members of the profession. With the rapidly changing health policies and the general dissatisfaction of consumers with health-care delivery, clearly stated expectations for services from each paradigm are a welcome change.

Just as in other disciplines, the nursing education and practice standards must be broad enough to encompass the possibility of practice within each paradigm. The totality paradigm frameworks and theories are more closely aligned with the medical model tradition. Nurses living the beliefs of this paradigm are concerned with participation of persons in health-care decisions but have specific regimes and goals to bring about change for the people they serve. Nurses living the simultaneity paradigm beliefs hold people's perspectives of their health situations and their desires to be primary. Nurses focus on knowing participation (Rogers, 1992) and bearing witness, as persons in their presence choose ways of changing health patterns (Parse, 1981, 1987, 1992, 1995, 1997a, 1998a). Human Becoming, a school of thought named such because it encompasses on ontology, epistemology, and methodologies, emanates from the simultaneity paradigm (Parse, 1997c).

A META-PERSPECTIVE OF PARSE'S HUMAN BECOMING SCHOOL OF THOUGHT

Parse's (1981) original work was named *Man-Living-Health: A Theory of Nursing*. When the term "mankind" was replaced with "male gender" in the dictionary definition of "man," the name of the theory was changed to "human becoming" (Parse, 1992). No aspect of the principles changed. With the 1998 publication of *The Human Becoming School of Thought*, Parse expanded the original work to include descriptions of three research methodologies and a unique practice methodology, thus classifying the science of Human Becoming as a school of thought (Parse, 1997c). As a school of thought, the philosophical ideas provide nurses and other health professionals with guides for their research and practice.

Human Becoming is a basic *human science* that has cocreated human experiences as its central

> *Human Becoming is a basic human science that has cocreated human experiences as its central focus.*

focus. The ontology—that is, the assumptions and principles—sets forth beliefs that are clearly different from other nursing frameworks and theories. Discipline-specific knowledge is articulated in unique language specifying a position on the phenomenon of concern for each discipline. The

Human Becoming language is unique to nursing. The three Human Becoming principles contain nine concepts written in verbal form with "ing" endings to make clear the importance of the ongoing process of change as basic to human-universe emergence. The fundamental idea that humans are unitary beings, as specified in the ontology, precludes any use of terms such as *physiological, biological, psychological,* or *spiritual,* because these terms describe the human in a particular way.

PHILOSOPHICAL ASSUMPTIONS

The assumptions of the human becoming school of thought are written at the philosophical level of discourse (Parse, 1998a). There are nine fundamental assumptions: four about the human and five about becoming (Parse, 1998a). Also, three assumptions about human becoming were synthesized from these nine assumptions (Parse, 1998a). The assumptions arose from a synthesis of ideas from Rogers' Science of Unitary Human Beings (Rogers, 1992) and from existential phenomenological thought (Parse, 1981, 1992, 1994a, 1995, 1997a, 1998a). In the assumptions, the author sets forth the view that unitary humans, in mutual process with the universe, are cocreating a unique becoming. The mutual process is the all-at-onceness of living freely chosen meanings that arise with multidimensional experiences. The chosen meanings are the value priorities cocreated in transcending with the possibles in unitary emergence (Parse 1998a, pp. 19–30).

Principles of Human Becoming

The principles and the assumptions of the human becoming school of thought make up the ontology. The principles are referred to as the theory. The principles of human becoming, which describe the central phenomenon of nursing (the human-universe-health process), arise from the three major themes of the assumptions: *meaning, rhythmicity,* and *transcendence*. Each principle describes a theme with three concepts. Each of the concepts explicates fundamental paradoxes of human becoming (Parse, 1998a, p. 58). The paradoxes are dimensions of the same rhythm lived all-at-once. Paradoxes are not opposites or problems to be solved but, rather, are ways humans live their chosen meanings. This way of viewing paradox is unique to the human becoming school of thought (Mitchell, 1993; Parse, 1981, 1994b).

With the first principle (see Parse, 1981, 1998a), the author explicates the idea that humans construct personal realities with unique choosings from multidimensional realms of the universe. Reality, the meaning given to the situation, is the individual human's ever-changing seamless symphony of becoming (Parse, 1996). The seamless symphony is the unique story of the human as mystery emerging with the explicit–tacit knowings of *imaging*. The human lives priorities of *valuing* in confirming–not confirming cherished beliefs, while *languaging* with speaking–being silent and moving–being still.

The second principle (Parse, 1981, 1998a) describes the rhythmical patterns of relating human with universe. The paradoxical rhythm "*revealing–concealing* is disclosing–not disclosing all-at-once" (Parse, 1998a, p. 43). Not all is explicitly known or can be told in the unfolding mystery of human becoming. "*Enabling-limiting* is living the opportunities-restrictions present in all choosings all-at-once" (Parse, 1998a, p. 44). There are opportunities and restrictions no matter what the choice. "*Connecting–separating* is being with and apart from others, ideas, objects and situations all-at-once" (Parse, 1998a, p. 45). It is coming together and moving apart, and there is closeness in the separation and distance in the closeness.

With the third principle (Parse, 1981, 1998a), the author explicates the idea that humans are ever-changing; that is, moving beyond with the possibilities, which are their intended hopes and dreams. A changing diversity unfolds as humans push and resist with *powering* in creating new ways of living the conformity-nonconformity and certainty-uncertainty of *originating*, while shedding light on the familiar-unfamiliar of *transforming*. "*Powering* is the pushing-resisting process of affirming–not affirming being in light of nonbeing" (Parse, 1998a, p. 47). The being-nonbeing rhythm is all-at-once living the ever-changing now moment as it melts with the not-yet. Humans, in *originating*, seek to conform–not conform; that is, to be like others and unique all-at-once, while living the ambiguity of the certainty-uncertainty embedded in all change. The changing diversity arises with *transforming* the familiar-unfamiliar as others, ideas, objects, and situations are viewed in a different light.

The three principles, along with the assumptions, make up the ontology of the Human Becoming School of Thought. The principles are referred to as the Human Becoming Theory. The concepts, with the paradoxes, describe the human-universe-health process. This ontological base gives rise to the epistemology and methodologies of Human Becoming. Epistemology refers to the focus of inquiry. Consistent with the Human Becoming School of Thought, the focus of inquiry is on humanly lived experiences.

HUMAN BECOMING RESEARCH METHODOLOGIES

Sciencing Human Becoming is the process of coming to know; it is an ongoing inquiry to discover and understand the meaning of lived experiences. The Human Becoming research tradition has three methods; two are basic research methods and the other is an applied research method (Parse, 1998a, pp. 59–68, 2001b). The methods flow from the ontology of the school of thought. The basic research methods are the Parse Method (Parse, 1987, 1990, 1992, 1995, 1997a, 1998a, 2001b) and the Human Becoming Hermeneutic Method (Cody, 1995c; Parse, 1995, 1998a, 2001b). The purpose of these two methods is to advance the science of Human Becoming by studying lived experiences from participants' descriptions (Parse Method) and from written texts and art forms (Human Becoming Hermeneutic Method). The phenomena for study with the Parse Method are universal lived experiences such as joy, sorrow, hope, grieving, and courage, among others. Written texts from any literary source or any art form may be the subject of research with the Human Becoming Hermeneutic Method. The processes of both methods call for a unique dialogue, a researcher with participant, or a researcher with text or art form. The researcher in the Parse Method is truly present as the participant moves through an unstructured discussion about the lived experience under study. The researcher in the Human Becoming Hermeneutic Method is truly present to the emerging possibilities in the horizon of meaning arising in dialogue with texts or art forms. True presence is an intense attentiveness to unfolding essences and emergent meanings. The researcher's intent with these research methods is to discover essences (Parse Method) and emergent meanings (Human Becoming Hermeneutic Method). The contributions of the findings from studies using these two methods is "new knowledge and understanding of humanly lived experiences" (Parse, 1998a, p. 62). Many studies have been conducted and some have been published in which nurse scholars used the Parse Method. Two studies have been published in which the author used the Human Becoming Hermeneutic Method (Cody, 1995c; Ortiz, 2003).

The applied research method is the descriptive qualitative preproject-process-postproject method. It is used when a researcher wishes to evaluate the changes, satisfactions, and effectiveness of health care when human becoming guides practice. A number of studies have been published in which the authors used this method (Jonas, 1995a; Mitchell, 1995; Northrup & Cody, 1998; Santopinto & Smith, 1995), and a synthesis of the findings of these and other such studies was written and published (Bournes, 2002b).

HUMAN BECOMING PRACTICE METHODOLOGY

From the human becoming perspective, the discipline's goal is quality of life. The goal of the nurse

> *The goal of the nurse living the human becoming beliefs is true presence in bearing witness and being with others in their changing health patterns.*

living the human becoming beliefs is true presence in bearing witness and being with others in their changing health patterns. True presence is lived through the human becoming dimensions and processes: illuminating meaning, synchronizing rhythms, and mobilizing transcendence (Parse, 1987, 1992, 1994a, 1995, 1997a, 1998a). The nurse with individuals or groups is truly present with the unfolding meanings as persons *explicate, dwell with,* and *move on* with changing patterns of diversity.

Living true presence is unique to the art of human becoming. It is sometimes misinterpreted as simply asking persons what they want and respecting their desires. This alone is not true presence. "True presence is an intentional reflective love, an interpersonal art grounded in a strong

knowledge base" (Parse, 1998a, p. 71). The knowledge base underpinning true presence is specified in the assumptions and principles of human becoming (Parse, 1981, 1992, 1995, 1997a, 1998a). True presence is a free-flowing attentiveness that arises from the belief that the human in mutual process with the universe is unitary, freely chooses in situations, structures personal meaning, lives paradoxical rhythms, and moves beyond with changing diversity (Parse, 1998a). Parse states: "To know, understand, and live the beliefs of human becoming requires concentrated study of the ontology, epistemology, and methodologies and a commitment to a different way of being with people. The different way that arises from the human becoming beliefs is true presence" (Parse, 1987, 1998b). Many papers are published explicating human becoming practice (Arndt, 1995; Banonis, 1995; Bournes, 2000, 2003; Bournes & Flint, 2003; Butler, 1988; Butler & Snodgrass, 1991; Chapman, Mitchell, & Forchuk, 1994; Hansen-Ketchum, 2004; Huchings, 2002; Jonas, 1994, 1995b; Lee & Pilkington, 1999; Liehr, 1989; Mattice & Mitchell, 1990; Mitchell, 1988, 1990b; Mitchell & Bournes, 2000; Mitchell & Copplestone, 1990; Mitchell & Pilkington, 1990; Norris, 2002; Paille & Pilkington, 2002; Quiquero, Knights, & Meo, 1991; Rasmusson, 1995; Rasmusson, Jonas, & Mitchell, 1991; Smith, 2002; Stanley & Meghani, 2001; among others).

True presence is a powerful human-universe connection experienced in all realms of the universe. It is lived in face-to-face discussions, silent immersions, and lingering presence (Parse, 1987, 1998a, pp. 71–80). Nurses may be with persons in discussions, imaginings, or remembrances through stories, films, drawings, photographs, movies, metaphors, poetry, rhythmical movements, and other expressions (Parse, 1998a, p. 72).

HUMAN BECOMING GLOBAL PRESENCE

The Human Becoming School of Thought is a guide for research, practice, education, and administration in settings throughout the world. Scholars from five continents have embraced the belief system and live Human Becoming in a variety of venues, including health-care centers and university nursing programs. The Human Becoming Community Change Concepts (Parse, 2003a), the Human Becoming Teaching-Learning Model

Themes, Assumptions, Principles, and Practice Dimensions of Parse's Theory

THEMES	ASSUMPTIONS	PRINCIPLES	PRACTICE DIMENSIONS	COMMENTS
Meaning	Human becoming is freely choosing personal meaning in situations in the intersubjective process of relating value priorities.	Structuring meaning multidimensionally is cocreating reality through the languaging of valuing and imaging.	Illuminating meaning is shedding light through uncovering the what was, is, and will be, as it is appearing now; it happens in explicating what is.	*People always participate in creating their realities through choosing how to understand and interpret experiences. Expressing oneself clarifies values and furthers understanding of experiences.*
Rhythmicity	Human becoming is cocreating rhythmical patterns of relating in open interchange with the universe.	Cocreating rhythmical patterns of relating is living the paradoxical unity of revealing-concealing, enabling-limiting, while connecting-separating.	Synchronizing rhythms happens in dwelling with the pitch, yaw, and roll of the interhuman cadence.	*People live potentialities with actualities all-at-once; the apparent opposite of what is in the fore of experience is always also present with us. Exploring options in the attentive, loving presence of another is a way of connecting-separating with others in the universe.*
Transcendence	Human becoming is transcending multidimensionally with the unfolding possibles.	Cotranscending with the possibles is powering originating in the process of transforming.	Mobilizing transcendence happens in moving beyond the meaning moment to what is not-yet.	*People live with change in chosen ways that evolve into patterns of living that also change over time. Coparticipating in change through one's choice affirms self and cocreates with the universe what will be. By exploring options in the presence of another, one moves beyond what is to what is not yet*

Explication of the Human Becoming Perspective of the Hermeneutic Processes of Discoursing, Interpreting, and Understanding

THEME EXPLICATION

Meaning "Discoursing is the interplay of shared and unshared meanings through which beliefs are appropriated and disappropriated. A text, as something written and read, is a form of discourse. Author and reader are discoursing whenever the text is read" (Cody, 1995, p. 275).

Rhythmicity "Interpreting is expanding the meaning moment through dwelling in situated openness with the disclosed and the hidden. Interpreting a text is constructing meanings with the text through the rhythmic movement between the language of the text and the language of the researcher" (Cody, 1995, p. 275).

Transcendence "Understanding is choosing from possibilities a unique way of moving beyond the meaning moment. Understanding a text is interweaving the meaning of the text with the pattern of one's life in a chosen way" (Cody, 1995c, p. 276).

(Parse, 2004), and the Human Becoming Synergistic Collaborating Leadership Model (Parse, in press) are being disseminated and utilized in several settings.

For example, in Toronto, Sunnybrook, and Women's College Health Science Centre's multidisciplinary standards of care arise from the beliefs and values of the Human Becoming School of Thought. University Health Network, also in Toronto, Canada, is in the process of conducting an 18-month study (Bournes & Ferguson-Paré, 2004) to evaluate implementation of human becoming as a guide to nursing practice on a unit where they are also evaluating the implementation of a staffing model in which registered nurses are spending 80 percent of their time in direct patient care and 20 percent of their time on professional development (80/20 model). It is believed that learning to use the human becoming theory in practice will enhance nurses' satisfaction and be responsive to health-care recipients' call for patient-centered care (Bournes, 2002b). The addition of the 80/20 nurse staffing model is to address issues raised in the nurse retention literature indicating that nurses want professional development opportunities, time to be involved in developing professional practice and research initiatives, demonstrated commitment and support from nurse leaders, and reductions in workload. There are other health centers throughout the world that have Human Becoming as a guide to health care (see, for example, the "Scholarly Dialogue" column in *Nursing Science Quarterly*, volume 17, numbers 3 and 4).

In South Dakota, a parish nursing model was built on the principles of human becoming to guide nursing practice at the First Presbyterian Church in Sioux Falls (Bunkers, Michaels, & Ethridge, 1997; Bunkers & Putnam, 1995). Also, the Board of Nursing of South Dakota has adopted a decisioning model based on the human becoming school of thought (Damgaard & Bunkers, 1998). Augustana College (in Sioux Falls) has human becoming as one central focus of the curricula for the baccalaureate and master's programs. It is the basis of Augustana's Health Action Model for Partnership in Community (Bunkers, Nelson, Leuning, Crane, & Josephson, 1999).

A research project on the lived experience of hope was conducted using the Parse method, with participants from Australia, Canada, Finland, Italy, Japan, Sweden, Taiwan, the United Kingdom, and the United States. The findings from these studies

and the stories of the participants are published in the book *Hope: An International Human Becoming Perspective* (Parse, 1999). Collaborating research projects also have been published on feeling very tired (Baumann, 2003; Huch & Bournes, 2003; Parse, 2003b).

Approximately 300 participants subscribe to Parse-L, an e-mail listserv where Parse scholars share ideas. There is a Parse home page on the World Wide Web that is updated regularly. Each year, most of the 100 or more members of the International Consortium of Parse Scholars meet in Canada for a weekend immersion in human becoming research and practice. Members of the consortium have prepared a set of teaching modules (Pilkington & Jonas-Simpson, 1996) and a video recording (International Consortium of Parse Scholars, 1996) of Parse nurses in true presence with persons in different settings. Parse scholars present lectures and symposia regularly at international forums.

The Institute of Human Becoming

The Institute of Human Becoming, founded in 1992, was created to offer interested nurses and others the opportunity to study, with the author, the ontological, epistemological, and methodological aspects of the human becoming school of thought. Toward that goal, the institute offers regular sessions devoted to the study of the ontology and the research and practice methodologies. There are also sessions on teaching-learning, leading-following, community, and family. All of the sessions have as their goal the understanding of the meaning of the human-universe-health process from a human becoming perspective.

SUMMARY

Through the efforts of Parse scholars, the Human Becoming School of Thought will continue to emerge as a major force in the twenty-first century evolution of nursing science. Knowledge gained from the basic research studies will continue to be synthesized to further explicate the meaning of lived experiences. The findings from applied research projects related to fostering understanding of

Human Becoming in practice also will continue to be synthesized and conclusions will be drawn. These syntheses will guide decisions for continually creating the vision for sciencing and living the art of the Human Becoming School of Thought for the betterment of humankind.

PART TWO:
Applications of Parse's Human Becoming School of Thought

Gail J. Mitchell, Sandra Schmidt Bunkers, & Debra Bournes

Applications

References

Applications

This section of the chapter describes the application of Parse's Theory of Human Becoming in practice, research, administration, education, and regulation.

PRACTICE

The human becoming practice methodology (Parse, 1987) helps nurses know how to be with

people as they speak about their personal realities, explore life options, ponder the possible outcomes of various choices, and select ways to move on amid life's unfolding consequences. The nurse guided by the human becoming perspective lives a commitment to honor persons as they disclose their realities in the presence of another who will not judge or try to control their processes of illuminating meaning, synchronizing rhythms, and mobilizing transcendence. The human becoming theory specifies relationships among particular values and beliefs about the human-universe process, quality of

> The human becoming theory specifies relationships among particular values and beliefs about the human-universe process, quality of life, and nursing.

life, and nursing. The nurse who embraces these particular values and beliefs expresses them with others who recognize the presence of human becoming nursing.

As Rosemarie Rizzo Parse (1998) has shown earlier in the chapter, the Theory of Human Becoming has given rise to a school of thought. The theory's assumptions and principles comprise the school of thought's ontology, which describes the person as freely choosing meaning in situation, coexisting and interrelating multidimensionally with the universe, and continuously cotranscending with the possibles in uniquely personal ways. Freely choosing meaning is cocreating reality through one's imaginings and self-expressions while living cherished values. Coexisting and interrelating with others generates rhythmical patterns and paradoxes that disclose the ups and downs of living. One continuously transcends with the possibles through shifting perspectives of unfolding events and committing to one course of action over another while never fully knowing the outcomes.

The human becoming practice methodology flows from these beliefs and delineates a way of authentically living these beliefs. The essence of the methodology is structured in the written dimensions and processes published by Parse in 1987; but less formal guidance was offered in the 1981 text introducing the human becoming theory, then called "man-living-health." The dimensions and processes are stated in the table on p. 192.

Since Parse's theory was first published, an increasing number of nurses have cited it as having

Table 14-1	**Extracted-Synthesized Essences and Language Art for Ben**

Ben's Language	Researcher's Language
Feeling confident is feeling good, calm, content, and secure, keeping up-to-date and being aware of what is going on; and knowing whatever happens, it should be okay.	Serene assuredness amid ambiguity surfaces with vigilant attentiveness.
Feeling confident is feeling important and worthwhile, encouraging others, getting psyched up, accomplishing something of interest, and staying mostly confident, except when intimidated by unfamiliar situations.	Cherished triumphs emerge with gratitude in the wavering buoyancy of pursuing sustaining-daunting engagements.

LANGUAGE ART

Feeling confident is serene assuredness amid ambiguity surfacing with vigilant attentiveness as cherished triumphs emerge with gratitude in the wavering buoyancy of pursuing sustaining-daunting engagements.

an important and lasting influence on their activities as a nurse. Nurses of multiple backgrounds, with different levels of preparation and in varied settings and countries, have found Parse's perspective to be closest to their own beliefs about nursing and have therefore chosen to use the theory to guide their practice and research.

The broad appeal of the theory and its meaningfulness in practice has been described in many publications too numerous to list. In several university-affiliated settings in Canada, human becoming practice has been evaluated, and the theory has provided underpinnings for standards of care (Bournes, 2002b; Legault & Ferguson-Paré, 1999; Mitchell, 1998a; Mitchell, Closson, Coulis, Flint, & Gray, 2000; Northrup & Cody, 1998) and nursing best practice guidelines (Nelligan, Grinspun, Jonas-Simpson, McConnell, Peter, Pilkington et al., 2002; RNAO, 2002).

On a smaller scale, the Center for Human Becoming was established in 1997 in Charlotte, North Carolina, as a milieu for the nurse-person process within a 25-unit housing complex for people living with HIV. The theory has guided practice in several community settings with various groups, including persons who have no home (Bunkers, Nelson, Leuning, Crane, & Josephson, 1999; Williamson, 2000).

Implementing the human becoming theory as the central guide to nursing practice is never easy for individuals or institutions. Adopting the Human Becoming Theory often means confronting doubts about one's knowledge, experiencing conflict and confusion in practice, and sometimes alienating coworkers committed to more traditional paradigms. Nurses may gain knowledge and encouragement from available texts and other media (Fitne, 1997; International Consortium of Parse Scholars, 1996), from the regular conferences of the International Consortium of Parse Scholars and its regional chapters, from sessions with Dr. Parse at the Human Becoming Institute in Pittsburgh, and from the annual conferences led by Parse at Loyola University in Chicago. It is difficult, though not impossible, to implement the theory in practice without the support of others.

In institutions, a dependable commitment of resources from top-level administration and the ready availability of well-prepared education and practice leaders are minimal essentials for implementing Parse's theory-guided practice (Bournes & DasGupta, 1997; Linscott, Spee, Flint, & Fisher, 1999; Mitchell et al., 2000). Shifting practice in an institutional setting from traditional biomedical to the human becoming perspective requires a radical paradigm shift within the local health-care culture. To adopt Parse's theory as the guide to practice is to adopt fundamentally different definitions of such key notions as health, family, community, presence, person, freedom, change, and reality. Parse's Theory of Human Becoming is not a model for nursing practice that can be imposed on unwilling workers. The Parse nurse lives the values and beliefs manifest and structured linguistically in the theory. Clearly, this can only become an actuality through individual study, reflection, choice, and action.

Fostering the art of true presence in nursing practice—which is living the values and beliefs underpinning Parse's practice methodology in the nurse-person process—requires the creation of spaces where nurses' choices to move with a new paradigm of nursing practice are honored, spaces where persons' individual meanings and choices are profoundly valued, and spaces where resources are dedicated to cocreating quality of life from each person's own perspective. In this section of the chapter, we present two detailed examples of practice guided by the Human Becoming Theory, illustrating a parish nursing model and a community action model.

Human Becoming as a Guide for Parish Nursing

A Human Becoming parish nursing practice model was developed at the First Presbyterian Church in Sioux Falls, South Dakota (Bunkers & Putnam, 1995). The central focus of this nursing theory–based health model is quality of life for the parish community (see Fig. 14–1). The nurse-community health process emphasizes lived experiences of health of individual parishioners and of the entire parish community. The eight beatitudes, being fundamental to the parish's belief system, are paralleled with concepts of the Human Becoming Theory to guide nursing practice in the parish. For example, true presence is paralleled with the beatitude, "Blessed are those who hunger and thirst for righteousness, for they shall be filled," which expresses the desire for a deep, loving relationship with people and with God (Ward, 1972). True presence, the cornerstone of human becoming nursing practice, is lived with the parish community in a loving, reflective way, bearing witness to others' living health and honoring each person's uniqueness without judging him or her. The nurse, in true presence, respects people as knowing their own way, a chosen personal way of being with the world. A further example of paralleling the beatitudes with the Human Becoming Theory is the beatitude, "Blessed are the pure in heart, for they shall see God," which describes a singleness of purpose for living an ethic of love and care for others (Ward, 1972). This ethic of love and care honors human freedom. The Parse nurse understands that humans are inherently free, and the nurse in parish nursing practice honors this freedom. "The nurse honors how others choose to create their world and seeks to know and understand the wholeness of their lived experiences of faith and health" (Bunkers,

1998b; Bunkers, Nelson, Leuning et al., 1999, p. 92). Living Parse's Theory of Human Becoming with parishioners holds the possibility of transforming community nursing practice and transforming ways of living health. Bunkers and Putnam (1995) state, "The nurse, in practicing from the human becoming perspective and emphasizing the teachings of the Beatitudes, believes in the endless possibilities present for persons when there is openness, caring, and honoring of justice and human freedom" (p. 210).

Human Becoming as a Guide for Nursing Education-Practice

The Health Action Model for Partnership in Community is a nursing education-practice model originating in the Department of Nursing at Augustana College in Sioux Falls, South Dakota, which addresses "the connections and disconnections existing in human relationship" (Bunkers, Nelson, Leuning et al., 1999, p. 92) (see Fig. 14–2). This collaborative community nursing practice model focuses on lived experiences of connection-disconnection "for persons homeless and low income who are challenged with the lack of economic, social and interpersonal resources" (Bunkers, Nelson, Leuning et al., 1999, p. 92). The

> *The Health Action Model, based on the human becoming school of thought, focuses on the primacy of the nurse's presence with others.*

Health Action Model, based on the human becoming school of thought, focuses on the primacy of the nurse's presence with others. The focus of the nurse-community health process is quality of life from the community's perspective. Quality of life, the central concept of the model, is elaborated on in the conceptualizations of health as human becoming, community interconnectedness, and

> *"The purpose of the model is to respond in a new way to nursing's social mandate to care for the health of society by gaining an understanding of what is wanted from those living these health experiences."*

First Presbyterian Church
Sioux Falls, South Dakota

CONGREGATIONAL HEALTH MODEL
Christ-Centered
Covenant

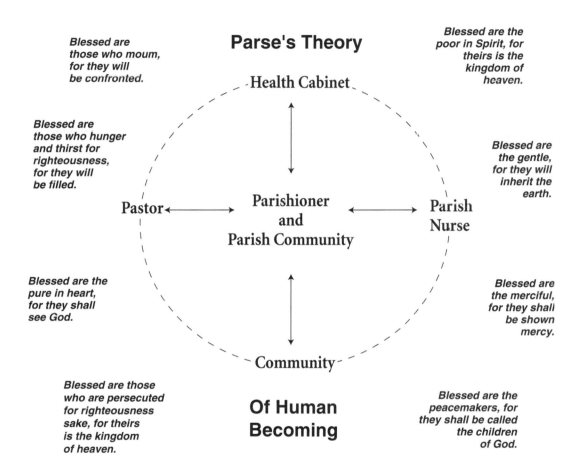

Blessed are those who mourn, for they will be confronted.

Blessed are the poor in Spirit, for theirs is the kingdom of heaven.

Blessed are those who hunger and thirst for righteousness, for they will be filled.

Blessed are the gentle, for they will inherit the earth.

Parse's Theory

Health Cabinet

Pastor ← → Parishioner and Parish Community ← → Parish Nurse

Community

Of Human Becoming

Blessed are the pure in heart, for they shall see God.

Blessed are the merciful, for they shall be shown mercy.

Blessed are those who are persecuted for righteousness sake, for theirs is the kingdom of heaven.

Blessed are the peacemakers, for they shall be called the children of God.

Cocreating Health in a Parish Community

- ❏ "Love one another as I have loved you." *John 13:34*
- ❏ "Health is a personal commitment to a lived value system; cocreating quality of life with the human-universe process." *R.R. Parse, 1992*
- ❏ "Go ye into the world..." *Matthew 25:31–46*
- ❏ "Qualtiy of life is whatever the person living the life says it is." *R.R. Parse, 1994*

© Bunkers, S. & Putnam, V., 1995

FIGURE 14–1   Congregational health model. *Reprinted with permission from the First Presbyterian Church, Sioux Falls, South Dakota.*

The Health Action Model For Partnership In Community

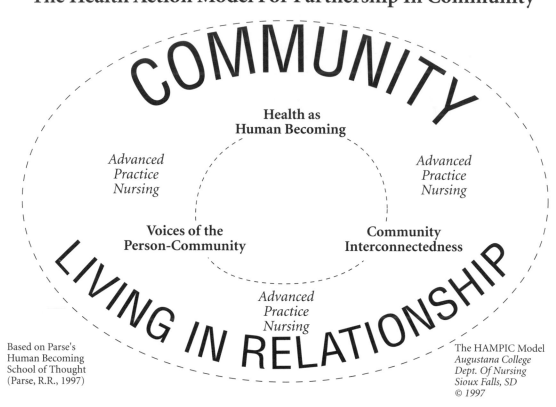

Based on Parse's
Human Becoming
School of Thought
(Parse, R.R., 1997)

The HAMPIC Model
Augustana College
Dept. Of Nursing
Sioux Falls, SD
© 1997

FIGURE 14–2   The health action model for partnership in community. *Reprinted with permission from the Augustana College, Department of Nursing, Sioux Falls, SD © 1997.*

voices of the person-community. "The purpose of the model is to respond in a new way to nursing's social mandate to care for the health of society by gaining an understanding of what is wanted from those living these health experiences" (Bunkers, Nelson, Leuning et. al, 1999, p. 94). Advanced practice nurses, a steering committee, and six "site communities" are moving together in seeking mutual understanding of human health issues while holding as important the unique perspectives presented by individuals and groups with complex health situations. The community of Sioux Falls, South Dakota, has embraced this theory-based nursing education-practice model by providing funding from many community sources.

In the Health Action Model, "advanced practice nurses work with persons and groups in the 'Site Communities' in creating a prototype of collaboration in addressing issues concerning quality of life" (Bunkers, Nelson, Leuning et al., 1999, p. 94). "Site communities" are agencies or places that seek to

respond to the health and social-welfare issues of those struggling with lack of resources (see Fig. 14–3). Issues of quality of life are addressed with nurses asking persons, families, and communities what their hopes for the future are and working with them to create personal health descriptions and health action plans. Personal health descriptions are written in the words of the person, family, or community and include: (1) what life is like for me now; (2) my health concerns are ___; (3) what's most important to me now; (4) my hopes for the future are ___; (5) my plans for the future are ___; (6) how I can carry out my plans; and (7) my specific health action plan is ___ (Bunkers, Nelson, Leuning et al., 1999). When a person or community identifies a health pattern they want to develop further or identifies a desire to change certain health patterns, the nurse explores how she or he can support that process.

Objectives of the Health Action Model include: (1) creating a nursing practice model to guide

THE HEALTH ACTION MODEL
FOR PARTNERSHIP IN COMMUNITY
Connections in Community

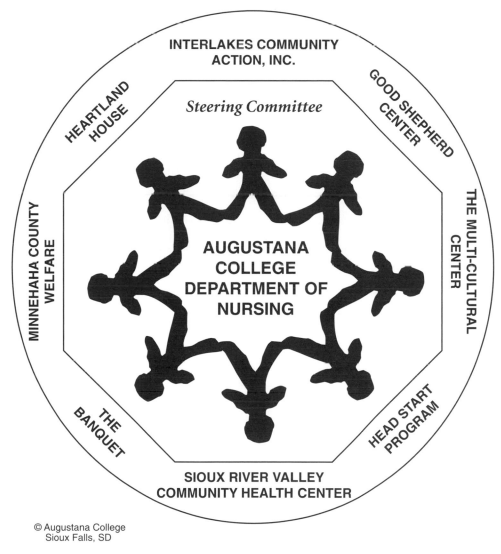

© Augustana College
Sioux Falls, SD

FIGURE 14–3   The health action model for partnership in community: Connections in community. *Reprinted with permission from ©
Augustana College, SD.*

provision of health services based on Human Becoming for families experiencing economic and social marginalization and/or homelessness; (2) using the Health Action Model to address health issues of "site communities"; (3) providing educational experiences for nursing and other health professional students, focusing on diversity; and (4) extending the Health Action Model beyond the local area and sharing it as a prototype for health care regionally, nationally, and internationally (Bunkers, Nelson, Leuning et al., 1999).

Parse's human becoming school of thought serves as the linchpin in this model for developing new ways of connecting person to person, agency to agency, and community to community. Bunkers and colleagues (1999) stated:

The interconnectedness of community involves relationship that transcends *separating differences*. There [is] no lack of spoken and written words about persons experiencing the *separating differences* of living with little or no money and no place to call home. What is missing in community is an intentional listening to the sound of these voices speaking and writing about their own hopes and meanings. To embrace *separating differences* involves listening and understanding others. The nurse-person-community health process involves being truly present with others with a listening receptivity to differing values. Nurses practicing in this model understand that community as process entails moving together in seeking mutual understanding.... Moving together in seeking mutual understanding calls for a type of listening to one another where both nurse and person-community engage in contributing to expanding choices for living health. (pp. 94–95)

Parse (1996) proposed that community in its most abstract sense is "the universe, the galaxy of human connectedness" (p. 4). Her most recent book offers new ways to think about community change and community connectedness (Parse, 2003a). The Health Action Model for Partnership in Community seeks to cultivate this human connectedness for the betterment of humankind.

RESEARCH

The published research that has been generated, inspired, and guided by the human becoming school of thought has been on the three research methods mentioned in Part 1 of this chapter: the Parse research method, the human becoming hermeneutic method, and the qualitative-descriptive preproject-process-postproject method.

Parse's Research Method

The essentials of Parse's phenomenological-hermeneutic research methodology were first published in the book *Nursing Science: Major Paradigms, Theories, and Critiques* (Parse, 1987). In 1990, Parse published a more detailed explication of the method, along with an illustration focusing on the lived experience of hope (Parse, 1990). A number of studies using the method have been published over the past 15 years (for example, see Bournes, 2002a; Bournes & Mitchell, 2002; Bunkers, 1998a, 2004; Cody, 1991, 1995a,b; Jonas-Simpson, 2003; Parse, 1994a, 1997b, 2001b, 2003b;

Pilkington, 1993). A previously unpublished example, drawn from a study of the lived experience of feeling confident with persons living with a spinal cord injury, follows.

Research guided by human becoming focuses on enhancing understanding of universal lived experiences such as *feeling confident.* Parse (1981, 1998a) posits that in all situations, and with every choice humans make, both certainty and uncertainty exist as a paradoxical, rhythmical pattern of human experience, since in every choice there is a sureness about what one wants to do, yet there is always ambiguity about how situations will unfold. People cannot predict how life will turn out, but they can imagine what is possible in light of what is familiar-unfamiliar, choose among imaged options, and live a commitment to what is important to them.

Consider, for example, a study of the lived experience of feeling confident of people living with a spinal cord injury. Participants in this study were three women and seven men between 22 and 42 years of age (mean 32.7 years) who agreed to speak with the researcher about their experience of feeling confident. The participants, all living in their own homes, had been living with a spinal cord injury for a period that ranged from 1.5 to 16 years (mean 7.9 years).

In the Parse research method, data-gathering happens through the process of *dialogical engagement*—an intersubjective process whereby the researcher lives true presence with the participant. The researcher moves in rhythm with the participant's description of the phenomenon (Parse, 1998, 2001a). In this study, the researcher asked the participants, "Please tell me about your experience of feeling confident." The researcher then attended to each participant's description. No other questions were planned—although the participants were sometimes encouraged to say more or to speak about how some things they said related to their experience of feeling confident. The dialogues, which lasted from 20 to 60 minutes, were all audiotaped and transcribed for the *extraction-synthesis* (data-analysis) process.

Extraction-synthesis is the process of moving the descriptions from the language of the participants across levels of abstraction to the language of science (Parse, 1998, 2001a). It includes: extracting and synthesizing stories and essences (core ideas and examples each participant shared about feeling confident) from the transcribed descriptions in the participants' language; conceptualizing the essences in the language of the researcher; synthesizing language art from the essences of each participant's description; extracting and synthesizing core concepts (core ideas about feeling confident that were described, in some way, by all participants); and synthesizing a structure of the lived experience (Parse, 1998, 2001a). The structure, as evolved, answers the research question. The extraction-synthesis process is illustrated here, beginning with Ben's story.

Ben at 42 years of age said that feeling confident is "an overall feeling good, like I have something to offer," and "like my thoughts and ideas have value and weight." It is "feeling useful and important and worthwhile." Ben described volunteer work he did with other people who have spinal cord injuries. He said, "speaking with somebody and helping strangers who seem motivated or encouraged by what I have to say, that's makes me feel good, like I have done something of value." Feeling confident is "not worrying or wondering about what is going to happen the next day, or the rest of your life." It is "being calm," "content," and "happy." It is "knowing that whatever happens, you will get through it." Ben said, "You can't know the answers ahead of time, or how you'll deal with things, but you know that you should be okay." He shared, feeling confident is "feeling comfortable about what I do, and if anyone wanted to argue about it, I could." It

is knowing "there's nothing about me that I have to feel insecure about, or feel like someone is going to look at me and judge me and think I am less than they are. I guess it is all self image." Ben said feeling confident is "getting psyched up" and "doing something that I am interested in accomplishing." It is "recognizing things around you and being aware of what is going on, rather than just aimlessly plodding along." It is having "a bigger sense of life and keeping up to date with the world and friends and people." Ben added, "my experience of feeling confident changes almost daily. Sometimes I have confidence and other times I don't, it depends on how familiar I am with the situation" and "on the feedback I get from the other person I am dealing with. If I feel intimidated then I don't always feel confident." (Table 14–2)

Three core concepts were extracted-synthesized from the language art of all participants: *buoyant assuredness amid unsureness, sustaining engagements,* and *persistently pursuing the cherished.* They were then synthesized into the structure. *Feeling confident is a buoyant assuredness amid unsureness that arises with sustaining engagements while persistently pursuing the cherished.* The structure was then woven with the principles of human becoming through the three processes of *heuristic interpretation:* structural transposition, conceptual integration, and artistic expression (Parse, 2003c). *Structural transposition* and *conceptual integration*

Table 14–2	**Progressive abstraction of the core concepts of the lived experience of feeling confident**	
Core Concept	**Structural Transposition**	**Conceptual Integration**
Buoyant assuredness amid unsureness	Elated certainty-uncertainty	Originating
Sustaining engagements	Emboldening involvements	Connecting-separating
Persistently pursuing the cherished	Pushing-resisting with the treasured	Powering-valuing

STRUCTURE

Feeling confident is a buoyant assuredness amid unsureness that arises with sustaining engagements while persistently pursuing the cherished.

STRUCTURAL TRANSPOSITION

Feeling confident is an elated certainty-uncertainty that arises with emboldening involvements while pushing-resisting with the treasured.

CONCEPTUAL INTEGRATION

Feeling confident is originating the connecting-separating of powering valuing.

are the processes of heuristic interpretation that move the discourse of the structure to the discourse of the theory. *Artistic expression* is "cocreating an artform incarnating the researcher's transfiguring moments with the researched. The artforms may be paintings, drawings, literary works, metaphors, music, and others" (Parse, 2003, p. 1). In the next section, the core concepts, structural transposition, and conceptual integration for this study are summarized (see Table 14–2) and described in detail, followed by the researcher's artistic expression.

Buoyant Assuredness Amid Unsureness

The first core concept, buoyant assuredness amid unsureness, captures the participants' descriptions of *feeling confident* as an enriching and exhilarating feeling of surety experienced together with the unsettling tentativeness of wavering with the ambiguity in their lives. As they spoke about their experiences, the participants described feeling confident as, for example, "an upward spiral of believing I can do just about anything"; "getting psyched up"; "a euphoric feeling"; "being happy and very, very positive"; "energizing"; and "being on a natural high." Simultaneously, all of the participants also described experiences of "not feeling confident." They talked, for instance, about feeling "intimidated," "insecure," "scared," "worried," and "terrified." For example, one participant, who injured her spinal cord in a car accident, shared, "There are times where I feel completely safe and completely confident. It's the moments when the injury totally goes away. I do not feel injured, I do not look injured, I do not think injured and it feels good, it provides energy. I am happy and very positive." The same participant went on to say:

> Sometimes I feel very unconfident. I am still lacking confidence in my ability to return to work. I can't work hands on any more and I am afraid of the pain of not being able to do the job that I love. A lot of experiences with health care people have degraded my confidence. When I was first trying to get off the ventilator, I was terrified. They plugged the trach, put a nasal cannula on me and said go to town. I remember anxiety over not being able to get enough oxygen. I was alone and I couldn't even yell for help. The nasal cannula had come out of my nose and the nurse came and shoved it back and said, 'You're fine, stop messing around.' That one experience scared me so badly.

Similarly, the notion of buoyant assuredness amid unsureness emerged with other participants' descriptions of their patterns of relating with others. For instance, one participant shared:

> Feeling confident is a euphoric feeling. I am not always confident. Many people don't know what I have accomplished and they are amazed by all that I do. But, that kind of stuff can erode away your confidence because it takes me getting into this situation to impress them, but I was flying before my accident. I was working, I had a house, I was going to start a family. Sometimes it can bleed your confidence away at times.

The core concept, buoyant assuredness amid unsureness, captures participants' descriptions of feeling confident as an uplifting experience of being certain, yet all-at-once uncertain about themselves and about the people and projects in their lives. At the structural transposition level, the ideas captured by buoyant assuredness amid unsureness are conceptualized as *elated certainty-uncertainty*. Elated certainty-uncertainty is conceptually integrated with human becoming as *originating*.

Originating is related to the ways humans create means of distinguishing and living their personal uniqueness while simultaneously designing ways to go along with and to be like others. As humans originate ways of being the same yet unique, they are both sure about the choices they make and unsure about what the outcomes will be (Parse, 1998). In this study, the participants' descriptions of their experiences of feeling confident that led to buoyant assuredness amid unsureness are an example of the way people continuously experience doubt and unsureness, even when they describe being energized and uplifted by a feeling of sureness about the people, projects, and possibilities that they choose to pursue. The descriptions that led to this core concept connect the participants' experiences of feeling confident with their having faith or trusting that, despite the continuous presence of unsureness, they will be fine.

The descriptions given by the participants in this study also demonstrate the ways others cocreate persons' experiences of certainty-uncertainty with feeling confident. The descriptions that contributed to the core concept of buoyant assuredness amid unsureness demonstrated the dimension of uncertainty that is emphasized with some patterns of relating with others. The core ideas about feeling confident represented by the next core concept, sustaining engagements, illuminate patterns of relating with others, ideas, and projects that are helpful for feeling confident.

Sustaining Engagements

The second core concept, sustaining engagements, signifies the participants' descriptions of feeling confident as feeling good about, and believing in, themselves in connection with their activities, accomplishments, and relationships that "reawakened" and "refueled" their confidence. Participants all shared details about, for example, feeling confident when they were "able to do things" both for themselves and for others. One participant shared, "I try to do things that make me feel good about myself. It has to do with building my confidence. I feel better about myself, because I am able to do more, smile more, that is confidence inspiring." Another participant said, "Accomplishing the tiniest little things, as small as being able to operate a door handle, gives me the confidence to keep on the healing path," while someone else described feeling confident as a "freedom to believe in myself that I get from motorcycling, water skiing, and boating."

The notion of sustaining engagements is also illuminated in the words of one participant who described feeling confident as the moments when she is either with someone, or she is doing something, and her injury "just disappears." She shared, "It could be when I am lying in bed with a friend or sitting in a restaurant. And those episodes usually happen when I am dealing with a challenge and I am managing it. I think that when it disappears for me, people around me see it less too, and that's directly related to confidence. I have learned to trust myself." For others, sustaining engagements is evident in their descriptions of feeling loved, supported, and cared for. One participant said, "Staying near the things I love, my friends and family having confidence in me, every experience I face, positive or negative, they all reawaken my confidence." Similarly, others described experiences that contributed to their feeling confident that included having: "huge support from friends and family"; "the support of a team and a doctor that called every day and showed they cared"; and "people that listen to what I have to say."

Several other participants described feeling confident in connection with sustaining engagements with objects or symbols of their confidence. For ex-

ample, one participant said, "Some old family photographs are a symbol of my confidence. I have pictures of when I am water-skiing and I was always very confident. Looking at pictures of water-skiing really gives me a whole new rush of confidence. Those pictures help refuel the fire." Another offered, "My bicycle is a symbol of my confidence. Being a quadriplegic and being able to walk and ride a bicycle is a really big feat. I have an intimate connection with my bicycle. The bicycle is a gauge to how I am doing."

The core concept of sustaining engagements signifies the participants' descriptions of feeling confident as *emboldening involvements* with others, activities, and objects. It is conceptually integrated with human becoming as *connecting-separating*— the paradoxical rhythm of being with and away from others, ideas, objects, and events (Parse, 1998). When the participants in this study spoke about feeling confident in ways that led the researcher to the core concept of sustaining engagements, they talked about the importance of being with and away from family, friends, health-care providers, activities, and objects in ways that helped them to feel confident. For example, one participant described confidence as inspiring connections with old photographs of himself and his family taking part in activities from which he was simultaneously separating, since he could no longer be involved with them in the same way. Others described connecting with people and activities— such as skiing, horseback riding, public speaking, teaching, or attending school—that helped them to feel confident, yet also separating from the way their relationships with those same people and activities were prior to their accidents. Participants described feeling confident in relation to connecting with either friends or health-care providers who were helpful and who inspired their confidence and separating from those who did not as they were persisting and striving to accomplish what was important to them.

Persistently Pursuing the Cherished

The third core concept, persistently pursuing the cherished, captures the participants' descriptions of feeling confident as a determined and ardent quest to achieve what was important to them. When they described their experiences of *feeling confident*, the participants talked about, for example, the "intensity" of "being focused on" and "making" their goals happen. They described feeling confident as "having drive," "just going ahead," "being willing to try again," and "standing up for what you believe in." For one participant, feeling confident was connected with "taking charge, moving forward, and focusing on buying a house, starting up a business, [and] getting my life back into shape." He recalled, "I did it with an intensity that even today I find a little bit hard to realize." Another participant shared:

> Feeling confident is pushing myself to do the things that I want to do. People think that I can afford this house because I had my accident. No, it's because I worked hard when I was sick, when I had a huge sciatic nerve problem in my legs and I used to crawl up ladders, dragging my leg up the ladder and that was because I had a goal in mind. In order to live the life I wanted to live, I had to work hard. You have just got to keep on going.

The core concept of persistently pursuing the cherished is structurally transposed as *pushing-resisting with the treasured* and conceptually integrated with human becoming as the theoretical construct *powering valuing*. Powering valuing is confirming-not confirming one's value priorities while continuously living the pushing-resisting rhythm of affirming-not affirming being with non-being (Parse, 1998). In this study, the descriptions of feeling confident that led to the core concept of persistently pursuing the cherished illuminated the participants' commitment to living in ways that confirmed and achieved what was most important to them. The notion of affirming being in spite of the possibility of non-being surfaced in all participants' descriptions of pushing and persisting with their priorities—even though there were people and circumstances that were not affirming and that made the possibility of non-being explicit. In affirming and moving with their value priorities, the participants were simultaneously not affirming the possibility of non-being, which for them meant consequences such as not getting better, not accomplishing things, and not standing up for what they wanted.

The implications of this study primarily relate to what can happen when health professionals have an enhanced understanding of human experience. For example, the descriptions of feeling confident as one dimension of the paradoxical rhythm, feeling confident–feeling unsure, underscore the importance of health professionals being available to bear witness to both dimensions of the rhythm should persons want to share them. It also helps nurses and others to understand that even though persons may describe feeling confident about something in the moment, the experience is dynamic and continuously shifting. What someone is confident about today may be a source of uncertainty tomorrow. The way professionals are with people as they live the shifting rhythm of feeling confident–feeling unsure can be helpful, or harmful.

Human Becoming Hermeneutic Method

The human becoming hermeneutic method (Cody, 1995c; Parse, 1998, 2001a) was developed in congruence with the assumptions and principles of Parse's theory, drawing on works by Bernstein (1983), Gadamer (1976, 1989), Heidegger (1962), Langer (1967), and Ricoeur (1976). Gadamer's work in particular guided the explication of the method. This method is intended to guide the interpretation of texts and art forms in light of the human becoming perspective, giving rise to new understandings of human experiences as manifest in the emergent meanings that are the findings of a hermeneutic study. In Cody's work in developing the method, the hermeneutic processes of *discoursing, interpreting,* and *understanding* were explicated within a human becoming perspective, informed by important works by the authors previously mentioned. Parse (1998, 2001a) further refined the processes and gave depth and clarity to their meaning. The processes are: *discoursing with penetrating engaging, interpreting with quiescent beholding,* and *understanding with inspiring envisaging*. To date, three studies (Cody, 1995c, 2001; Ortiz, 2003) using this method have been published.

Qualitative-Descriptive Preproject-Process-Postproject Method

The qualitative-descriptive preproject-process-postproject method is described in detail in Parse's (1998, 2001a) works. This method's purpose is to understand what happens when human becoming is lived in the nurse-person/family/community process. It has been used in multiple settings (Bournes, 2002b).

NURSING LEADERSHIP

The Human Becoming school of thought (Parse, 1981, 1998) prepares nurses to assume positions of leadership for the purpose of enhancing the quality of human care in all settings. The knowledge base of the theory enables leaders to create and nurture opportunities for staff to change their attitudes, values, and approaches in practice and research. Parse's Theory of Human Becoming helps professionals move toward a more participative, client-centered model of service delivery (see for discussion, Bournes, 2002b). Knowledge framed by human becoming constitutes the leader's unique contribution to a community of health-care professionals. The nurse leader's views coexist with multiple other views and beliefs about health care. It is precisely the diversity of ideas and purposes that generate the dynamic culture of comprehensive and compassionate human care.

In the broadest sense, leadership guided by the human becoming theory means working toward creating a particular culture of care. *Culture of care,* as defined here, refers to the assumptions, values, and meanings expressed and shared in the language patterns of a group of people. The changes that are invited include changing from telling and teaching to listening and dialoguing, changing from trying to control patients' decisions to facilitating choices, and changing from judging and labeling differences among people to respecting and representing differences. Like all cultures, the human becoming culture coexists with other cultures of the community. For instance, in hospital settings, other cultures that coexist and complement the human becoming beliefs include those of medicine and management.

The Human Becoming Theory provides the foundation for leaders to invite others to explore the values, intentions, and desires that shape human

> Leading is about a process of guided discovery that surfaces insights about self and human becoming—the insights are the windows of change.

care and professional practice. The leading process is not about educating staff—meaning it is not about giving information. Rather, leading is about a process of guided discovery that surfaces insights about self and human becoming—the insights are the windows of change. Personal insights coupled with new knowledge can dramatically change practice and the quality of relationships that staff have with individuals, families, and groups (Bournes, 2002b; Mitchell, Closson, Coulis et al., 2000).

Processes of Leading in Change

Leading in a community involves processes of explicating, visioning, discovering, confirming, and disclosing. These processes happen in the context of discussions about human care and meaningful service.

Explicating involves a process of examining the assumptions, values, and meanings embedded in current practices. For example, this includes examination of the assumptions and values of the traditional nursing process multisystem assessments, and prescription. Nurses require opportunities to consider the meanings of words like "dysfunctional," "manipulative," "unrealistic," and "noncompliant." The Human Becoming school of thought offers an alternative framework for all professionals to think about the human-universe process and its connections with practice and human care. The outcome of explicating includes clarification of the values and assumptions of different processes of care and service.

Visioning is the process whereby staff imagine the forms and patterns that could constitute human care. The predominant questions that invite discourse and insight here are "what if" questions: What if individuals were considered to be the experts about their own health and quality of life? What if nurses were required to listen to individuals' meanings and values in order to know how to care and be helpful? What if records were kept at the bedside and patients and families were the ones who monitored access to the record, documented their experiences, and evaluated care? These sorts of questions invite staff to think outside of familiar patterns of practice.

Discovering happens as staff see the familiar in a new light. Nurses glimpse contrasting realities and views in discourse with others who discuss alternative ideas. Insights occur in flashes that shed light on how reality in practice could be shaped. The process of discovery can be both exciting and unsettling. There is risk in opening oneself to see things in a new way. Discovery changes everything in a cascading flow of understanding. Leaders can invite and nurture discovery, but ultimately it is a self-directed process that is lived by each person considering and choosing or not choosing to change.

Confirming is a process of seeking personal and organizational coherence with the values clarified in the process of visioning. Nurses seek coherence with cherished values in dialogue with others. Confirming new values is facilitated in standards of practice that specify expectations in the nurse-person process. As members of a self-regulating discipline, nurses have the authority to study and define the knowledge that will guide their practice and research activities. Standards make concrete the values chosen to guide practice and clarify the purpose of nursing in any organization.

Disclosing happens through actions taken and words spoken as staff integrate and share their new realities in the context of day-to-day relationships with patients and families. Disclosing is about presenting self to colleagues and to patients and families as a professional with intent and direction. Disclosing also happens through storytelling as staff members share their experiences with others. Telling stories of changing realities in practice and research perpetuates the living of new values and is the primary way nurses and other professionals propel the ongoing journey of change. The way these processes get lived out in any community of professionals will be unique, yet common patterns are recognizable.

Common patterns include explicit commitment and communication on the part of leaders in an organization where expectations are changing in the direction of a new way that is consistent with the human becoming school of thought. Patterns emerge that reflect the pushing-resisting with the central message from leaders and with the core ideas of the human becoming theory. Professionals can experience interest, anger, excitement, apathy, and resistance to ideas expressed. As new ideas and processes of care are described and explored, staff begin to discourse about the possibilities. Leaders are required in order to present the alternative views that inspire reflection and creative tension as new ideas about patient care are tossed about. Leaders facilitate patterns of discovery in the pushing-

resisting of change (Bournes & DasGupta, 1997; Linscott, Spee, Flint, & Fisher, 1999).

A necessary pattern to keep introducing into the process of changes is the pattern of reality linked with patients'/families' lived experiences in healthcare systems. Patient and family experiences are critical to sustaining the impetus for change. Valuable video resources on the topic of patient experiences include "Not My Home" (Deveaux & Babin, 1994), "Real Stories" (Deveaux & Babin, 1996), "The Grief of Miscarriage" (Pilkington, 1987), and "Handle with Care" (Gray, 2000; Gray & Sinding, 2002), to name several. Simply stated, people want to be listened to, to be regarded as knowing participants, to be respected for their unique lives and meanings, to have meaningful dialogue, and to have their choices and wishes integrated in plans of care. These basic requests are consistent with what the human becoming theory offers professional staff.

Patterns of thinking and acting, as well as patterns of attitude and intention, are complex and multidimensional. Nursing practice encompasses multiple realms of responsibility, yet there is with human becoming an identifiable coherence amid the apparent dissonance of diverging paradigms. Nurses who practice human becoming describe being more vigilant and attentive to the medical and technological responsibilities, because they are concerned in a different way about the person as a unitary human being who is illuminating meaning, synchronizing rhythms, and mobilizing transcendence. Leaders in large systems know that serious mishaps can sometimes be avoided if professionals truly listened to people and trusted their knowing of potential or impending danger and concern.

Organizational structures and systems must change if professional staff are to be supported to practice in ways consistent with the human becoming theory. For example, documentation of patient care changes from a stance of observed interpretation of patient behavior to a representation of the patient's experience from the patient/family perspective. This change in documentation is dramatic. For instance, a record in the problem-based, observed behavior model may include a notation like, "Patient refusing to take medications; confused, upset, and occasionally yelling out." In a culture in which patients are respected as leaders of their care, the same occasion might prompt this note: "Mr. B. states he is 'feeling sick from taking his pills.' He would like to speak with the doctor but does not know how to reach him; requests nurse to contact doctor. Mr. B. states that he 'wants to lie quietly but is too uncomfortable to do so.'" Professionals guided by standards of practice consistent with human becoming record the patient's experiences and the actions taken based on the person's concerns and wishes.

Practice consistent with the Human Becoming Theory is transformative. Some staff choose to study the theory so that the source of their transforming can continue in more depth and with more clarity. At the very least, persons who have the opportunity to learn human becoming will learn something about their own values and intentions as a person and as a professional. Whether or not the journey will continue on any particular path is not known. The professionals who accept the invitation to think and be different become the leaders for change. One consistent pattern over time has been that if the theory does help, if it does enhance quality of care and quality of work life, then it also has the power to resist the pressure to return to the status quo.

EDUCATION

A process model of teaching-learning is supported by Parse's human becoming school of thought. From a human becoming perspective, Bunkers defined *teaching-learning* as "an all at once process of engaging with others in coming to know" (1999, p. 227). Eight teaching-learning processes, emphasizing the notion that teaching-learning is a dynamic interactive human encounter with ideas, places, people, and events, are listed in Figure 14–4. These eight teaching-learning processes include "expanding imaginal margins, naming the new, going with content-process shifts, abiding with paradox, giving meaning, inviting dialogue, noticing the now, and growing story" (Bunkers, 1999, p. 227).

Bunkers (1999) wrote:

- *Expanding imaginal margins* involves focusing on the imaging process. Expanding imaginal margins while engaging with others in coming

The Teaching-Learning Process and the Theory of Human Becoming

The teaching-learning process confronts the familiar-unfamiliar all-at-once. From a human becoming perspective, teaching-learning is a **process of engaging with others in coming to know.** The **Seeker,** in engaging with others, participates in simultaneous processes of coming to know at an explicit-tacit level. These processes include:

E Expanding Imaginal Margins
N Naming the New
G Going with Content-Process Shifts
A Abiding with Paradox
G Giving Meaning
I Inviting Dialogue
N Noticing the Now
G Growing Story

WITH OTHERS IN THE PROCESS OF COMING TO KNOW

FIGURE 14–4 The teaching-learning process and the theory of human becoming. *Reprinted with permission from Bunkers, S. S., 1999. The teaching process and the theory of human becoming. Nursing Quarterly, 11, 56–63.*

to know coshapes what one will learn. In imaging valued possibilities, one is already moving with those possibilities.

- *Naming the new* concerns itself with languaging. Naming the new in the process of engaging with others in coming to know cocreates the meaning of the moment.
- *Going with content-process shifts* involves a synthesis of ideas with action. Going with content-process shifts while engaging with others in coming to know involves the intentionality of focusing on the unity of idea-action while participating in relationship.
- *Abiding with paradox* involves recognizing the contradictions in life. . . . Abiding with paradox in the process of engaging with others in coming to know involves honoring the tensions of contradiction and living in the questions.
- *Giving meaning* involves ascribing value to ideas and lived experiences. Giving meaning in the process of engaging with others in coming to know involves creating one's personal reality in light of choosing a personal stance toward ideas and experience. Giving meaning forms the purpose of one's life.
- *Inviting dialogue* consists of generating an atmosphere for conversation while being attentive to offered information. Inviting dialogue in the process of engaging with others in coming to know involves participating in discerning discourse while focusing on understanding unique patterns of evolving. Such understanding uncovers diverse realities.
- *Noticing the now* means being present to what was, is, and will be in human evolving. This presence involves an attentive, being with the other. Noticing the now in the process of engaging with others in coming to know involves living an attentive presence with others as possibility becoming actuality. It involves reflecting on how one moves moment to moment in relationship with others as transforming occurs.
- *Growing story* involves giving meaning to abstract concepts with narrative description. Storytelling reflects the unity and multidimensionality of human experience. Growing story in the process of engaging with others in coming to know immerses the community in meaning-making and comprehending personal realities. Meaning-making with storytelling unveils the wholeness of lived experience.

People who embrace this human becoming perspective of teaching-learning participate in fostering "the unique unfolding of human potential" (Bunkers, 1999).

References

Allchin-Petardi, L. (1996). *Weathering the storm: Persevering through a difficult time.* Unpublished doctoral dissertation, Loyola University, Chicago.

Arndt, M. J. (1995). Parse's theory of human becoming in practice with hospitalized adolescents. *Nursing Science Quarterly, 8,* 86–90.

Banonis, B. C. (1995). Metaphors in the practice of the human becoming theory. In Parse, R. R. (Ed.), *Illuminations: The human becoming theory in practice and research* (pp. 87–95). New York: National League for Nursing Press.

Baumann, S. L. (1996). Feeling uncomfortable: Children in families with no place of their own. *Nursing Science Quarterly, 9,* 152–159.

Baumann, S. L. (2003). The lived experience of feeling very tired: A study of adolescent girls. *Nursing Science Quarterly, 16,* 326–333.

Beauchamp, C. (1990). *The lived experience of struggling with making a decision in a critical life situation.* Unpublished doctoral dissertation, University of Miami, FL.

Blanchard, D. (1996). *The lived experience of intimacy: A study using Parse's theory and research methodology.* Unpublished doctoral dissertation, Wayne State University, Detroit, MI.

Bournes, D. A. (2000). A commitment to honoring people's choices. *Nursing Science Quarterly, 13,* 18–23.

Bournes, D. A. (2002a). Having courage: A lived experience of human becoming. *Nursing Science Quarterly, 15,* 220–229.

Bournes, D. A. (2002b). Research evaluating human becoming in practice. *Nursing Science Quarterly, 15,* 190–195.

Bournes, D. A. (2003). Stories of courage and confidence: Interpretation with the human becoming community change concepts. In Parse, R. R., *Community: A human becoming perspective* (pp. 131–145). Sudbury, MA: Jones & Bartlett.

Bournes, D. A., & DasGupta, D. (1997). Professional practice leader: A transformational role that addresses human diversity. *Nursing Administraton Quarterly, 21*(4), 61–68.

Bournes, D. A., & Ferguson-Paré, M. (2004). Innovations in nurse retention and patient centered care. Unpublished manuscript, University Health Network, Toronto, Canada.

Bournes, D. A., & Flint, F. (2003). Mistakes: Mistakes in the nurse-person process. *Nursing Science Quarterly, 16,* 127–130.

Bournes, D. A., & Mitchell, G. J. (2002). Waiting: The experience of persons in a critical care waiting room. *Research in Nursing & Health, 25,* 58–67.

Bunkers, S. S. (1998). Considering tomorrow: Parse's theory-guided research. *Nursing Science Quarterly, 11,* 56–63.

Bunkers, S. S. (1998a). A nursing theory-guided model of health ministry: Human becoming in parish nursing. *Nursing Science Quarterly, 11,* 7–8.

Bunkers, S. S. (1998b). Translating nursing conceptual frameworks and theory for nursing practice in the parish community. In Solari-Twadell, A., & McDermott, M. (Eds.), *Parish nursing* (pp. 205–214). Thousand Oaks, CA: Sage.

Bunkers, S. S. (2004). The lived experience of feeling cared for: A human becoming perspective. *Nursing Science Quarterly, 17,* 63–71.

Bunkers, S. S., Michaels, C., & Ethridge, P. (1997). Advanced practice nursing in community: Nursing's opportunity. *Advanced Practice Nursing Quarterly, 2*(4), 79–84.

Bunkers, S. S., Nelson, M. L., Leuning, C. J., Crane, J. K., & Josephson, D. K. (1999). The health action model: Academia's partnership with the community. In Cohen, E. L., & DeBack, V. (Eds.), *The outcomes mandate: Case management in health care today* (pp. 92–100). St. Louis: Mosby.

Bunkers, S. S., & Putnam, V. (1995). A nursing theory based model of health ministry: Living Parse's theory of human becoming in the parish community. In *Ninth Annual Westberg Parish Nurse Symposium: Parish nursing: Ministering through the arts*. Northbrook, IL: International Parish Nursing Resource Center—Advocate Health Care.

Butler, M. J. (1988). Family transformation: Parse's theory in practice. *Nursing Science Quarterly, 1,* 68–74.

Butler, M. J., & Snodgrass, F. G. (1991). Beyond abuse: Parse's theory in practice. *Nursing Science Quarterly, 4,* 76–82.

Chapman, J. S., Mitchell, G. J., & Forchuk, C. (1994). A glimpse of nursing theory-based practice in Canada. *Nursing Science Quarterly, 7,* 104–112.

Cody, W. K. (1991). Grieving a personal loss. *Nursing Science Quarterly, 4,* 61–68.

Cody, W. K. (1995a). The lived experience of grieving, for families living with AIDS. In Parse, R. R. (Ed.), *Illuminations: The human becoming theory in practice and research* (pp. 197–242). New York: National League for Nursing Press.

Cody, W. K. (1995b). The meaning of grieving for families living with AIDS. *Nursing Science Quarterly, 8,* 104–114.

Cody, W. K. (1995c). Of life immense in passion, pulse, and power: Dialoguing with Whitman and Parse, a hermeneutic study. In Parse, R. R. (Ed.), *Illuminations: The human becoming theory in practice and research* (pp. 269–307). New York: National League for Nursing Press.

Daly, J. (1995). The lived experience of suffering. In Parse, R. R. (Ed.), *Illuminations: The human becoming theory in practice and research* (pp. 243–268). New York: National League for Nursing Press.

Damgaard, G., & Bunkers, S. S. (1998). Nursing science-guided practice and education: A state board of nursing perspective. *Nursing Science Quarterly, 11,* 142–144.

Gouty, C. A. (1996). *Feeling alone while with others.* Unpublished doctoral dissertation, Loyola University, Chicago.

Hansen-Ketchum, P. (2004). Parse's theory in practice. *Journal of Holistic Nursing, 22,* 57–72.

Huch, M. H., & Bournes, D. A. (2003). Community dwellers' perspectives on the experience of feeling very tired. *Nursing Science Quarterly, 16,* 334–339.

Huchings, D. (2002). Parallels in practice: Palliative nursing practice and Parse's theory of human becoming. *American Journal of Hospice and Palliative Care, 19,* 408–414.

International Consortium of Parse Scholars. (1996). *The human becoming theory: Living true presence in nursing practice.* Available from ICPS, c/o Pat Lyon, The Rehabilitation Institute of Toronto, 550 University Avenue, Toronto, Ontario, Canada M5G 2A2.

Jonas, C. M. (1994). True presence through music. *Nursing Science Quarterly, 7,* 102–103.

Jonas, C. M. (1995a). Evaluation of the human becoming theory in family practice. In Parse, R. R. (Ed.), *Illuminations: The human becoming theory in practice and research* (pp. 347–366). New York: National League for Nursing Press.

Jonas, C. M. (1995b). True presence through music for persons living their dying. In Parse, R. R. (Ed.), *Illuminations: The human becoming theory in practice and research* (pp. 97–104). New York: National League for Nursing Press.

Jonas-Simpson, C. (2001). Feeling understood: A melody of human becoming. *Nursing Science Quarterly, 14,* 222–230.

Jonas-Simpson, C. M. (2003). The experience of being listened to: A human becoming study with music. *Nursing Science Quarterly, 16,* 232–238.

Kelley, L. S. (1991). Struggling to go along when you do not believe. *Nursing Science Quarterly, 4,* 123–129.

Kruse, B. (1996). *The lived experience of serenity: Using Parse's research method.* Unpublished doctoral dissertation, University of South Carolina at Columbia.

Lee, O. J., & Pilkington, F. B. (1999). Practice with persons living their dying: A human becoming perspective. *Nursing Science Quarterly, 12,* 324–328.

Legault, F., & Ferguson Paré, M. (1999). Advancing nursing practice: An evaluation study of Parse's theory of human becoming. *Canadian Journal of Nursing Leadership, 12*(1), 30–35.

Liehr, P. R. (1989). The core of true presence: A loving center. *Nursing Science Quarterly, 2,* 7–8.

Linscott, J., Spee, R., Flint, F., & Fisher, A. (1999). Creating a culture of patient-focused care through a learner-centred philosophy. *Canadian Journal of Nursing Leadership, 12*(4), 5–10.

Lui, S. L. (1993). *The meaning of health in hospitalized older women in Taiwan.* Unpublished doctoral dissertation, University of Colorado Health Sciences Center, Denver.

Mattice, M., & Mitchell, G. J. (1990). Caring for confused elders. *The Canadian Nurse, 86*(11), 16–18.

Milton, C. (1998). *Making a promise.* Unpublished doctoral dissertation, Loyola University, Chicago.

Mitchell, G. J. (1988). Man-living-health: The theory in practice. *Nursing Science Quarterly, 1,* 120–127.

Mitchell, G. J. (1990a). The lived experience of taking life day-by-day in later life: Research guided by Parse's emergent method. *Nursing Science Quarterly, 3,* 29–36.

Mitchell, G. J. (1990b). Struggling in change: From the traditional approach to Parse's theory-based practice. *Nursing Science Quarterly, 3,* 170–176.

Mitchell, G. J. (1993). Living paradox in Parse's theory. *Nursing Science Quarterly, 6,* 44–51.

Mitchell, G. J. (1995). The lived experience of restriction-freedom in later life. In Parse, R. R. (Ed.), *Illuminations: The human becoming theory in practice and research* (pp. 159–195). New York: National League for Nursing Press.

Mitchell, G. J. (1998). Standards of nursing and the winds of change. *Nursing Science Quarterly, 11,* 97–98.

Mitchell, G. J., & Bournes, D. A. (2000). Nurse as patient advocate? In search of straight thinking. *Nursing Science Quarterly, 13,* 204–209.

Mitchell, G. J., & Copplestone, C. (1990). Applying Parse's theory to perioperative nursing: A nontraditional approach. *AORN Journal, 51*(3), 787–798.

Mitchell, G. J., & Heidt, P. (1994). The lived experience of wanting to help another: Research with Parse's method. *Nursing Science Quarterly, 7,* 119–127.

Mitchell, G. J., & Pilkington, B. (1990). Theoretical approaches in nursing practice: A comparison of Roy and Parse. *Nursing Science Quarterly, 3,* 81–87.

Northrup, D. (1995). Exploring the experience of time passing for persons with HIV disease: Parse's theory-guided research. Doctoral dissertation, the University of Austin, 1995. University Microfilms International, 9534912.

Northrup, D. (2002). Time passing: A Parse research method study. *Nursing Science Quarterly, 15,* 318–326.

Northrup, D., & Cody, W. K. (1998). Evaluation of the human becoming theory in practice in an acute care psychiatric setting. *Nursing Science Quarterly, 11,* 23–30.

Norris, J. R. (2002). One-to-one teleapprenticeship as a means for nurses teaching and learning Parse's theory of human becoming. *Nursing Science Quarterly, 15,* 113–116.

Ortiz, M. R. (2003). Lingering presence: A study using the human becoming hermeneutic method. *Nursing Science Quarterly, 16,* 146–154.

Paille, M., & Pilkington, F. B. (2002). The global context of nursing: A human becoming perspective. *Nursing Science Quarterly, 15,* 165–170.

Parse, R. R. (1974). *Nursing fundamentals.* Flushing, NY: Medical Examination.

Parse, R. R. (1981). *Man-living-health: A theory of nursing.* New York: Wiley.

Parse, R. R. (1987). *Nursing science: Major paradigms, theories, and critiques.* Philadelphia: Saunders.

Parse, R. R. (1990). Parse's research methodology with an illustration of the lived experience of hope. *Nursing Science Quarterly, 3,* 9–17.

Parse, R. R. (1992). Human becoming: Parse's theory of nursing. *Nursing Science Quarterly, 5,* 35–42.

Parse, R. R. (1994a). Laughing and health: A study using Parse's research method. *Nursing Science Quarterly, 7,* 55–64.

Parse, R. R. (1994b). Quality of life: Sciencing and living the art of human becoming. *Nursing Science Quarterly, 7,* 16–21.

Parse, R. R. (Ed.). (1995). *Illuminations: The human becoming theory in practice and research.* New York: National League for Nursing Press.

Parse, R. R. (1996). Reality: A seamless symphony of becoming. *Nursing Science Quarterly, 9,* 181–183.

Parse, R. R. (1997a). The human becoming theory: The was, is, and will be. *Nursing Science Quarterly, 10,* 32–38.

Parse, R. R. (1997b). Joy-sorrow: A study using the Parse research method. *Nursing Science Quarterly, 10,* 80–87.

Parse, R. R. (1997c). The language of nursing knowledge: Saying what we mean. In Fawcett, J., & King, I. M. (Eds.), *The language of theory and metatheory* (pp. 73–77). Sigma Theta Tau monograph.

Parse, R. R. (1998a). *The human becoming school of thought.* Thousand Oaks, CA: Sage.

Parse, R. R. (Summer, 1998b). On true presence. *Illuminations, 7*(3), 1.

Parse, R. R. (1999). *Hope: An international human becoming perspective.* Sudbury, MA: Jones & Bartlett.

Parse, R. R. (2001a). The lived experience of contentment: A study using the Parse research method. *Nursing Science Quarterly, 14,* 330–338.

Parse, R. R. (2001b). *Qualitative inquiry: The path of sciencing.* Sudbury, MA: Jones and Bartlett.

Parse, R. R. (2003a). *Community: A human becoming perspective.* Sudbury, MA: Jones and Bartlett.

Parse, R. R. (2003b). The lived experience of feeling very tired: A study using the Parse research method. *Nursing Science Quarterly, 17,* 33–35.

Parse, R. R. (2004). A human becoming teaching-learning model. *Nursing Science Quarterly, 17,* 33–35.

Parse, R. R. (in press). The human becoming synergistic collaborating leadership model. *Nursing Science Quarterly.*

Parse, R. R., Coyne, B. A., & Smith, M. J. (1985). *Nursing research: Qualitative methods.* Bowie, MD: Brady.

Pilkington, F. B. (1993). The lived experience of grieving the loss of an important other. *Nursing Science Quarterly, 6,* 130–139.

Pilkington, F. B. (1997). *Persisting while wanting to change: Research guided by Parse's theory.* Unpublished doctoral dissertation, Loyola University, Chicago.

Pilkington, F. B., & Jonas-Simpson, C. (1996). *The human becoming theory: A manual for the teaching-learning process.* The International Consortium of Parse Scholars.

Quiquero, A., Knights, D., & Meo, C. O. (1991). Theory as a guide to practice: Staff nurses choose Parse's theory. *Canadian Journal of Nursing Administration, 4*(1), 14–16.

Rasmusson, D. L. (1995). True presence with homeless persons. In Parse, R. R. (Ed.), *Illuminations: The human becoming theory in practice and research* (pp. 105–113). New York: National League for Nursing Press.

Rasmusson, D. L., Jonas, C. M., & Mitchell, G. J. (1991). The eye of the beholder: Parse's theory with homeless individuals. *Clinical Nurse Specialist, 5*(3), 139–143.

Rogers, M. E. (1992). Nursing science and the space age. *Nursing Science Quarterly, 5,* 27–34.

Santopinto, M. D. A., & Smith, M. C. (1995). Evaluation of the human becoming theory in practice with adults and children. In Parse, R. R. (Ed.), *Illuminations: The human becoming theory in practice and research* (pp. 309–346). New York: National League for Nursing Press.

Smith, M. C. (1990a). *The lived experience of hope in families of critically ill persons.* Paper presented at UCLA National Nursing Theory Conference, Los Angeles, CA.

Smith, M. C. (1990b). Struggling through a difficult time for unemployed persons. *Nursing Science Quarterly, 3,* 18–28.

Smith, M. K. (2002). Human becoming and women living with violence. *Nursing Science Quarterly, 15,* 302–307.

Stanley, G. D., & Meghani, S. H. (2001). Reflections on using Parse's theory of human becoming in a palliative care setting in Pakistan. *Canadian Nurse, 97,* 23–25.

Thornburg, P. D. (1993). *The meaning of hope in parents whose infants died from Sudden Infant Death Syndrome.* Doctoral dissertation, University of Cincinnati, OH. University Microfilms International No. 9329939.

Wang, C. E. H. (1997). *Mending a torn fishnet: Parse's theory-guided research on the lived experience of hope.* Unpublished doctoral dissertation, Loyola University, Chicago.

Ward, W. (1972). Matthew. In Paschall, H., & Hobbs, H. (Eds.), *The teacher's bible commentary* (pp. 586–616). Nashville, TN: Broadman Press.

Williamson, G. J. (2000). The test of a nursing theory: A personal view. *Nursing Science Quarterly, 13,* 124–128.

Bibliography

Arrigo, B., & Cody, W. K. (2004). A dialogue on existential-phenomenological thought in psychology and in nursing. *Nursing Science Quarterly, 17,* 6–11.

Banonis, B. C. (1989). The lived experience of recovering from addiction. A phenomenological study. *Nursing Science Quarterly, 2,* 37–43.

Baumann, S. (1994). No place of their own: An exploratory study. *Nursing Science Quarterly, 7,* 162–169.

Baumann, S. (1995). Two views of children's art: Psychoanalysis and Parse's human becoming theory. *Nursing Science Quarterly, 8,* 65–70.

Baumann, S. (1996). Parse's research methodology and the nurse-researcher-child process. *Nursing Science Quarterly, 2,* 27–32.

Baumann, S. (1997). Contrasting two approaches in a community-based nursing practice with older adults: The medical model and Parse's nursing theory. *Nursing Science Quarterly, 10,* 124–130.

Baumann, S. L. (2000). The lived experience of feeling loved: A study of mothers in a parolee program. *Nursing Science Quarterly, 13,* 332–338.

Baumann, S. L., & Carroll, K. (2001). Human becoming practice with children. *Nursing Science Quarterly, 14,* 120–125.

Bernardo, A. (1998). Technology and true presence in nursing. *Holistic Nursing Practice, 12*(4), 40–49.

Bernstein, R. J. (1983). *Beyond objectivism and relativism: Science, hermeneutics, and praxis.* Menlo Park, CA: Addison-Wesley.

Bournes, D. A. (2000). Concept inventing: A process for creating a unitary definition of having courage. *Nursing Science Quarterly, 13,* 143–149.

Bunkers, S. S. (1999). The teaching-learning process and the theory of human becoming. *Nursing Science Quarterly, 12,* 227–232.

Bunkers, S. S. (1999b). Emerging discoveries and possibilities in nursing. *Nursing Science Quarterly, 12,* 26–29.

Bunkers, S. S. (2002). Lifelong learning: A human becoming perspective. *Nursing Science Quarterly, 15,* 294–300.

Bunkers, S. S. (2003a). Comparison of three Parse method studies on feeling very tired. *Nursing Science Quarterly, 16,* 340–344.

Bunkers, S. S. (2003b). Understanding the stranger. *Nursing Science Quarterly, 16,* 305–309.

Bunkers, S. S., Damgaard, G., Hohman, M., & Vander Woude, D. (1998). *The South Dakota Nursing Theory–Based Regulatory Decision-Making Model.* Unpublished manuscript. Sioux Falls, SD: Augustana College.

Bunkers, S. S., & Putnam, V. (1995). A nursing theory based model of health ministry: Living Parse's theory of human becoming in the parish community. In *Ninth Annual Westberg Parish Nurse Symposium: Parish nursing: Ministering through the arts.* Northbrook, IL: International Parish Nursing Resource Center—Advocate Health Care.

Cody, W. K. (1991). Multidimensionality: Its meaning and significance. *Nursing Science Quarterly, 4,* 140–141.

Cody, W. K. (1995). True presence with families living with HIV disease. In Parse, R. R. (Ed.), *Illuminations: The human becoming theory in practice and research* (pp. 115–133). New York: National League for Nursing Press.

Cody, W. K. (1995). The view of the family within the human becoming theory. In Parse, R. R. (Ed.), *Illuminations: The human becoming theory in practice and research* (pp. 9–26). New York: National League for Nursing Press.

Cody, W. K. (1995). The lived experience of grieving for families living with AIDS. In Parse, R. R. (Ed.), *Illuminations: The human becoming theory in practice and research* (pp. 197–242). New York: National League for Nursing Press.

Cody, W. K. (1996). Drowning in eclecticism. *Nursing Science Quarterly, 9,* 86–88.

Cody, W. K. (1996). Occult reductionism in the discourse of theory development. *Nursing Science Quarterly, 9,* 140–142.

Cody, W. K. (2000). The lived experience of grieving for persons living with HIV who have used injection drugs. *Journal of the Association of Nurses in AIDS Care, 11,* 82–92.

Cody, W. K. (2000). Parse's human becoming school of thought and families. *Nursing Science Quarterly, 13,* 281–284.

Cody, W. K. (2001). Mendacity as the refusal to bear witness: A human becoming hermeneutic study of a theme from Tennessee Williams' *Cat on a Hot Tin Roof.* In Parse, R. R., *Qualitative inquiry: The path of sciencing* (pp. 205–220). Sudbury, MA: Jones and Bartlett.

Cody, W. K. (2003). Diversity and becoming: Implications of human existence as coexistence. *Nursing Science Quarterly, 16,* 195–200.

Cody, W. K., Hudepohl, J. H., & Brinkman, K. S. (1995). True presence with a child and his family. In Parse, R. R. (Ed.), *Illuminations: The human becoming theory in practice and research* (pp. 135–146). New York National League for Nursing Press.

Cody, W. K., & Mitchell, G. J. (1992). Parse's theory as a model for practice: The cutting edge. *Advances in Nursing Science, 15*(2), 52–65.

Costello-Nickitas, D. M. (1994). Choosing life goals: A phenomenological study. *Nursing Science Quarterly, 7,* 87–92.

Daly, J. (1995). The view of suffering within the human becoming theory. In Parse, R. R. (Ed.), *Illuminations: The human becoming theory in practice and research* (pp. 45–59). New York: National League for Nursing Press.

Daly, J., Mitchell, G. J., & Jonas-Simpson, C. M. (1996). Quality of life and the human becoming theory: Exploring discipline-specific contributions. *Nursing Science Quarterly, 9,* 170–174.

Davis, C., & Cannava, E. (1995). The meaning of retirement for communally-living retired performing artists. *Nursing Science Quarterly, 8,* 8–16.

Deveaux, B., & Babin, S. (1994). [Review of the Canadian Broadcasting Corporation documentary *Not My Home.*] Deveaux-Babin Productions.

Deveaux, B., & Babin, S. (1996). [Review of the Canadian Ministry of Health video *Real Stories.*] Deveaux-Babin Productions.

Fawcett, J. (2001). The nurse theorists: 21st-century updates—Rosemarie Rizzo Parse. *Nursing Science Quarterly, 14,* 126–131.

Fisher, M. A., & Mitchell, G. J. (1998). Patients' views of quality of life: Transforming the knowledge base of nursing. *Clinical Nurse Specialist, 12*(3), 99–105.

Fitne, Inc. (1997). *The nurse theorists: Portraits of excellence: Rosemarie Rizzo Parse* [CD-ROM]. Athens, OH: Author.

Futrell, M., Wondolowski, C., & Mitchell, G. J. (1994). Aging in the oldest old living in Scotland: A phenomenological study. *Nursing Science Quarterly, 6,* 189–194.

Gadamer, H-G. (1976). *Philosophical hermeneutics* (D. E. Linge, Trans. & Ed.). Berkeley: University of California Press.

Gadamer, H-G. (1989). *Truth and method* (2nd rev. ed.). (Translation revised by J. Weinsheimer & D. G. Marshall.) New York: Crossroad. (Original work published 1960.)

Gates, K. M. (2000). The experience of caring for a loved one: A phenomenological study. *Nursing Science Quarterly, 13,* 54–59.

Gray, R. (2000). [Review of *Handle with Care.*] © Psychosocial & Behavioural Research Unit, Toronto-Sunnybrook Regional Cancer Centre, Toronto, Canada.

Gray, R., & Sinding, C. (2002). Standing ovation: Performing social science research about cancer. Walnut Creek, CA: AltaMira.

Heidegger, M. (1962). *Being and time.* (J. Macquarrie & E. Robinson, Trans.). San Francisco: Harper & Row. (Original work published 1927.)

Heine, C. (1991). Development of gerontological nursing theory: Applying man-living-health theory of nursing. *Nursing & Health Care, 12,* 184–188.

Jacono, B. J., & Jacono, J. J. (1996). The benefits of Newman and Parse in helping nurse teachers determine methods to enhance student creativity. *Nursing Education Today, 16,* 356–362.

Janes, N. M., & Wells, D. L. (1997). Elderly patients' experiences with nurses guided by Parse's theory of human becoming. *Clinical Nursing Research, 6,* 205–224.

Jonas, C. M. (1992). The meaning of being an elder in Nepal. *Nursing Science Quarterly, 5,* 171–175.

Jonas, C. M. (1995). Evaluation of the human becoming theory in family practice. In Parse, R. R. (Ed.), *Illuminations: The human becoming theory in practice and research* (pp. 347–366). New York: National League for Nursing Press.

Jonas, C. M. (1995). True presence through music for persons living their dying. In Parse, R. R. (Ed.), *Illuminations: The human becoming theory in practice* (pp. 97–104). New York: National League for Nursing Press.

Jonas-Simpson, C. (1997). Living the art of the human becoming theory. *Nursing Science Quarterly, 10,* 175–179.

Jonas-Simpson, C. (2001). From silence to voice: Knowledge, values, and beliefs guiding healthcare practices with persons living with dementia. *Nursing Science Quarterly, 14,* 304–310.

Jonas-Simpson, C. M. (1996). The patient focused care journey: Where patients and families guide the way. *Nursing Science Quarterly, 9,* 145–146.

Jonas-Simpson, C. M. (1997). The Parse research method through music. *Nursing Science Quarterly, 10,* 112–114.

Kelley, L. S. (1995). The house-garden-wilderness metaphor: Caring frameworks and the human becoming theory. In Parse, R. R. (Ed.), *Illuminations: The human becoming theory in practice and research* (pp. 61–76). New York: National League for Nursing Press.

Kelley, L. S. (1995). Parse's theory in practice with a group in the community. *Nursing Science Quarterly, 8,* 127–132.

Langer, S. (1967). *Philosophy in a new key: A study in the symbolism of reason, rite, and art* (3rd ed.). Cambridge, MA: Harvard University Press.

Lui, S. L. (1994). The lived experience of health for hospitalized older women in Taiwan. *Journal of National Taipei College of Nursing, 1,* 1–84.

Mattice, M. (1991). Parse's theory of nursing in practice: A manager's perspective. *Canadian Journal of Nursing Administration, 4*(1), 11–13.

Melnechenko, K. L. (2003). To make a difference: Nursing presence. *Nursing Forum, 38,* 18–24.

Milton, C. L. (2003). A graduate curriculum guided by human becoming: Journeying with the possible. *Nursing Science Quarterly, 16,* 214–218.

Milton, C. L. (2003). The American Nurses Association code of ethics: A reflection on the ethics of respect and human dignity with nurse as expert. *Nursing Science Quarterly, 16,* 301–304.

Milton, C. L., & Buseman, J. (2002). Cocreating anew in public health nursing. *Nursing Science Quarterly, 15,* 113–116.

Mitchell, G. J. (1986). Utilizing Parse's theory of man-living-health in Mrs. M's neighborhood. *Perspectives, 10*(4), 5–7.

Mitchell, G. J. (1990). Struggling in change: From the traditional approach to Parse's theory-based practice. *Nursing Science Quarterly, 3,* 170–176.

Mitchell, G. J. (1991). Diagnosis: Clarifying or obscuring the nature of nursing. *Nursing Science Quarterly, 4,* 52–53.

Mitchell, G. J. (1991). Distinguishing practice with Parse's theory. In Goertzen, I. E. (Ed.), *Differentiating nursing practice into the twenty-first century* (pp. 55–58). New York: ANA Publication.

Mitchell, G. J. (1991). Human subjectivity: The cocreation of self. *Nursing Science Quarterly, 4,* 144–145.

Mitchell, G. J. (1991). Nursing diagnosis: An ethical analysis. *IMAGE: Journal of Nursing Scholarship, 23*(2), 99–103.

Mitchell, G. J. (1992). Parse's theory and the multidisciplinary team: Clarifying scientific values. *Nursing Science Quarterly, 5,* 104–106.

Mitchell, G. J. (1993). Parse's theory in practice. In Parker, M. E. (Ed.), *Patterns of nursing theories in practice* (pp. 62–80). New York: National League for Nursing Press.

Mitchell, G. J. (1993). The same-thing-yet-different phenomenon: A way of coming to know—or not? *Nursing Science Quarterly, 6,* 61–62.

Mitchell, G. J. (1993). Time and a waning moon: Seniors describe the meaning to later life. *Canadian Journal of Nursing Research, 25*(1), 51–66.

Mitchell, G. J. (1994). The meaning of being a senior: A phenomenological study and interpretation with Parse's theory of nursing. *Nursing Science Quarterly, 7,* 70–79.

Mitchell, G. J. (1995). Evaluation of the human becoming theory in practice in an acute care setting. In Parse, R. R. (Ed.), *Illuminations: The human becoming theory in practice and research* (pp. 367–399). New York: National League for Nursing Press.

Mitchell, G. J. (1995). The lived experience of restriction-freedom in later life. In Parse, R. R. (Ed.), *Illuminations: The human becoming theory in practice and research* (pp. 159–195). New York: National League for Nursing Press.

Mitchell, G. J. (1995). The view of freedom within the human becoming theory. In Parse, R. R. (Ed.), *Illuminations: The human becoming theory in practice and research* (pp. 27–43). New York: National League for Nursing Press.

Mitchell, G. J. (1996). Clarifying contributions of qualitative research findings. *Nursing Science Quarterly, 9,* 143–144.

Mitchell, G. J. (1996). Pretending: A way to get through the day. *Nursing Science Quarterly, 9,* 92–93.

Mitchell, G. J. (1997). Retrospective and prospective of practice applications: Views in the fog. *Nursing Science Quarterly, 10,* 8–9.

Mitchell, G. J. (1998). Living with diabetes: How understanding expands theory for professional practice. *Canadian Journal of Diabetes Care, 22*(1), 30–37.

Mitchell, G. J. (2003). Abstractions and particulars: Learning theory for practice. *Nursing Science Quarterly, 16,* 310–314.

Mitchell, G. J., Bernardo, A., & Bournes, D. (1997). Nursing guided by Parse's theory: Patient views at Sunnybrook. *Nursing Science Quarterly, 10,* 55–56.

Mitchell, G. J., & Bournes, D. A. (1998). Finding the way: A video guide to patient focused care [videotape]. Available from Sunnybrook & Women's Health Science Centre, 2075 Bayview Avenue, Toronto, Ontario, 4N 3M5.

Mitchell, G. J., & Bunkers, S. S. (2003). Engaging the abyss: A mis-take of opportunity? *Nursing Science Quarterly, 16,* 121–125.

Mitchell, G. J., Closson, T., Coulis, N., Flint, F., & Gray, B. (2000). Patient-focused care and human becoming thought: Connecting the right stuff. *Nursing Science Quarterly, 13,* 216–224.

Mitchell, G. J., & Cody, W. K. (1992). Nursing knowledge and human science: Ontological and epistemological considerations. *Nursing Science Quarterly, 5,* 54–61.

Mitchell, G. J., & Cody, W. K. (2002). Ambiguous opportunity: Toiling for truth of nursing art and science. *Nursing Science Quarterly, 15,* 71–79.

Mitchell, G. J., & Copplestone, C. (1990). Applying Parse's theory to perioperative nursing: A nontraditional approach. *AORN Journal, 51*(3), 787–798.

Mitchell, G. J., & Santopinto, M. D. A. (1988). An alternative to nursing diagnosis. *The Canadian Nurse, 84*(10), 25–28.

Mitchell, G. J., & Santopinto, M. D. A. (1988). The expanded role nurse: A dissenting viewpoint. *Canadian Journal of Nursing Administration, 4*(1), 8–14.

Mitchell, M. G. (2002). Patient-focused care on a complex continuing care dialysis unit: Rose's story. *CAANT Journal— Canadian Association of Nephrology Nurses & Technicians, 12,* 48–49.

Nelligan, P., Grinspun, D., Jonas-Simpson, C., McConnell, H., Peter, E., Pilkington, F. B., Balfour, J., Connolly, L., Lefebre, N., Reid-Haughian, C., & Sherry, K. (2002). Client-centred care: Making the ideal real. *Hospital Quarterly,* Summer, 70–76.

Noh, C. H. (2004). Meaning of quality of life for persons with serious mental illness: Human becoming practice with groups. *Nursing Science Quarterly, 17.*

Nokes, K. M., & Carver, K. (1991). The meaning of living with AIDS: A study using Parse's theory of man-living-health. *Nursing Science Quarterly, 4,* 175–179.

BOOKS

Parse, R. R. (1974). *Nursing fundamentals.* Flushing, NY: Medical Examination.

Parse, R. R. (1985). *Nursing research: Qualitative methods.* Bowie, MD: Brady.

Parse, R. R. (Ed.). (1995). *Illuminations: The human becoming theory in practice and research.* New York: National League for Nursing Press.

Parse, R. R. (1998). *The human becoming school of thought: A perspective for nurses and other health professionals.* Thousand Oaks, CA: Sage.

Parse, R. R. (1999). *Hope: An international human becoming perspective.* Sudbury, MA: Jones & Bartlett Publishers.

Parse, R. R. (2001). *Qualitative inquiry: The path of sciencing.* Sudbury, MA: Jones & Bartlett.

Parse, R. R. (2003). *Community: A human becoming perspective.* Sudbury, MA: Jones & Bartlett.

BOOK CHAPTERS, ARTICLES, AND EDITORIALS

Parse, R. R. (1978). Rights of medical patients. In Fischer, C. T., & Brodsky, S. L. (Eds.), *Client participation in human services.* New Brunswick, NJ: Transaction.

Parse, R. R. (1981). Caring from a human science perspective. In Leininger, M. M. (Ed.), *Caring: An essential human need.* Thorofare, NJ: Slack.

Parse, R. R. (1988). Beginnings. *Nursing Science Quarterly, 1.*

Parse, R. R. (1988). Creating traditions: The art of putting it together. *Nursing Science Quarterly, 1,* 45.

Parse, R. R. (1988). The mainstream of science: Framing the issue. *Nursing Science Quarterly, 1,* 93.

Parse, R. R. (1988). Scholarly dialogue: The fire of refinement. *Nursing Science Quarterly, 1,* 141.

Parse, R. R. (1989). Essentials for practicing the art of nursing. *Nursing Science Quarterly, 2,* 111.

Parse, R. R. (1989). Making more out of less. *Nursing Science Quarterly, 2,* 155.

Parse, R. R. (1989). Man-living-health: A theory of nursing. In Riehl-Sisca, J. (Ed.), *Conceptual models for nursing practice* (3rd ed.). Norwalk, CT: Appleton & Lange.

Parse, R. R. (1989). Martha E. Rogers: A birthday celebration. *Nursing Science Quarterly, 2,* 55.

Parse, R. R. (1989). Parse's man-living-health model and administration of nursing service. In Henry, B., Arndt, C., DiVincenti, M., & Marriner-Tomey, A. (Eds.), *Dimensions of nursing administration: Theory, research, education, and practice.* Cambridge, MA: Blackwell Scientific.

Parse, R. R. (1989). The phenomenological research method: Its value for management science. In Henry, B., Arndt, C., DiVincenti, M., & Marriner-Tomey, A. (Eds.), *Dimensions of nursing administration: Theory, research, education, and practice.* Cambridge, MA: Blackwell Scientific.

Parse, R. R. (1989). Qualitative research: Publishing and funding. *Nursing Science Quarterly, 2,* 1.

Parse, R. R. (1990). Health: A personal commitment. *Nursing Science Quarterly, 3,* 136–140.

Parse, R. R. (1990). Nurse theorist conference comes to Japan. *Japanese Journal of Nursing Research, 23*(3), 99.

Parse, R. R. (1990). Nursing theory-based practice: A challenge for the 90s. *Nursing Science Quarterly, 3,* 53.

Parse, R. R. (1990). Promotion and prevention: Two distinct cosmologies. *Nursing Science Quarterly, 3,* 101.

Parse, R. R. (1990). A time for reflection and projection. *Nursing Science Quarterly, 3,* 143.

Parse, R. R. (1991). Electronic publishing: Beyond browsing. *Nursing Science Quarterly, 4,* 1.

Parse, R. R. (1991). Growing the discipline of nursing. *Nursing Science Quarterly, 4,* 139.

Parse, R. R. (1991). Mysteries of health and healing: Two perspectives. *Nursing Science Quarterly, 4,* 93.

Parse, R. R. (1991). Nursing knowledge for the 21st century. *Japanese Journal of Nursing Research, 24*(3), 198–202.

Parse, R. R. (1991). Parse's Theory of Human Becoming. In Goertzen, I. E. (Ed.), *Differentiating nursing practice: Into the twenty-first century* (pp. 51–53). Kansas City: American Academy of Nursing.

Parse, R. R. (1991). Phenomenology and nursing. *Japanese Journal of Nursing, 17*(2), 261–269.

Parse, R. R. (1991). The right soil, the right stuff. *Nursing Science Quarterly, 4,* 47.

Parse, R. R. (1992). Moving beyond the barrier reef. *Nursing Science Quarterly, 5,* 97.

Parse, R. R. (1992). Nursing knowledge for the 21st century: An international commitment. *Nursing Science Quarterly, 5,* 8–12.

Parse, R. R. (1992). The performing art of nursing. *Nursing Science Quarterly, 5,* 147.

Parse, R. R. (1992). The unsung shapers of nursing science. *Nursing Science Quarterly, 5,* 47.

Parse, R. R. (1993). Cartoons: Glimpsing paradoxical moments. *Nursing Science Quarterly, 6,* 1.

Parse, R. R. (1993). Critical appraisal: Risking to challenge. *Nursing Science Quarterly, 6,* 163.

Parse, R. R. (1993). Critique of critical phenomena of nursing science suggested by O'Brien, Reed, and Stevenson. *Proceedings of the 1993 Annual Forum on Doctoral Nursing Education: A Call for Substance: Preparing Leaders for Global Health* (pp. 71–81). St. Paul, MN: University of Minnesota School of Nursing.

Parse, R. R. (1993). The experience of laughter: A phenomenological study. *Nursing Science Quarterly, 6,* 39–43.

Parse, R. R. (1993). Nursing and medicine: Two different disciplines. *Nursing Science Quarterly, 6,* 109.

Parse, R. R. (1993). Parse's human becoming theory: Its research and practice implications. In Parker, M. E. (Ed.), *Patterns of nursing theories in practice* (pp. 49–61). New York: National League for Nursing Press.

Parse, R. R. (1993). Plant now; reap later. *Nursing Science Quarterly, 6,* 55.

Parse, R. R. (1993). Scholarly dialogue: Theory guides research and practice. *Nursing Science Quarterly, 6,* 12.

Parse, R. R. (1994). Charley Potatoes or mashed potatoes? *Nursing Science Quarterly, 7,* 97.

Parse, R. R. (1994). Martha E. Rogers: Her voice will not be silenced. *Nursing Science Quarterly, 7,* 47.

Parse, R. R. (1994). Scholarship: Three essential processes. *Nursing Science Quarterly, 7,* 143.

Parse, R. R. (1995). Again: What is nursing? *Nursing Science Quarterly, 8,* 143.

Parse, R. R. (1995). Building the realm of nursing knowledge. *Nursing Science Quarterly, 8,* 51.

Parse, R. R. (1995). Commentary: Parse's theory of human becoming: An alternative to nursing practice for pediatric oncology nurses. *Journal of Pediatric Oncology Nursing, 12*(3), 128.

Parse, R. R. (1995). Foreword. In Frey, M. A., & Sieloff, C. L. (Eds.), *Advancing King's systems framework and theory of nursing.* Thousand Oaks, CA: Sage.

Parse, R. R. (1995). Man-living-health. A theory of nursing. In Mischo-Kelling, M., & Wittneben, K. (Eds.), *Auffassungen von pflege in theorie und praxis* (pp. 114–132). Munchen: Urban & Schwarzenberg.

Parse, R. R. (1995). Nursing theories and frameworks: The essence of advanced practice nursing. *Nursing Science Quarterly, 8,* 1.

Parse, R. R. (1996). Building knowledge through qualitative research: The road less traveled. *Nursing Science Quarterly, 9,* 10–16.

Parse, R. R. (1996). Critical thinking: What is it? *Nursing Science Quarterly, 9,* 138.

Parse, R. R. (1996). Hear ye, Hear ye: Novice and seasoned authors! *Nursing Science Quarterly, 9,* 1.

Parse, R. R. (1996). The human becoming theory: Challenges in practice and research. *Nursing Science Quarterly, 9,* 55–60.

Parse, R. R. (1996). Nursing theories: An original path. *Nursing Science Quarterly, 9,* 85.

Parse, R. R. (1996). Quality of life for persons living with Alzheimer's disease: A human becoming perspective. *Nursing Science Quarterly, 9,* 126–133.

Parse, R. R. (1996). [Review of the book *Martha E. Rogers: Her life and her work.*] *Visions: The Journal of Rogerian Science, 2,* 52–53.

Parse, R. R. (1997). Concept inventing: Unitary creations. *Nursing Science Quarterly, 10,* 63–64.

Parse, R. R. (1997). The human becoming theory and its research and practice methodologies. In Osterbrink, J. (Ed.), *Pflegetheorien—eine Zusammenfassung der 1st International Conference.* Freiburg, Germany: Verlag Hans Huber.

Parse, R. R. (1997). Investing the legacy: Martha E. Rogers' voice will not be silenced. *Visions: The Journal of Rogerian Science, 5,* 7–11.

Parse, R. R. (1997). The language of nursing knowledge: Saying what we mean. In Fawcett, J., & King, I. M. (Eds.), *The Language of theory and metatheory* (pp. 73–77). Sigma Theta Tau monograph.

Parse, R. R. (1997). Leadership: The essentials. *Nursing Science Quarterly, 10,* 109.

Parse, R. R. (1997). New beginnings in a quiet revolution. *Nursing Science Quarterly, 10,* 1.

Parse, R. R. (1997). [Review of the book *Quality of life in behavioral medicine.*] *Women and Health, 25*(3), 83–86.

Parse, R. R. (1997). Transforming research and practice with the human becoming theory. *Nursing Science Quarterly, 10,* 171–174.

Parse, R. R. (1998). The art of criticism. *Nursing Science Quarterly, 11,* 43.

Parse, R. R. (1998). Moving on. *Nursing Science Quarterly, 11,* 135.

Parse, R. R. (1998). Will nursing exist tomorrow? A reprise. *Nursing Science Quarterly, 11,* 1.

Parse, R. R. (1999). Authorship: Whose responsibility? *Nursing Science Quarterly, 12,* 99.

Parse, R. R. (1999). Community: An alternative view. *Nursing Science Quarterly, 12,* 119–121.

Parse, R. R. (1999). Expanding the vision: Tilling the field of nursing knowledge. *Nursing Science Quarterly, 12,* 3.

Parse, R. R. (1999). Integrity and the advancement of nursing knowledge. *Nursing Science Quarterly, 12*(3).

Parse, R. R. (1999). Nursing Science: The transformation of practice. *Journal of Advanced Nursing, 30*(6), 1383–1387.

Parse, R. R. (1999). Nursing: The discipline and the profession. *Nursing Science Quarterly, 12,* 275.

Parse, R. R. (1999). Witnessing as true presence. *Illuminations. Newsletter for the International Consortium of Parse Scholars, 8*(3), 1.

Parse, R. R. (2000). Enjoy your flight: Health in the new millennium. *Visions, 8*(1), 26–31.

Parse, R. R. (2000). Into the new millennium. *Nursing Science Quarterly, 13,* 3.

Parse, R. R. (2000). Language: Words reflect and cocreate meaning. *Nursing Science Quarterly, 13,* 187.

Parse, R. R. (2000). Obfuscating: The persistent practice of misnaming. *Nursing Science Quarterly, 13,* 91–92.

Parse, R. R. (2000). Paradigms: A reprise. *Nursing Science Quarterly, 13,* 275–276.

Parse, R. R. (2000). Prolegomenon. In Bunkers, S. S., *Simple things: Writings of human becoming.* Sioux Falls, SD: Pine Hills Press.

Parse, R. R. (2000). Quiescence. *Illuminations: Newsletter for the International Consortium of Parse Scholars, 9*(1), 1.

Parse, R. R. (2000). Vigilance. *Illuminations: Newsletter for the International Consortium of Parse Scholars, 9*(2), 1.

Parse, R. R. (2001). Contributions to the discipline. *Nursing Science Quarterly, 14,* 5.

Parse, R. R. (2001). Forward for the Taiwanese translation of Parse, R. R. (1998), *The human becoming school of thought.*

Parse, R. R. (2001). Language and the sow-reap rhythm. *Nursing Science Quarterly, 14,* 273.

Parse, R. R. (2001). Mourning. *Illuminations: Newsletter for the International Consortium of Parse Scholars, 10*(2), 1.

Parse, R. R. (2001). Nursing: Still in the shadow of medicine. *Nursing Science Quarterly, 14,* 181.

Parse, R. R. (2001). Rosemarie Rizzo Parse: The human becoming school of thought. In Parker, M. E. (Ed.), *Nursing theories and nursing practice* (pp. 227–238). Philadelphia, PA: F. A. Davis.

Parse, R. R. (2001). The lived experience of contentment: A study using the Parse research method. *Nursing Science Quarterly, 14,* 330–338.

Parse, R. R. (2001). Thoughts on valuing. *Illuminations: Newsletter for the International Consortium of Parse Scholars, 9*(3), 1.

Parse, R. R. (2001). The universe is flat. *Nursing Science Quarterly, 14,* 93.

Parse, R. R. (2002). 15th anniversary celebration. *Nursing Science Quarterly, 15,* 3.

Parse, R. R. (2002). Aha! Ah! HaHa! Discovery, wonder, laughter. *Nursing Science Quarterly, 15,* 273.

Parse, R. R. (2002). Mentoring moments. *Nursing Science Quarterly, 15,* 97.

Parse, R. R. (2002). Transforming health care with a unitary view of the human. *Nursing Science Quarterly, 15,* 46–50.

Parse, R. R. (2002). Words, words, words: Meanings, meanings, meanings! *Nursing Science Quarterly, 15,* 183.

Parse, R. R. (2003). A call for dignity in nursing. *Nursing Science Quarterly, 16,* 193–194.

Parse, R. R. (2003). Advocacy and human becoming. *Illuminations: Newsletter for the International Consortium of Parse Scholars, 12*(1), 1.

Parse, R. R. (2003). Qualitative research in nursing. *Japanese Journal of Nursing Research, 36*(2), 79–87.

Parse, R. R. (2003). Reflections on change. *Illuminations: Newsletter for the International Consortium of Parse Scholars, 11*(3/4), 1.

Parse, R. R. (2003). Research approaches: Likenesses and differences. *Nursing Science Quarterly, 16,* 5.

Parse, R. R. (2003). Silos and schools of thought. *Nursing Science Quarterly, 16,* 101.

Parse, R. R. (2003). The lived experience of feeling very tired: A study using the Parse research method. *Nursing Science Quarterly, 16,* 319–325.

Parse, R. R. (2003). What constitutes nursing research? *Nursing Science Quarterly, 16,* 287.

Parse, R. R. (2003). Wisdom. *Illuminations: Newsletter for the International Consortium of Parse Scholars, 12*(2), 1.

Parse, R. R. (2004). A human becoming teaching-learning model. *Nursing Science Quarterly, 17,* 33–35.

Parse, R. R. (2004). New directions. *Nursing Science Quarterly, 17,* 5.

Parse, R. R. (2004). Power in position. *Nursing Science Quarterly, 17,* 101.

Parse, R. R., & Bournes, D. A. (1997). Interview with Dr. Rosemarie Parse. *Illuminations: Newsletter for the International Consortium of Parse Scholars, 6*(4), 1–3.

Parse, R. R., Bournes, D. A., Barrett, E. A. M., Malinski, V. M., & Phillips, J. R. (1999). A better way: 10 things health professionals can do to move toward a more personal and meaningful system. *On Call: A Magazine for Nurses and Health Care Professionals, 2*(8), 14–17.

Pickrell, K. D., Lee, R. E., Schumacher, L. P., & Twigg, P. (1998). Rosemarie Rizzo Parse: Human becoming. In Tomey, A. M., & Alligood, M. R. (Eds.), *Nursing theorists and their work* (4th ed). New York: Mosby.

Pilkington, F. B. (1987). The grief of miscarriage [videotape]. Available from City Communications, 3011 Markham Rd., Unit 60, Scarborough, Ontario, M1X 1L7.

Pilkington, F. B. (1993). The lived experience of grieving the loss of an important other. *Nursing Science Quarterly, 6,* 130–139.

Pilkington, F. B. (1999). An ethical framework for nursing practice: Parse's human becoming theory. *Nursing Science Quarterly, 12,* 21–25.

Registered Nurses Association of Ontario (2002). Client Centred Care. Toronto, ON: Registered Nurses Association of Ontario.

Rendon, D. C., Sales, R., Leal, I., & Pique, J. (1995). The lived experience of aging in community-dwelling elders in Valencia, Spain: A phenomenological study. *Nursing Science Quarterly, 8,* 152–157.

Ricoeur, P. (1976). *Interpretation theory: Discourse and the surplus of meaning.* Fort Worth: Texas Christian University Press.

Saltmarche, A., Kolodny, V., & Mitchell, G. J. (1998). An educational approach for patient-focused care: Shifting attitudes and practice. *Journal of Nursing Staff Development, 14*(2), 81–86.

Santopinto, M. D. A. (1989). The relentless drive to be ever thinner: A study using the phenomenological method. *Nursing Science Quarterly, 2,* 29–36.

Thornburg, P. (2002). "Waiting" as experienced by women hospitalized during the antepartum period. *MCN, American Journal of Maternal Child Nursing, 27,* 245–248.

Wondolowski, C., & Davis, D. K. (1988). The lived experience of aging in the oldest old: A phenomenological study. *American Journal of Psychoanalysis, 48,* 261–270.

Wondolowski, C., & Davis, D. K. (1991). The lived experience of health in the oldest old: A phenomenological study. *Nursing Science Quarterly, 4,* 113–118.

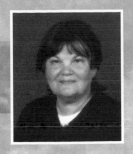

CHAPTER 15

Margaret A. Newman

PART ONE: Margaret A. NEWMAN's Theory of Health as Expanding Consciousness and Its Applications

Margaret Dexheimer Pharris

*I don't like controlling, manipulating other people.
I don't like deceiving, withholding, or treating people
as subjects or objects.
I don't like acting as an objective non-person.
I do like interacting authentically, listening, under-
standing, communicating freely.
I do like knowing and expressing myself in mutual
relationships.*

—**Margaret Newman (1985)**

Introducing the Theorist

The foundation for the theory of Health as Expanding Consciousness was laid prior to the time Margaret Newman entered nursing school at the University of Tennessee in 1959 (Newman, 1997c). After graduating from Baylor University, Newman went home to Memphis to work and care for her mother, who had amyotrophic lateral sclerosis (ALS), a degenerative neurological disease that progressively diminishes the movement of all muscles except those of the eyes. Caring for her mother was transformative for Margaret Newman. This experience provided her with two profound realizations: that simply having a disease does not make you unhealthy, and that time, movement, and space are in some way interrelated with health, which can be manifested by increased connectedness and quality of relationships. The restrictions of movement that Margaret Newman's mother experienced due to the ALS altered her experience of time, space, and consciousness. In caring for her physically immobilized mother, Newman experienced similar alterations in movement, space, time, and consciousness (Newman, 1997c). In the midst of this terminal disease, both mother and daughter experienced a greater sense of connectedness and increased insight into the meaning of their experience and into the meaning of health.

Later, when Newman decided to pursue doctoral studies in nursing, she was drawn to New York University (NYU), where she would be able to study with Martha Rogers, whose Science of Unitary Human Beings theory resonated with Newman's conceptualizations of nursing and health (Newman, 1997b). In her doctoral work at NYU, Newman (1982, 1987) began studying movement, time, and space as parameters of health, but she did so out of a logical positivist scientific paradigm. She designed an experimental study that manipulated participants' movement and then measured their perception of time. Her results showed a changing perception of time across the life span, with subjective time (as compared to objective time) increasing with age. Although her results seemed to support what she later would term "health as expanding consciousness," at that time she felt they did little to inform or shape nursing practice (Newman, 1997a).

Introducing the Theory

Newman's theory is a composite of her early influences and life and practice experiences.

EARLY INFLUENCES AND DEBUT OF THEORY

Newman's paradigmatic transformation occurred as she delved into the works of Martha Rogers and Itzhak Bentov, while at the same time reflecting on her own personal experience (Newman, 1997b). Several of Martha Rogers' assumptions became central in enriching Margaret Newman's theoretical perspective (Newman, 1997b). First and foremost, Rogers saw health and illness not as two separate realities, but rather as a unitary process. This was congruent with Margaret Newman's earlier experience with her mother and with her patients. On a very deep level, Newman knew that people can experience health even when they are physically or mentally ill. Health is not the opposite of illness, but rather health and illness are both manifestations of a greater whole. One can be very healthy in the midst of a terminal illness.

Second, Rogers argued that all of reality is a unitary whole and that each human being exhibits a unique pattern. Rogers (1970) saw energy fields to be the fundamental unit of all that is living and nonliving, and she posited that there is interpenetration between the fields of person, family, and environment. Person, family, and environment are not separate entities, but rather are an interconnected, unitary whole. In defining *field*, Rogers wrote: "Field is a unifying concept. Energy signifies the dynamic nature of the field. A field is in continuous motion and is infinite" (Rogers, 1990, p. 29).

> *Rogers defined the unitary human being as "[a]n irreducible, indivisible, pandimensional energy field identified by pattern and manifesting characteristics that are specific to the whole and which cannot be predicted from knowledge of the parts."*

Rogers defined the *unitary human being* as "[a]n irreducible, indivisible, pandimensional energy field identified by pattern and manifesting characteristics that are specific to the whole and which cannot be predicted from knowledge of the parts" (Rogers, 1990, p. 29). Finally, Rogers saw the life process as showing increasing complexity. This assumption, along with the work of Itzhak Bentov (1978), which viewed life as a process of expanding consciousness, helped to enrich Margaret Newman's conceptualization of health and eventually her theory (1997b).

In 1977, when teaching nursing theory development at Penn State, Margaret Newman received an invitation to speak at a nursing theory conference in New York. It was in preparing for that presentation, entitled "Toward a Theory of Health," that the theory of Health as Expanding Consciousness (HEC) began to take shape. In her address (Newman, 1978) and in a written overview of the address (Newman, 1979), Newman outlined the basic assumptions that were integral to her theory. Drawing on the work of Martha Rogers and Itzhak Bentov and on her own experience and insight, she proposed that:

• health encompasses conditions known as disease as well as states where disease is not present;
• disease, when it manifests itself, can be considered a manifestation of the underlying pattern of the person;
• the pattern of the person manifesting itself as disease was present prior to the structural and functional changes of disease; and
• health is the expansion of consciousness (Newman, 1979).

Newman's presentation drew thunderous applause as she ended with "[t]he responsibility of the

> "[t]he responsibility of the nurse is not to make people well, or to prevent their getting sick, but to assist people to recognize the power that is within them to move to higher levels of consciousness."

nurse is not to make people well, or to prevent their getting sick, but to assist people to recognize the power that is within them to move to higher levels of consciousness" (Newman, 1978).

Although Margaret Newman never set out to become a nursing theorist, in that 1978 presentation in New York City she articulated a theory that resonated with what was meaningful in the practice of nurses in many countries throughout the world. Nurses wanted to go beyond combating diseases; they wanted to accompany their patients in the process of discovering meaning and wholeness in their lives. Margaret Newman's proposed theory would serve as a guide for them to do so.

After identifying the basic assumptions of the HEC theory, the next step for Margaret Newman was to focus on how to test the theory with nursing research and how the theory could inform nursing practice. Newman began to concentrate on:

• the mutuality of the nurse-client interaction in the process of pattern recognition,
• the uniqueness and wholeness of the pattern in each client situation,
• the sequential configurations of pattern evolving over time,
• insights occurring as choice points of action potential, and
• the movement of the life process toward expanded consciousness (Newman, 1997a).

A NEW PARADIGM EMERGES

In an attempt to acknowledge and define the various scientific paradigmatic perspectives and to eliminate some of the confusion regarding the nature of the discipline of nursing, Margaret Newman, Marilyn Sime, and Sheila Corcoran-Perry (1991) collaborated on an article to define the overarching focus of the nursing discipline and its prevailing paradigms. They defined the focus of the nursing discipline to be *caring in the human health experience*, which they saw as the common umbrella under which three distinct paradigmatic perspectives fell: the particulate-deterministic, the interactive-integrative, and the unitary-transformative (with the first word indicating the nature of reality and the second word indicating the nature of change in each paradigm).

The particulate-deterministic paradigm holds that phenomena are isolatable, reducible entities with definable, measurable properties. Relationships between entities are seen as orderly, predictable, linear, and causal (i.e., A causes B, or atherosclerotic plaque causes heart attacks). In this perspective, health is dichotomized with clearly defined characteristics that are either healthy or unhealthy, and change occurs in a manner that is predictable and causal in nature.

The interactive-integrative perspective, which stems from the particulate-deterministic, views reality as multidimensional and contextual. Multiple antecedents and probabilistic relationships are believed to bring about change in a phenomenon (i.e., A + B + C + D are interrelated in their affect on E; or diet, exercise, smoking, family history, and lifestyle are interconnected in their affect on heart attacks). Relationships may be reciprocal, and subjective data are seen as legitimate.

The unitary-transformative perspective is distinct from the other two. Here a phenomenon is seen as a "unitary, self-organizing field embedded in a larger self-organizing field. It is identified by pattern and by interaction with the larger whole" (Newman, Sime, & Corcoran-Perry, 1991, p. 4). Change is unpredictable and unidirectional, always moving toward a higher level of complexity. Knowledge is arrived at through pattern recognition and reflects both the phenomenon viewed and the viewer.

Margaret Newman (1979, 1986, 1994a), like Martha Rogers (1970, 1990), sees human beings as unitary energy fields that are inseparable from the larger unitary field that combines person, family, and community all at once. A nurse operating out of the unitary-transformative paradigm does not think of mind, body, spirit, and emotion as separate entities, but rather sees them as an undivided whole.

Newman's theory (1979, 1990, 1994a, 1997a, 1997b) proposes that we cannot isolate, manipulate, and control variables in order to understand the whole of a phenomenon. The nurse and client form a mutual partnership to attend to the pattern of meaningful relationships and experiences in the client's life. In this way, a patient who has had a heart attack can understand the experience of the heart attack in the context of all that is meaningful in his or her life, and through the insight gained, experience expanding consciousness. Newman's (1994a, 1997a, 1997b) methodology does not divide people's lives into fragmented variables, but rather attends to the nature and meaning of the whole, which becomes apparent in the nurse-patient dialogue.

Paradigmatic view shapes nursing theory and research methodologies. The old paradigm proposes methods that are analogous to trying to appreciate a loaf of warm bread by analyzing flour, water, salt, yeast, and oil. No matter how much we come to know these ingredients separately, we will not know the texture, smell, taste, and essence of the loaf of bread that has just come out of the oven. The whole is greater than the sum of its parts and exhibits unique qualities that cannot be fully comprehended by looking at parts. Individual qualities of the whole, however, do give us some understanding of the nature of the whole. For example, the smell of the loaf of bread provides one insight into its nature, the texture provides another, and so on. A nurse practicing out of the HEC theoretical

perspective possesses multifaceted levels of awareness and is able to sense how physical signs, emotional conveyances, spiritual insights, physical appearances, and mental insights are all meaningful manifestations of a person's underlying pattern.

Newman, Sime, and Corcoran-Perry (1991) concluded that the knowledge generated by the particulate-deterministic paradigm and the interactive-integrative was relevant to nursing but that the knowledge gained by using the unitary-transformative paradigm was *essential* to the nursing discipline. In a later work, Newman (1997a) asserted that knowledge emanating from the unitary-transformative paradigm is the knowledge of the discipline and that the focus, philosophy, and theory of the discipline must be consistent with each other and therefore cannot flow out of different paradigms. Newman states:

> The paradigm of the discipline is becoming clear. We are moving from attention on the other as object to attention to the we in relationship, from fixing things to attending to the meaning of the whole, from hierarchical one-way intervention to mutual process partnering. It is time to break with a paradigm of health that focuses on power, manipulation, and control and move to one of reflective, compassionate consciousness. The paradigm of nursing embraces wholeness and pattern. It reveals a world that is moving, evolving, transforming—a process. (1997a, p. 37)

The unitary-transformative paradigm transcends, yet includes, knowledge from the particulate-deterministic and the integrative-interactive paradigms; it is a more inclusive level of wholeness (Newman, 2002a). Newman's call for nurses to practice and conduct research out of a unitary-participatory paradigm, which sees the process of the nursing partnership as integral to the evolving definition of health for the patient (Litchfield, 1993, 1999; Newman, 1997a) and is synchronous with participatory philosophical thought (Skolimowski, 1994) and research methodology (Heron & Reason, 1997).

SEQUENTIAL CONFIGURATIONS OF PATTERN EVOLVING OVER TIME

Essential to Margaret Newman's theory is the belief that each person exhibits a distinct pattern, which is constantly unfolding and evolving as the person

> *Each person exhibits a distinct pattern, which is constantly unfolding and evolving as the person interacts with the environment. Pattern is information that depicts the whole of a person's relationship with the environment.*

interacts with the environment. Pattern is information that depicts the whole of a person's relationship with the environment and gives an understanding of the meaning of the relationships all at once (Endo, 1998; Newman, 1994a). Pattern is a manifestation of consciousness, which Newman (1994a) defines as the informational capacity of the system to interact with its environment.

To describe the nature of pattern, Newman draws on the work of David Bohm (1980) who said that anything *explicate* (that which we can hear, see, taste, smell, touch) is a manifestation of the *implicate* (the unseen underlying pattern) (Newman, 1997b). In other words, there is information about the underlying pattern of each person in all that we sense about them, such as their movements, tone of voice, interactions with others, activity level, genetic pattern, vital signs. There is also information about their underlying pattern in all that they tell us about their experiences and perceptions, including stories about their life, recounted dreams, and portrayed meanings.

The HEC perspective sees disease, disorder, disconnection, and violence as an explication of the underlying implicate pattern of the person, family, or community. Reflecting on the meaning of these conditions can be part of the process of expanding consciousness (Newman, 1994a, 1997a, 1997b).

Pattern recognition is a profound act of nurse caring in that it focuses on *knowing* the patient, family, and/or community at a very deep level (Newman, 2002b). Pattern recognition happens in the context of a caring nurse partnership, which is centered on exploring that which is considered most meaningful.

INSIGHTS OCCURRING AS CHOICE POINTS OF ACTION POTENTIAL

The disruption of disease and other traumatic life events may be critical points in the expansion of consciousness. To explain this phenomenon, Newman (1994a, 1997b) draws on the work of Ilya Prigogine (1976), whose theory of Dissipative Structures asserts that a system fluctuates in an orderly manner until some disruption occurs, and the system moves in a seemingly random, chaotic, disorderly way until at some point it chooses to move into a higher level of organization (Newman, 1997b). Nurses see this all the time—the patient who is lost to his work and has no time for his family or himself, and then suddenly has a heart attack, an experience that leaves him open to reflecting on how he has been using his energy. Insights gained through this reflection give rise to transformation of his life pattern, which becomes more creative, relational, and meaningful. Nurses also see this in people diagnosed with a terminal illness that causes them to reevaluate what is really important, attend to it, and then to state that for the first time they feel as though they are really living. The expansion of consciousness is an innate tendency of human beings; however, some experiences and processes precipitate more rapid transformations. Nurse researchers operating out of the HEC theory have clearly demonstrated how nurses can create a mutual partnership with their patients to reflect on their evolving pattern. The insights gained in this process lead to an awakening and transformation to a higher level of consciousness (Endo, 1998; Endo, Minegishi, & Kubo, 2004; Endo, Nitta, Inayoshi, Saito, Takemura, et al., 2000; Jonsdottir, 1998; Jonsdottir, Litchfield, & Pharris, 2003; Kiser-Larson, 2002; Lamendola, 1998; Lamendola & Newman, 1994; Litchfield, 1993, 1999, 2004; Moch, 1990; Neill, 2002a, 2002b; Newman, 1995; Newman & Moch, 1991; Noveletsky-Rosenthal, 1996; Pharris, 2002, 2004; Picard, 2000, 2004; Tommet, 2003).

Newman (1999) points out that nurse-client relationships often begin during periods of disruption, uncertainty, and unpredictability in patients' lives. When patients are in a state of chaos because of disease, trauma, loss, etc., they often cannot see their past or future clearly. In the context of the nurse-patient partnership, which centers on the meaning the patient gives to the health predicament, insight for action arises and it becomes clear to the patient how to get on with life (Jonsdottir, Litchfield, & Pharris, 2003, 2004; Litchfield, 1999; Newman, 1999). Litchfield (1993, 1999) sees this as experiencing an expanding present that connects to the past and creates an extended horizon of action potential for the future.

Endo (1998) in her work in Japan with women with cancer, Noveletsky-Rosenthal (1996) in her work in the United States with people with chronic obstructive pulmonary disease, and Pharris (2002) in her work with U.S. adolescents convicted of murder, found that it is when patient's lives are in the greatest states of chaos, disorganization, and uncertainty that the HEC nursing partnership and pattern-recognition process is perceived as most beneficial to patients (Figure 15–1).

Many nurses who encounter patients in times of chaos strive for stability; they feel they have to *fix* the situation, not realizing that this disorganized time in the patient's life presents an opportunity for growth. Newman (1999) states:

> The "brokenness" of the situation . . . is only a point in the process leading to a higher order. We need to join in partnership with clients and dance their dance, even though it appears arrhythmic, until order begins to emerge out of chaos. We know, and we can help clients know, that there is a basic, underlying pattern

evolving even though it might not be apparent at the time. The pattern will be revealed at a higher level of organization. (p. 228)

The disruption brought about by the presence of disease, illness, and traumatic or stressful events creates an opportunity for transformation to a higher, expanded level of consciousness (Newman, 1997b, 1999) and represents a time when patients most need nurses who are attentive to that which is most meaningful. Newman (1999, p. 228) states, "Nurses have a responsibility to stay in partnership with clients as their patterns are disturbed by illness or other disruptive events." This disrupted state presents a *choice point* for the person to either continue going on as before, even though the old rules are not working, or to shift into a new way of being. To explain the concept of a *choice point* more clearly, Newman draws on Arthur Young's (1976) theory of the Evolution of Consciousness. Young suggests that there are seven stages of binding and unbinding, which begin with total freedom and unrestricted choice, followed by a series of losses of freedom. After these losses comes a choice point

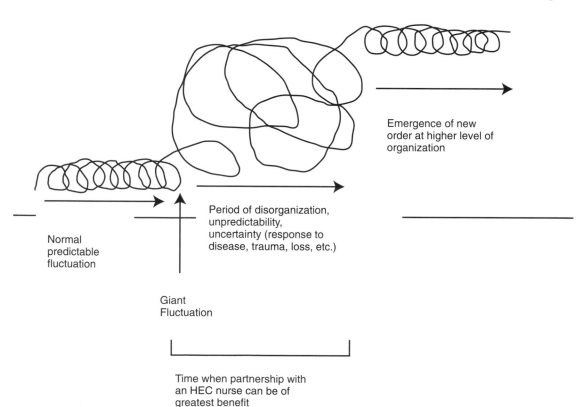

FIGURE 15–1 Prigogine's theory of dissipative structures applied to HEC nursing.

and a reversal of the losses of freedom, ending with total freedom and unrestricted choice. These stages can be conceptualized as seven equidistant points on a V shape (see Figure 15–2). Beginning at the uppermost point on the left is the first stage, *potential freedom*. The next stage is *binding*. In this stage, the individual is sacrificed for the sake of the collective, with no need for initiative because everything is being regulated for the individual. The third stage, *centering*, involves the development of an individual identity, self-consciousness, and self-determination. "Individualism emerges in the self's break with authority" (Newman, 1994b). The fourth stage, *choice*, is situated at the base of the V. In this stage the individual learns that the old ways of being are no longer working. It is a stage of self-awareness, inner growth, and transformation. A new way of being becomes necessary. Newman (1994b) describes the fifth stage, *decentering*, as being characterized by a shift

> from the development of self (individuation) to dedication to something greater than the individual self. The person experiences outstanding competence; their works have a life of their own beyond the creator. The task is transcendence of the ego. Form is transcended, and the energy becomes the dominant feature—in terms of animation, vitality, a quality that is somehow infinite. Pattern is higher than form; the pattern can manifest itself in different forms. In this stage the person experiences the power of unlimited growth and has learned how to build order against the trend of disorder. (pp. 45–46)

Newman (1994b) goes on to state that few experience the sixth stage, *unbinding*, or the seventh stage, *real freedom*, unless they have had these experiences of transcendence characterized by the fifth stage. It is in the moving through the choice point and the stages of decentering and unbinding that a person moves on to higher levels of consciousness (Newman, 1999). Newman proposes a corollary between her theory of Health as Expanding Consciousness and Young's theory of the Evolution of Consciousness in that we "come into being from a state of potential consciousness, are bound in time, find our identity in space, and through movement we learn 'the law' of the way things work and make choices that ultimately take us beyond space and time to a state of absolute consciousness" (Newman, 1994b, p. 46) (see Figure 15–2).

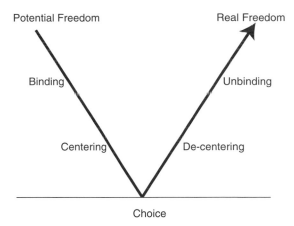

FIGURE 15–2 Young's spectrum of the evolution of consciousness.

EXPANDING CONSCIOUSNESS

Ultimate consciousness has been equated with love, which embraces all experience equally and unconditionally: pain as well as pleasure, failure as well as success, ugliness as well as beauty, disease as well as nondisease.

—**M. A. Newman (2003, p. 241)**

The process of expanding consciousness is characterized by the evolving pattern of the person-environment interaction (Newman, 1994a). Consciousness is much more than just cognitive thought. Margaret Newman (1994a) defines consciousness as

> the information of the system: The capacity of the system to interact with the environment. In the human system the informational capacity includes not only all the things we normally associate with consciousness, such as thinking and feeling, but also all the information embedded in the nervous system, the immune system, the genetic code, and so on. The information of these and other systems reveals the complexity of the human system and how the information of the system interacts with the information of the environmental system. (p. 33)

To illustrate consciousness as the interactional capacity of the person-environment, Newman (1994a) draws on the work of Bentov (1978), who presents consciousness on a continuum ranging from rocks on one end of the spectrum (which have little interaction with their environment), to plants (which draw nutrients and provide carbon dioxide), to animals (which can move about and interact freely), to humans (who can reflect and make in-depth plans regarding how they want to interact with their environment), and ultimately to spiritual beings on the spectrum's other end. Newman sees death as a transformation point, with a person's consciousness continuing to develop beyond the physical life, becoming a part of a universal consciousness (Newman, 1994a).

Nurses and their clients know that there has been an expansion of consciousness when there is a richer, more meaningful quality to their relationships. Relationships that are more open, loving, caring, connected, and peaceful are a manifestation of expanding consciousness. These deeper, more meaningful relationships may be interpersonal, or they may be relationships with the wider community. The nurse and client may also see movement through Young's spectrum of evolving consciousness, where people transcend their own egos, dedicate their energy to something greater than the individual self, and learn to build order against the trend of disorder.

THE MUTUALITY OF THE NURSE-CLIENT INTERACTION IN THE PROCESS OF PATTERN RECOGNITION

We come to the meaning of the whole not by viewing the pattern from the outside, but by entering into the evolving pattern as it unfolds.

—M. A. Newman

Nursing out of the HEC perspective involves being fully present to the patient without judgments, goals, or intervention strategies. It involves

> *Nursing out of the HEC perspective involves being fully present to the patient without judgments, goals, or intervention strategies. It involves being with rather than doing for.*

being with rather than *doing for*. It is caring in its deepest, most respectful sense. It is a mutual process of attending to that which is meaningful. The nurse-patient interaction becomes like a pure reflection pool through which both the nurse and the patient get a clear picture of their pattern and come away transformed by the insights gained.

To illustrate the mutually transforming effect of the nurse-patient interaction, Newman (1994a) offers the image of a smooth lake into which two stones are thrown. As the stones hit the water, concentric waves circle out until the two patterns reach one another and interpenetrate. The new pattern of their interaction ripples back and transforms the two original circling patterns. Nurses are changed by their interactions with their patients, just as patients are changed by their interactions with nurses. This mutual transformation extends to the surrounding environment and relationships of the nurse and patient.

In the process of doing this work, it is important that the nurse sense his or her own pattern. Newman states: "We have come to see nursing as a process of relationship that co-evolves as a function of the interpenetration of the evolving fields of the nurse, client, and the environment in a self-organizing, unpredictable way. We recognize the need for process wisdom, the ability to come from the center of our truth and act in the immediate moment" (Newman, 1994b, p. 155). Sensing one's own pattern is an essential starting point for the nurse. In her book *Health as Expanding Consciousness,* Newman (1994a, pp. 107–109) outlines a process of focusing to assist nurses as they begin working in the HEC perspective. It is important that the nurse be able to practice from the center of his or her own truth and be fully present to the patient. The nurse's consciousness, or pattern, becomes like the vibrations of a tuning fork that resonate at a centering frequency, and the client has the opportunity to resonate and tune to that clear frequency during their interactions (Newman, 1994a; Quinn, 1992). The nurse-patient relationship ideally continues until the patient finds his or her own rhythmic vibrations without the need of the stabilizing force of the nurse-patient dialogue. Newman (1999) points out that the partnership demands that nurses develop tolerance for uncertainty, disorganization, and dissonance, even though it may be quite uncomfortable. It is in the state of disequilibrium that the potential for growth exists. She states, "The rhythmic relating of nurse with client at this critical boundary is a window of opportunity for transformation in the health experience" (Newman, 1999, p. 229).

PART TWO

Applications

Margaret Newman's Theory of Health as Expanding Consciousness is being used throughout the world, but it has been more quickly embraced and understood by nurses from indigenous and Eastern cultures, who are less bound by linear, three-dimensional thought and physical concepts of health and who are more immersed in the metaphysical, mystical aspect of human existence. Increasingly, however, the theory is being enthusiastically embraced by nurses in industrialized nations who are finding it increasingly difficult to nurse in the modern technologically driven and intervention-oriented health-care system, which is dependent on diagnosing and treating diseases (Jonsdottir, Litchfield, & Pharris, 2003, 2004). Practicing from an HEC perspective places what is meaningful to patients back at the center of the nurse's focus.

RESEARCH

Margaret Newman (1994a) describes her research methodology as hermeneutic dialectic—*hermeneutic* in that it focuses on meaning, interpretation, and understanding; and *dialectic* in that both the process and content are dialectic (Newman, 1997b). Guba and Lincoln (1989, p. 149) describe the dialectic process as representing "a comparison and contrast of divergent views with a view to achieving a higher synthesis of them all in the Hegelian sense." Hegel proposed that opposite points of view can come together and fuse into a new, synthesized view of reality (Newman, 1994a). It is in the contrast that pattern can be appreciated.

For example, one cannot fully comprehend joy unless one has fully comprehended sorrow, and vice versa. Although they seem to be opposites, these two emotions are two manifestations of human connectedness. If you want to see a dark pattern more clearly, you would put it against a light background. The dialectic aspect of this methodology permits a nurse to be present to a client whose life circumstances are very different from those of the nurse. For example, the pattern-recognition interaction for a homeless 16-year-old

teenage boy from Solna, Sweden, with a female nurse from a very intact, loving family in Somalia may provide clearer insight than with a young Swedish male nurse from Solna, who himself had been homeless, because less will be assumed and taken for granted. The Somali nurse will have to ask more clarifying questions and seek to understand that which has not been her experience. No matter what the background of the nurse and patient, the clarifying process, if done in an open, caring, and nonjudging manner, provides great insight for both participants in the pattern-recognition process as the nurse and the patient realize their interconnectedness. When the nurse-patient interaction is focused on attending to meaning, it transcends barriers of culture, gender, age, class, race, education, and ethnicity. The HEC theory focuses on the interconnectedness and common humanity of all people, and research from the HEC perspective seeks to understand the whole, rather than predict cause and effect (Newman, 2002).

The Health as Expanding Consciousness Research Process

After several years of positivist research (Engle, 1986; Newman, 1976, 1982), which attempted to isolate and manipulate variables seen as basic to HEC theory (movement, time, consciousness), Susan Moch, who was working as a research assistant with Margaret Newman, suggested they ask participants about the most meaningful experiences in their lives (Newman & Moch, 1991). In a pilot study, Margaret Newman, Jim Vail, and Richard Cowling devised a method of pattern identification by asking people to describe meaningful people and events in their lives. They then looked at sequential patterns of people's lives, which facilitated recognition and insight into pattern, and involved the nurse-researcher-practitioner in the movement toward higher consciousness (Newman, 1997b). The pilot study informed the methodology used by Newman and Moch (1991) in their research with people with cardiovascular disease.

Susan Diemert Moch (1990) went on to interview 20 women diagnosed with breast cancer, centering the nurse-patient dialogue on the pattern of the whole. Moch asked the women in her study to describe what was meaningful to them and found that in talking about meaningful people and events, the sequential patterns of interaction between people and their environment become apparent. The explicate patterns give insight into the implicate, and expanding consciousness becomes a reality.

In the second edition of her book, *Health as Expanding Consciousness,* Newman, (1994a, pp. 147–149) summarizes the research methodology as follows:

The interview: After the study has been explained and informed consent obtained, the data collection process begins with the nurse asking the participant a simple, open-ended question such as, "Tell me about the most meaningful people and events in your life." If the researcher asks simply about meaningful events, the meaningful relationships usually arise as the stories are told. The interview proceeds in a nondirective manner, with the nurse asking clarifying questions if necessary. The nurse researcher focuses on being fully present and sensing intuitively what to say or ask. Pauses are respected and attended to.

Transcription: Soon after the interview is completed, the nurse researcher transcribes the tape of the interview, including only the information that seems relevant to the participant's life pattern, but noting separately any information that was omitted, in case it becomes relevant after subsequent interviews. Not all HEC researchers have found audiotaping the interview necessary.

The narrative: The nurse researcher then organizes the narrative data into chronological order, taking note of sequential patterns of relationships and ways of relating with the environment.

Diagram: A diagram is drawn of the sequential patterns of relationships and transformation points. Although optional, this step has been found to be helpful by many HEC researchers and participants in visualizing the pattern of the whole.

Follow-up: At the second interview, the diagram (or other visual portrayal) is shared with the participant without any causal interpretation. The participant is given the opportunity to comment on what has been portrayed. This dialectic process is repeated in subsequent interviews, with data added to the narrative and the diagram redrawn until no further insight can be reached about the pattern of person-environment interaction. The pattern emerges in terms of the energy flow (e.g., blocked, diffused, disorganized, and repetitive). It is important not to force pattern recognition; sometimes no signs of

pattern recognition emerge, and if so, that characterizes the pattern for that particular person.

Application of the theory: The HEC theory is active throughout the process and is explicated by the process. It is the theory that guides the interaction. The theory is pervasive in the unfolding and grasping of insights. After completion of the interviews, the data are analyzed more intensely in light of the theory of health as expanding consciousness. Young's spectrum of consciousness is applied, and the quality and complexity of the sequential patterns of interaction are evaluated. If the intent of the research is to look at a group of people or at a community, similarities of pattern among participants are identified.

HEC Research as Praxis

Research from the HEC perspective is *research as praxis,* meaning that the researcher is an active

> *Research from the HEC perspective is research as praxis, meaning that the researcher is an active participant in the research and engages with the participant in understanding the meaning of his or her situation and its potential for action.*

participant in the research and engages with the participant in understanding the meaning of his or her situation and its potential for action (Connor, 1998; Litchfield, 1993, 1999; Newman, 1990, 1994b, 1997a). In HEC research, the researcher is also a practitioner. Litchfield (1999) refers to the "researcher-as-if-practitioner" in what she terms "practice wisdom" in which caring and health are seen as dialectically related and merging together in the process of health as expanding consciousness. Newman states: "Not only is our science a *human science,* but, within the context of a practice discipline, it is a science of *praxis.* This kind of theory is *embodied* in the investigator-nurse. It informs the situation being addressed by making a difference in the situation, as well as being informed by the data of the situation" (Newman, 1994b, p. 155).

Research Identifying Patterns of People with Common Conditions

Although the intent of HEC research is to understand the nature of the nurse-patient relationship in the process of expanding consciousness (Newman, 1994), the early HEC pattern-recognition studies sought to identify similarities and variations of pattern among individuals with the same medical disease diagnosis or with similar life circumstances (Newman, 1994). HEC researchers reported common themes of experiences and transformation in the quality and connectedness of relationships. More recent HEC research focuses on the process of pattern recognition and the evolving nature of the nurse-patient partnership.

Moch (1990) found U.S. women with breast cancer to experience changes in relatedness with significant others and to identify meaning in their experience of living with cancer, which added new perspectives about health as expanding consciousness. In discussing the implications her research holds for nursing practice, Moch stressed that incorporating a "health-within-illness experience" view has the potential to drastically change the way nurses practice as they would shift their focus from simply fighting illness to helping patients learn about themselves through the illness experience.

Moch later collaborated with Newman (Newman & Moch, 1991) to look at the person-environment pattern of people with coronary heart disease. They found three common themes: the *need to excel,* the *need to please others,* and *feelings of being alone.* These findings were consistent with the literature on coronary artery disease and personality type. When applying Young's (1976) theory to the participants, they found that most participants were caught in a repetitive cycle characteristic of the centering stage. Blocks to movement along the spectrum were seen as being mirrored by the blocks in the disease process. Newman and Moch (1991) concluded, "If they reached the choice point early enough and still had enough resources to confront their pattern and allow the meaning of their pattern to unfold, they had the potential of transcending the physical limitations and moving beyond themselves to a higher level of consciousness. If they had reached the limits of their resources, death was the 'transformative door' to higher consciousness" (Moss, 1981, p. 101, 166). Newman and Moch stress that nurses could help patients get in touch with their pattern and express themselves more fully.

Newman (1995) further demonstrated the importance of nurses being fully present, seeking to know about the most meaningful experiences in patients' lives, mirroring the story so that insights can be gained into the evolving pattern, and being sensitive to the fact that thoughts and feelings that arise within the nurse are manifestations of their interpenetration of the nurse-patient field. In addressing long-term implications of this study, Newman pointed to the increasing societal need for connectedness and nurturing as manifested by heightening rates of homelessness and poverty. She posed the challenge that "people should not have to wait until the manifestation of disease brings them to the attention of 'caring and concerned help'" (p. 169).

Helga Jonsdottir (1998) conducted a study with people in Iceland with chronic obstructive pulmonary disease (COPD). She characterized the overall pattern to be one of *isolation and being closed in* because participants isolated themselves from situations they were unable to deal with and avoided any stimuli that could threaten their pulmonary status. Jonsdottir (1998) maintained that for people with COPD, the threatened exchange of essential elements between the human body and the environment resembles "the participants' difficulty in open interactions between themselves and other people, in finding effective approaches to facing adversities, in their mental and physical activity restrictions, and in their inability to pursue what they need and want" (p. 164). Noveletsky-Rosenthal (1996) conducted a similar study in the United States and found a relationship between pattern recognition and evolving consciousness to be related to a sense of connectedness, with the participants who manifested a sense of connectedness being able to utilize pattern recognition to transcend their illness. She found timing of the nurse-patient partnership to be an important aspect of potential for transformation, with greater insight gained immediately after diagnosis as opposed to after years of living with COPD.

Yamashita (1998, 1999) studied caregivers of people with schizophrenia in Japan and in Canada. She (Yamashita, 1999) described a process whereby caregivers moved through *struggling alone* and feeling alienated from those around them as the schizophrenia was first manifested, and feeling a *lack of connectedness,* particularly with health-care professionals. Yamashita reported that in the process of pattern recognition, participants were able to recognize turning points in their lives and discover new rules as they started to move beyond the binding stage in Young's spectrum of consciousness. They eventually deepened connections with important others, including the person with schizophrenia.

Carol Picard (2000) brought the HEC research full circle to a place where movement is again explicitly central. Picard utilized the HEC hermeneutic dialectic process with midlife women. Picard's research methodology was unique in that it expanded the narrative/diagram pattern-recognition process to include an intentional creative movement group experience for each participant and a piece of reflective art conceptualized by Picard to illuminate the participant's pattern. Participants were asked to put the sequential patterns of meaningful events to movement. Picard found congruence between the narratives and the expressions of creative movement. Participants revealed an integrated embodiment of emotion when expressing themselves in movement, which they had not previously experienced. Picard reports that participants expressed the awareness of the past within the present and experienced a deep sense of healing in their movement. Participants reported valuing: being known, feeling accepted, not being diagnosed, and having enough time to tell their stories.

In another study, Picard (2004) utilized HEC to understand the experience of parents of persons with bipolar disorder. Picard met with each participant for two interview/dialogue sessions and then did one creative movement experience in which the parents demonstrated a movement or gesture that captured the essence of the meaning of their experience. In a presentation of this research, Picard did a slide presentation of her study's findings and then performed a choreographed dance made up of the combined movements of all of the parents in her study (Jonsdottir, Litchfield, Pharris, & Picard, 2001). Participants at the session could feel on a very deep level what the experience of being a parent of a person with bipolar disorder might be like. It was a different and deeper way of knowing the experience from that gained by reading the common themes and quotes on the overhead screen.

In Australia, HEC nurse researcher, Jane Neill conducted pattern recognition with women with rheumatoid arthritis (2002a) and other chronic illnesses (2002b). She followed the HEC protocol outlined by Newman (1994a); in addition, when she went back the second time with the diagrammatic depiction of sequential patterns, she brought a disposable camera and asked the women to take photos as a continued reflection on what was mean-

ingful to them. She told them the images could be symbolic or not. New interpretations evolved in the dialogue as the women reviewed the photos with Neill and reflected on what was most important to them. Neill (2002b) concludes that pattern recognition and practicing from an HEC perspective is essential even in short nurse-patient encounters, stating, "I remain convinced that the exclusive focus on technical work and practical nursing knowledge fails to address the central concern of nursing with the whole person and his or her environment, and is ultimately unsatisfying" (p. 53).

Focusing on the Process of Health Patterning and the Nurse-Patient Partnership

Merian Litchfield (1993), from New Zealand, was the first HEC researcher to apply the HEC theory to a nursing partnership with families. Litchfield (1993, 1997, 1999, 2004) has led the way in focusing on the process of the nursing partnership with patients and families. In her first study, Litchfield (1993) described health patterning as "a process of nursing practice whereby, through dialogue, families with researcher as practitioner, recognise pattern in the life process providing opportunity for insight as the potential for action; a process by which there may be increased self-determination as a feature of health" (p. 10). Litchfield (1993) describes HEC research as a "shared process of inquiry through which participants are empowered to act to change their circumstances" (p. 20). Through her research over several years with families with complex health predicaments requiring repeated hospitalizations, Litchfield (1993, 1999, 2004) found that she could not stand outside of the process of recognizing pattern to observe a fixed health pattern of the family. She sees the pattern as continuously evolving dialectically in the dialogue within the nursing partnership. The findings are literally created in the participatory process of the partnership (Litchfield, 1999). For this reason, Litchfield did not use diagrams to reflect pattern, as she thought they would imply that the pattern is static rather than continually evolving. As the family reflects on the pattern, insight into action may involve a transformative process, with the same events being seen in a new light. Family health is seen as a function of the nurse-family relationship. Many of the families in partnership with Litchfield gained insight into their own predicaments in such a way that they required less interaction and service from traditional health-care services (1999, 2004).

Exploring Pattern Recognition as a Nursing Intervention

Emiko Endo (1998) explored HEC pattern recognition as a nursing intervention in Japan with women living with ovarian cancer. She asked, "When a person with cancer has an opportunity to share meaning in the life process within the nurse-client relationship, what changes may occur in the evolving pattern?" Attending to the flow of meaningful thoughts for each participant and building on the previous work of Litchfield (1993, 1997), Endo found four common phases of the process of expanding consciousness for all participants: client-nurse mutual concern, pattern recognition, vision and action potential, and transformation. Participants differed in the pace of evolving movement toward a turning point and in the characteristics of personal growth at the turning point. The characteristics of growth ranged from assertion of self, to emancipation of self, to transcendence of self. Reflecting on her experience, Endo (1998) put forth that pattern recognition is "not intended to fix clients' problems from a medical diagnostic standpoint, but to provide individuals with an opportunity to know themselves, to find meaning in their current situation and life, and to gain insight for the future."

Endo, Nitta, Inayoshi, Saito, Takemura, et al. (2000) carried out a similar study with Japanese families in which the wife-mother was hospitalized because of a cancer diagnosis. Families found meaning in their patterns and reported increased understanding of their present situation. In the pattern-recognition process, most families reconfigured from being a collection of separated individuals to trustful, caring relationships as a family unit, showing more openness and connectedness. The researchers concluded that pattern recognition as a nursing intervention was a "meaning-making transforming process in the family-nurse partnership" (p. 604).

Early research emanating from Margaret Newman's HEC theoretical perspective added to understanding the interrelatedness of time, movement, space, and consciousness as manifestations of health. These studies pointed to the need to look at health as expanding consciousness using a research methodology that acknowledges, under-

stands, and honors the undivided wholeness of the human health experience. They pointed to a need to *step inside* to view the whole from within. These studies cleared away the murky waters so that what previously appeared as separate islands became clearly visible as mountaintops on one undivided piece of land, newly emerged but always there as a whole. As a result, a new generation of qualitative HEC research has emerged, and a deeper understanding of health has surfaced.

PRACTICE

Patricia Tommet (2003) used the HEC hermeneutic dialectic methodology to explore the pattern of nurse-parent interaction in families faced with choosing an elementary school for their children who were medically fragile. She found a pattern of *living in uncertainty* to exist for the families in the intense period of disruption and disorganization following the birth of their medically fragile child through the first few years. After two to three years, the families exhibited a pattern of *order in chaos* where they learned how to live in the present, letting go of the way they lived in the past. Tommet found that "families changed from being passive recipients to active participants in the care of their children" (p. 90) and that the "experience of their children's birth and life transformed these families and through them, transformed systems of care" (p. 86). Tommet demonstrated insights gained in family pattern recognition and concluded that a nurse-parent partnership could have had a more profound impact on these families, and hence the services they used, during the first three years of their children's lives.

Working with colleagues in New Zealand, Litchfield undertook a pilot project that included 19 families in a predicament of strife (Litchfield & Laws, 1999). The goal of the pilot project, which built on Litchfield's previous work (1993, 1999), was to explore a model of nurse case management incorporating the use of a family nurse trained in HEC theory. In the context of a family–family nurse partnership, the unfolding pattern of family living was attended to. Family nurses shared their stories of the families with the research group, who reflected together on the families' changing predicaments and the whole picture of family living in terms of how each family moved in time and place. Subsequent visits with the families focused on recognition of pattern and potential for action. The family nurse mobilized relief services if necessary and orchestrated services as needs emerged in the process of pattern recognition. The research group found that families became more open and spontaneous through the process of pattern recognition, and their interactions evidenced more focus, purposefulness, and cooperation. In analyzing costs of medical care for one participating family, it was estimated that a 3 to 13 percent savings could be seen by employing the model of family nursing, with greater savings being possible when family nurses are available immediately after a family disruption takes place. Based on Litchfield's work with families with complex health predicaments, the government has funded a large demonstration project where family nurses are employed to nurse from an HEC perspective and partner with families without having predetermined goals and outcomes that the families and nurses must achieve. These nurses are free to focus on family health as defined and experienced by the families themselves.

Endo and colleagues (Endo, Minegishi, & Kubo, 2004; Endo, Miyahara, Suzuki, & Ohmasa, 2004) in Japan have expanded their work to incorporate the pattern-recognition process at the hospital nursing unit level. After engaging the professional nursing staff in reading and dialogue about the HEC theory, nurses are encouraged to incorporate the exploration of meaningful events and people into their practice with their patients. Nurses keep journals and come together to reflect on the experience of expanding consciousness in their patients and in themselves. Endo, Miyahara, Suzuki, and Ohmasa (2004) conclude: "Retrospectively it was found through dialogue in the research/project meetings that in the usual nurse-client relationships, nurses were bound by their responsibilities within the medical model to help clients get well, but in letting go of the 'old rules,' they encountered an amazing experience with clients' transformations. The nurses' transformation occurred concomitantly, and they were free to follow the clients' paths and incorporate all realms of nursing interventions in everyday practice into the unitary perspective."

Jane Flanagan (2004) transformed the practice of presurgical nursing by developing the preadmission nursing practice model, which is based on HEC. The nursing practice model shifted from a disease focus to a process focus, with attention being given to the nurses knowing their patients and that which is meaningful to them, so that the surgery experience could be put in proper context and appropriate care provided. Nursing presurgical visits were emphasized. Flanagan reported that the nursing staff was exuberant to be free to be a nurse once again, and patients frequently stopped by to comment on their preoperative experience and evolving life changes.

Similarly, Susan Ruka (2004) made HEC pattern recognition the foundation of care at a long-term-care nursing facility, transforming the nursing practice and the sense of connectedness among staff, families, and residents—each became more peaceful, relaxed, and loving.

Application of HEC at the Community Level

Pharris (2002, 2004) attempted to understand a community pattern of rising youth homicide rates by conducting a study with incarcerated teens convicted of murder participating as coinvestigators. When the experiences of meaningful events and relationships were compared across participants, the pattern of disconnection with the community became evident and various aspects of the community (youth workers, juvenile detention staff, emergency hospital staff, pediatric nurses and physicians, social workers, educators, etc.) were engaged in dialogues reflecting on the youths' stories and the community pattern. Insights transformed community responses to youths at risk for violent perpetration. The youth in the study reported the pattern-recognition process to be transformative, and expanding consciousness was visible in changed behaviors, increased connectedness, and more loving attention to meaningful relationships. Alterations in movement, time, and space inherent in the jail system can intensify the process of expanding consciousness. Pharris (2004) and colleagues are extending the community pattern-recognition process in a partnership with a multiethnic community interested in understanding and transforming patterns of racism and health disparities.

Pharris (1999) gives the example of a 16-year-old young man placed in an adult correctional facility after a murder conviction. This young man was constantly getting into fights and generally feeling lost. As he and the nurse researcher met over several weeks to gain insight into patterns of meaningful people and events in his life, the process seemed to be blocked, with the pattern not emerging and little insight being gained. He spoke of how he felt he had lost himself several years back when he went from being a straight A student from a stable family to stealing cars, drinking, getting into fights, and eventually murdering someone. One week he walked into the room where the nurse was waiting and his movements seemed more controlled and labored; he sat with his arms tightly cradling his rounded abdomen, and his chest was expanded as though it were about to explode. His palms were glistening with sweat. His face was erupting with acne. He talked as usual in a very detached manner, but his words came out in bursts. The nurse chose to give him feedback about what she was seeing and sensing from his body. She reflected that he seemed to be exerting a great deal of energy holding back something that was erupting within him. With this insight, he was quiet for a few minutes and tears began rolling down his cheeks. Suddenly he began talking about a very painful family history of sexual abuse that had been kept secret for many years. It became obvious that the experience of covering up the abuse had been so all-encompassing that it was suppressing his pattern. This young man had reached a choice point at which he realized his old ways of interacting with others were no longer serving him, and he chose to interact with his environment in a different way. By the next meeting, his movements had become smooth and sure, his complexion had cleared up, he was now able to reflect on his insights, and he no longer was involved in the chaos and fighting in his cellblock. He was able to let go of his need to control everything and was able to connect with the emotions of his childhood experiences; he was also able to cry for the first time in years. In their subsequent work together, this young man and the nurse were able to distinguish between his implicit pattern, which had now become clear through their dialogue, and the impact that keeping the abusive experience a secret had had on him and on other members of his family. Since that time, the young man has been able to transcend previous limitations and has become involved in several efforts to help others, both in and out of the prison environment. He has entered into several warm and loving relationships with family members and friends and has achieved academic success. This was evidence

of expanding consciousness for the young man. He reflected that he wished he had had a nurse to talk with prior to "catching his case" (being arrested for murder). He had been seen by a nurse in the juvenile detention center, who did a physical exam and gave him aspirin for a headache. A few days before the murder, he saw a nurse practitioner in a clinic who wrote a prescription for antibiotics and talked with him about safe sex. These interactions are explicate patterns of the implicate order of the U.S. health-care system and the increasingly task-oriented role that nursing is being pressured to take (Jonsdottir, Litchfield, & Pharris, 2003, 2004).

That which is underlying makes itself known in the physical realm, and nurses operating out of the HEC theory are able to be in relationship with patients, families, and communities in such a way that insights arising in their dialogue shed light on an expanded horizon of potential actions (Newman, 1997a; Litchfield, 1999).

Another example, at the community level, arises out of the work of Frank Lamendola and Margaret Newman (1994) with people with HIV/AIDS. They found that the experience of HIV/AIDS opened the participants to suffering and physical deterioration and at the same time introduced greater sensitivity and openness to themselves and to others. Drawing on the work of cultural historian William Irwin Thompson, systems theorist Will McWhinney, and musician David Dunn, Lamendola and Newman, state:

> They [Thompson, McWhinney, and Dunn] see the loss of membranal integrity as a signal of the loss of autopoetic unity analogous to the breaking down of boundaries at a global level between countries, ideologies, and disparate groups. Thompson views HIV/AIDS not simply as a chance infection but part of a larger cultural phenomenon and sees the pathogen not as an object but as heralding the need for living together characterized by a symbiotic relationship. (Lamendola & Newman, 1994, p. 14)

In making the appeal that AIDS calls us to a reconceptualization of the nature of the self and greater interconnectedness on the interpersonal, community, and global level, Lamendola and Newman quote Thompson (1989, p. 99), who states that we need to "learn to tolerate aliens by seeing the self as a cloud in a clouded sky and not as a lord in a walled-in fortress."

Sharon Falkenstern (2003) found the community pattern to emerge as significant when she studied the process of HEC nursing with families with a child with special health-care needs. She found that the nursing partnership was very important to the families as they struggled to make sense of their experiences and tried to discern how to get on with their lives. The evolving pattern of these families included the social and political forces within the educational, disabilities support, and health care systems, as well as community patterns of caring, prejudice, and racism (Falkenstern, 2003).

The pattern of the community is visible in the stories of individuals and families. Nurses can play an important role in engaging communities in dialogue as these stories are shared and reflected upon. More work needs to be done on methods of engaging communities in dialogue about what is meaningful. For example, if an HEC nurse were to take on the task of engaging her or his country's nurses in a dialogue about what is meaningful in their practice, expanding consciousness would be manifest as the profession reorganizes at a higher level of functioning. In the process, the public would no doubt experience an expanded sense of health.

a process of becoming more of oneself, of finding greater meaning in life, and of reaching new dimensions of connectedness with other people and the world" (1). HEC nurses attend to that process.

SUMMARY

Margaret Newman's theory of Health as Expanding Consciousness (HEC) calls nurses to focus on that which is meaningful in their practice and in the lives of their patients. It is a philosophy of *being with* rather than *doing for*. The HEC nurse brings to the patient encounter all that she or he has learned in school and in practice, but begins by attending to the patient's definition of health and seeing it in the context of the patient's expression of meaningful relationships and events. The focus is not on predetermined outcomes mandated by the health system or on *fixing* the patient, but rather is on partnering with the patient in his or her experience of health. Rather than simply using technological tools, we are using ourselves as instruments in our patient's evolving experience of health. Newman (n.d., HEC Web site) states, "The theory asserts that every person in every situation, no matter how disordered and hopeless it may seem, is part of the universal process of expanding consciousness—

References

Bentov, I. (1978). *Stalking the wild pendulum.* New York: E. P. Dutton.

Bohm, D. (1980). *Wholeness and the implicate order.* London: Routledge & Kegan Paul.

Connor, M. (1998). Expanding the dialogue on praxis in nursing research and practice. *Nursing Science Quarterly, 11*(2), 51–55.

Endo, E. (1998). Pattern recognition as a nursing intervention with Japanese women with ovarian cancer. *Advances in Nursing Science, 20*(4), 49–61.

Endo, E., Minegishi, H., & Kubo, S. (2004). Creating action research teams: A praxis model of care. In Picard, C., & Jones, D. (Eds.), *Giving voice to what we know: Margaret Newman's theory of health as expanding consciousness in research, theory, and practice* (pp. 143–152). Boston: Jones & Bartlett.

Endo, E., Miyahara, T., Suzuki, S., & Ohmasa, T. (2004). Partnering of researcher and practicing nurses for transformative nursing. *Nursing Science Quarterly, 15*(2), p. 609.

Endo, E., Nitta, E., Inayoshi, M., Saito, R., Takemura, K., Minegishi, H., Kubo, S., & Kondo, M. (2000). Pattern recognition as a caring partnership in families with cancer. *Journal of Advanced Nursing, 32*(3), 603–610.

Engle, V. (1986). The relationship of movement and time to older adults' functional health. *Research in Nursing and Health, 9,* 123–129.

Flanagan, J. (2004). Creating a healing environment for staff and patients in a pre-surgery clinic. In Picard, C., & Jones, D. (Eds.), *Giving voice to what we know: Margaret Newman's theory of health as expanding consciousness in research, theory, and practice* (pp. 53–64). Boston: Jones & Bartlett.

Guba, E. G., & Lincoln, Y. S. (1989). *Fourth generation evaluation.* Newbury Park, CA: Sage Publications.

Heron, J., & Reason, P. (1997). A participatory inquiry paradigm. *Qualitative Inquiry, 3*(3), 274–294.

Jonsdottir, H. (1988). Life problems of people with chronic pulmonary obstructive disease: Isolation and being closed in. *Nursing Science Quarterly, 11*(4), 160–166.

Jonsdottir, H. (1998). Life patterns of people with chronic obstructive pulmonary disease: Isolation and being closed in. *Nursing Science Quarterly, 11*(4), 160–166.

Jonsdottir, H., Litchfield, M., & Pharris, M. D. (2003). Partnership in practice. *Research and Theory for Nursing Practice, 17*(3), 51–63.

Jonsdottir, H., Litchfield, M., & Pharris, M. D. (2004). The relational core of nursing practice. *Journal of Advanced Nursing, 47*(3), in press.

Jonsdottir, H., Litchfield, M., Pharris, M. D., & Picard, C. L. (2001). *Partnership as a nursing intervention?* Symposium presentation at the International Council of Nurses 22nd Quadrennial Congress, Copenhagen, Denmark. June 11, 2001.

Kiser-Larson, N. (2002). Life pattern of native women experiencing breast cancer. *International Journal for Human Caring, 6*(2), 61–68.

Lamendola, F. (1998). *Patterns of the caregiver experiences of selected nurses in hospice and HIV/AIDS care.* Unpublished doctoral thesis, University of Minnesota, Minneapolis.

Lamendola, F., & Newman, M. A. (1994). The paradox of HIV/AIDS as expanding consciousness. *Advances in Nursing Science, 16*(3), 13–21.

Litchfield, M. C. (1993). *The process of health patterning in families with young children who have been repeatedly hospitalized.* Unpublished master's thesis, University of Minnesota, Minneapolis.

Litchfield, M. C. (1997). *The process of nursing partnership in family health.* Unpublished doctoral thesis, University of Minnesota, Minneapolis.

Litchfield, M. (1999). Practice wisdom. *Advances in Nursing Science, 22*(2), 62–73.

Litchfield, M. C. (2004). The nursing praxis of family health. In Picard, C., & Jones, D. (Eds.), *Giving voice to what we know: Margaret Newman's theory of health as expanding consciousness in research, theory, and practice* (pp. 73–83). Boston: Jones & Bartlett.

Litchfield, M., & Laws, M. (1999). Achieving family health and cost-containment outcomes. In Cohen, E. L., & De Back, V. (Eds.), *The outcomes mandate: Case management in health care today* (pp. 306–314). St. Louis: Mosby.

Moch, S. D. (1990). Health within the experience of breast cancer. *Journal of Advanced Nursing, 15,* 1426–1435.

Moss, R. (1991). *The I that is we.* Millbrae, CA: Celestial Arts.

Neill, J. (2002a). Transcendence and transformation in the life patterns of women living with rheumatoid arthritis. *Advances in Nursing Science, 24*(4), 27–47.

Neill, J. (2002b). From practice to caring praxis through Newman's theory of health as expanding consciousness: A personal journey. *International Journal for Human Caring, 6*(2), 48–54.

Newman, M. A. (n.d.). *Health as expanding consciousness* Web site. Available at: http://healthasexpandingconsciousness.org.

Newman, M. A. (1976). Movement tempo and the experience of time. *Nursing Research, 25,* 173–179.

Newman, M. A. (1978). *Nursing theory.* (Audiotape of an address to the 2nd National Nurse Educator Conference in New York.) Chicago: Teach'em, Inc.

Newman, M. A. (1979). *Theory development in nursing.* Philadelphia: F. A. Davis.

Newman, M. A. (1982). Time as an index of expanding consciousness with age. *Nursing Research, 31,* 290–293.

Newman, M. A. (1986). *Health as expanding consciousness.* St. Louis, MO: Mosby.

Newman, M. A. (1987). Aging as increasing complexity. *Journal of Gerontological Nursing, 12,* 16–18.

Newman, M. A. (1990). Newman's theory of health as praxis. *Nursing Science Quarterly, 3,* 37–41.

Newman, M. A. (1994a). *Health as expanding consciousness* (2nd ed.). Boston: Jones & Bartlett (NLN Press).

Newman, M. A. (1994b). Theory for nursing practice. *Nursing Science Quarterly, 7*(4), 153–157.

Newman, M. A. (1995). Recognizing a pattern of expanding consciousness in persons with cancer. In *A developing discipline* (pp. 159–171). Boston: Jones & Bartlett (formerly, New York: National League for Nursing Press).

Newman, M. A. (1997a). Experiencing the whole. *Advances in Nursing Science, 20*(1), 34–39.

Newman, M. A. (1997b). Evolution of the theory of health as expanding consciousness. *Nursing Science Quarterly, 10*(1), 22–25.

Newman, M. A. (1997c). Margaret Newman: Health as expanding consciousness. In Fuld Institute for Technology in Nursing Education, *The nurse theorists: Portraits of excellence* [CD-ROM]. Athens, OH: FITNE, Inc.

Newman, M. A. (1997d). A dialogue with Martha Rogers and David Bohm about the science of unitary human beings. In Madrid, M. (Ed.), *Patterns of Rogerian knowing* (pp. 3–10). New York: National League for Nursing Press.

Newman, M. A. (1999). The rhythm of relating in a paradigm of wholeness. *Image: Journal of Nursing Scholarship, 31*(3), 227–230.

Newman, M. A. (2002a). The pattern that connects. *Advances in Nursing Science, 24*(3), 1–7.

Newman, M. A. (2002b). Caring in the human health experience. *International Journal for Human Caring, 6*(2), 8–11.

Newman, M. A. (2003). A world with no boundaries. *Advances in Nursing Science, 26*(4), 240–245.

Newman, M. A., & Moch, S. D. (1991). Life patterns of persons with coronary heart disease. *Nursing Science Quarterly, 4,* 161–167.

Newman, M. A., Sime, A. M., & Corcoran-Perry, S. A. (1991). The focus of the discipline of nursing. *Advances in Nursing Science, 14*(1), 1–6.

Noveletsky-Rosenthal, H. T. (1996). *Pattern recognition in older adults living with chronic illness.* Unpublished doctoral thesis, Boston College.

Pharris, M. D. (1999). *Pattern recognition as a nursing intervention with adolescents convicted of murder.* Unpublished doctoral thesis, University of Minnesota, Minneapolis.

Pharris, M. D. (2002). Coming to know ourselves as community through a nursing partnership with adolescents convicted of murder. *Advances in Nursing Science, 24*(3), 21–42.

Pharris, M. D. (2004). Engaging with communities in a pattern recognition process. In Picard, C., & Jones, D. (Eds.), *Giving voice to what we know: Margaret Newman's theory of health as expanding consciousness in research, theory, and practice* (pp. 83–94). Boston: Jones & Bartlett.

Picard, C. (2000). Pattern of expanding consciousness in midlife women: Creative movement and the narrative as modes of expression. *Nursing Science Quarterly, 13*(2), 150–158.

Picard, C. (2004). Parents of persons with bipolar disorder and pattern recognition. In Picard, C., & Jones, D. (Eds.), *Giving voice to what we know: Margaret Newman's theory of health as expanding consciousness in research, theory, and practice* (pp. 133–141). Boston: Jones & Bartlett.

Picard, C., & Jones, D. (Eds.). (2004). *Giving voice to what we know: Margaret Newman's theory of health as expanding consciousness in research, theory, and practice.* Boston: Jones & Bartlett.

Prigogine, I. (1976). Order through fluctuation: Self-organization and social system. In Jantsch, E., & Waddington, C. H. (Eds.), *Evolution and consciousness* (pp. 93–133). Reading, MA: Addison-Wesley.

Quinn, J. F. (1992). Holding sacred space. The nurse as healing environment. *Holistic Nursing Practice, 6*(4), 26–36.

Rogers, M. E. (1970). *An introduction to the theoretical basis of nursing.* Philadelphia: F. A. Davis.

Rogers, M. E. (1990). Nursing science and the space age. *Nursing Science Quarterly, 5*(1), 27–34.

Ruka, S. (2004). Creating balance, rhythm and patterns in people with dementia living in a nursing home. In Picard, C., & Jones, D. (Eds.). *Giving voice to what we know: Margaret Newman's theory of health as expanding consciousness in research, theory, and practice* (pp. 59–104). Boston: Jones & Bartlett.

Skolimowski, H. (1994). *The participatory mind.* London: Arkana.

Thompson, W. I. (1989). *Imaginary landscape: Making worlds of myth and science.* New York: St. Martin's Press.

Tommet, P. (2003). Nurse-parent dialogue: Illuminating the evolving pattern of families with children who are medically fragile. *Nursing Science Quarterly, 16*(3), 239–246.

Weingourt, R. (1998). Using Margaret A. Newman's theory of health with elderly nursing home residents. *Perspectives in Psychiatric Care, 34*(3), 25–30.

Yamashita, M. (1998). Newman's theory of health as expanding consciousness: Research of family caregiving in mental illness in Japan. *Nursing Science Quarterly, 11*(3), 110–115.

Yamashita, M. (1999). Newman's theory of health as expanding consciousness: Research of family caregiving in mental illness in Japan. *Nursing Science Quarterly, 12*(1), 73–79.

Young, A. M. (1976). *The reflexive universe: Evolution of consciousness.* San Francisco, CA: Robert Briggs Associates.

CHAPTER 16

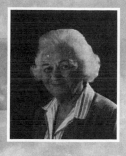

Imogene M. King

PART ONE: Imogene M. King's Theory of Goal Attainment

Imogene M. King

Introducing the Theorist
Introducing the Theory
Use of King's Conceptual System and Theory
Summary

Introducing the Theorist

My postsecondary education experiences included a diploma in nursing from St. John's Hospital School of Nursing in St. Louis, baccalaureate and master's degrees in nursing from St. Louis University, and a doctor of education from Teachers College, Columbia University, New York. Postdoctoral study included work in advanced statistics, systems research, and computers. Continuing education is an ongoing process. My avocation includes nursing history in the context of world history, and philosophy with emphasis on science and ethics.

The majority of my nursing experience, which spans over 50 years, included clinical practice of nursing adults in hospitals. While working my way through college, I worked in a physician's office as a school nurse and as an occupational health nurse. I have always believed that as a teacher one must also be an excellent practitioner, so my experience as a teacher of nursing at undergraduate and graduate levels included practice. I taught at Loyola University, Chicago; the Ohio State University; and the University of South Florida, advancing from assistant professor to full professor and now as professor emeritus.

I have received multiple honors and awards. The most recent are the Jessie Scott Award for Leadership, presented by the American Nurses' Association at the 100th anniversary convention in 1996, and an honorary doctor of science degree in 1998.

My peers at the house of delegates at the Florida Nurses Association voted in 1996 to give me life-time membership. The University of Tampa Department of Nursing named the annual research award given to students the "Imogene M. King Research Award." I was honored at the 75th anniversary convention of Sigma Theta Tau International with a research grant named for me and with a program that presented a description of me as a caring individual. I also appear in *Who's Who in America, American Women,* and *Who's Who in Nursing.*

Introducing the Theory

Continuous discoveries in telecommunications and technology, and a daily bombardment of information about world events bring complexity to one's life that is unprecedented in history. Instant communication reminds us that we live in an information-processing world of systems: "A system is defined as a series of functional components connected by communication links exhibiting purposeful goal-directed behavior" (King, 1996). As individuals, we are born, grow, and develop within each nation. Nations make up the world society. A sense of a global community can be understood as we view the interactions of individuals and groups with linguistic, ethnic, and religious differences. The commonality in this worldview is the human being. How is this global community and health care related to theory construction and testing in research in nursing?

The commonality in my worldview is human beings who communicate and interact in their small groups within their nations' social systems; that is, human environments as well as physical environments. Three dynamic interacting systems, shown in Figure 16–1, represent individuals as personal systems, groups as interpersonal systems, and large groups as social systems that make up most societies in the world (King, 1981). These systems represent interconnected links for information processing in a high-tech world of health care and nursing. This conceptual system provides one approach to structure a world community of human beings, who are the recipients of nursing care.

This chapter presents a review of my ideas about developing theoretical knowledge for nursing. A

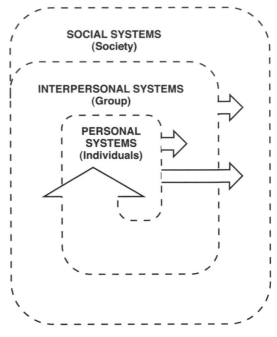

FIGURE 16–1   King's conceptual system.

process for developing a conceptual system is explained. The method used to derive a theory of goal attainment from my conceptual system is demonstrated. The application of this conceptual system and Theory of Goal Attainment is discussed in Part 2 of this chapter.

INITIAL IDEAS

My first theory publication pronounced the problems and prospect of knowledge development in nursing (King, 1964). Over 30 years ago, the problems were identified as (1) lack of a professional nursing language; (2) atheoretical nursing phenomena; and (3) limited concept development. Today, theories and conceptual frameworks have identified theoretical approaches to knowledge development and utilization of knowledge in practice. Concept development is a continuous process in the nursing science movement (King, 1988).

My rationale for developing a schematic representation of nursing phenomena was influenced by the Howland Systems Model (Howland, 1976) and the Howland and McDowell conceptual framework (Howland & McDowell, 1964). The levels of interaction in those works influenced my ideas relative to organizing a conceptual frame of reference for nursing, as shown in Figure 16–1. Because concepts offer one approach to structure knowledge for nursing, a comprehensive review of nursing literature provided me with ideas to identify five comprehensive concepts as a basis for a conceptual system for nursing. The overall concept is a human being, commonly referred to as an "individual" or a "person." Initially, I selected abstract concepts of perception, communication, interpersonal relations, health, and social institutions (King, 1968). These ideas forced me to review my knowledge of philosophy relative to the nature of human beings (ontology) and to the nature of knowledge (epistemology).

PHILOSOPHY OF SCIENCE

In the late 1960s, while auditing a series of courses in systems research, I was introduced to a philosophy of science called General System Theory (Von Bertalanffy, 1968). This philosophy of science gained momentum in the 1950s, although its roots date to an earlier period. This philosophy refuted logical positivism and reductionism and proposed the idea of isomorphism and perspectivism in knowledge development. Von Bertalanffy, credited with originating the idea of General System Theory, defined this philosophy of science movement as a "general science of wholeness: systems of elements in mutual interaction" (Von Bertalanffy, 1968, p. 37).

My philosophical position is rooted in General System Theory, which guides the study of organized complexity as whole systems. This philosophy gave me the impetus to focus on knowledge development as an information-processing, goal-seeking, and decision-making system. General System Theory provides a holistic approach to study nursing phenomena as an open system and frees one's thinking from the parts-versus-whole dilemma. In any discussion of the nature of nursing, the central ideas revolve around the nature of human beings and their interaction with internal and external environments. During this journey, I began to conceptualize a theory for nursing. However, because a manuscript was due in the publisher's office, I organized my ideas into a conceptual system (formerly called a "conceptual framework"), and the result was the publication of a book entitled *Toward a Theory of Nursing* (King, 1971).

DESIGN OF A CONCEPTUAL SYSTEM

A conceptual system provides structure for organizing multiple ideas into meaningful wholes. From my initial set of ideas in 1968 and 1971, my conceptual framework was refined to show some unity and relationships among the concepts. In addition, the next step in this process was to review the research literature in the discipline in which the concepts had been studied. For example, the concept of perception has been studied in psychology for many years. The literature indicated that most of the early studies dealt with sensory perception. Around the 1950s, psychologists began to study interpersonal perception, which related to my ideas about interactions. From this research literature, I identified the characteristics of perception and defined the concept for my framework. I continued searching literature for knowledge of each of the concepts in my framework. An update on my conceptual system was published in 1995 (King, 1995).

Process for Developing a Concept

"Searching for scientific knowledge in nursing is an ongoing dynamic process of continuous identification, development, and validation of relevant concepts" (King, 1975). What is a concept? A *concept* is an organization of reference points. Words are the verbal symbols used to explain events and things in our environment and relationships to past experiences. Northrop (1969) noted: "[C]oncepts fall into different types according to the different sources of their meaning.... A concept is a term to which meaning has been assigned." Concepts are the categories in a theory.

The concept development and validation process is as follows:

1. Review, analyze, and synthesize research literature related to the concept.
2. From the above review, identify the characteristics (attributes) of the concept.
3. From the characteristics, write a conceptual definition.
4. Review literature to select an instrument or develop an instrument.

5. Design a study to measure the characteristics of the concept.
6. Decisions are made on selection of the population to be sampled.
7. Collect data.
8. Analyze and interpret data.
9. Write results of findings and conclusions.
10. State implications for adding to nursing knowledge.

Concepts that represent phenomena in nursing are structured within a framework and a theory to show relationships.

King's Conceptual System

Twelve concepts—self, body image, role, perception, communication, interaction, transaction, growth and development, power, authority, organization, and decision making—were identified from my analysis of nursing literature (King, 1981). The concepts that provided substantive knowledge about human beings were placed within the personal system, those related to groups were placed within the interpersonal system, and those related to large groups that make up a society were placed within the social system. However, knowledge from all of the concepts is used in nurses' interactions with individuals and groups within social organizations, such as the family, the educational system, and the political system. Knowledge of these concepts came from my synthesis of research in many disciplines. Concepts, when defined from research literature, give nurses knowledge that can be applied in the concrete world of nursing. The concepts represent basic knowledge that nurses use in their role and functions either in practice, education, or administration. In addition, the concepts provide ideas for research in nursing.

One of my goals was to identify what I call the essence of nursing. That brought me back to the question, What is the nature of human beings? A vicious circle? Not really! Because nurses are first and foremost other human beings who give nursing care to other human beings, my philosophy of the nature of human beings has been presented along with assumptions I have made about individuals (King, 1989a). Recognizing that a conceptual system represents structure for a discipline, the next step in the process of knowledge development was to derive one or more theories from this

structure. Lo and behold, a theory of goal attainment was developed (King, 1981, 1992). More recently, several dissertations by Frey (1995), Sieloff (1995), and Killeen (1996) have derived theories from my conceptual system.

THEORY OF GOAL ATTAINMENT

Generally speaking, nursing care's goal is to help individuals maintain health or regain health (King, 1990). Concepts are essential elements in theories. When a theory is derived from a conceptual system, concepts are selected from that system. Remember my question: What is the essence of nursing?

> *Concepts of self, perception, communication, interaction, transaction, role, and decision making were selected.*

The concepts of self, perception, communication, interaction, transaction, role, and decision making were selected. Self is an individual whose perception and role influence that person's communication, interaction, and decision making in small and large groups. So, what is the health-care system within which nurses function? Is it a social system of individuals and groups interacting to achieve goals related to health? A transaction model, shown in Figure 16–2, was developed that represented the process whereby individuals interact to set goals that result in goal attainment (King, 1981).

As the twenty-first century begins, cost containment appears to be the primary goal of health-care administrators and insurance companies. If the goals and the means to achieve them are mutually agreed upon by nurses and patients, 99 percent of the time, goals will be achieved (King, 1989b). Goal attainment represents outcomes. Outcomes indicate effective nursing care. Nursing care is a critical element to provide quality care that is also cost-effective. Using the transaction process model is one way to achieve this goal.

Transaction Process Model

The model shown in Figure 16–2 is a human process that can be observed in many situations when two or more people interact, such as in the family and in social events (King, 1996). As nurses, we bring knowledge and skills that influence our

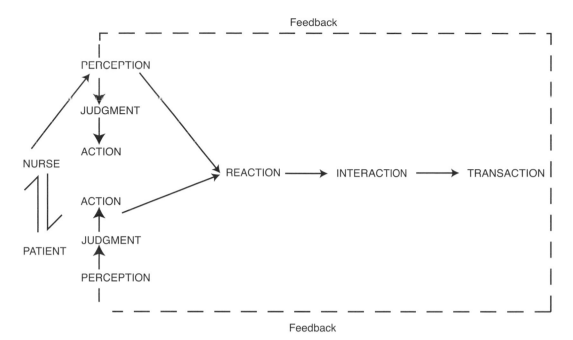

FIGURE 16–2 Transaction process model. From King, I. M. (1981). *A theory for nursing: Systems, concepts, process* (p. 145) New York: John Wiley & Sons, Inc.

perceptions, communications, and interactions in performing the functions of the role. In your role as a nurse, after interacting with a patient, sit down and write down your behavior and that of the patient. It is my belief that you can identify your perceptions, mental judgments, mental action, and reaction (negative or positive). Did you make a transaction? That is, did you exchange information and set a goal with the patient? Did you explore the means for the patient to use to achieve the goal? Was the goal achieved? If not, why? It is my opinion that most nurses use this process but are not aware that it is based in a nursing theory. With knowledge of the concepts and of the process, nurses have a scientific base for practice that can be articulated clearly and documented to show quality care. How can a nurse document this transaction model in practice?

Documentation System

A documentation system was designed to implement the transaction process that leads to goal attainment (King, 1984a). Most nurses use the nursing process of assess, diagnose, plan, implement, and evaluate, which I call a method. My transaction process provides the theoretical knowl-

edge base to implement this method. For example, as one assesses the patient and the environment and makes a nursing diagnosis, the concepts of perception, communication, and interaction represent knowledge the nurse uses to gather information and make a judgment. A transaction is made when the nurse and patient decide mutually on the goals to be attained, agree on the means to attain goals that represent the plan of care, and then implement the plan. Evaluation determines whether or not goals were attained. If not, you ask why, and the process begins again. The documentation is recorded directly in the patient's chart. The patient's record indicates the process used to achieve goals. On discharge, the summary indicates goals set and goals achieved. One does not need multiple forms to complete when this documentation system is in place, and the quality of nursing care is recorded. Why do nurses insist on designing critical paths, various care plans, and other types of forms when, with knowledge of this system, the nurse documents nursing care directly on the patient's chart? Why do we use multiple forms to complicate a process that is knowledge-based and also provides essential data to demonstrate outcomes and to evaluate quality nursing care?

Federal laws have been passed that indicate that patients must be involved in decisions about their care and about dying. This transaction process provides a scientifically based process to help nurses implement federal laws such as the Patient Self-Determination Act.

Goal Attainment Scale

Analysis of nursing research literature in the 1970s revealed that very few instruments were designed for nursing research. In the late 1980s, the faculty at the University of Maryland, experts in measurement and evaluation, applied for and received a grant to conduct conferences to teach nurses to design reliable and valid instruments. I had the privilege of participating in this two-year continuing education conference, where I developed a Goal Attainment Scale (King, 1989b). This instrument may be used to measure goal attainment. It may also be used as an assessment tool to provide patient data to plan and implement nursing care.

Use of King's Conceptual System and Theory

Over the years of presenting my ideas at theory conferences throughout the world, nurses have asked many excellent questions, which I have tried to answer. Initially, the questions pertained to, How does one implement this in practice? This motivated me to design the documentation system to show the relationship between the nursing process as method and my nursing process as theory. Prior to presenting this at a national meeting, several staff nurses tested this and suggested this system be implemented in practice. I reminded the nurses that they were not applying a theory, but were applying the knowledge of the theory's concepts. This has become a repetitive statement of mine; that is, one cannot apply an abstraction, which is what conceptual frameworks, models, and theories represent. What one applies is the knowledge of the concepts of the structure and process proposed in the abstractions. Before retiring from a full-time teaching position, the last thing I had to do was design an instrument to measure goal attainment. The use of my ideas in practice, education, administration,

and research is overviewed here and is detailed in Part 2 of this chapter.

NURSING EDUCATION

My first faculty position was as an assistant professor at Loyola University, Chicago. Because my area of study was curriculum and instruction, I was selected to chair a faculty committee to develop a curriculum leading to a master of science degree in nursing. This was one of the first master's programs that used a nursing framework to design a curriculum. The theoretical model was designed by a nurse as part of a dissertation from the University of California (Kaufman, 1958). The model was composed of three concepts—time, stress, and perception. Needless to say, this approach to develop a new graduate program was revolutionary in 1961. This activity provided the impetus for me to reflect on my knowledge of curriculum and instruction, and also to think about structure for organizing undergraduate and graduate nursing programs. The rest is history and is recorded in my books and articles over the past 30 years (King, 1986a).

In the 1970s, the professional nursing staff at the National League for Nursing conducted conferences to disseminate information about the curriculum process for developing or revising a baccalaureate nursing program (King, 1978). The major components in a curriculum discussed at these conferences were "a philosophy, conceptual framework, course objectives, and evaluation of the curriculum" (National League for Nursing, 1978).

The scope of knowledge is so vast that it is impossible to teach students everything they need to learn to begin to practice nursing today and tomorrow. It is imperative that nursing curricula be based on a conceptual framework. Such curricula must be structured to provide students with the essential concepts, skills, and values that serve as foundations and as catalysts to continue to learn after graduation (National League for Nursing, 1978).

As a participant observer who provided administrative support for a faculty engaged in constructing a new undergraduate curriculum, I witnessed the development of a curriculum that moved nursing education into the future (Daubenmire & King, 1973). This baccalaureate nursing curriculum, based on my conceptual framework, was published in 1989. According to Daubenmire (1989, p. 167), "[T]he curriculum model and conceptual framework implemented in 1970 based on King's theory have remained essentially the same for about 15 years except for updating knowledge from year to year. King's framework continues to provide a viable curriculum strategy. A curriculum model which is conceptually based allows for updating content and skills without the necessity for major curriculum change."

One of the criteria used to develop nursing curricula in colleges and universities is a clear statement of a philosophy consistent with the institution offering the nursing program. The philosophy is essential for faculty to identify a conceptual framework and program objectives. A study was conducted in order to identify the major terms used in stated philosophies in nursing programs to attempt to describe the philosophical foundations of nursing. A random sample of nursing schools, stratified by program type and by region of the country, was selected from the National League for Nursing's published list of accredited baccalaureate, associate degree, and diploma nursing programs. A pilot study was conducted from which a classification resulted in the formation of 12 categories (King, 1984b). A table of random numbers was used to select 20 percent of the schools within each category and were distributed according to region and type of program. The conclusion reported differences in use of the terms *man, health, perception, role, social systems,* and *God* by program type and by location of the program in a university, community college, and hospital. The findings of this national survey provided some information about similarities and differences in major terms used in statements of philosophy. The terms *nursing, environment,* and *interpersonal relations* did not differ significantly, which indicated a few commonalities in those three programs. However, differences in statements of philosophy imply differences in curricula, which in turn provide different kinds of education for different kinds of nursing practice. This study, done over 15 years ago, raised the questions, What is the philosophy of nursing education? Has a philosophy of nursing education changed historically?

A publishing company asked me to write a curriculum book. In the 1980s, articulation between associate degree nursing programs and baccalaureate programs seemed to be a problem. Using my conceptual framework, I designed a hypothetical baccalaureate degree program and an associate degree program to begin to identify differences and commonalities, because the same structure was used. My idea was to show clear and reasonable articulation between the two programs when the same conceptual framework is used. It would be interesting for a faculty group to design a curriculum in a university today that offers both a baccalaureate and an associate degree program to test out this hypothetical curriculum (King, 1986b).

When curricula are developed that identify common concepts (knowledge), skills, and professional values, the practice of professional nursing will be the center of health care in the twenty-first century. Increased technology and knowledge require a conceptually based curriculum for the future (Gulitz & King, 1988).

PRACTICE

In the past 10 years, nurses have published their use of my conceptual system and Theory of Goal Attainment in practice. Some nurses have used knowledge of the concepts to implement theory-based practice (Coker & Schreiber, 1989; Hanna, 1995; Messmer, 1995; Smith, 1988).

Nursing's goal is to help individuals and groups attain, maintain, and regain a healthy state: "In

> *Nursing's goal is to help individuals and groups attain, maintain, and regain a healthy state.*

nursing situations where life and health goals are influenced by a severe illness, nurses give care and help persons to die with dignity. My systems framework has described a holistic view of the complexity in nursing within various groups, in different types of health-care systems. This framework differs from other conceptual schema in that it is concerned not with fragmenting human beings and the environment but with human transactions in different types of environments (King, 1995). A few examples from the literature are given.

Family Health

The use of my conceptual system and Theory of Goal Attainment in family health was suggested (King, 1983). The family is usually the immediate social environment in which individuals grow and develop and learn through interactions to set goals. Nurses work with families and with individual family members. The family is seen as a social system, a group of interacting individuals. The family is also viewed as an interpersonal system. For example, nurses' perceptions of family members and family members' perceptions of the nurse influence their responses in situations and their openness in giving information. Congruence in perceptions of nurse and family members helps in assessing a situation to identify concerns and/or problems in the interpersonal system. Knowledge of a concept or role is essential and related to growth and development and to stress in family environments. Two cases were presented and the use of the Theory of Goal Attainment was described in each situation.

Community Health

Community health nursing involves a variety of populations within a variety of social systems. For example, school nurses must understand the education system. Occupational health nurses must understand the political system, the economic system, and the belief system in a community. Some nurses have used the Transaction Process Model in the Theory of Goal Attainment in community health programs as they interact and set goals with interdisciplinary teams to manage health care (Hampton, 1994; Sowell & Fuszard, 1989; Sowell & Lowenstein, 1994). Nurses in community health focus on different populations. In this sense, they are relating to the interpersonal systems in the framework. This is done within a variety of social systems in the community. Although the focus is groups, nurses work with individuals for whom they provide services. My conceptual system (Fig. 16–1) shows the interactions of the three systems in community health.

Use in Hospitals

Two case studies were presented to demonstrate nurses' use of the transaction process and knowledge of the concepts of perception, communication, interaction, and role (King, 1986b). Nurses in a Canadian hospital used the framework to structure the delivery of nursing care. They determined that nurses could identify the published nursing diagnoses in 1990 with the concepts in the framework (Coker et al., 1990). Nurses in Canada, in which two hospitals were involved at a distance from each other, used the conceptual framework to design a system for delivery of nursing care (Fawcett, Vaillancourt, & Watson, 1995). A director of nursing research and education in a large municipal hospital in the United States reported the implementation of theory-based nursing practice using my conceptual system (Messmer, 1995). Theory-based practice in an emergency department used my framework and Theory of Goal Attainment (Benedict & Frey, 1995). The Theory of Goal Attainment was used in adult orthopedic nursing (Alligood, Evans, & Wilt, 1995).

The transaction process was used in short-term group psychotherapy settings. Laben, Dodd, and Sneed (1991) stated that my interactive systems approach of goal attainment is an ideal basis for short-term group psychotherapy. This group used my theory with inpatient juvenile sexual offenders, offenders in maximum security, and community parolees.

Continuous Quality Improvement

Continuous quality improvement in nursing and health care is a reality. Three major categories have been suggested as a way to develop a program. These elements are: (1) structure, (2) process, and (3) outcomes. *Structure* provides an overall organization of the program. *Process* relates to nursing activities. *Outcomes* are separate from but related to performance criteria for evaluation of nursing care and nurses' performance. My conceptual system provides structure for a continuous quality-improvement program (King, 1994). The Transaction Process Model in my Theory of Goal Attainment gives a process that leads to goal attainment that represents outcomes. Outcomes indicate effective nursing care. An example was given to document effectiveness of nursing care if one uses a goal-oriented nursing record (King, 1984a). The record system is an information system based on my Theory of Goal Attainment. The record system can be designed and adapted to most health-care systems. For nurses, it was designed to gather data from assessments of the patient, make a nursing diagnosis, construct a goal list, write orders for nursing care, and write mutually agreed-upon goals and means to attain them. Goals that are achieved are outcomes and represent effective nursing care. Elements in the goal-oriented nursing record are: (1) data base, (2) goal list, (3) nursing orders, (4) flow sheets, (5) progress notes, and (6) discharge summary. This information system can be designed for any patient population and for current and future computerization of records in a health-care system.

RESEARCH

Several nurses have tested the theory in research on aging, parenting, psychiatric-mental health, and ambulatory care (Alligood et al., 1995; Benedict & Frey, 1995; Norris & Hoyer, 1993; Woods, 1994). Nurses in Japan, Sweden, and Canada have conducted studies in their cultures to test the Theory of Goal Attainment (Coker et al., 1990; Kameoka, 1995; Rooke, 1995).

Sieloff (1995) developed a theory of power for nursing administration. Frey (1995) proposed a theory of family, children, and chronic illness and continues to test it in research. Killeen's dissertation (1996) studied patient-consumer perceptions and responses to professional nursing care that resulted in an instrument that measures patient satisfaction.

VISION FOR THE FUTURE

My vision for the future of nursing is that nursing will provide access to health care for all citizens. The United States' health-care system will be structured using my conceptual system. Entry into the system will be via nurses' assessment so individuals are directed to the right place in the system for nursing care, medical care, social services information, health teaching, or rehabilitation. My transaction process will be used by every practicing nurse so that goals can be achieved to demonstrate quality care that is cost-effective. My conceptual system, Theory of Goal Attainment, and Transaction Process Model will continue to serve a useful purpose in delivering professional nursing care. The ideas have been tested in research and in practice, and nurses in education and practice have used the knowledge of the concepts. The relevance of evidence theory–based practice, using my theory, has been shown to join the art of nursing of the twentieth century to the science of nursing in the twenty-first century.

SUMMARY

The U.S. health-care system is in constant flux in an attempt to restructure health-care delivery. How can a conceptual system and the Theory of Goal Attainment provide the structure, process, and outcomes that represent a way to manage and deliver quality health care for all citizens? My conceptual system and transaction process in the Theory of Goal Attainment provides one approach to accomplish the goal of access and quality in the following ways:

1. For interaction between nurses and health-care professionals and between health-care agencies for continuity of care, respect for roles, and responsibilities of each health profession; for case management and collaborative and integrated practice.
2. Essential knowledge to assess, diagnose, plan, implement, and evaluate care.
3. For common discourse among health professionals and between nurses and nursing personnel.
4. A framework within health-care systems and between health-care providers and agencies.
5. Direct measure of outcomes resulting in quality care and cost-effective care; that is, goals are set and goals are attained.
6. A systematic and efficient documentation system.
7. One valid and reliable assessment instrument to assess activities of daily living as a basis for goal-setting.
8. For continuity of care within and between health-care agencies.
9. Results in satisfaction for patients, families, physicians, and administrators.

When knowledge of the concepts and the transaction process has been used in hospitals, homes, nursing homes, and community health agencies, nurses have been motivated to seek additional knowledge in formal educational programs.

PART TWO: Applications of King's Theory of Goal Attainment

Christina Leibold Sieloff, Maureen Frey, & Mary Killeen

Application of Interacting Systems Framework

Concept Development Within the Framework

Theory of Goal Attainment

Recommendations for Knowledge Development Related to King's Framework and Theory

Summary

References

Since the first publication of Dr. Imogene King's work (1971), nursing's interest in the application of her work to practice has grown. The fact that she was one of the few theorists who generated both a framework and a midrange theory further expanded her work. Today, new publications related to Dr. King's work are a frequent occurrence. Additional middle-range theories have been generated and tested, and applications to practice have expanded. Since her retirement, Dr. King continues to publish and examine new applications of her work. The purpose of this part of the chapter is to

provide an updated review of the state of the art in terms of the application of King's Interacting Systems Framework and midrange theory in a variety of areas: practice, administration, education, and research. Publications, including Frey & Sieloff (1995), identified from a review of the literature, will be summarized and briefly discussed. Finally, recommendations will be made for future knowledge development in relation to King's Interacting Systems Framework and midrange theory, particularly in relation to the importance of their application within an evidence-based practice environment.

Application of Interacting Systems Framework

In conducting the literature review, the authors began with the broadest category of application—application within the Interacting Systems Framework to nursing care situations. Because a con-

> *In conducting the literature review, the authors began with the broadest category of application—application within the Interacting Systems Framework to nursing care situations.*

ceptual framework is, by nature, very broad and abstract, it can only serve to guide, rather than prescriptively direct, nursing practice.

King's Interacting Systems Framework has been used to guide nursing practice in several ways. For example, Coker et al. (1995) used the framework to guide the implementation of nursing diagnosis in a large community hospital. Fawcett, Vaillancourt, and Watson (1995) used the framework to guide nursing practice in a large tertiary care hospital. In contrast, several authors used the framework to guide nursing practice with specific patient populations. Doornbos (2002) explored family health in families with chronically mentally ill family members. Hobdell (1995) examined the "relationship between chronic sorrow and accuracy of perception of a child's cognitive development in parents of children with neural tube defects" (p. 132). Table 16–1 delineates other applications related to King's Interacting Systems Framework.

Table 16–1	**Application of the Interacting Systems Framework**	
TOPIC	**AUTHOR(S)**	**YEAR**
Anxiety	LaFontaine	1989
Autonomy	Glenn*	1989
Change	DeFeo	1990
Child health	Steele	1981
Chronic mental illness	Doornbos	1995
Communication	Daubenmire, Searles, and Ashton	1978
Community assessment	Hanchett	1988
Community	Hanchett	1990
	Myks Babb, Fouladbakhsh, and Hanchett	1988
	King	1984
	Asay and Ossler	1984
Continuing education	Brown and Lee	1980
Education	Daubenmire	1989
	King	1989
	Gulitz and King	1988
	King	1986
	Froman and Sanderson	1985
	Daubenmire and King	1973
Family therapy	Gonot	1986
Menopause	Sharts-Hopko	1995
	Heggie and Gangar	1992
Neural tube defect	Hobdell	1995
Nursing administration	Elberson	1989
	Sieloff	1995
Nursing diagnosis	Byrne-Coker, Fradley, Harris, Tomarchio, and Caron	1990
Operating room	Gill, Hopwood-Jones, Tyndall, Gregoroff, LeBlance, Lovett, Rasco, and Ross	1995
Patient education	Spees	1991
	Martin	1990
	King and Tarsitano	1982
Perception	Bunting	1988
Reproductive health	Davis and Dearman	1991
Smoking	Kneeshaw	1990
Social support	Frey	1989
Theory-based practice	Messmer	1995
		1992
	West	1991
	Byrne and Schreiber	1990

*Indicates thesis or dissertation

Concept Development Within the Framework

Concept development within a conceptual framework is particularly valuable, as it often explicates concepts more clearly than a theorist may have done in his or her original work. Concept development may also demonstrate how other concepts, of interest to nursing, can be examined through a "nursing lens." Such explication further assists the development of nursing knowledge by enabling the nurse to better understand the application of the concept within specific practice situations. Examples of concepts developed from within King's work include the following: empathy (Alligood, Evans, & Wilt, 1995), health of a social

Table 16–2	Concept Development within the Framework	
TOPIC	**AUTHOR(S)**	**YEAR**
Advocacy	Bramlett, Gueldner, and Sowell	1990
Autonomy	Glenn*	1989
Coping	King	1983
Empathy	Alligood, Evans, and Wilt	1995
Health	King	1990
Health (social system)	Sieloff	1995
Health (systems)	Winker	1995
Power	Hawkes	1991
Quality of life	King	1993
Social support	Frey	1989
Space	Rooke	1995
Transaction	Binder*	1992

*Indicates thesis or dissertation

system (Sieloff, 1995b), health of systems (Winker, 1995), and space (Rooke, 1995b). Table 16–2 further details applications related to concept development within King's framework (1981).

Theory of Goal Attainment

Dr. King's work is unique in that, in addition to the Interacting Systems Framework, she developed the midrange Theory of Goal Attainment (1981) from concepts within the Interacting Systems Framework.

PRACTICE

This midrange theory has found great application to nursing practice, since the theory focuses on concepts relevant to all nursing situations—the attainment of client goals. The application of the midrange Theory of Goal Attainment (King, 1981) is documented in several categories: (1) general application of the theory, (2) exploring a particular concept within the context of the Theory of Goal Attainment, (3) exploring a particular concept related to the Theory of Goal Attainment, and (4) application of the theory in nonclinical nursing situations. For example, King (1997) described the

use of the Theory of Goal Attainment in nursing practice. Alligood (1995) applied the theory to orthopedic nursing with adults. Short-term group psychotherapy was the focus of theory application for Laben, Sneed, and Seidel (1995). In contrast, Benedict and Frey (1995) examined the use of the theory within the delivery of emergency care.

The midrange Theory of Goal Attainment (King, 1981) is also used when nurses wish to explore a particular concept within a theoretical context. Temple and Fawdry (1992) examined caregiver role strain while perceptual congruency between nurses and clients was explored by Froman (1995).

Nurses also use the Theory of Goal Attainment (King, 1981) to examine concepts related to the theory. This application was demonstrated by Kameoka (1995) as she analyzed nurse-patient interactions in Japan.

Finally, the theory has been applied in nonclinical nursing situations. Messmer (1995) used the theory in implementing theory-based nursing practice. And Jolly and Winker (1995) applied the theory to organizations. In summary, Table 16–3 chronicles applications of King's midrange Theory of Goal Attainment.

Nursing Process and Related Languages

Within the nursing profession, the nursing process has consistently been used as the basis for nursing practice. King's framework and midrange Theory of Goal Attainment have been linked to the process of nursing. Although many published applications have broad reference to the nursing process, several deserve special recognition. First, Dr. King herself (1981) clearly linked the Theory of Goal Attainment to nursing process as theory and to nursing process as method. Application of King's work to nursing curricula further strengthened this link. Other explicit examples of integration with the nursing process are those by Woods (1994), and Frey and Norris (1997). Additionally, Frey and Norris also drew parallels between the processes of critical thinking, nursing, and transaction.

In addition, over time, nursing has developed standardized nursing languages (SNL) that are used to assist the profession to improve communication both within, and external to, the profession. These languages include the Nursing Diagnoses, Nursing Interventions, and Nursing Outcomes. Although these languages were developed after many of the original nursing theorists had completed their

Table 16–3	**Application of the Theory of Goal Attainment**	
TOPIC	**AUTHOR(S)**	**YEAR**
Adolescent health behavior	Hanna	1995
	Hanna	1993
Anxiety	La Fontaine	1989
	Swindale	1989
Birth	Smith	1988
Cardiac rehabilitation	McGirr, Rukhorm, Salmoni, O'Sullivan, and Koren	1990
Case management	Sowell and Lowenstein	1994
Coma	Ackerman, Brink, Clanton, Jones, Moody, Pirlech, Price, and Prusinsky	1989
Diabetes	Husband	1988
Emergency room	Benedict and Frey	1995
	Hughes	1983
Family	Rawlins, Rawlins, and Horner	1990
	King	1989
		1986
		1983
Group psychotherapy	Laben, Sneed, and Seidel	1995
	Laben, Dodd, and Sneed	1991
Health promotion	Calladine	1996
Hospitals	Messmer	1995
HIV	Kemppainen	1990
Interactions	Kameoka	1995
Managed care	Hampton	1993
Neurofibromatosis	Messmer and Neff Smith	1986
Nursing care effectiveness	King	1984
Nursing situations	Nagano and Funashima	1995
	Rooke and Norberg	1988
Oncology	Lockhart*	1992
	Porter	1991
Organ donation	Richard-Hughes	1997
Organizations	Jolly and Winker	1995
Parenting	Norris and Hoyer	1994
Perceptual congruence	Froman	1995
Psychosis	Kemppainen	1990
Psychotherapy	DeHowitt	1992
Quality of life	King	1993
Recovery	Hanucharurnkui and Vinya-nguag	1991
Reproductive health	Hanna	1993
Role strain	Temple and Fawdrey	1992
Senior adults	Woods	1994
	Jonas	1987
Theory-based practice	Messmer	1992
	West	1991
Transactions	Monti*	1992
Transcultural critique	Husting	1997

*Indicates thesis or dissertation

Table 16–4	Development of Middle-Range Theories within the Framework	
TOPIC	**AUTHOR(S)**	**YEAR**
Departmental power (revised to group power)	Sieloff	1998* 1996* 1995
Families, children, and chronic illness	Frey	1995 1993
Family health	Wicks	1995
Family health (families with young chronic mentally ill individuals)	Doornbos	1995
Perceptual awareness	Brooks and Thomas	1997
Satisfaction, client	Killeen*	1996

*Indicates thesis or dissertation or research in progress

works, nursing frameworks such as King's Interacting Systems Framework (1981) can still find application and use in the SNLs. And, it is this type of application that further demonstrates the framework's utility across time. For example, Coker et al. (1995) implemented nursing diagnoses within the context of King's framework. Table 16–4 provides a listing of applications of King's work in relation to the nursing process and to nursing languages.

DEVELOPMENT OF MIDDLE-RANGE THEORIES WITHIN THE FRAMEWORK

Development of middle-range theories is a natural extension of a conceptual framework. Middle-range theories, clearly developed from within a conceptual framework, accomplish two goals: (1) Such theories can be directly applied to nursing situations, whereas a conceptual framework is usually too abstract for such direct application; and (2) validation of middle-range theories, clearly developed within a particular conceptual framework, lends validation to the conceptual framework itself.

In addition to the midrange Theory of Goal Attainment (King, 1981), several other midrange theories have been developed from within King's Interacting Systems framework. In terms of the personal system, Brooks and Thomas (1997) used

Several other midrange theories have been developed from within King's Interacting Systems framework.

King's framework to derive a theory of perceptual awareness. The focus was to develop the concepts of judgment and action as core concepts in the personal system. Other concepts in the theory included communication, perception, and decision making.

In relation to the interpersonal system, several middle-range theories have been developed regarding families. Doornbos (2000) addressed family health in terms of families with young chronically mentally ill individuals. Frey (1995) developed a middle-range theory regarding families, children, and chronic illness; and Wicks (1995) delineated a middle-range theory regarding the broader concept of family health. In relation to social systems, Sieloff (1995a) developed the Theory of Departmental Power to assist in explaining the power of groups within organizations. Table 16–5 further lists middle-range theories developed within King's framework (1981).

Instrument Development

Instrument development in nursing is needed in order to measure relevant nursing concepts. However, instruments developed for a research study rarely undergo the rigor of research undertaken for the purpose of instrument development.

However, review of the literature identified instruments specifically designed within King's framework. King (1988a) developed the Health Goal Attainment instrument, designed to detail the level of attainment of health goals by individual clients. The Family Needs Assessment Tool was developed by Rawlins, Rawlins, and Horner (1990). Table 16–6 provides a listing of instruments developed in relation to King's work.

Clients Across the Life Span

Additional evidence of the scope and usefulness of King's framework and theory is its use with clients across the life span. Several applications have targeted high-risk infants (Frey & Norris, 1997; Norris & Hoyer, 1993; Syzmanski, 1991). Frey (1993, 1995, 1996) developed and tested relationships among

Table 16–5	**Instrument Development Related to King's Work**	
TOPIC	**AUTHOR(S)**	**YEAR**
Family Needs Assessment Tool	Rawlins, Rawlins, and Horner	1990
Health goal attainment	King	1988
Nursing Care Survey (client-consumer perceptions and responses to professional nursing care)	Killeen	1996
Sieloff-King assessment of group power within organizations	Sieloff	1998

multiple systems with children, youth, and young adults. Hanna (1993) investigated the effect of nurse-client interactions on oral-contraceptive adherence in adolescent females. Interestingly, these studies considered personal systems (infants), interpersonal systems (parents, families), and social systems (the nursing staff and hospital environment). Clearly, a strength of King's framework and theory is their utility in encompassing complex settings and situations.

Table 16–6	**Application to Clients across the Life Span**	
TOPIC	**AUTHOR(S)**	**YEAR**
Infants	Frey and Norris	1997
	Norris and Hoyer	1993
	Syzmanski	1991
Children	Scott	1998
	Frey	1996
		1995
	Hobdell	1995
	Frey	1993
		1989
	Steele	1981
Adolescents	Hanna	1995
		1993
	Binder*	1992
	Laben, Dodd, and Sneed	1991
	Hughes	1983
	Daubenmire, Searles, and Ashton	1978
Adults, young	Doornbos	1995
Adults	Ollsson and Forsdahl	1996
	Alligood	1995
	Froman	1995
	Jones, Clark, Merker, and Palau	1995
	Kameoka	1995
	Nagano and Funashima	1995
	Rooke	1995
	Sharts-Hopko	1995
	Norris and Hoyer	1994
	Hanna	1993
	DeHowitt	1992
	Heggie and Gangar	1992
	Hobdell	1992

(Continued on the following page)

Table 16–6	**Application to Clients across the Life Span** *(Continued)*	
TOPIC	**AUTHOR(S)**	**YEAR**
Adults *(continued)*	Lockhart*	1992
	Laben, Dodd, and Sneed	1991
	Hanucharurnkui and Vinya-nguag	1990
	Kemppainen	1990
	McGirr, Rukholm, Salmoni, O'Sullivan, and Koren	1990
	Martin	1990
	Glenn*	1989
	O'Shall*	1989
	Sirles and Selleck	1989
	Swindale	1989
	Husband	1988
	Smith	1988
	Laben, Sneed, and Seidel	1986
	Jonas	1987
	Pearson and Vaughan	1986
	King and Tarsitano	1982
	King	1984
	Strauss	1981
	Brown and Lee	1980
	Daubenmire, Searles, and Ashton	1978
Adults, mature	Allan*	1995
	Jones, Clark, Merker, and Palau	1995
	Rooke	1995
	Woods	1994
	Tawil*	1993
	Temple and Fawdry	1992
	Zurakowski*	1991
	Kenny	1990
	Miller	1990
	Kohler	1988
	Jonas	1987
	King	1983
	Rosendahl and Ross	1982

*Indicates thesis or dissertation

The Interacting Systems Framework and midrange Theory of Goal Attainment have also been used to guide practice with adults (young adults, adults, mature adults) with a broad range of concerns. Doornbos (1995) used King's work in her study of young adults experiencing chronic mental illness.

Examples of applications focusing on adults include cardiac disease (McGirr, Rukholm, Salmoni, O'Sullivan, & Koren, 1990), chemical dependence (McKinney & Dean, 2000), diabetes (Husband, 1988), and renal procedures (Hanucharurnkui & Vinya-nguag, 1990). Gender-specific work included Sharts-Hopko's (1995) use of concepts within the Interacting Systems Framework to study the health status of women during menopause transition and Martin's (1990) application of the framework toward cancer awareness among males.

Several of the applications with adults have targeted the mature adult, thus demonstrating contributions to the nursing specialty of gerontology. Kohler (1988) used the framework to increase elderly clients' sense of shared control over health and health behaviors. Kenny (1990) also studied the role of the elderly in their care. Milne (2000) studied the "impact of information on the health behaviors of older adults" (p. 161). In addition,

Woods (1994) proposed that the Theory of Goal Attainment can be used to decrease chronic health problems among nursing home residents. Clearly, these applications, and others, show how the complexity of King's framework and midrange theory increases its usefulness for nursing (refer to Table 16–7).

Client Systems

A major strength of King's work is that it can be used with virtually all client populations. In addition to discussing client populations across the life span, client populations can be identified by focus of care (client system) and/or focus of health problem (phenomenon of concern). The focus of care, or interest, can be an individual (personal system) or group (interpersonal or social system). Thus, application of King's work, across client systems, would be divided into the three systems identified within King's Interacting Systems Framework (1981): personal (the individual), interpersonal (small groups), and social (large groups/society).

Table 16–7	**Application to Various Client Systems**	
TOPIC	**AUTHOR(S)**	**YEAR**
Personal systems	Brooks and Thomas	1997
	Frey and Norris	1997
	Hanna	1993
	Jackson, Pokorny, and Vincent	1993
	DeHowitt	1992
	Hanucharurnkui and Vinya-nguag	1990
	Kemppainen	1990
	Kenny	1990
	McGirr, Rukholm, Salmoni, O'Sullivan, and Koren	1990
	Husband	1988
	Kohler	1988
	Levine, Wilson, and Guido	1988
	Smith	1988
	Jonas	1987
	Pearson and Vaughan	1986
	King	1984
	Hughes	1983
	King and Tarsitano	1982
Interpersonal systems	O'Shall*	1989
Interpersonal systems (families)	Frey and Norris	1997
	Norris and Hoyer	1994
	Frey	1993
	Temple and Fawdry	1992
	Spees	1991
	Syzmanski	1991
	Dispenza*	1990
	Rawlins, Rawlins, and Horner	1990
	Sirles and Selleck	1989
	Frey	1989
	Davis	1987
	Gonot	1986
	Messmer and Neff Smith	1986
	King	1983
	Strauss	1981
Interpersonal systems (groups)	Woods	1994
	Monti*	1992
	Laben, Dodd, and Sneed	1991

(Continued on the following page)

Table 16–7	**Application to Various Client Systems** *(Continued)*	
TOPIC	**AUTHOR(S)**	**YEAR**
Interpersonal systems (nurse-client)	Nagano and Funashima	1995
	DeHowitt	1992
	Houfek	1992
	Temple and Fawdry	1992
	Rundell	1991
	Martin	1990
	Swindale	1989
	Kohler	1988
	Messmer and Smith	1986
	Daubenmire, Searles, and Ashton	1978
Interpersonal systems (stepfamilies)	Omar*	1990
Social systems	Brown and Lee	1980
Social systems (aggregates)	Norgan, Ettipio, and Lasome	1995
Social systems (communities)	Temple and Fawdry	1992
	Hanchett	1990
	Hanchett	1988
	Myks Babb, Fouladbakhsh, and Hanchett	1988
	Asay and Ossler	1984
	King	1984
Social systems (education)	Daubenmire	1989
	Gulitz and King	1988
	Froman and Sanderson	1985
	Brown and Lee	1980
	Daubenmire and King	1973
Social systems (nursing unit)	Rundell	1991
Social systems (organizations)	Tritsch	1996
	Fawcett, Vaillancourt, and Watson	1995
	Jolly and Winker	1995
	Messmer	1995
	Sieloff	1995
	Fitch, Rogers, Ross, Shea, Smith, and Tucker	1991
	Schreiber	1991
	West	1991
	Byrne-Coker, Fradley, Harris, Tomarchio, and Caron	1990
	Kenny	1990
	Byrne and Schreiber	1989
	Elberson	1989
	Hampton	1989
	LaFontaine	1989

*Indicates thesis or dissertation

Use with personal systems has included both patients and nurses. Patients as personal systems were the focus of applications by DeHowitt (1992). Levine, Wilson, and Guido (1988) considered critical care nurses as the personal system of interest, as did Brooks and Thomas (1997).

When the focus of interest moves from an individual to include interaction between two people, the interpersonal system is involved. Interpersonal systems often include clients and nurses. Examples of an application to a nurse-client dyad and larger groups is Messmer and Neff Smith's (1986) approach to nursing with clients with neurofibromatosis, and Campbell-Begg (2000) studied "animal-assisted therapy to promote abstinence from the use of chemicals by groups" (p. 31).

In relation to interpersonal systems, or small groups, many publications focus on the family. Gonot (1986) proposed the Interacting Systems Framework as a model for family therapy. Frey and Norris (1997) used both the Interacting Systems Framework and Theory of Goal Attainment in planning care with families of premature infants.

King's Interacting Systems Framework and midrange Theory of Goal Attainment have a long history of application with large groups or social systems (organizations, communities). The earliest applications involved the use of the framework and theory to guide continuing education (Brown & Lee, 1980) and nursing curricula (Daubenmire, 1989; Gulitz & King, 1988). More contemporary applications address models of care. For example, the framework served as the basis for practice in an acute-care setting (Byrne & Schreiber, 1989). In addition, applications proposed the Theory of Goal Attainment as the practice model for case management (Hampton, 1994; Tritsch, 1996). These latter applications are especially important, as they may be the first use of the framework by other disciplines.

Within organizations, a midrange theory of departmental power has been developed (Sieloff, 1995a) and revised into a Theory of Group Power within Organizations (2003). Educational settings, also considered as social systems, have also been the focus of application of King's work (Bello, 2000; Froman & Sanderson, 1985). Table 16–8

Table 16–8	**Application to Client Concerns**	
TOPIC	**AUTHOR(S)**	**YEAR**
Care of self	Hanucharurnkui and Vinya-nguag	1991
Autonomy	Glenn*	1989
	Husband	1988
Birth	Smith	1988
Goal-setting	Tritsch	1996
Health promotion	Calladine	1996
	Hanna	1995
Body weight	Sharts-Hopko	1995
Menopause	Hanna	1993
	Heggie and Gangar	1992
Morale	Kohler	1988
Parenting	Norris and Hoyer	1993
Reproductive health	Hanna	1993
Role	O'Shall*	1989
Sexual counseling	Villeneuve and Ozolins*	1991
Stress	DeHowitt	1992
	Dispenza*	1990
Health status	Frey	1996
		1995
	Doornbos	1995
	Woods	1994
	Smith	1988
Illness management		
Asthma	Frey	1995
Anxiety	Swindale	1989
Bronchopneumonia	Pearson and Vaughan	1986
Cardiac rehabilitation	McGirr, Rukhorm, Salmoni, O'Sullivan, and Koren	1990
Cardiovascular	Sirles and Selleck	1989
Carpal tunnel syndrome	Norgan, Ettipio, and Lasome	1995
Chronic illness	Wicks	1995
Chronic obstructive pulmonary disorder	Wicks	1995

(Continued on the following page)

Table 16–8	**Application to Client Concerns** *(Continued)*	
TOPIC	**AUTHOR(S)**	**YEAR**
Illness management *(continued)*		
Coma	Ackerman, Brink, Clanton, Jones, Moody, Pirlech, Price, and Prusensky	1989
Diabetes	Frey	1995
		1988
	White-Linn*	1994
	Husband	1988
	Jonas	1987
End-stage renal disease	King	1984
HIV	Kemppainen	1990
	Syzmanski	1991
High-risk infants	Woods	1994
Hypertension	Hanucharurnkui and Vinya-nguag	1991
Nephrology	Hobdell	1995
	Messmer and Neff Smith	1986
Neural tube defects	Nagano and Funashima	1995
Neurofibromatosis	Lockhart*	1992
Oncology	Temple and Fawdry	1992
	Porter	1991
	Martin	1990
	Alligood	1995
Orthopedic	Kameoka	1995
	Jackson, Pokorny, and Vincent	1993
Ostomy	Temple and Fawdry	1992
Pain management	Hanucharurnkui and Vinya-nguag	1991
	Murray and Baier	1996
	Doornbos	1995
Psychiatric	Laben, Sneed, and Seidel	1995
	DeHowitt	1991
	Gonot	1990
	Schreiber	1990
	Kemppainen	1982
	Rosendahl and Ross	1982
Terminal illness	Woods	1994
Risky health behaviors	Frey	1996
Smoking	Kneeshaw	1990
Well-being	DeHowitt	1992

*Indicates thesis or dissertation

consolidates applications of King's work to various client systems.

Phenomena of Concern to Clients

Within King's work, it is critically important for the nurse to focus on, and address, the phenomenon of concern to the client. Without this emphasis on the client's perspective, mutual goal-setting cannot occur. Hence, a client's phenomena of concern was selected as neutral terminology that clearly demon-strated the broad application of King's work to a wide variety of practice situations. Table 16–9 sum-marizes applications related to clients' phenomena of concern; the table also groups these applications, primarily identified by disease or medical diagno-sis, as illness management.

Health is one area that certainly binds clients and nurses. Improved health is clearly the desired end point, or outcome, of nursing care and something to which clients aspire. Review of the

Table 16–9	**Application within Nursing Specialties**	
TOPIC	**AUTHOR(S)**	**YEAR**
Administration	Olsson and Forsdahl	1996
	Winker*	1996
	Sieloff	1995
	Batchelor*	1994
	Hampton	1994
	Elberson	1989
	Glenn*	1989
	King	1989
	O'Shall*	1989
Cardiovascular	Woods	1994
Case management	Sowell and Lowenstein	1994
Chronic illness	White-Linn*	1994
Continuing education	Brown and Lee	1980
Critical care	Scott	1998
	Norris and Hoyer	1994
Education	Brooks*	1995
	Rooke	1995
	Daubenmire	1989
	King	1986
	Froman and Sanderson	1985
	Asay and Ossler	1984
	Brown and Lee	1980
	Daubenmire and King	1973
Education, client	King and Tarsitano	1982
Endocrinology	Frey	1989
	Husband	1988
	Jonas	1987
Forensic	Laben, Dodd, and Sneed	1991
Genetics	Messmer and Neff Smith	1988
Gerontology	Rooke	1995
	Woods	1994
	Temple and Fawdry	1992
	Kenny	1990
	Jonas	1987
Hospice	Woods	1994
Medical-surgical	Froman	1995
	Rooke	1995
Mother-child	Dawson*	1996
	Omar*	1990
Nephrology	King	1984
Oncology	Nagano and Funashima	1995
	Lockhart*	1992
	Porter	1991
Orthopedics	Alligood	1995
	Kameoka	1995
Neurology	Messmer and Neff Smith	1986
Nurses	Olsson and Forsdahl	1996
	Kneeshaw	1990
Political action	Krassa*	1994

(Continued on the following page)

Table 16–9	**Application within Nursing Specialties** (Continued)	
TOPIC	**AUTHOR(S)**	**YEAR**
Psychiatric/Mental health	Murray and Baier	1996
	Doornbos	1995
	Laben, Sneed, and Seidel	1995
	DeHowitt	1992
	Schreiber	1991
	Kemppainen	1990
	Gonot	1986
Quality improvement	Killeen* (client satisfaction)	1996
	O'Connor* (client satisfaction)	1990
Respiratory	Davis and Dearman	1991
	Pearson and Vaughan	1986
Reproductive health	Hanna	1993
Surgery	Gill, Hopwood-Jones, Tyndall, Gregoroff, LeBlanc, Lovett, Rasco, and Ross	1995
	Rooke	1995
	Porteous and Tyndall	1994
	King and Tarsitano	1982
	Daubenmire, Searles, and Ashton	1978

*Indicates thesis or dissertation

outcome of nursing care, as addressed in published applications, tends to support the goal of improved health directly and/or indirectly, as the result of the application of King's work. Health status is explicitly the outcome of concern in practice applications by Smith (1988). Several applications used health-related terms. For example, Kohler (1988) focused on increased morale and satisfaction, and DeHowitt (1992) studied well-being.

Health promotion has also been an emphasis for the application of King's ideas. Sexual counseling was the focus of work by Villeneuve and Ozolins (1991). The experience of parenting was studied by Norris and Hoyer (1993), and health behaviors were Hanna's (1995) focus of study.

King (1981) stated that individuals act to maintain their own health. Although not explicitly stated, the converse is probably true as well: Individuals often do things that are not good for their health. Accordingly, it is not surprising that the Interacting Systems Framework and related midrange theory are often directed toward patient and group behaviors that influence health. Frey (1997), Frey and Denyes (1989), and Frey and Fox (1990) looked at both health behaviors and illness management behaviors in several groups of children with chronic conditions. In addition, Frey (1996) expanded her research to include risky behaviors.

As stated previously, diseases or diagnoses are often identified as the focus for the application of nursing knowledge. Pearson and Vaughan (1986) conducted research with patients with bronchopneumonia, while patients with end-stage renal disease were the focus of Jonas' (1987) work. In addition, clients with chronic inflammatory bowel disease were involved in research by Daniel (2002).

Clients experiencing a variety of psychiatric concerns have also been the focus of work, using King's conceptualizations (Murray & Baier, 1996; Schreiber, 1991). Clients' concerns ranged from psychotic symptoms (Kemppainen, 1990) to families experiencing chronic mental illness (Doornbos, 2002) to clients in short-term group psychotherapy (Laben, Sneed, & Seidel, 1995). Table 16–9 delineates applications related to clients' phenomena of concern.

Multicultural Applications

Multicultural applications of King's Interacting Systems Framework and related theories are many. Such applications are particularly critical as a frequent limitation expressed regarding theoretical formulations are their culture-bound nature. Several authors specifically addressed the utility of King's framework and theory for transcultural nursing. Spratlen (1976) drew heavily from King's framework and theory to integrate ethnic cultural factors into nursing curricula and to develop a culturally oriented model for mental health care. Key elements derived from King's work were the focus on perceptions and communication patterns that motivate action, reaction, interaction, and transaction. Rooda (1992) derived propositions from the midrange Theory of Goal Attainment as the framework for a conceptual model for multicultural nursing.

Cultural relevance has also been demonstrated in reviews by Frey, Rooke, Sieloff, Messmer, and Kamcoka (1995) and Husting (1997). Although Husting identified that cultural issues were implicit variables throughout King's framework, particular attention was given to the concept of health, which, according to King (1990), acquires meaning from cultural values and social norms.

Undoubtedly, the strongest evidence for the cultural utility of King's conceptual framework and midrange Theory of Goal Attainment (1981) is the extent of work that has been done in other cultures. Applications of the framework and related theories have been documented in the following countries beyond the United States: Canada (Coker et al., 1995), Japan (Funashima, 1990; Kameoka & Sugimori, 1992), Portugal (Moreira & Arajo, 2002; Viera & Rossi, 2000), and Sweden (Rooke, 1995a, 1995b). In Japan, a culture very different from the United States with regard to communication style, Kameoka (1995) used the classification system of nurse-patient interactions identified within the Theory of Goal Attainment (King, 1981) to analyze nurse-patient interactions. In addition to research and publications regarding the application of King's work to nursing practice internationally, publications by and about Dr. King have been translated into other languages, including Japanese (King, 1976, 1985; Kobayashi, 1970). Therefore, perception and the influence of culture on perception were identified as strengths of King's theory. Table 16–10 lists applications of King's work in countries outside the United States.

Table 16–10	**Application within Nursing Work Settings**	
TOPIC	**AUTHOR(S)**	**YEAR**
Clinics	Hanna	1993
	DeHowitt	1992
	Porter	1991
	Kemppainen	1990
	Frey	1989
	Husband	1988
	Gonot	1986
Community	Sowell and Lowenstein	1994
	Temple and Fawdry	1992
	King	1984
Home health	Rosendahl and Ross	1982
Hospitals	Frey and Norris	1997
	Olsson and Forsdahl	1996
	Tritsch	1996
	Gill, Hopwood-Jones, Tyndall, Gregoroff, LeBlanc, Lovett, Rasco, and Ross	1995
	Jones, Clark, Merker, and Palau	1995
	Nagano and Funashima	1994
	Sowell and Lowenstein	1993
	Hampton	1993
	Jackson, Pokorny, and Vincent	1993
	Norris and Hoyer	1993

(Continued on the following page)

Table 16–10	Application within Nursing Work Settings *(Continued)*	
TOPIC	**AUTHOR(S)**	**YEAR**
Hospitals *(continued)*	Messmer	1992
	Fitch, Rogers, Ross, Shea, Smith, and Tucker	1991
	West	1991
	Kemppainen	1990
	Kenny	1990
	LaFontaine	1989
	Levine, Wilson, and Guido	1988
	Jonas	1987
	Pearson and Vaughan	1986
	King	1984
	Rosendahl and Ross	1982
	Daubenmire, Searles, and Ashton	1978
Hospitals, community	Coker, Fradley, Harris, Tomarchio, Chan, and Caron	1995
	Byrne-Coker, Fradley, Harris, Tomarchio, Chan, and Caron	1990
	Byrne and Schreiber	1989
	Schreiber	1991
Hospitals, public	Messmer	1995
Hospitals, urban	Messmer	1995
	King and Tarsitano	1982
Intensive care units	Scott	1998
	Rooke	1995
	Norris and Hoyer	1994
	Jacono, Hicks, Antontoni, O'Brien, and Rasi	1990
Nursing homes	Woods	1994
	Zurakowski*	1991
Step-down units	Rundell	1991

*Indicates thesis or dissertation

ADMINISTRATION

The theory and conceptual model also can apply in various situations relevant to nursing work and administration.

Nursing Specialties

A topic that frequently divides nurses is their area of specialty. However, by using a consistent framework across specialties, nurses would be able to focus more clearly on their commonalities, rather than highlighting their differences. A review of the literature clearly demonstrates that Dr. King's framework and related theories have application within a variety of nursing specialties (see Table 16–11). This application is evident whether one is reviewing a "traditional" specialty, such as medical-surgical nursing (Gill et al., 1995; King & Tarsitano, 1982; Porteous & Tyndall, 1994), or in the nontraditional specialties of forensic nursing (Laben, Dodd, & Sneed, 1991) and/or nursing administration (Elberson, 1989).

Work Settings

An additional source of division within the nursing profession is the work sites where nursing is practiced and care is delivered. As the delivery of health care moves from the more traditional site of the acute care hospital to community-based agencies and clients' homes, it is important to highlight commonalities across these settings, and it is important to identify that King's framework and midrange Theory of Goal Attainment continue to

> *Although many applications tend to be with nurses and clients in traditional settings, successful applications have been shown across other, including newer and nontraditional, settings.*

Table 16–11	Application within the Nursing Process and Related Languages		
TOPIC	**AUTHOR(S)**		**YEAR**
Documentation	King		1984
Nursing diagnoses	Gill, Hopwood-Jones, Tyndall, Gregorott, LeBlanc, Lovett, Rasco, and Ross		1995
	Byrne-Coker, Fradley, Harris, Tomarchio, Chan, and Caron		1990
Nursing process	Frey and Norris		1997
	Calladine		1996
	Woods		1992
	Schreiber		1991

be applicable. Although many applications tend to be with nurses and clients in traditional settings, successful applications have been shown across other, including newer and nontraditional, settings. From hospitals (Jacono, Hicks, Antonioni, O'Brien, & Rasi, 1990; Lockhart, 2000) to nursing homes (Zurakowski, 2000), King's framework and related theories provide a foundation on which nurses can build their practice interventions. Table 16–12 lists applications within a variety of nursing work settings.

HEALTH CARE BEYOND NURSING

When originally developing the Interacting Systems Framework, King (1981) borrowed from knowledge external to nursing and used a systems framework perspective to assist in explaining nursing phenomena. This use of knowledge across disciplines occurs frequently and can be very appropriate if both disciplines' perspectives are similar and reformulation occurs. Because of King's emphasis on the attainment of goals and the relevancy of goal attainment to many disciplines, both within and external to health care, it is reasonable to expect that King's work could find application

beyond nursing-specific situations. Two specific examples of this include the application of King's work to case management (Hampton, 1994; Sowell & Lowenstein, 1994) and to managed care (Hampton, 1994). Both case management and managed care incorporate multiple disciplines as they work to improve the overall quality and cost efficiency of the health care provided. These applications also address the continuum of care, a priority in today's health-care environment. Table 16–13 details applications of King's work beyond nursing.

Recommendations for Knowledge Development Related to King's Framework and Theory

Obviously, new nursing knowledge has resulted from applications of King's framework and theory. However, nursing, as are all sciences, is evolving. Additional work continues to be needed. Based on a review of the applications previously discussed, recommendations for future knowledge development focus on (1) the need for evidenced-based

Table 16–12	Application to Health Care beyond Nursing		
TOPIC	**AUTHOR(S)**		**YEAR**
Advocacy	Bramlett, Gueldner, and Sowell		1990
Case management	Tritsch		1996
	Hampton		1994
	Sowell and Lowenstein		1994
Managed care	Hampton		1994

Table 16–13	**Multicultural Application**	
TOPIC	**AUTHOR(S)**	**YEAR**
Documentation	King	1984
African-American	Richard-Hughes	1997
Canada	Gill, Hopwood-Jones, Tyndall, Gregoroff, LeBlanc, Lovett, Rasco, and Ross	1995
	Porteous and Tyndall	1994
	Byrne-Coker, Fradley, Harris, Tomarchio, Chan, and Caron	1990
	Fitch, Rogers, Ross, Shea, Smith, and Tucker	1991
	Porter	1991
	Schreiber	1991
	Byrne and Schreiber	1989
England	Pearson and Vaughan	1986
Japan	Kameoka	1995
	Nagano and Funashima	1995
	Kusaka	1991
Norway	Olsson and Forsdahl	1996
Sweden	Rooke	1995
		1995
	Rooke and Norberg	1988
Multicultural approach	Frey, Rooke, Sieloff, Messmer, and Kameoka	1995
	Rooda	1992
	King	1990
	Spratlen	1976

nursing practice that is theoretically derived; (2) the integration of King's work in evidence-based nursing practice; (3) the integration of King's concepts within standardized nursing language (SNLs); (4) analyzing the future impact of managed care, continuous quality improvement, and technology on King's concepts; (5) identification, or development and implementation, of relevant instruments; and (6) clarification of effective nursing interventions, including identification of relevant NICs, based on King's work.

EVIDENCE-BASED PRACTICE DERIVED FROM THEORY

What is evidence-based practice and how will evidence-based nursing practice evolve? Even though Florence Nightingale realized the importance of using evidence to guide practice 135 years ago, the field of medicine takes credit for the current trend of evidence-based practice.

However, nursing, as a discipline, has continued to evolve in the use of scientific evidence. Titler (1998), a nurse, defines evidence-based practice as

"the conscientious and judicious use of current best evidence to guide health care decisions" (p. 1). Similar to evidence-based medicine, nursing must attend to what is critical for effective nursing care. The questions practicing nurses address, and the types of research that provide these answers, are likely to be different from the questions of other disciplines.

From an evidence-based practice and King's perspective, the profession must implement three strategies to apply theory-based research findings effectively. First, nursing as a discipline must develop rules of evidence in evaluation of quality research that reflect the unique contribution of nursing to health care. Second, the nursing rules of evidence must include heavier weight for research that is derived from, or adds to, nursing theory. Third, the nursing rules of evidence must reflect higher scores when nursing's central beliefs are affirmed in the choice of variables. King's (1981) work on the concepts of client and nurse perceptions, and the achievement of mutual goals, has been assimilated and accepted as core beliefs of the discipline. This third strategy of the use of concepts central to nursing has clear relevance for evidence-based practice when using King's (1981) concepts, such as perception.

Research conducted with a King theoretical base is well positioned for application by nurse caregivers, nurse administrators (Sieloff, 2003), and client-consumers (Killeen, 1996) as part of an evolving definition of evidence-based nursing practice. For example, King (1971) addressed client preference, a possible part of an evidence-based nursing definition, as satisfaction. In an update of the concept of satisfaction, King submits that satisfaction is a subset of her central concept of perceptions (Killeen, 1996).

KING'S CONCEPTS, THE NURSING PROCESS, AND STANDARDIZED NURSING LANGUAGES

The steps of the nursing process have long been integrated within King's interacting systems framework and midrange Theory of Goal Attainment (Daubenmire & King, 1973; Husband, 1988; Woods, 1994). In these process applications, assessment, diagnosis, and goal-setting occur, followed by actions based on the nurse-client goals. The evaluation component of the nursing process consistently refers back to the original goal statement(s). With the use of standardized nursing languages (SNLs), the nursing process is further refined. Standardized terms for diagnoses, interventions, and outcomes potentially improve communication among nurses.

Using SNLs enables the development of middle-range theory by building on concepts unique to nursing, such as those concepts of King that can be directly applied to the nursing process: action, reaction, interaction, transaction, goal-setting, and goal attainment. Biegen and Tripp-Reimer (1997) suggested middle-range theories be constructed from the concepts in the taxonomies of the nursing languages focusing on outcomes. Alternatively, King's framework and theory may be used as a theoretical basis for these phenomena and may assist in knowledge development in nursing in the future.

With the advent of SNLs, "outcome identification" is identified as a step in the nursing process following assessment and diagnosis (McFarland & McFarland, 1997, p. 3). King's (1981) concept of mutual goal-setting is analogous to the outcomes identification step, because King's concept of goal attainment is congruent with the evaluation of client outcomes.

In addition, King's concept of perception (1981) lends itself well to the definition of client outcomes. Johnson and Maas (1997) define a nursing-sensitive client outcome as "a measurable client or family caregiver state, behavior, or perception that is conceptualized as a variable and is largely influenced and sensitive to nursing interventions" (p. 22). This is fortuitous since the development of nursing knowledge requires the use of client outcome measurement. The use of standardized client outcomes as study variables increases the ease with which research findings could be compared across settings and contributes to knowledge development. Therefore, King's concept of mutually set goals could be studied as "expected outcomes." In addition, using SNLs, King's (1981) midrange Theory of Goal Attainment could be conceptualized as "attainment of expected outcomes" as the evaluation step in the application of the nursing process.

IMPACT OF MANAGED CARE AND TECHNOLOGY ON KING'S CONCEPTS

Both managed care and increasing use of technology have challenged existing conceptual frameworks of nursing, requiring adaptation and evolution. The following is an overview of the ways that King's concepts have evolved within this changing health-care climate.

Managed Care

With managed care, nursing is increasingly involved with collaboratively developing evidence-based care planning tools and critical pathways, protocols, and guidelines with other disciplines. King (1981) has always promoted cooperation and collaboration among disciplines.

In the managed care environment, personal, interpersonal, and social systems need to include an expanded conceptualization of King's concept of goal-setting. Personal and professional goal-setting, nurse-client/consumer dyad goal-setting, nurse task force and team goal-setting, and nurse leader-organization goal-setting are examples of broader applications common in nursing situations.

Multidisciplinary care conferences, an example of a situation where goal-setting among professionals occurs, is a label for an indirect nursing intervention within the Nursing Interventions Classification (Dochterman & Bulechek, 2000). Some of the activities listed under this label reflect King's (1981) concepts: "establish mutually agreeable goals; solicit input for client care planning; revise client care plan, as necessary; discuss progress toward goals; and provide data to facilitate evaluation of client care plan" (p. 460).

Technology

King (1997) is keeping pace with the changing world of technology by exploring the impact of nursing knowledge on technology, positing that her conceptual system provides the structure for health-care informatics. Specifically, she recommends using her concepts of self, role, power, authority, decisions, time, space, communication, and interaction with an emphasis on goal-setting and goal attainment as the theoretical basis for nursing informatics. With this forward-looking direction set by the theorist, nurse scholars need to further evaluate the use of King's concepts, and possibly, redefine them in relation to future contexts. For example, the concepts of interactions and transactions now occur without visual perceptions in the emerging area of telenursing.

SUMMARY

An essential component in the analysis of conceptual frameworks and theories is the consideration of their adequacy (Ellis, 1968). Adequacy depends on the three interrelated characteristics of scope, usefulness, and complexity. Conceptual frameworks are broad in scope and are sufficiently complex to be useful for many situations. Theories, on the other hand, are narrower in scope, usually addressing less abstract concepts, and are more specific in terms of the nature and direction of relationships and focus.

King fully intended her Interacting Systems Framework for nursing to be useful in all nursing situations. Likewise, the midrange Theory of Goal Attainment (King, 1981) has broad scope because interaction is a part of every nursing encounter.

Although evaluation of the scope of King's framework and midrange theory has resulted in mixed reviews (Austin & Champion, 1983; Carter & Dufour, 1994; Frey, 1996; Jonas, 1987; Meleis, 1985), the nursing profession has clearly recognized their scope and usefulness. In addition, the variety of practice applications evident in the literature clearly attest to the complexity of King's work. As researchers continue to integrate King's theory and framework with the dynamic health-care environment, future applications involving evidence-based practice will continue to demonstrate the adequacy of King's work in terms of nursing practice.

References

Alligood, M. R. (1995). Theory of goal attainment: Application to adult orthopedic nursing. In Frey, M. A., & Sieloff, C. L. (Eds.), *Advancing King's systems framework and theory of nursing* (pp. 209–222). Thousand Oaks, CA: Sage Publications.

Alligood, M. R., Evans, G. W., & Wilt, D. L. (1995). King's interacting systems and empathy. In Frey, M. A., & Sieloff, C. L., (Eds.), *Advancing King's systems framework and theory of nursing* (pp. 66–78). Thousand Oaks, CA: Sage Publications.

Austin, J. K., & Champion, V. L. (1983). King's theory for nursing: Explication and evaluation. In Chinn, P. L. (Ed.), *Advances in nursing theory development* (pp. 49–61). Rockville, MD: Aspen.

Baumann, S. L. (2000). Research issues: Family nursing: Theory-anemic, nursing theory-derived. *Nursing Science Quarterly, 13*(4), 285–290.

Bello, I. T. R. (2000). Imogene King's theory as the foundation for the set of a teaching-learning process with undergrauation [sic] students [Portuguese]. *Texto & Contexto Enfermagem, 9*(2 part 2), 646–657.

Benedict, M., & Frey, M. A. (1995). Theory-based practice in the emergency department. In Frey, M. A., & Sieloff, C. L. (Eds.), *Advancing King's systems framework and theory of nursing* (pp. 317–324). Thousand Oaks, CA: Sage Publications.

Biegen, M. A., & Tripp-Reimer, T. (1997). Implications of nursing taxonomies for middle-range theory development. *Advances in Nursing Science, 19*(3), 37–49.

Bramlett, M. H., Gueldner, S. H., & Sowell, R. L. (1989). Consumer centric advocacy: Its connection to nursing frameworks. *Nursing Science Quarterly, 3*(4), 156–161.

Brooks, E. M., & Thomas, S. (1997). The perception and judgement of senior baccalaureate student nurses in clinical decision making. *Advances in Nursing Science, 19*(3), 50–69.

Brown, S. T., & Lee, B. T. (1980). Imogene King's conceptual framework: A proposed model for continuing nursing education. *Journal of Advanced Nursing, 5,* 467–473.

Bunting, S. M. (1988). The concept of perception in selected nursing theories. *Nursing Science Quarterly, 1*(4), 168–174.

Byrne, E., & Schreiber, R. (1989). Concept of the month: Implementing King's conceptual framework at the bedside. *Journal of Nursing Administration, 19*(2), 28–32.

Calladine, M. L. (1996). Nursing process for health promotion using King's theory. *Journal of Community Health Nursing, 13*(1), 51–57.

Campbell-Begg, T. (2000). A case study using animal-assisted therapy to promote abstinence in a group of individuals who are recovering from chemical addictions. *Journal of Addictions Nursing, 12*(1), 31–35.

Carter, K. F., & Dufour, L. T. (1994). King's theory: A critique of the critiques. *Nursing Science Quarterly, 7*(3), 128–133.

Coker, E. A., & Schreiber, R. (1989). King at the bedside. *The Canadian Nurse,* 24.

Coker, E., Fradley, T., Harris, J., Tomarchio, D., Chan, V., & Caron, C. (1995). Implementing nursing diagnoses within the context of King's conceptual framework. In Frey, M. A., & Sieloff, C. L. (Eds.), *Advancing King's systems framework and theory of nursing* (pp. 161–176). Thousand Oaks, CA: Sage Publications.

Daniel, J. M. (2002). Young adults' perceptions of living with chronic inflammatory bowel disease. *Gastroenterology Nursing, 25*(3), 83–94.

Daubenmire, M. J. (1989). A baccalaureate nursing curriculum based on King's conceptual framework. In Riehl-Sisca, J. P. (Ed.), *Conceptual models for nursing practice* (3rd ed., pp. 167–178). Norwalk, CT: Appleton & Lange.

Daubenmire, M. J., & King, I. M. (1973). Nursing process models: A systems approach. *Nursing Outlook, 21,* 512–517.

Daubenmire, M. J., Searles, S. S., & Ashton, C. A. (1978). A methodologic framework to study nurse patient communication. *Nursing Research, 27*(5), 303–310.

Davis, D. C. (1987). A conceptual framework for infertility. *Journal of Obstetric, Gynecologic, and Neonatal Nursing, 16,* 30–35.

Davis, D. C., & Dearman, C. N. (1991). Coping strategies of infertile women. *Journal of Obstetric, Gynecologic, and Neonatal Nursing, 20,* 221–228.

DeFeo, D. J. (1990). Change: A central concern of nursing. *Nursing Science Quarterly, 3*(2), 88–94.

DeHowitt, M. C. (1992). King's conceptual model and individual psychotherapy. *Perspectives in Psychiatric Care, 28*(4), 11–14.

Dochterman, J. M., & Bulechek, G. M. (2000). *Nursing interventions classification (NIC)* (3rd ed.). St Louis: Mosby.

Doornbos, M. M. (1995). Using King's systems framework to explore family health in the families of the young chronically mentally ill. In Frey, M. A., & Sieloff, C. L. (Eds.), *Advancing King's systems framework and theory of nursing* (pp. 192–205). Thousand Oaks, CA: Sage Publications.

Doornbos, M. M. (2000). King's systems framework and family health: The derivation and testing of a theory. *Journal of Theory Construction & Testing, 4*(1), 20–26.

Doornbos, M. M. (2002). Predicting family health in families with young adults with severe mental illness. *Journal of Family Nursing, 8*(3), 241–263.

Elberson, K. (1989). Applying King's model to nursing administration. In Henry, B., DiVicenti, M., Arndt, C., & Marriner, A. (Eds.), *Dimensions of nursing administration: Theory, research, education and practice* (pp. 47–53). Boston: Blackwell Scientific Publications.

Ellis, R. (1968). Characteristics of significant theories. *Nursing Research, 17,* 217–222.

Fawcett, J. (1978). The relationship between theory and research: A double helix. *Advances in Nursing Science, 1*(1), 49–62.

Fawcett, J. M., Vaillancourt, V. M., & Watson, C. A. (1995). Integration of King's framework into nursing practice. In Frey, M. A., & Sieloff, C. L. (Eds.), *Advancing King's systems framework and theory of nursing* (pp. 176–191). Thousand Oaks, CA: Sage Publications.

Fitch, M., Rogers, M., Ross, E., Shea, H., Smith, I., & Tucker, D. (1991). Developing a plan to evaluate the use of nursing conceptual frameworks. *Canadian Journal of Nursing Administration, 4*(1), 22–28.

Frey, M. A. (1989). Social support and health: A theoretical formulation derived from King's conceptual framework. *Nursing Science Quarterly, 2*(2), 138–148.

Frey, M. A. (1993). A theoretical perspective of family and child health derived from King's conceptual framework of nursing: A deductive approach to theory building. In Feetham, S. L., Meister, S. B., Bell, J. M., & Gillis, C. L. (Eds.), *The nursing of families: Theory/research/education/practice* (pp. 30–37). Newbury Park, CA: Sage Publications.

Frey, M. A. (1995). Toward a theory of families, children, and chronic illness. In Frey, M. A., & Sieloff, C. L. (Eds.), *Advancing King's systems framework and theory of nursing* (pp. 109–125). Thousand Oaks, CA: Sage Publications.

Frey, M. A. (1996). Behavioral correlates of health and illness in youths with chronic illness. *Advanced Nursing Research, 9*(4), 167–176.

Frey, M. A. (1997). Health promotion in youth with chronic illness: Are we on the right track? *Quality Nursing, 3*(5), 13–18.

Frey, M. A., & Denyes, M. J. (1989). Health and illness self-care in adolescents with IDDM: A test of Orem's theory. *Advances in Nursing Science, 12*(1), 67–75.

Frey, M. A., & Fox, M. A. (1990). Assessing and teaching self-care to youths with diabetes mellitus. *Pediatric Nursing, 16,* 597–599.

Frey, M. A., & Norris, D. M. (1997). King's systems framework and theory in nursing practice. In Marriner-Tomey, A. (Ed.), *Nursing theory utilization and application* (pp. 71–88). St. Louis: Mosby.

Frey, M. A., Rooke, L., Sieloff, C. L., Messmer, P., & Kameoka, T. (1995). King's framework and theory in Japan, Sweden, and the United States. *Image: Journal of Nursing Scholarship, 27*(2), 127–130.

Frey, M. A., & Sieloff, C. L. (1995). *Advancing King's systems framework and theory of nursing.* Thousand Oaks, CA: Sage Publications.

Froman, D. (1995). Perceptual congruency between clients and nurses: Testing King's theory of goal attainment. In Frey, M. A., & Sieloff, C. L. (Eds.), *Advancing King's systems framework and theory of nursing* (pp. 223–238). Thousand Oaks, CA: Sage Publications.

Froman, D., & Sanderson, H. (1985). *Application of Imogene King's framework.* Paper presented at the Nursing Theory in Action Conference, Edmonton, Alberta, Canada.

Funashima, N. (1990). King's goal attainment theory. *Knago MOOK, 35,* 56–62.

Gill, J., Hopwood-Jones, L., Tyndall, J., Gregoroff, S., LeBlanc, P., Lovett, C., Rasco, L., & Ross, A. (1995). Incorporating nursing diagnosis and King's theory in the O. R. documentation. *Canadian Operating Room Nursing Journal, 13*(1), 10–14.

Gonot, P. J. (1986). Family therapy as derived from King's conceptual model. In Whall, L. (Ed.), *Family therapy for nursing:*

Four approaches (pp. 33–48). Norwalk, CT: Appleton-Century-Crofts.

Goodwin, Z., Kiehl, E. M., & Peterson, J. Z. (2002). King's theory as foundation for an advanced directive decision-making model. *Nursing Science Quarterly, 15*(3), 237–241.

Gulitz, E. A., & King, I. M. (1988). King's general systems model: Application to curriculum development. *Nursing Science Quarterly, 1,* 128–132.

Hampton, D. C. (1994). King's theory of goal attainment as a framework for managed care implementation in a hospital setting. *Nursing Science Quarterly, 7*(4), 170–173.

Hanchett, E. S. (1988a). Community assessment: King's conceptual framework dynamic interacting systems. In Hanchett, E. S. (Ed.), *Nursing frameworks and community as client: Bridging the gap* (pp. 89–107). Norwalk, CT: Appleton & Lange.

Hanchett, E. S. (1988b). King's general system framework. In Hanchett, E. S. (Ed.), *Nursing frameworks and community as client: Bridging the gap* (pp. 83–87). Norwalk, CT: Appleton & Lange.

Hanchett, E. S. (1990). Nursing models and community as client...public health/community health nursing. *Nursing Science Quarterly, 3*(2), 67–72.

Hanna, K. (1993). Effect of nurse-client transaction on female adolescents' oral contraceptive use. *Image, 25*(4), 285–290.

Hanna, K. M. (1995). Use of King's theory of goal attainment to promote adolescents' health behavior. In Frey, M. A., & Sieloff, C. L. (Eds.), *Advancing King's systems framework and theory of nursing* (pp. 239–250). Thousand Oaks, CA: Sage Publications.

Hanucharurnkui, S., & Vinya-nguag, P. (1991). Effects of promoting patients' participation in self-care on postoperative recovery and satisfaction with care. *Nursing Science Quarterly, 4,* 14–20.

Hawks, J. H. (1991). Power: A concept analysis. *Journal of Advanced Nursing, 16,* 754–762.

Heggie, M., & Gangar, E. (1992). A nursing model for menopause clinics. *Nursing Standard, 6*(21), 32–34.

Hobdell, E. F. (1995). Using King's interacting systems framework for research on parents of children with neural tube defects. In Frey, M. A., & Sieloff, C. L. (Eds.), *Advancing King's systems framework and theory of nursing* (pp. 126–136). Thousand Oaks, CA: Sage Publications.

Houfek, J. F. (1992). Nurses' perceptions of the dimenions of nursing care episodes. *Nursing Research, 41,* 280–285.

Howland, D. (1976). An adaptive health system model. In Werley, H. H., et al. (Ed.), *Health systems research: The systems approach* (p. 109). New York: Springer Publishing.

Howland, D., & McDowell, W. (1964). A measurement of patient care: A conceptual framework. *Nursing Research, 13*(4), 320–324.

Hughes, M. M. (1983). Nursing theories and emergency nursing. *Journal of Emergency Nursing, 9,* 95–97.

Husband, A. (1988). Application of King's theory of nursing to the care of the adult with diabetes. *Journal of Advanced Nursing, 13,* 484–488.

Husting, P. M. (1997). A transcultural critique of Imogene King's theory of goal attainment. *Journal of Multicultural Nursing & Health, 3*(3), 15–20.

Jackson, A. L., Pokorny, M. E., & Vincent, P. (1993). Relative satisfaction with nursing care of patients with ostomies. *Journal of ET Nursing, 20*(6), 233–238.

Jacono, J., Hicks, G., Antonioni, C., O'Brien, K., & Rasi, M. (1990). Comparison of perceived needs of family members between registered nurses and family members of critically ill patients in intensive care and neonatal intensive care units. *Heart and Lung: Journal of Critical Care, 19*(1), 72–78.

Jacox, A. (1993). Addressing variations in nursing practice/technology through clinical practice guidelines methods. *Nursing Economics, 11*(3), 170–172.

Johnson, M., & Maas, M. (1997). *Nursing outcomes classification (NOC).* St. Louis: Mosby-Year Book.

Jolly, M. L., & Winker, C. K. (1995). Theory of goal attainment in the context of organizational structure. In Frey, M. A., & Sieloff, C. L. (Eds.), *Advancing King's systems framework and theory of nursing* (pp. 305–316). Thousand Oaks, CA: Sage Publications.

Jonas, C. M. (1987). King's goal attainment theory: Use in gerontological nursing practice. *Perspectives: Journal of the Gerontological Nursing Association, 11*(4), 9–12.

Jones, S., Clark, V. B., Merker, A., & Palau, D. (1995). Changing behaviors: Nurse educators and clinical nurse specialists design a discharge planning program. *Journal of Nursing Staff Development, 11*(6), 291–295.

Kameoka, T. (1995). Analyzing nurse-patient interactions in Japan. In Frey, M. A., & Sieloff, C. L. (Eds.), *Advancing King's systems framework and theory of goal attainment* (pp. 251–260). Thousand Oaks, CA: Sage Publications.

Kameoka, T., & Sugimori, M. (1992). *Application to King's goal attainment theory in Japanese clinical setting: Part 2.* Paper presented at the First International Nursing Research Conference, Japan.

Kemppainen, J. K. (1990). Imogene King's theory: A nursing case study of a psychotic client with human immunodeficiency virus infection. *Archives of Psychiatric Nursing, 4*(6), 384–388.

Kenny, T. (1990). Erosion of individuality in care of elderly people in hospital—an alternative approach. *Journal of Advanced Nursing, 15,* 571–576.

Killeen, M. (1996). Patient-consumer perceptions and responses to professional nursing care: Instrument development. *Dissertation Abstracts International, 57-04B,* 2479.

Kilo, C. M., Kabcenell, A., & Berwick, D. (1998). Beyond survival: Toward continuous improvement in medical care. *New Horizons, 61*(1), 3–11.

King, I. M. (1964). Nursing theory: Problems and prospect. *Nursing Science Quarterly, 2,* 294.

King, I. M. (1968). A conceptual frame of reference for nursing. *Nursing Research, 17,* 27–31.

King, I. M. (1971). *Toward a theory for nursing: General concepts of human behavior.* New York: Wiley.

King, I. M. (1975). A process for developing concepts for nursing through research. In Verhonick, P. J. (Ed.), *Nursing Research* (p. 25). Boston: Little, Brown.

King, I. M. (1976). *Toward a theory of nursing: General concepts of human behavior* (Sugimori, M., Trans.). Tokyo: Igaku-Shoin.

King, I. M. (1978). How does the conceptual framework provide structure for the curriculum? In *Curriculum process for developing or revising a baccalaureate nursing program.* New York: National League for Nursing, pp. 23–34.

King, I. M. (1981). *A theory of goal attainment: Systems, concepts, process.* New York: Wiley.

King, I. M. (1983a). King's theory of goal attainment. In

Clements, I. W., & Roberts, F. B. (Eds.), *Family health: A theoretical approach to nursing care* (p. 177). New York: Wiley.

King, I. M. (1983b). The family coping with a medical illness: Analysis and application of King's theory of goal attainment. In Clements, I. W. R., & Roberts, F. B. (Eds.), *Family health: A theoretical approach to nursing care* (pp. 383–385). New York: John Wiley & Sons.

King, I. M. (1983c). The family with an elderly member: Analysis and application of King's theory of goal attainment. In Clements, I. W. R., & Roberts, F. B. (Eds.), *Family health: A theoretical approach to nursing care* (pp. 341–345). New York: John Wiley & Sons.

King, I. M. (1984a). Effectiveness of nursing care: Use of a goal oriented nursing record in end stage renal disease. *American Association of Nephrology Nurses and Technicians Journal, 11*(2), 11–17, 60.

King, I. M. (1984b). A theory for nursing: King's conceptual model applied to community health nursing. In *Conceptual models of nursing applications in community health nursing* (p. 14). Chapel Hill, NC: Department of Public Health Nursing.

King, I. M. (1984c). Philosophy of nursing education. A national survey. *Western Journal of Nursing Research, 6*, 387.

King, I. M. (1985). *A theory for nursing: Systems, concepts, process* (Sugimori, M., Trans.). Tokyo: Igaku-Shoin.

King, I. M. (1986a). *Curriculum and instruction in nursing: Concepts and process.* Norwalk, CT: Appleton-Century-Crofts.

King, I. M. (1986b). King's theory of goal attainment. In Fry, P. (Ed.), *Case studies in nursing theory* (p. 197). New York: National League for Nursing.

King, I. M. (1988a). Measuring health goal attainment in patients. In Waltz, C. F., & Strickland, O. L. (Eds.), *Measurement of nursing outcomes* (Vol. 1, pp. 108–127). New York: Springer.

King, I. M. (1988b). Concepts: Essential elements of theories. *Nursing Science Quarterly, 1*(1), 22–24.

King, I. M. (1989a). King's general systems framework and theory. In Riehl-Sisca, J. P. (Ed.), *Conceptual models for nursing practice* (p. 149). Norwalk, CT: Appleton & Lang.

King, I. M. (1989b). King's systems framework for nursing administration. In Henry, B., et al. (Eds.), *Dimensions of nursing administration: Theory, research, education* (p. 35). Cambridge, England: Blackwell Scientific.

King, I. M. (1989c). Measuring health goal attainment in patients. In Waltz, C. F., & Strickland, O. L. (Eds.), *Measurment of nursing outcomes* (p. 108). New York: Springer Publishing.

King, I. M. (1990). Health as a goal for nursing. *Nursing Science Quarterly, 3*, 123–128.

King, I. M. (1992). King's theory of goal attainment. *Nursing Science Quarterly, 5*, 19.

King, I. M. (1993). Quality of life and goal attainment. *Nursing Science Quarterly, 7*(1), 29–32.

King, I. M. (1994). Quality of life and goal attainment. *Nursing Science Quarterly, 7*, 29.

King, I. M. (1995). The theory of goal attainment. In Frey, M., & Sieloff, C. (Eds.), *Advancing King's systems framework and theory of goal attainment* (p. 23). Thousand Oaks, CA: Sage.

King, I. M. (1996). The theory of goal attainment in research and practice. *Nursing Science Quarterly, 9*, 61.

King, I. M. (1997). King's theory of goal attainment in practice. *Nursing Science Quarterly, 10*(4), 180–185.

King, I. M. (1998). Nursing informatics: A universal nursing language. *The Florida Nurse, 46*, 1.

King, I. M., & Tarsitano, B. (1982). The effect of structured and unstructured pre-operative teaching: A replication. *Nursing Research, 31*(6), 324–329.

Kneeshaw, M. F. (1990). Nurses' percpeption of co-worker responses to smoking cessation attempts. *Journal of the New York State Nurses Association, 21*(1), 9–13.

Kobayashi, F. T. (1970). A conceptual frame of reference for nursing. *Japanese Journal of Nursing Research, 3*(3), 199–204.

Kohler, P. (1988). Model of shared control. *Journal of Gerontological Nursing, 14*(7), 21–25.

Kusaka, T. (1991). Application to the King's goal attainment theory in Japanese clinical setting. *Journal of the Japanese Academy of Nursing Education, 1*(1), 30–31.

Laben, J. K., Dodd, D., & Sneed, L. (1991). King's theory of goal attainment applied in group therapy for inpatient juvenile offenders, maximum security state offenders, and community parolees, using visual aids. *Issues in Mental Health Nursing, 12*(1), 51–64.

Laben, J. K., Sneed, L. D., & Seidel, S. L. (1995). Goal attainment in short-term group psychotherapy settings: Clinical implications for practice. In Frey, M. A., & Sieloff, C. L. (Eds.), *Advancing King's systems framework and theory of nursing* (pp. 261–277). Thousand Oaks, CA: Sage Publications.

LaFontaine, P. (1989). Alleviating patient's apprehension and anxieties. *Gastroenterology Nursing, 11*, 256–257.

Laramee, A. (1999). The building blocks of successful relationships. *Journal of Care Management, 5*(4), 40, 42, 44–45.

Lawler, J., Dowswell, G., Hearn, J., Forster, A., & Young, J. (1999). Recovering from stroke: A qualitative investigation of the role of goal setting in late stroke recovery. *Journal of Advanced Nursing, 30*(2), 401–409.

Levine, C. D., Wilson, S. F., & Guido, G. W. (1988). Personality factors of critical nurses. *Heart and Lung, 17*(4), 392–398.

Lockhart, J. S. (2000). Nurses' perceptions of head and neck oncology patients after surgery: Severity of facial disfigurement and patient gender. *Plastic Surgical Nursing, 20*(2), 68–80.

Martin, J. P. (1990). Male cancer awareness: Impact of an employee education program. *Oncology Nursing Forum, 17*, 59–64.

Mayer, B. W. (2000). Female domestic violence victims: Perspectives on emergency care. *Nursing Science Quarterly, 13*(4), 340–346.

McFarland, G. K., & McFarland, E. A. (1997). *Nursing diagnosis and intervention: Planning for patient care.* St. Louis: Mosby-Year Book.

McGirr, M., Rukholm, E., Salmoni, A., O'Sullivan, P., & Koren, I. (1990). Perceived mood and exercise behaviors of cardiac rehabilitation program referrals. *Canadian Journal of Cardiovascular Nursing, 1*(4), 14–19.

McKinney, N. L., & Dean, P. R. (2000). Application of King's theory of dynamic interacting systems to the study of child abuse and the development of alcohol use/dependence in adult females. *Journal of Addictions Nursing, 12*(2), 73–82.

Meleis, A. (1985). *Theoretical nursing: Developments and progress* (2nd ed.). Philadelphia: J. B. Lippincott.

Messmer, P. R. (1992). Implementing theory based nursing practice. *Florida Nurse, 40*(3), 8.

Messmer, P. R. (1995). Implementation of theory-based nursing practice. In Frey, M. A., & Sieloff, C. L. (Eds.), *Advancing King's systems framework and theory of nursing* (pp. 294–304). Thousand Oaks, CA: Sage Publications.

Messmer, R., & Neff Smith, M. N. (1986). Neurofibromatosis: Relinquishing the masks: A quest for quality of life. *Journal of Advanced Nursing, 11*, 459–464.

Milne, J. (2000). The impact of information on health behaviors of older adults with urinary incontinence. *Clinical Nursing Research, 9*(2), 161–176.

Moorhead, S., Johnson, M., & Maas, M. (Eds.) (2004). *Nursing outcomes classification (NOC): Iowa outcomes project* (3rd ed.) St. Louis: Mosby.

Moreira, T. M. M., & Arajo, T. L. (2002). The conceptual model of interactive open systems and the theory of goal attainment by Imogene King [Portuguese]. *Revista Latino-Americana de Enfermagem, 10*(1), 97–103.

Murray, R. L. E., & Baier, M. (1996). King's conceptual framework applied to a transitional living program. *Perspectives in Psychiatric Care, 32*(1), 15–19.

Myks Babb, B. A., Fouladbakhsh, J. M., & Hanchett, E. S. (1988). Interactions on main street. In Hanchett, E. S. (Ed.), *Nursing frameworks and community as client: Bridging the gap* (pp. 109–115). Norwalk, CT: Appleton & Lange.

Nagano, M., & Funashima, N. (1995). Analysis of nursing situations in Japan: Using King's goal attainment theory. *Quality Nursing, 1*(1), 74–78.

National League for Nursing. (1978). *Curriculum process for developing or revising a baccalaureate nursing program.* New York: National League for Nursing.

Norgan, G. H., Ettipio, A. M., & Lasome, C. E. M. (1995). A program plan addressing carpal tunnel syndrome: The utility of King's goal attainment theory. *American Association of Occupational Health Nurses Journal, 43*(8), 407–411.

Norris, D. M., & Hoyer, P. J. (1993). Dynamism in practice: Parenting within King's framework. *Nursing Science Quarterly, 6*(2), 79–85.

Northrop, F. C. S. (1969). *The logic of the sciences and the humanities.* Cleveland: Meridian.

Olsson, H., & Forsdahl, T. (1996). Expectations and opportunities of newly employed nurses at the University Hospital, Tromso, Norway. *Social Sciences in Health: International Journal of Research and Practice, 2*(1), 14–22.

Pearson, A., & Vaughan, B. (1986). *Nursing models for practice.* London: William Heinemann Medical Books.

Petrich, B. (2000). Medical and nursing students' perceptions of obesity. *Journal of Addictions Nursing, 12*(10), 3–16.

Porteous, A., & Tyndall, J. (1994). Yes, I want to talk to the OR. *Canadian Operating Room Nursing, 12*(2), 15–16, 18–19.

Porter, H. (1991). A theory of goal attainment and ambulatory oncology nursing: An introduction. *Canadian Oncology Nursing, 1*(4), 124–126.

Rawlins, P. S., Rawlins, T. D., & Horner, M. (1990). Development of the family needs assessment tool. *Western Journal of Nursing Research, 12*, 201–214.

Richard-Hughes, S. (1997). Attitudes and beliefs of Afro-Americans related to organ and tissue donation. *International Journal of Trauma Nursing, 3*(4), 119–123.

Riggs, C. J. (2001). A model of staff support to improve retention in long-term care. *Nursing Administration Quarterly, 25*(2), 43–54.

Rooda, L. A. (1992). The development of a conceptual model for multicultural nursing. *Journal of Holistic Nursing, 10*(4), 337–347.

Rooke, L. (1995a). The concept of space in King's systems framework: Its implications for nursing. In Frey, M. A., & Sieloff, C. L. (Eds.), *Advancing King's systems framework and theory of nursing* (pp. 79–96). Thousand Oaks, CA: Sage Publications.

Rooke, L. (1995b). Focusing on King's theory and systems framework in education by using an experiential learning model: A challenge to improve the quality of nursing care. In Frey, M. A., & Sieloff, C. L. (Eds.), *Advancing King's systems framework and theory of nursing* (pp. 278–293). Thousand Oaks, CA: Sage Publications.

Rooke, L., & Norberg, A. (1988). Problematic and meaningful situations in nursing interpreted by concepts from King's nursing theory and four additional concepts. *Scandinavian Journal of Caring Sciences, 2*(2), 80–87.

Rosendahl, P. B., & Ross, V. (1982). Does your behavior affect your patient's response? *Journal of Gerontological Nursing, 8*, 572–575.

Rundell, S. (1991). A study of nurse patient interaction in a high dependency unit. *Intensive Care Nursing, 7*, 171–178.

Schorr, T. M., & Zimmerman, A. (1990). *Making Choices, Taking Chances.* St. Louis: Mosby-Year Book, Inc.

Schreiber, R. (1991). Psychiatric assessment— "A la King." *Nursing Management, 22*(5), 90, 92, 94.

Scott, L. D. (1998). Perceived needs of parents of critically ill children. *Journal of the Society of Pediatric Nurses, 3*(1), 4–12.

Sharts-Hopko, N. C. (1995). Using health, personal, and interpersonal system concepts within the King's systems framework to explore perceived health status during the menopause transition. In Frey, M. A., & Sieloff, C. L. (Eds.), *Advancing King's system framework and theory of nursing* (pp. 147–160). Thousand Oaks, CA: Sage Publications.

Sieloff, C. L. (1995a). Development of a theory of departmental power. In Frey, M. A., & Sieloff, C. L. (Eds.), *Advancing King's systems framework and theory of nursing* (pp. 46–65). Thousand Oaks, CA: Sage Publications.

Sieloff, C. L. (1995b). Defining the health of a social system within Imogene King's framework. In Frey, M. A., & Sieloff, C. L. (Eds.), *Advancing King's systems framework and theory of nursing* (pp. 137–146). Thousand Oaks, CA: Sage Publications.

Sieloff, C. L. (1996). Development of an instrument to estimate the actualized power of a nursing department. *Dissertation Abstracts International, 57-04B*, 2484.

Sieloff, C. L. (2003). Measuring nursing power within organizations. *Journal of Nursing Scholarship, 35*(2), 183–187.

Sirles, A. T., & Selleck, C. S. (1989). Cardiac disease and the family: Impact, assessment, and implications. *Journal of Cardiovascular Nursing, 3*(2), 23–32.

Smith, M. C. (1988). King's theory in practice. *Nursing Science Quarterly, 1*, 145–146.

Sowell, R. L., & Lowenstein, A. (1994). King's theory: A framework for quality; linking theory to practice. *Nursing Connections, 7*(2), 19–31.

Spees, C. M. (1991). Knowledge of medical terminology among clients and families. *Image: Journal of Nursing Scholarship, 23*(4), 225–229.

Spratlen, L. P. (1976). Introducing ethnic-cultural factors in models of nursing: Some mental health care applications. *Journal of Nursing Education, 15*(2), 23–29.

Stanley, J. M. (2000). Nurses' perceptions of hypnosis. *Masters Abstracts International, 38-03*, 685.

Steele, S. (1981). *Child health and the family: Nursing concepts and management.* New York: Masson.

Strauss, S. S. (1981). Abuse and neglect of parents by professionals. *Maternal/Child Nursing, 6,* 157–160.

Swindale, J. E. (1989). The nurse's role in giving pre-operative information to reduce anxiety in patients admitted to hospital for elective minor surgery. *Journal of Advanced Nursing, 14,* 899–905.

Syzmanski, M. E. (1991). Use of nursing theories in the care of families with high-risk infants: Challenges for the future. *Journal of Perinatal and Neonatal Nursing, 4*(4), 71–77.

Temple, A. F., & Fawdry, M. K. (1992). King's theory of goal attainment: Resolving filial caregiver role strain. *Journal of Gerontological Nursing, 18*(3), 11–15.

Titler, M. G. (1998, June). Evidence-based practice and research utilization: One and the same? Paper presented at the ANA Council for Nursing Research's 1998 Pre-Convention Research Utilization Conference, Evidence-based Practice, San Diego, CA.

Tritsch, J. M. (1996). Application of King's theory of goal attainment and the Carondelet St. Mary's case management model. *Nursing Science Quarterly, 11*(2), 69–73.

Viera, C. S., & Rossi, L. (2000). Nursing diagnoses from NANDA's taxonomy in women with a hospitalized preterm child and King's conceptual system [Portuguese]. *Revista Latin-Americana de Enfermagem, 8*(6), 110–116.

Villeneuve, M. J., & Ozolins, P. H. (1991). Sexual counselling in the neuroscience setting: Theory and practical tips for nurses. *AXON, 12*(3), 63–67.

Von Bertalanffy, L. (1968). *General system theory.* New York: Braziller.

Wadensten, B., & Carlsson, M. (2003). Nursing theory views on how to support the process of aging. *Journal of Advanced Nursing, 42*(2), 118–124.

Walker, K. M., & Alligood, M. R. (2001). Empathy from a nursing perspective: Moving beyond borrowed theory. *Archives of Psychiatric Nursing, 15*(3), 140–147.

Walton, M. (1986). *The Deming management method.* New York: Putnam.

West, P. (1991). Theory implementation: A challenging journey. *Canadian Journal of Nursing Administration, 4*(1), 29–30.

Wicks, M. N. (1995). Family health as derived from King's framework. In Frey, M. A., & Sieloff, C. L. (Eds.), *Advancing King's systems framework and theory of nursing* (pp. 97–108). Thousand Oaks, CA: Sage Publications.

Wilkinson, C. R., & Williams, M. (2002). Strengthening patient-provider relationships. *Lippincott's Case Management, 7*(3), 86–102.

Williams, L. A. (2001). Imogene King's interacting systems theory—Application in emergency and rural nursing. *Online Journal of Rural Nursing and Health Care, 2*(1). Retrieved January 8, 2004, from CINAHL.

Winker, C. K. (1995). A systems view of health. In Frey, M. A., & Sieloff, C. L. (Eds.), *Advancing King's systems framework and theory of nursing* (pp. 35–45). Thousand Oaks, CA: Sage Publications.

Woods, E. C. (1994). King's theory in practice with elders. *Nursing Science Quarterly, 7*(2), 65–69.

Zurakowski, T. L. (2000). The social environment of nursing homes and the health of older residents. *Holistic Nursing Practice, 14*(4), 12–23.

CHAPTER 17

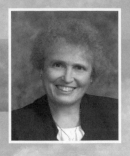

Sister Callista Roy

Sister Callista Roy's Adaptation Model and Its Applications

Sister Callista Roy & Lin Zhan

Introducing the Theorist

Sister Callista Roy is a highly respected nurse theorist, writer, lecturer, researcher, and teacher who currently holds the position of professor and nurse theorist at the Boston College William F. Connell School of Nursing. It is often said that her name is the most recognized name in the field of nursing today, worldwide, and she is one of our greatest living thinkers. Dr. Roy shakes her head on hearing these premature epitaphs and notes that her best work is yet to come. As a theorist, Dr. Roy often emphasizes her primary commitment to define and develop nursing knowledge and regards her work with the Roy Adaptation Model as one rich source of knowledge for clinical nursing. Early in the new century, Dr. Roy has provided an expanded, values-based concept of adaptation based on insights related to the place of the person in the universe. She hopes her redefinition of adaptation, with its cosmic philosophical and scientific assumptions, will become the basis for developing knowledge that will make nursing a major social force in the century to come.

Dr. Roy credits her major influences in personal and professional growth as her family, her religious commitment, and her teachers and mentors. Dr. Roy was born in Los Angeles, California, on October 14, 1939. Her mother was a licensed vocational nurse and instilled the values of always seeking to know more about people and their care, and of selfless giving as a nurse. At age 14 she began working at a large general hospital, first as a pantry girl, then as a maid, and finally as a nurse's aid. After soul-searching, she entered the Sisters of Saint Joseph of Carondelet, of which she has been a member for more than 40 years. Her college education began with a bachelor of arts degree with a major in nursing at Mount St. Mary's College, Los Angeles, followed by master's degrees in pediatric nursing and sociology at the University of California, Los Angeles, and a PhD in sociology at the same school. Later, Dr. Roy had the opportunity to be a clinical nurse scholar in a two-year postdoctoral program in neuroscience nursing at the University of California at San Francisco. Important mentors in her life have included Dorothy E. Johnson, Ruth Wu, Connie Robinson, and Barbara Smith Moran.

Dr. Roy is still best known for developing and continually updating the Roy Adaptation Model as a framework for theory, practice, administration, and research in nursing. Books on the model have been translated into many languages, including French, Italian, Spanish, Finnish, Chinese, Korean, and Japanese. Two recent publications that Dr. Roy considers of great significance are *The Roy Adaptation Model* (2nd edition), written with Heather Andrews (Appleton & Lange); and *The Roy Adaptation Model-Based Research: Twenty-Five*

Years of Contributions to Nursing Science, published as a research monograph by Sigma Theta Tau. The latter is a critical analysis of the 25 years of model-based literature, which includes 163 studies published in 46 English-speaking journals, dissertations, and theses. This project was completed by the Boston-Based Adaptation Research Society in Nursing (BBARSN), a group of scholars founded by Dr. Roy in the interest of advancing nursing practice by developing basic and clinical nursing knowledge based on the Roy Adaptation Model.

One of Dr. Roy's major recent activities was cochairing the annual Knowledge Conferences hosted by the Boston College School of Nursing between 1996 and 2001, which developed into a book on knowledge for practice and was coauthored with Dr. Dorothy Jones. Being a teacher and a mentor to doctoral students in nursing is another role that she cherishes, and she extends that influence by serving on the Board of the International Network for Doctoral Education in Nursing. Dr. Roy has been a major speaker on topics related to nursing theory, research, curriculum, clinical practice, and professional trends for the future.

Dr. Roy has played a major role in at least 35 research projects, including the development and testing of a measure of Coping and Adaptation Processing (CAPS). Results of research and papers on nursing knowledge have appeared in *Image: Journal of Nursing Scholarship, Nursing Science Quarterly, Scholarly Inquiry for Nursing Practice, Biological Research for Nursing,* and other journals. During 2000, two papers were published in *Nursing Administration Quarterly* that focused on looking to the future of nursing. Dr. Roy's current clinical research continues her long-time interest in neuroscience. She is currently continuing her research on cognitive recovery and is working with families to use information processing practice to help patients who have sustained mild head injuries, as well as promoting adaptation of patients with acute and chronic health challenges.

Introducing the Theory

The Roy Adaptation Model has been in use for approximately 35 years, providing direction for nursing practice, education, administration, and research. Extensive implementation efforts around the world, and continuing philosophical and scientific developments by the theorist, have contributed to model-based knowledge for nursing practice. The purpose of this chapter is to describe the use of the model in developing knowledge for practice, with particular emphasis on research with the elderly. A study of coping, adaptation, and self-consistency in the elderly with hearing impairment provides an example of some of the key concepts of the model, as well as a research design to test the relationships among the concepts. Specifically, the study provides a test of a generic proposition derived from the Roy Adaptation Model. But first, a brief review of the Roy Adaptation Model is provided, with emphasis on recent developments of the theoretical work and its use in nursing research. Then, the theoretical and empirical concepts of coping and adaptation processing and self-consistency are described in greater detail.

Applications: Research Framework

The Roy Adaptation Model (Roy, 1984, 1988a, 1988b; Roy & Andrews, 1991, 1999; Roy & Roberts, 1981) provides the framework for programs of nursing research, particularly the constructs for the research exemplar involving elderly patients with hearing impairment.

ASSUMPTIONS

The model's philosophical assumptions are rooted in the general principles of humanism and in what Roy has termed "veritivity and cosmic unity" (Roy & Andrews, 1999). Scientific assumptions for the model have been based on general systems theory and adaptation-level theory (Roy & Corliss, 1993). More recently, the assumptions have been extended to include Roy's redefinition of adaptation for the twenty-first century (Roy & Andrews, 1999). The cosmic unity stressed in Roy's vision for the future emphasizes the principle that people and the earth have common patterns and integral relationships. Rather than the system acting to maintain itself, the emphasis shifts to the purposefulness of human existence in a universe that is creative.

MAJOR CONCEPTS

People, both individually and in groups, are viewed as holistic adaptive systems, with coping processes acting to maintain adaptation and to promote per-

son and environment transformations. The coping processes are broadly described within the regulator and cognator subsystems for the individual and within the stabilizer and innovator subsystems for groups. Through coping processes, persons as holistic adaptive systems interact with the internal and external environment, transform the environment, and are transformed by it. A particular aspect of the internal environment is the adaptation level. This is the name given to the three possible conditions of the life processes of the human adaptive system: integrated, compensatory, and compromised (Roy & Andrews, 1999). Processing of the internal and external environment by the coping subsystems results in human behavior. Four categories for assessing behaviors are termed "adaptive modes." Initially developed to describe persons as individuals (Roy, 1971), the modes have been expanded to include groups and are termed physiologic-physical, self-concept-group identity, role function, and interdependence (Roy & Andrews, 1999). Central to Roy's theoretical model is the belief that adaptive responses support *health,*

> *Adaptive responses support health, which is defined as a state and a process of being and becoming integrated and whole.*

which is defined as a state and a process of being and becoming integrated and whole.

USES IN RESEARCH

Roy has described strategies for knowledge development based on the model and a structure of knowledge to guide research (Roy & Andrews, 1999). Knowledge-development strategies that she has integrated through decades of work include model construction; theory development (including concept analysis, synthesis, and derivation of propositional statements); philosophic explication; and research, qualitative, quantitative, and instrument development. The structure for knowledge includes the broad categories of the basic and clinical science of nursing.

Basic nursing science discovers knowledge about persons and groups from a nursing perspective that can provide understandings for practice. The clinical science of nursing investigates specifically the role of the nurse in promoting adaptation and human and environment transformations. Within the basic science, the investigator studies the person or group as an adaptive system, including (1) the adaptive processes; that is, cognator and regulator activity, stabilizer and innovator activity, stability of adaptation level patterns, and dynamics of evolving adaptive patterns; (2) the adaptive modes; that is, their development, interrelatedness, and cultural and other influences; and (3) adaptation related to health, particularly person and environment interaction and integration of the adaptive modes. Topics for research in the clinical science of nursing include (1) changes in cognator-regulator or stabilizer-innovator effectiveness; (2) changes within and among the adaptive modes; and (3) nursing care to promote adaptive processes, particularly in times of transition, during environmental changes, and during acute and chronic illness, injury, treatment, and technologic threats.

Roy has summarized her own research within the structure of knowledge (Roy & Andrews, 1999). In her early work, Roy used three methods to explore how the cognator coping processes act to promote adaptation and how they relate to the adaptive modes. Two inductive processes involved content analysis of patient interviews before diagnostic tests and recordings of the nursing process done by students in 10 schools where the Roy Adaptation Model was the basis of their curricula. This data was used in the development of the Coping and Adaptation Processing Scale (CAPS) described below. The second major research effort, again within the basic science of nursing, used a systematic controlled comparison of survey data collected in six hospitals across the United States. One purpose within the larger study aims was to examine levels of wellness in relation to levels of adaptation. For the 208 patients of the sample, some of the measures of physiologic adaptation were related to levels of wellness, but no evidence was found of a relationship between psychosocial adaptation and measures of levels of wellness. There was, however, such a relationship in the least acute care setting and for patients with longer hospital stays. Thus, it was suggested that adaptation is a process that takes place over time. Further, Roy (1977) noted that the measures of levels of wellness were limited and not entirely consistent with the dynamic and holistic concept of health as defined by the model.

Roy's more recent research is related to clinical nursing science. A model of cognitive information processing was developed (Roy, 1988b, 2001), and a program of research was initiated to contribute to

further understanding of cognitive processes; that is, how people take in and process environmental interactions and how nurses can help people use these processes to positively affect their health status. Cognitive recovery from head injury was the focus of the research. The first study used a repeated measures design to describe changes in cognitive performance over six months of recovery for 50 patients (Roy, 1985). Nursing intervention protocols were then developed for use during the first month, which is considered the critical period for recovery. The initial pilot study of nine matched pairs shows some promising trends. Graphs of recovery curves on all nine measures showed earlier improvement of performance in the treated group as compared with the matched group that did not receive the planned nursing interventions to promote cognitive recovery from head injury (Roy & Hanna, 1999). The intervention has been extended to involve family members as study partners with the nurse to practice the information processing protocol. Another funded research project in clinical progress focuses on nurse coaching for symptom management and recovery after same-day surgery.

The use of the Roy Adaptation Model for nursing research is strikingly demonstrated by a research synthesis project conducted by the Boston-Based Adaptation Research Society in Nursing (BBARSN). Roy worked with seven other scholars for about four years to develop a method to conduct a review and synthesis of research, based on the Roy Adaptation Model, to identify and locate the literature from a 25-year period, to conduct the critical analysis, and to present the findings in a research monograph (Roy et al., 1999). From 1970 through 1994, a total of 163 studies met the inclusion criteria. Only English-language publications were included. The sample included 94 articles in 44 different research and specialty journals from five continents. In addition, there were 77 dissertations and theses from a total of 35 universities and colleges in the United States and Canada that were retrieved and included in the synthesis review. The major concepts of the model were used to organize the presentation of the review of this extensive use of the Roy Adaptation Model in nursing research. Although studies focused on more than one model concept, it was possible to group the studies by their major topic, as follows: multiple adaptive modes and processes; physiologic, self-concept, role function, and interdependence modes; stimuli; and intervention.

The critical analysis involved evaluating each study according to predetermined criteria for the quality of the research and for the linkages of the research to the model. The studies that met the established criteria for adequacy of the quality of the research and links to the model were used to test propositions derived from the model. They were based on 12 generic propositions from Roy's published work. As the studies were analyzed, the findings were used to state ancillary and practice propositions. ("Ancillary propositions" are special instances of the general propositions and sometimes are stated in terms directly relevant to practice and thus are referred to as "practice propositions.") Significant research support for the ancillary propositions lent support to the theoretical statements of the generic propositions. This process is demonstrated in the exemplar study reported here.

The BBARNS reviewers also examined the application of findings to nursing practice. They used three categories to assess the potential of research findings for use in practice: Category 1—high potential for implementation based on positive findings with methodologic adequacy and without risk to patients; Category 2—need further clinical evaluation before implementation (for example, by teams of advanced practice nurses in the practice area to evaluate potential effectiveness relative to risk); and Category 3—further research warranted before implementation; designation used in cases where findings were negative or equivocal or that were promising but posed a risk to patients and thus needed replication and clarification before being recommended for practice. This review showed the breadth and depth of the Roy model's use in nursing research in qualitative and quantitative research and in instrument development studies, using populations of individuals and groups (of all ages, both in health and in illness, and in all areas of nursing practice). A review of the next five years of research, including 57 identified studies, is underway, along with a critique, examples, and recommendations for the use of instruments to measure concepts of the Roy Adaptation Model (visit the Roy Adaptation Association Web site at: http://www2.bc.edu/~royca/htm/raa.htm).

COPING AND ADAPTATION PROCESSING

Two constructs of the model—coping and adaptation processing and self-consistency—are discussed

in greater detail as a basis for applying the model in the research exemplar with the elderly. The Roy Adaptation Model focuses on enhancing the basic

> *The Roy Adaptation Model focuses on enhancing the basic life processes of the individual and group.*

life processes of the individual and group. The cognator and regulator of the individual, and the innovator and stabilizer of the group, have basic abilities to promote adaptation; that is, the process and outcome whereby thinking and feeling are used in conscious awareness and choice to create human and environmental integration (Roy & Andrews, 1999). A major concentration of nursing activity is to assist people in using their cognitive abilities to handle their internal and external environment effectively. Given the priority of this notion, Roy focused efforts on further conceptual and empirical work to understand this human ability and nursing practice based on that understanding.

Conceptual Development

The conceptual basis for coping and adaptation processing lies in Roy's work on understanding the cognator and regulator as processors of adaptation (Roy & Andrews, 1999), on the development of a nursing model for cognitive processing (Roy, 1988a, 1988b), and on understanding of Das and Luria's model of simultaneous and successive information processing (Das, 1984; Luria, 1980). Drawing from knowledge in the neurosciences, her early theory development and research on the model, and her observations in neuroscience nursing practice, Roy proposed a nursing model for cognitive processing (Roy, 1988b, 2001). Cognitive processes in human adaptation are described as follows: input processes (arousal and attention, sensation and perception), central processes (coding, concept formation, memory, language), output processes (planning and motor responses), and emotion. Through these cognitive processes, adaptive responses occur.

Taylor (1983), in a study of cancer patients, proposed a related theory of cognitive adaptation. According to Taylor, cognitive adaptation is centered on three themes: a search for a meaning in the experience, an attempt to regain mastery over the event, and an effort to restore self-esteem through self-enhancing evaluation. Taylor's propositions are in concert with Roy's assumptions of cognitive adaptation, in which individuals make cognitive efforts to understand the purpose of their lives, maintain their sense of self, and enhance their well-being.

Instrument Development

In developing a new instrument, Roy sought to address issues in the measurement of coping as identified by Aldwin (1994) and Schwarzer & Schwarzer (1996). Further, it was important to have a tool that is useful for nursing assessment and intervention. Based on the cognator subsystem of the grand theory, Roy developed a middle-range theory of Coping and Adaptation Processing (Roy & Chayaput, 2004; Roy, in review). The theory identifies how adaptation is manifested in the four adaptive modes, which provides for multidimensionality and is accomplished by the three stages of information processing that are hierarchical, from input to central to output processes. Items of coping strategies within these categories were generated by patient interviews and nursing care plans based on the Roy model, as well as by deductively derived categories of information processing, with related patient observations to identify related strategies. A total of 73 items were developed using these approaches. For the tool, 47 items met all criteria for inclusion and represented all dimensions and processes of the constructs of the middle-range theory.

The psychometric properties were established with a data set that included 349 subjects from nonprobability purposive samples from national mailing lists of patient support groups for persons with long-term neurologic deficits. The Thai translation of the CAPS was conducted, and the psychometric properties were established by Roy & Chayaput (2004) with a sample of 580 medical and surgical Thai patients with acute illnesses from three hospitals in Thailand. The five factors of the CAPS were extracted in five iterations. Factor 1, *resourceful and focused,* contained 10 items with factor loadings ranging from .71 to .49 and explained 26.6 percent of the variance. Factor 2, *physical and fixed,* had 14 items with factor loadings from .72 to .43 and explained 8.4 percent of the variance. Factor 3, *alert processing,* had nine items with loadings from .61 to .49 and explained 3.8 percent of the variance. Factor 4, *systematic processing,* contained six items with

loadings from .71 to .31 and explained 3.3 percent of the variance. Finally, Factor 5, *knowing and relating,* had eight items whose loadings ranged from .63 to .31 and explained 3.2 percent of the variance. The Thai version was considered comparable to a large extent.

A 48-item CAPS for the elderly had been selected from the longer set of items. This version of the scale was used in the research exemplar described in this chapter. The items retained were inclusive of the inferred coping strategies, and the categories were derived from the nursing model for cognitive processing. Content-validity of the CAPS was based on both the strong theoretical-empirical basis for its development and the review by content experts. Internal consistency reliability for the total scale was .85 (Zhan, 1993a). The conceptual clarification of this version of the CAPS was further examined by using a principal component factor extraction with a varimax rotation, resulting in five factors that accounted for 48 percent of variances among the scores (Zhan, 1993b). At that time, Roy termed these five factors (1) cognitive processing of self-perception, (2) clear focus and method, (3) knowing awareness, (4) sensory regulation, and (5) selective focus. The scores on this version of the CAPS can range from 48 to 192; a total high score represents a greater use of cognitive adaptation strategies.

Cognitive processing of self-perception refers to self-awareness, self-analysis, emotion, and consciousness (Carver & Scheier, 1991). It serves to signal needs for cognitive efforts, to help the person to attend, and to interfere with cognition. Examples of items were "keep in touch with emotions," "put things into perspective," "rechannel feelings," and "be aware of self-limits." Cognitive processing of clear focus and method refers to programming, attention, thinking, reasoning, problem solving, concept formation, and cognitive coding. It involves systematic thinking. The real process of systematic thinking lacks full understanding. However, it can be viewed in part as a process in which people classify the problem, organize information to accomplish some desired end, and weigh the benefits and risks of their efforts to their self-structure (Das, 1984; Luria, 1980; Roy, 1988b, 2001). The thinking process requires knowledge of the adaptation encounter, perceptions of one's thoughts, action tendencies, and bodily changes. Items included: "give self time to grasp situations," "be objective about what happened," "identify the situation," and "follow directions." Cognitive processing of knowing awareness involves retrieving information from one's mind and recognizing what has worked for the person in the past. It can be viewed as a self-regulating process (Carver & Scheier, 1991). The overall function of such cognitive processing is to minimize discrepancies between a desirable sense of self and a present perception of self. It includes cognitive input processing of receiving, analyzing, storing, memory, successive processing, and arousal-attention (Roy, 1988b, 2001). Example items were "gather information," "recall past strategies," "keep eyes and ears open," "get more resources," "learn from others," "feel alert and active," and "be creative."

Cognitive processing of sensory regulation involves immediate sensory experience, output processing, motor response, movement, and regulating tone (Roy & Hanna, 1999). Examples of items include "try to maintain balance," "change physical activity," "picture actions," and "share concerns with others." Cognitive processing of selective focus refers to one's cognitive efforts to select attention and focus in coping with stressful encounters. Some examples of items were "useful to focus," "tend not to blame self," "get away by self," and "put the events out of mind." These five cognitive processes form subscales of the CAPS. Internal consistency reliability of these five subscales ranged from .56 to .89 (Zhan, 1993b). Later development of the tool improved the reliability of the subscales (Roy, in review).

SELF-CONSISTENCY

Roy (Roy & Andrews, 1999) describes "self-concept" as one adaptive mode of the individual within an adaptive system. The self-concept mode for the individual has two subareas: the physical self and the personal self. The physical self includes two components: body sensation and body image; and the personal self has three components: selfconsistency, self-ideal, and moral-ethical-spiritual self.

Conceptual Development

Self-consistency was introduced during the development of the Roy Adaptation Model based on the work of Coombs and Snyggs (1959). These authors noted that people strive to maintain a consistent self-organization and thus avoid disequilibrium

(Coombs & Snyggs, 1959; Lecky, 1961; Roy & Andrews, 1991). Lecky (1961) proposed the Theory of Self-consistency to conceptualize a person as a holistic and consistent structure. Central to Lecky's Self-consistency Theory is that people are motivated to act in a way that is congruent with their sense of self and thereby maintain intactness when facing potentially challenging situations. To maintain self-consistency in the transaction between the person and the environment (Elliot, 1986, 1988; Lecky, 1961; Rogers, 1961; Roy & Roberts, 1981), one initiates cognitive and emotional responses (Roy & Andrews, 1991).

An individual's sense of self may influence the person's ability to heal and to do what is necessary

> *An individual's sense of self may influence the person's ability to heal and to do what is necessary to maintain health.*

to maintain health. In particular, related to the application exemplar in this chapter, previous studies (Atchley, 1988; Kaufman, 1987; Klarkowska & Klarkowska, 1987; Ahan and Zhan, 1994) report that older persons with greater self-consistency had more positive levels of well-being. Further, they coped better with physical and psychosocial changes in aging than did those who had less consistency of self-perceptions. Being old does not necessarily mean one forms a new self-concept. Instead, older people carry their sense of self and personality with them into the later stage of their lives and adapt to a given situation as best as they can (Gove, Ortage, & Style, 1989). Lieberman and Tobin (1988) examined how older people coped with certain stressful life events such as the loss of loved ones, relocation, the experience of chronic conditions, and the approach of death. Their findings suggested that the older people who had a stability of self-concept coped well in stressful encounters. Therefore, the critical task for older

> *The critical task for older people is to maintain self-consistency by transcending internal and external losses in the aging process.*

people is to maintain self-consistency by transcending internal and external losses in the aging process.

They further assert that central to understanding how well a person can cope with any stressful condition in aging is understanding how one maintains consistency of self and whether one is able to achieve that goal.

Instrument Development

Based on extensive literature review on theories of self-concept and self-consistency (Andrews, 1990; Beck, 1976; Elliot, 1986; Goffman, 1959; Lecky, 1961; Mead, 1934; Rogers, 1961; Rosenberg, 1979; Roy & Andrews, 1991; Wylie, 1989), Zhan developed the Self-Consistency Scale (SCS). A measure of self-consistency is based on the assumption that an individual has the capacity for self-examination and evaluation. Therefore, self-perception and self-evaluation are consciously available and can be reported by the individual. Twenty-seven items in the SCS reflect the concepts of self-esteem, private consciousness, social anxiety, and stability of self-concept.

Self-esteem was measured by a global index containing six items that were originally developed by Rosenberg (1979, 1989). Elliot (1986, 1988), in examining the relationship between self-esteem and self-consistency among a sample of 2,625 young people (ages 8 to 19), found that self-esteem was highly correlated with self-consistency. An example item reflecting the concept of self-esteem in the SCS was: "I feel that I am a person of worth, at least on an equal with others." Private self-consciousness measures how preoccupied the individual is with his or her personal characteristics or the individual's tendency to be the focus of his or her own attention. Being excessively focused on one's own characteristics is likely to lead to negative affect, as the individual becomes increasingly aware that he or she does not meet those "standards of correctness" set for the self (Elliot, 1986). Therefore, excessive private consciousness leads to less self-consistency. A sample item in the SCS was: "I spend a lot of time thinking about what I am like."

Stability of self-concept refers to the sameness of self-concept across time and space (Elliot, 1988). It measures the continuity of self-concept. A sample item in the SCS was: "I feel I know just who I am." Social anxiety is viewed as one's reaction to social stimuli. It measures one's worry about others' appraisals in social settings. High social anxiety leads to less self-consistency (Elliot, 1986). A sample item in the SCS was: "I think about how others are looking at me when I am talking to someone." Private self-consciousness and social anxiety could be viewed as mediating factors in self-consistency.

Each item of the SCS was scored on an ordinal scale from 1 to 4, with 1 indicating "never" and 4 indicating "always." Positive and negative items were ordered in a way to reduce the responsive set. For analysis, all negative items were reverse scored, so that a higher score would indicate a greater self-consistency. An example of a reverse-scored item was: "I feel mixed up about what I am really like." The SCS was administered to a sample of 130 older people. Psychometric evaluations of the SCS revealed an internal consistency reliability of .89, with a score range from 51 to 104, a mean total score of 85.10 and standard deviations of 11.04 (Zhan & Shen, 1994). Content validity was supported by extensive and concurrent literature research in the field of self-consistency and self-theory and by an expert panel consisting of four university faculty members who validated each item in the SCS. Convergent validity was supported by a significantly positive correlation between a Visual Analog Scale, "A Sense of Self," and the SCS, $r = .60, p < .01$. Divergent validity was supported by a significantly negative correlation between the SCS and the Geriatric Depression Scale (GDS), $r = 2.57, p < .01$. Using the GDS was based on the theoretical proposition that a lack of self-consistency leads to certain affective disorders, including depression (Beck, 1976; Lecky, 1961; Rosenberg, 1979, 1989). Therefore, the effects of its absence can perhaps best assess the strength of self-consistency.

APPLICATION OF THE MODEL USING A RESEARCH EXEMPLAR TO STUDY ELDERLY PATIENTS WITH HEARING IMPAIRMENT

It has been noted that the Roy Adaptation Model is useful in all areas of nursing practice and has been the basis of research questions to develop basic and clinical nursing science for people of all ages in health and illness (Roy & Andrews, 1999). Several authors have noted the model's particular relevance to assessment and intervention during the changes that occur across the life span. Particular changes within human development are the physical changes experienced in aging. Thus, research with elderly adults who are adapting to physical changes can provide an exemplar of use of the Roy Adaptation Model in nursing research.

Problem and Significance

Hearing loss is one of the most common conditions affecting older adults. One in three people older than 60 and a half of those older than 85 have hearing loss (National Institute on Deafness and Other Communication Disorders, 2001). The degree and types of hearing loss in older persons vary, ranging from decreased sensitivity to high frequency tones, to peripheral loss, sensorineural loss, presbycusis, or tinnitus (Maguire, 1985; Ritter, 1991). Older persons with presbycusis, for example, have more difficulty filtering out background noises (Von Wedel, Von Wedel, & Streppel, 1990). Tinnitus, a common hearing problem, is characterized by the symptoms of ringing, buzzing, hissing, whistling, or swishing sounds arising in the ear, and it affects nearly 11 percent of the elderly population (American Tinnitus Association, 1996).

Hearing serves as a sensory input necessary for one's interaction with the changing environment and for a number of critical adaptive functions. It provides the individual with cues of oncoming threats that can be heard only. The sense of hearing augments visual cues for orienting individuals in space and for locating other people and objects. Loss of hearing can have profound psychological effects on one's life, including feeling insecure, rejected, and depressed; family stress; social isolation; and a decline in one's overall self-concept (Chen, 1994; Salomon, 1986; Whitbourne, 1985; Zhan, 1993b). One elderly man described that "the greatest annoyance of hearing loss is in the subtle aspect of daily living with a partner who also has a hearing loss. You have to constantly repeat what you said; you have to raise your voice since your partner cannot hear well; after all, you are in your own silent world" (Zhan, 1992).

The core problem of hearing loss lies in communication failures and relationship stress, which in turn affects one's self-concept and well-being. Older people with hearing loss therefore face a major task that involves coping with and adapting to hearing impairment so as to maintain their senses of self. Roy & Andrews (1991) indicates that either sensory deprivation or overload can initiate one's cognitive efforts or cognator subsystem. It is through cognitive efforts that effective adaptation takes place. One effective adaptive response,

as described by Roy, is the maintenance of self-consistency. Roy's basic theoretical premises are that individuals are rarely passive in the face of what happens to them. They are adaptive, self-protective, and functional in the face of setbacks, and seek higher levels of adaptation by enhancing person and environment interactions. People seek to change things if they can, and when they cannot, they may use cognitive adaptation processes to change the meaning of the situation in order to protect themselves and enhance their selves and their world (Lazarus, 1991; Roy & Andrews, 1999; Taylor, 1983). To empirically validate Roy's generic theoretical proposition relating the cognator processes to adaptation, the author conducted a quantitative study to examine the relationship between cognitive adaptation processes and the maintenance of self-consistency in older persons with impaired hearing.

Study Design

Based on Roy's Adaptation Model—specifically, on the cognator subsystem of the individual—hearing loss in this study was viewed as a focal stimulus. In the elderly person, hearing loss during aging initiates cognitive coping efforts to bring about the effective adaptation: the maintenance of self-consistency. Personal characteristics and social, cultural, and environmental factors influence maintenance of self-consistency through coping and adaptation processes.

Research Hypotheses

The usefulness of a model for research depends on the model's ability to generate testable hypotheses. Within a larger study, the following hypothesis was tested: There will be a positive correlation between coping and adaptation processes and self-consistency in older persons with hearing impairment.

Sample

The nonprobability sample consisted of 130 subjects who were age 64 or older, who manifested hearing loss (defined for this study as an elevated threshold equal to or larger than 26 dB in the speech frequencies of 1000, 2000, and 3000 Hertz), with the onset at age 40 or older, who had no cognitive impairment, and who resided in the northeastern part of the United States. Subjects were drawn from two nonprofit organizations for hard-of-hearing people and from several community senior centers. Informed consents were obtained, and the study was approved by the appropriate institutional review board. The mean age of this sample was 74, with a range from 64 to 94. Forty-five percent of the sample were men, and 55 percent were women.

Major Variables

Coping and adaptation processing referred to cognitive and emotional efforts made by individuals to cope with hearing loss. These efforts were operationalized by the Coping and Adaptation Processing Scale (form for elders) (Roy & Kazanowski, in press). *Self-consistency* was defined as an organized set of congruent self-perceptions, including stability of self-concept, self-esteem, private consciousness, and social anxiety. It was operationalized by the Self-Consistency Scale (Zhan & Shen, 1994).

Data Collection and Analysis

Data were collected through mailed and hand-delivered survey questionnaires; for the entire study, these included the Coping and Adaptation Processing Scale (CAPS) (Roy & Kazanowski, in press), the Self-Consistency Scale (SCS), the Geriatric Depression Scale (Sheikh & Yesavage, 1986), the Visual Analog Scale, the Demographic Profile, and the Health Status Questionnaire (SF–36) (Inter-Study Outcome Management System, 1991).

Findings

The research hypothesis examined whether a positive relationship existed between coping and adaptation processing and self-consistency. This relationship was tested via Pearson's product moment correlation on the total scores of the CAPS and the SCS, resulting in a positive, moderately strong correlation of .65, $p < .01$. The research hypothesis was supported. To describe the effect of coping and adaptation processing on self-consistency, a liner regression equation using the least square criterion was supported. To describe the effect of coping and adaptation processing on self-consistency, a liner regression equation using the least square criterion was performed. The result of $R2 = .48$ indicated that coping and adaptation processing accounted for 48 percent of the variance in self-consistency, suggesting that the coping and adaptation processing may be a significant predictor for self-consistency.

Empirical evidence of this study supports the generic proposition of the Roy Adaptation Model that the adequacy of cognator and regulator processes affects adaptive responses (Roy & Andrews, 1999, p. 547). Further, the following ancillary proposition is derived: Patterns of unique cognator processing identified in a given patient group are related to effective adaptation. In particular, a practice proposition derived for elderly persons with hearing impairment states that the coping and adaptation processes of self-perception, clear focus and method, and knowing awareness are related to the maintenance of self-consistency.

The Roy Adaptation Model provides a useful framework for research inquiry. The theoretical and empirical study of coping and adaptation processing continues to develop. The processes used to maintain self-consistency may be highly variable. Specific coping processes may be functionally overlapping. Understanding coping and adaptation processes, though often challenging, can help nurses in their efforts to restore hope for patients in sometimes hopeless situations and to help them find new meaning in their lives, to empower themselves, and to promote their well-being.

Model in Practice

Because in this sample, coping and adaptation processing explained 48 percent of the variances in self-consistency, it is suggested that coping and adaptation processing plays an active role in keeping one's self-system in balance in the face of physical changes such as hearing loss. Further, coping processes of clear focus and method, knowing awareness, and self-perception contributed most to the maintenance of self-consistency in this sample.

Understanding these coping processes can help nurses to promote individuals' coping and adaptation processing in the context of health and illness, particularly with elderly patients.

Understanding these coping processes can help nurses to promote individuals' coping and adaptation processing in the context of health and illness, particularly with elderly patients.

Coping processes of clear focus and method has

to do with the internal restructuring of the person in challenging encounters. It involves mental construction of concept formation (Roy, 1988a, 1988b, 2001). Concepts allow the person to organize information into manageable units or related data. For example, an understanding of the relationships among the concepts of hearing loss, aging, and self guides the person's behavior in a given situation. In the situation of hearing loss, the person may modify or change the meaning of the term "hearing loss," which may in turn reduce the threat to the person and to his or her sense of self. Realistic concept formation results in effective coping. Therefore, to promote this adaptive coping process, nursing interventions need to identify how the person represents the problem, what meaning and concepts are attached to the person's experience, and what strategies can be used for effective adaptation.

Coping processes of knowing awareness involves individuals' efforts in searching for coping resources and strategies, retrieving information, recognizing workable methods or experience in the past, and learning from or comparing with others who have experienced similar or different encounters. Taylor (1983) viewed downward and upward social comparison as one effort of coping and adaptation. In using an upward comparison, the person may select a physically disadvantaged person who adapts effectively as a role model for the purpose of self-enhancement. Cognitively, a person may use downward comparison to compare his or her hearing problem to the more serious problems of other individuals, so as to reduce the threat of hearing loss and to enhance a sense of self. Such cognitive comparisons may serve the purpose of preventing discrepancies between a desired sense of self and the current self-perception. Another source of the knowing-awareness dimension of coping and adaptation processing in older persons is how they address and integrate their historical self into their current life. This coping strategy provides a source of pride for older persons. Nurses can facilitate older people's adaptation to chronic conditions by encouraging them to review the course of their lives in perspective, to draw on sources of positive life experiences, and to identify relevant information that promotes effective coping.

Coping processes of self-perception refers to self-awareness, self-analysis, emotion, and consciousness (Zhan, 1993a). This processing serves three functions in adaptation. First, self-awareness signals the need for adaptive efforts. A case in point is the inability to discriminate pain. In such cases, in order to survive, the person must be trained to recognize and react to strong stimuli, such as the danger of handling sharp objects. Maintenance of self-consistency involves efforts of self-adjustment as the person interacts with the environment. If a discrepancy is sensed, cognitive processes of self-awareness, analysis, and emotions are activated to reduce that discrepancy.

Second, self-analysis and emotions interrupt ongoing behavior patterns, so that the person can attend to a more salient danger in order to deal with it. For example, keeping in touch with emotion directs the person's attention and efforts toward goals imperative and important for the person in a given situation. In a study of coping strategies, Folkman and Lazarus (1988) found that stressful health events elicited greater use of emotion-focused coping responses than use of problem-focused coping strategies. Keeping in touch with emotions creates a sense of the emergency, without which adaptive reactions would be too pallid.

Third, self-consciousness and self-analysis involve a person's efforts to restore a sense of self through self-enhancing evaluation (Taylor, 1983). Self-enhancing evaluation may involve how an individual perceives the encounter. If older people view hearing loss as a challenge rather than as a threat, the anxiety associated with hearing loss may be minimized. Emotionally, older people with hearing loss may be less overwhelmed, and their self-structure hence would be protected. However, the relationship between perceiving the encounter as a threat or as a challenge can shift as an encounter unfolds (Lazarus & Folkman, 1984). The individual's coping resources and personality may influence how he or she views the encounter. Therefore, nursing intervention needs first to assess how the person affected perceives the stressful encounter and then to develop strategies that encourage perceptions of being challenged rather than being threatened. It is critical to keep in mind that the relationship between the threat and the challenge is recursive, in part depending on the individual's interaction with the external environment. As the environment is altered, cognitive perception may be changed. For example, as a supportive environment is given and a person searches for more resources, the perceived encounter can be changed from negative to positive.

This study, though limited by the sample size and representation, provided knowledge related to the cognator conceptualization of the Roy Adaptation Model. Maintenance of self-consistency is a task that engages older persons. It can be achieved through coping and adaptation processes and can be influenced by multiple factors. It can be viewed as a health indicator of how well a person copes with stress in the aging process. Self-consistency is a complex multidimensional construct. Maintenance of self-consistency is not necessarily a rigid, never-changing self-concept. Modifications of the self-concept are expected. Maturation and social learning provide the instance of a naturally changing self-concept. However, these changes need not imply inconsistency of self (Elliot, 1986, 1988; Roy & Andrews, 1999).

This empirical study provided support for the Roy Adaptation Model and for the theoretical proposition that cognitive processing brings about adaptive responses such as the maintenance of self-consistency. Coping and adaptation theory asserts that cognitive processing is an essential feature of a complete analysis of human responses to stressful conditions of life (Roy, in review; Roy & Andrews, 1999; Taylor, 1983). Coping and adaptation processing is not just information processing per se, although it partakes of such a process. Rather, it is largely evaluative, focusing on meaning and significance attached to each individual's lived experience. Further, coping and adaptation processing takes place continuously in the transaction between the person and the environment.

SUMMARY

This chapter focused on the Roy Adaptation Model as a basis for developing knowledge for clinical practice. There is extensive literature on both the theoretical development of the model and the use of the model in research. A brief review of the model focused on recent developments in theory and research. Two major constructs of the model were elaborated: coping and adaptation processing and self-consistency. The derived middle-range theory of coping and adaptation processing combined inferred coping strategies with observed cognitive behavior to provide the basis for an application of the

model in a research exemplar with elderly patients. The exemplar research project served to demonstrate support for a generic theoretical proposition based on the model. Further, the study illustrated how a hypothesis based on the model, with adequate conceptual and empirical development of the variables, can be used to derive clinical knowledge for a given patient population.

References

Aldwin, C. M. (1994). *Stress, coping, and development: An integrative perspective.* New York: The Guilford Press.

American Tinnitus Association. (1996). *Information about tinnitus.* Portland, OR: American Tinnitus Association.

Andrews, J. D. W. (1990). Interpersonal self-confirmation and challenge in psychotherapy. *Psychotherapy, 27*(4), 485–504.

Atchley, R. C. (1988). *Social forces and aging: An introduction to social gerontology* (5th ed.). Belmont, CA: Wadsworth.

Beck, T. (1976). *Cognitive therapy and the emotional disorder.* New York: International Psychiatry.

Boston-Based Adaptation Research in Nursing Society. (1999). *The Roy Adaptation Model-Based Research: Twenty-Five Years of Contributions to Nursing Science.* Indianapolis, IN: Center Nursing Press.

Carver, C. S., & Scheier, M. F. (1991). Self-regulation and the self. In Strauss, J., & Goethals, G. R. (Eds.), *The self: Interdisciplinary approaches* (pp. 172–207). New York: Springer-Verlag.

Chen, H. L. (1994). Relation of hearing loss, loneliness and self esteem. *Journal of Gerontological Nursing, 20*(6), 22.

Coombs, A., & Snyggs, D. (1959). *Individual behavior—A perceptual approach to behavior.* New York: Harper Brothers.

Das, J. P. (1984). Intelligence and information integration. In Kirby, J. (Ed.), *Cognitive strategies and educational performance* (pp. 13–31). New York: Academic Press.

Elliot, G. C. (1986). Self-esteem and self-consistency: A theoretical and empirical link between two primary motivations. *Social Psychology Quarterly, 49*(3), 207–218.

Elliot, G. C. (1988). Gender differences in self-consistency: Evidence from an investigation of self-concept structure. *Journal of Youth and Adolescence, 17*(1), 41–57.

Folkman, S., & Lazarus, R. (1988). *Manual for the ways of coping questionnaire.* Palo Alto, CA: Consulting Psychologists Press.

Goffman, E. (1959). *The presentation of self in everyday life.* New York: Anchor.

Gove, W. R., Ortage, S. T., & Style, C. B. (1989). The maturation and role perspective on aging and self through the adult years: An empirical evaluation. *American Journal of Sociology, 94,* 1117–1145.

InterStudy Outcome Management System. (1991). The health status questionnaire (SF–36). *Interstudy Quality Edge, 1*(1).

Kaufman, S. (1987). *The ageless self.* Madison: University of Wisconsin Press.

Klarkowska, G. H., & Klarkowska, A. (1987). Perceived self-concept discontinuity as a determinant of defensive information processing in conditions of threat to self. *Psychological Bulletin, 19,* 21–29.

Lazarus, R. S. (1991). *Emotion and adaptation.* New York: Oxford University Press.

Lazarus, R. S., & Folkman, S. (1984). *Stress, appraisal, and coping.* New York: Springer Publishing Co.

Lecky, P. (1961). *Self-consistency: A theory of personality.* Frederisk, CT: Shoe String Press.

Lieberman, M. A., & Tobin, S. S. (1988). *The experience of old age: Stress, coping and survival.* New York: Basic Books.

Luria, A. R. (1973). *The working brain: An introduction to neuropsychology.* New York: Basic Books.

Luria, A. R. (1980). *The working brain: An introduction to neuropsychology.* New York: Basic Books.

Maguire, G. (1985). The changing realm of senses. In Lewis, C. (Ed.), *Aging: The health care challenge* (pp. 101–116). Philadelphia: F. A. Davis.

Mead, G. (1934). *Mind, self, and society.* Chicago: University of Chicago Press.

National Institute on Deafness and Other Communication Disorders. (2001). http://www.nidcd.nih.gov/health/hearing/older.asp. National Institute of Health. Retreived May 14, 2004.

Ritter, M. (1991). Study suggested men losing hearing earlier. *Erie Daily Times,* November 26, 2.

Rogers, C. (1961). *On becoming a person.* Boston: Houghton Mifflin.

Rosenberg, M. (1979). *Conceiving self.* New York: Basic Books.

Rosenberg, M. (1989). *Society and adolescent self-image.* Princeton, NJ: Princeton University Press.

Roy, C. (1971). Adaptation: A basis for nursing practice. *Nursing Outlook, 19*(4), 254–257.

Roy, C. (1975). *Psycho-social adaptation and the coping mechanisms.* Unpublished manuscript.

Roy, C. (1977). Decision-making by the physically ill and adaptation during illness. Doctoral dissertation, University of California, Los Angeles. University Microfilms International.

Roy, C. (1984). *Introduction to nursing: An adaptation model* (2nd ed.). Englewood Cliffs, NJ: Prentice-Hall.

Roy, C. (1985). *Cognitive processing in patients with closed head injury.* Poster session, 18th Annual Communicating Nursing Research Conference. Seattle, Washington. Western Society for Research in Nursing.

Roy, C. (1988a). Altered cognition: An information processing approach. In Mitchell, P. H., Hodges, L. C., Muwaswes, M., & Walleck, C. A., (Eds.), *AANN's neuroscience nursing: Phenomenon and practice: Human responses to neurological health problems* (pp. 185–211). Norwalk, CT: Appleton & Lange.

Roy, C. (1988b). Human information processing. In Fitzpatrick, J. J., Taunton, R. L., & Benoliel, J. Q. (Eds.), *Annual review of nursing research* (pp. 237–261). New York: Springer Publishing.

Roy, C. (2001). Alterations in cognitive processing. In C. Stewart-Amidei & J. A. Kunkel (Eds). *AANN's neuroscience nursing: Human responses to neurologic dysfunction* (2nd ed., pp. 275–323). Philadelphia: Saunders.

Roy, C., & Andrews, H. (1991). *The Roy Adaptation Model: The definitive statement.* Norwalk, CT: Appleton & Lange.

Roy, C., & Andrews, H. (1999). *The Roy adaptation model* (2nd ed.). Norwalk, CT: Appleton & Lange.

Roy, C., & Chayaput, P. (2004). Coping and Adaptation Processing Scale—English and Thai versions. *RAA Review Newsletter, 6*(2), 4, 6.

Roy, C., & Corliss, P. (1993). The Roy adaptation model: Theoretical update and knowledge for practice. In Parker, M. E. (Ed.), *Patterns for nursing theories in practice* (pp. 215–229). New York: National League for Nursing Press.

Roy, C., & Hanna, D. (1999, April 9–11). *Acute phase nursing interventions for improving cognitive functional status in patients with closed head injury.* 11th Annual ENRS scientific sessions. New York.

Roy, C., & Kazanowski, M. (in press). *Cognitive adaptation processing scale: Instrument development.*

Roy, C., Pollock, S., Massey, V., Lauchner, K., Whetsel, V., Frederickson, K., Barone, S., & Carson, M. (1999). *The Roy adaptation model-based research: Twenty-five years of contributions to nursing science.* Indianapolis: Sigma Theta Tau International.

Roy, C., & Roberts, S. (1981). *Theory construction in nursing: An adaptation model.* Englewood Cliffs, NJ: Prentice-Hall.

Salomon, C. (1986). Hearing problems and the elderly. *Danish Medical Bulletin, 33*(Suppl. 3), 1–21.

Schwarzer, R., & Schwarzer, C. (1996). A critical survey of coping instruments. In Zeidner, M. & Endler, N. S. (Eds.), *Handbook of coping: Theory, research, applications,* (pp. 107–132). New York: John Wiley & Sons, Inc.

Sheikh, J. L., & Yesavage, J. A. (1986). A geriatric depression scale: Recent evidence and development of a shorter version. *Clinical Gerontologist, 5*(1/2), 165–173.

Taylor, C. (1983). Adjustment to threatening events: A theory of cognitive adaptation. *American Psychologists,* November 16, 1161–1173.

Von Wedel, H., Von Wedel, U. C., & Streppel, M. (1990). Selective hearing in the aged in regard to speech perception in quiet and in noise. *Acta Otolaryngol, 476* (Suppl.), 131.

Whitbourne, S. (1985). *The aging body: Physiological changes and psychological consequences.* New York: Springer-Verlag.

Wylie, R. (1989). *Measures of self-concept.* Lincoln: University of Nebraska Press.

Zhan, L. (1992). Interviewing with hearing impaired older persons. Unpublished paper, Boston College, Chestnut Hill, MA.

Zhan, L. (1993a). *Coping with hearing loss.* Unpublished paper, Boston College, Chestnut Hill, MA.

Zhan, L. (1993b). *Cognitive adaptation process in hearing impaired elderly.* Doctoral dissertation, Boston College, Chestnut Hill, MA.

Zhan, L., & Shen, C. (1994). The development of an instrument to measure self-consistency. *Journal of Advanced Nursing, 20,* 509–516.

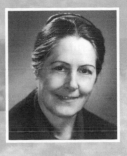

Betty Neuman

CHAPTER 18

Betty Neuman: The Neuman Systems Model and Global Applications

Patricia Deal Aylward

Introducing the Theorist

Betty Neuman developed the Neuman Systems Model in 1970 to "provide unity, or a focal point, for student learning" (Neuman, 1995, p. 674) at the School of Nursing, University of California at Los Angeles. Neuman recognized the need for educators and practitioners to have a framework to view nursing comprehensively within various contexts. While she developed the model strictly as a teaching aid, the model is now used globally as a nursing conceptual model. Dr. Neuman has been a pioneer in several areas within and outside of nursing. One example of Dr. Neuman's pioneering work is she was one of the first nurses to be licensed as a marriage, family, and child counselor in the state of

California in 1970. She is an author, lecturer, and independent nursing curriculum consultant. Neuman has published numerous books and journal articles in response to requests for support in applying the model to education, practice, research, and administration. Dr. Neuman received honorary doctorates from Grand Valley State University in Allendale, Michigan, in 1998, and from Neuman College in Aston, Pennsylvania, in 1992. Dr. Neuman is an honorary fellow in the American Academy of Nursing.

The Neuman Systems Model

The Neuman Systems Model provides a comprehensive, flexible, holistic, and systems-based perspective for nursing. This conceptual model of nursing focuses attention on the response of the client system to actual or potential environmental stressors, and the use of primary, secondary, and tertiary nursing prevention interventions for retention, attainment, and maintenance of optimal client system wellness.

—Betty Neuman (1996)

As its name suggests, the Neuman Systems Model is classified as a systems model or a systems category of knowledge. Neuman (1995) defined

> **Neuman (1995) defined system as a pervasive order that holds together its parts.**

system as a pervasive order that holds together its parts. With this definition in mind, she writes that nursing can be readily conceptualized as a complete whole, with identifiable smaller wholes or parts. The complete whole structure is maintained by interrelationships among identifiable smaller wholes or parts through regulations that evolve out of the dynamics of the open system. In the system there is dynamic energy exchange, moving either toward or away from stability. Energy moves toward negentropy or evolution as a system absorbs energy to increase its organization, complexity, and development when it moves toward a steady or wellness state. An open system of energy exchange is never at rest. The open system tends to move cyclically toward differentiation and elaboration for further growth and survival of the organism. With the

dynamic energy exchange, the system also can move away from stability. Energy can move toward extinction (entropy) by gradual disorganization, increasing randomness, and energy dissipation.

The Neuman Systems Model illustrates a client-client system and presents nursing as a field primarily concerned with defining appropriate nursing actions in stressor-related situations or in possible reactions of the client-client system. The client and environment may be positively or negatively affected by each other. There is a tendency within any system to maintain a steady state or balance among the various disruptive forces operating within or upon it. Neuman has identified these forces as stressors and suggests that possible reactions and actual reactions with identifiable signs or symptoms may be mitigated through appropriate early interventions (Neuman, 1995).

PROPOSITIONS

Neuman has identified 10 propositions inherent within her model. Fawcett (1995a, p. 2) defined *propositions* as "statements that describe or link concepts." She provided additional clarity to the term "proposition" by adding that some propositions are general descriptions or definitions of the conceptual model concepts, whereas other propositions state the relationships among conceptual model concepts in a general manner. In Fawcett's (1995a) analysis of the Neuman Systems Model, she acknowledged that Neuman's propositions that link person, environment, health, and nursing leave no gaps between these concepts. Fawcett believes that Neuman's primary, secondary, and tertiary preventions provide the required linkages among the concepts of the model (1995a). The following propositions describe, define, and connect concepts essential to understanding the conceptual model that is presented in the next section of this chapter.

1. Although each individual client or group as a client system is unique, each system is a composite of common known factors or innate characteristics within a normal, given range of response contained within a basic structure.
2. Many known, unknown, and universal environmental stressors exist. Each differs in its potential for disturbing a client's usual stability

level or normal line of defense. The particular interrelationships of client variables—physiological, psychological, sociocultural, developmental, and spiritual—at any point in time can affect the degree to which a client is protected by the flexible line of defense against possible reaction to a single stressor or a combination of stressors.

3. Each individual client-client system has evolved a normal range of response to the environment that is referred to as a normal line of defense, or usual wellness/stability state. It represents change over time through coping with diverse stress encounters. The normal line of defense can be used as a standard from which to measure health deviation.

4. When the cushioning, accordion-like effect of the flexible line of defense is no longer capable of protecting the client-client system against an environmental stressor, the stressor breaks through the normal line of defense. The interrelationships of variables—physiological, psychological, sociocultural, developmental, and spiritual—determine the nature and degree of system reaction or possible reaction to the stressor.

5. The client, whether in a state of wellness or illness, is a dynamic composite of the interrelationships of variables—physiological, psychological, sociocultural, developmental, and spiritual. Wellness is on a continuum of available energy to support the system in an optimal state of system stability.

6. Implicit within each client system are internal resistance factors know as lines of resistance, which function to stabilize and return the client to the usual wellness state (normal line of defense) or possibly to a higher level of stability following an environmental stressor reaction.

7. Primary prevention relates to general knowledge that is applied in client assessment and intervention in identification and reduction or mitigation of possible or actual risk factors associated with environmental stressors to prevent possible reaction. The goal of health promotion is included in primary prevention.

8. Secondary prevention relates to symptomatology following a reaction to stressors, appropriate ranking of intervention priorities, and treatment to reduce their noxious effects.

9. Tertiary prevention relates to the adaptive processes taking place as reconstitution begins and maintenance factors move the client back in a circular manner toward primary prevention.

10. The client as a system is in a dynamic, constant energy exchange with the environment (Neuman, 1995, pp. 20–21, with permission).

THE CONCEPTUAL MODEL

Neuman's original diagram of her model is illustrated in Figure 18–1. The conceptual model was developed to explain the client-client system as an individual person for the discipline of nursing. Neuman chose the terms "client" or "client system" instead of "human" to show respect for collaborative relationships that exist between the client and the caregiver in Neuman's model. Neuman now believes the model can be equally well applied to a group, larger community, or social issue and is appropriate for nursing and other health disciplines (Neuman, 1995).

The Neuman Systems Model provides a way of looking at the domain of nursing: humans, environment, health, and nursing. Figures 18–2, 18–3, and 18–4 are included to help focus on the client-client system, environment, and nursing aspects of the nursing domain.

CLIENT-CLIENT SYSTEM

The structure of the client-client system is illustrated in Figure 18–2. The client-client system consists of the flexible line of defense, the normal line of defense, lines of resistance, and the basic structure energy resources (shown at the core of the concentric circles in Figure 18-2). Five client variables—physiological, psychological, sociocultural, developmental, and spiritual—occur and are considered simultaneously in each concentric circle that makes up the client-client system (Neuman, 1995).

Flexible Line of Defense

Stressors must penetrate the flexible line of defense before they are capable of penetrating the rest of the client system. Neuman described this line of defense as an accordion-like mechanism that acts like a protective buffer system to help prevent stressor invasion of the client system. The flexible line of

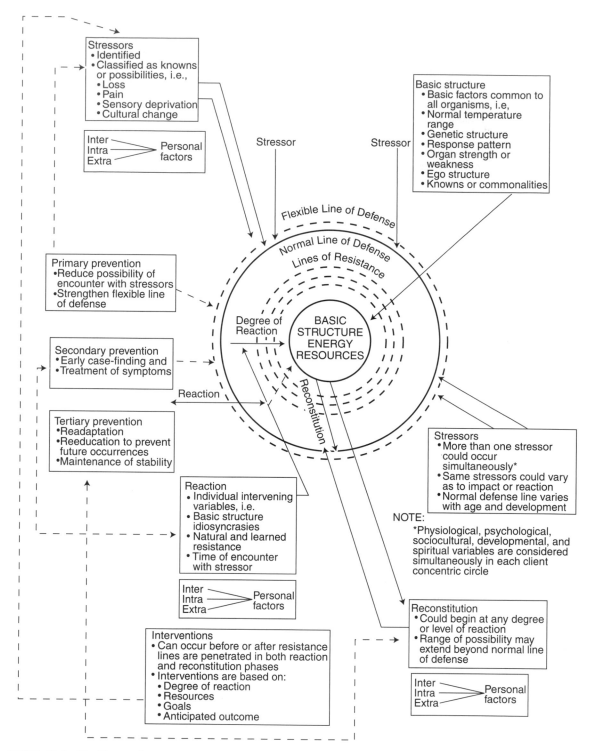

FIGURE 18–1 The Neuman Systems Model. Original diagram copyright 1970 by Betty Neuman. A holistic view of a dynamic open client-client system interacting with environmental stressors, along with client and caregiver collaborative participation in promoting an optimum state of wellness. From Neuman, 1995, p. 17, with permission.

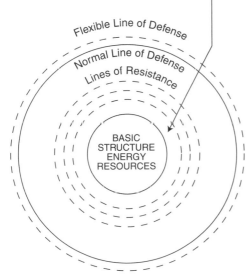

Basic structure
- Basic factors common to all organisms, i.e,
- Normal temperature range
- Genetic structure
- Response pattern
- Organ strength or weakness
- Ego structure
- Knowns or commonalities

Flexible Line of Defense
Normal Line of Defense
Lines of Resistance

BASIC
STRUCTURE
ENERGY
RESOURCES

NOTE:
Physiological, psychological, sociocultural, developmental, and spiritual variables occur and are considered simultaneously in each client concentric circle.

FIGURE 18–2   Client-client system. The structure of the client-client system, including the five variables that are occurring simultaneously in each client concentric circle. From Neuman, 1995, p. 26, with permission.

the latter examples. What are the effects of short-term loss of sleep, poor nutrition, or dehydration on a client's normal state of wellness? Will these situations increase the possibility for stressor penetration? The answer is that the possibility for stressor penetration may be increased. The actual response depends upon the accordion-like mechanism previously described, along with the other components of the client system.

Normal Line of Defense

The normal line of defense represents what the client has become over time, or the usual state of

> *The normal line of defense represents what the client has become over time, or the usual state of wellness.*

wellness. The nurse should determine the client's usual level of wellness in order to recognize a change in the level of wellness. The normal line of defense is considered dynamic by Neuman, because it can expand or contract over time. She demonstrated this dynamic state by giving an example in which the usual wellness level or system stability decreases, remains the same, or improves following treatment of a stressor reaction. Neuman also considers the normal line of defense dynamic because of its ability to become and remain stabilized with life stresses over time. The basic structure and system integrity are protected (Neuman, 1995).

Lines of Resistance

Neuman identified the series of concentric circles that surround the basic structure as lines of resistance for the client. When the normal line of defense is penetrated by stressors, a degree of reaction, or signs and/or symptoms, will occur. Lines of resistance are activated following invasion of the normal line of defense by environmental stressors. Each line of resistance contains known and unknown internal and external resource factors. These factors support the client's basic structure and the normal line of defense, resulting in protection of system integrity. Examples of the factors that support the basic structure and normal line of defense include the body's mobilization of white blood cells and activation of the immune system mechanisms. There

defense protects the normal line of defense. The client has more protection from stressors when the flexible line expands away from the normal line of defense. The opposite is true when the flexible line moves closer to the normal line of defense. The effectiveness of the buffer system can be reduced by single or multiple stressors. The flexible line of defense can be rapidly altered over a relatively short time period. States of emergency, or short-term conditions, such as loss of sleep, poor nutrition, or dehydration, are examples of what the client is like in the temporary state that is represented by the flexible line of defense (Neuman, 1995). Consider

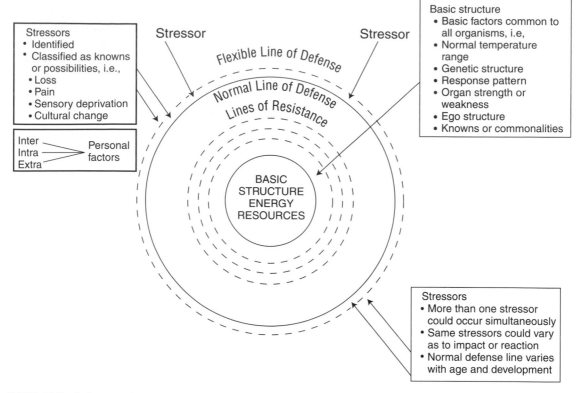

Stressors
• Identified
• Classified as knowns or possibilities, i.e.,
  • Loss
  • Pain
  • Sensory deprivation
  • Cultural change

Inter
Intra
Extra — Personal factors

Stressor

Flexible Line of Defense

Normal Line of Defense

Lines of Resistance

BASIC STRUCTURE ENERGY RESOURCES

Stressor

Basic structure
• Basic factors common to all organisms, i.e,
• Normal temperature range
• Genetic structure
• Response pattern
• Organ strength or weakness
• Ego structure
• Knowns or commonalities

Stressors
• More than one stressor could occur simultaneously
• Same stressors could vary as to impact or reaction
• Normal defense line varies with age and development

FIGURE 18–3   Environment. Internal and external factors surrounding the client-client system. From Neuman, 1995, p. 27, with permission.

Primary prevention
• Reduce possibility of encounter with stressors
• Strengthen flexible line of defense

Secondary prevention
• Early case-finding and
• Treatment of symptoms

Tertiary prevention
• Readaptation
• Reeducation to prevent future occurrences
• Maintenance of stability

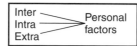

Inter
Intra
Extra — Personal factors

Interventions
• Can occur before or after resistance lines are penetrated in both reaction and reconstitution phases
• Interventions are based on:
  • Degree of reaction
  • Resources
  • Goals
  • Anticipated outcome

FIGURE 18–4   Nursing. Accurately assessing the effects and possible effects of environmental stressors (inter-, intra-, and extrapersonal factors) and using appropriate prevention by interventions to assist with client adjustments for an optimal level of wellness. From Neuman, 1995, p. 29, with permission.

is a decrease in the signs or symptoms, or a reversal of the reaction to stressors, when the lines of resistance are effective. The system reconstitutes itself or system stability is returned. The level of wellness may be higher or lower than it was prior to the stressor penetration. When the lines of resistance are ineffective, energy depletion and death occur (Neuman, 1995).

Basic Structure

The basic structure at the central core structure consists of factors that are common to all organisms. Neuman offered the following examples of basic survival factors: temperature range, genetic structure, response pattern, organ strength or weakness, ego structure, and commonalities (Neuman, 1995).

Five Client Variables

Neuman has identified five variables that are contained in all client systems: physiological, psychological, sociocultural, developmental, and spiritual. These variables are present in varying degrees of development and in a wide range of interactive styles and potential. Neuman offers the following definitions for each variable:

Physiological refers to bodily structure and function.
Psychological refers to mental processes and relationships.
Sociocultural refers to combined social and cultural functions.
Developmental refers to life-developmental processes.
Spiritual refers to spiritual belief influence. (Neuman, 1995, p. 28)

Neuman elaborated on the spiritual variable in order to assist readers in understanding that the variable is an innate component of the basic structure. While this variable may or may not be acknowledged or developed by the client or client system, Neuman views the spiritual variable as being on a continuum of development that penetrates all other client system variables and supports the client's optimal wellness. The client-client system can have a complete unawareness of the spiritual variable's presence and potential, deny its presence, or have a conscious and highly developed spiritual understanding that supports the client's optimal wellness.

Neuman explained that the spirit controls the mind, and the mind consciously or unconsciously controls the body. The spiritual variable affects or is affected by a condition and interacts with other variables in a positive or negative way. She gave the example of grief or loss (psychological state), which may inactivate, decrease, initiate, or increase spirituality. There can be movement in either direction of a continuum (Neuman, 1995). Neuman believes that spiritual variable considerations are necessary for a truly holistic perspective and for a truly caring concern for the client-client system.

Fulton (1995) has studied the spiritual variable in depth. She elaborated on research studies that extend our understanding of the following aspects of spirituality: spiritual well-being, spiritual needs, spiritual distress, and spiritual care. She suggested that spiritual needs include (1) the need for meaning and purpose in life; (2) the need to receive love and give love; (3) the need for hope and creativity; and (4) the need for forgiving, trusting relationships with self, others, and God or a deity, or a guiding philosophy.

ENVIRONMENT

The second concept identified by Neuman is the environment. Figure 18–3 illustrates this. Neuman defined *environment* broadly as "all internal and external factors or influences surrounding the identified client or client system" (Neuman, 1995, p. 30). Neuman has identified and defined the following environmental typology or classification of types for her model:

Internal environment—intrapersonal in nature.
External environment—inter- and extrapersonal in nature.
Created environment—intra-, inter-, and extrapersonal in nature. (Neuman, 1995, p. 31)

The internal environment consists of all forces or interactive influences contained within the boundaries of the client-client system. Examples of intrapersonal forces are presented for each variable.

Physiological variable—degree of mobility, range of body function.
Psychological and sociocultural variables—attitudes, values, expectations, behavior patterns, coping patterns.

Developmental variable—age, degree of normalcy, factors related to the present situation.

Spiritual variable—hope, sustaining forces. (Neuman, 1995)

The external environment consists of all forces or interactive influences existing outside the client-client system. Interpersonal factors in the environment are forces between people or client systems. These factors include the relationships and resources of family, friends, or caregivers. Extrapersonal factors include education, finances, employment, and other resources (Neuman, 1995).

Neuman (1995) has identified a third environment as the "created environment." The client unconsciously mobilizes all system variables, including the basic structure of energy factors toward system integration, stability, and integrity to create a safe environment. This safe, created environment offers a protective coping shield that helps the client to function. A major objective of the created environment is to stimulate the client's health. Neuman pointed out that what was originally created to safeguard the health of the system may have a negative outcome effect because of the binding of available energy. This environment represents an open system that exchanges energy with the internal and external environments. The created environment supersedes or goes beyond the internal and external environments while encompassing both. The created environment provides an insulating effect to change the response or possible response of the client to environmental stressors. Neuman (1995) gave the following examples of responses: use of denial or envy (psychological), physical rigidity or muscle constraint (physiological), life-cycle continuation of survival patterns (developmental), required social space range (sociocultural), and sustaining hope (spiritual).

Neuman believes the caregiver, through assessment, will need to determine (1) what has been created (nature of the created environment), (2) the outcome of the created environment (extent of its use and client value), and (3) the ideal that has yet to be created (the protection that is needed or possible, to a lesser or greater degree). This assessment is necessary to best understand and support the client's created environment (Neuman, 1995). Neuman suggested that nursing may wish to pursue and further develop an understanding of the client's awareness of the created environment and

its relationship to health. Neuman believes that as the caregiver recognizes the value of the client-created environment and purposefully intervenes, the interpersonal relationship can become one of important mutual exchange (Neuman, 1995).

HEALTH

Health is the third concept in Neuman's model. Neuman believes that wellness and illness are on opposite ends of the continuum and that *health* is the best possible wellness at any given time. Wellness exists when more energy is built and stored than expended, whereas death occurs when more energy is needed than is available to support life. Neuman views health as a manifestation of living energy available to preserve and enhance system integrity. Health is seen as varying levels within a normal range, rising and falling throughout the life span. These changes are in response to basic structure factors and reflect satisfactory and unsatisfactory adjustment by the client system to environmental stressors (Neuman, 1995).

NURSING

Nursing is the fourth concept in Neuman's model and is depicted in Figure 18–4. Nursing's major

> *Nursing's major concern is to keep the client system stable by (1) accurately assessing the effects and possible effects of environmental stressors, and (2) assisting client adjustments required for optimal wellness.*

concern is to keep the client system stable by (1) accurately assessing the effects and possible effects of environmental stressors, and (2) assisting client adjustments required for optimal wellness. Neuman defined *optimal* as the best possible health state achievable at a given point in time. Nursing actions, which she labels as prevention by intervention, are initiated to keep the system stable. Neuman has created a typology for her prevention by intervention nursing actions. They include primary prevention by intervention, secondary prevention by intervention, and tertiary prevention by intervention. All of these actions are initiated to best retain, attain, and maintain optimal client health or wellness. Neuman (1995) believes the nurse creates a linkage among the client, the environment, health, and nursing in the process of keeping the system stable.

PREVENTION AS INTERVENTION

Primary prevention as intervention involves the nurse's actions that promote client wellness by stressor prevention and reduction of risk factors. These interventions can begin at any point a stressor is suspected or identified, before a reaction has occurred. They protect the normal line of defense and strengthen the flexible lines of defense. Health promotion is a significant intervention. The goal of these interventions is to "retain" optimal stability or wellness. The nurse should consider primary prevention along with secondary and tertiary preventions as interventions. Once a reaction occurs from a stressor, the nurse can use secondary prevention as intervention to protect the basic structure by strengthening the internal lines of resistance. The goal of these interventions is to "attain" optimal client-system stability, or wellness, and energy conservation. The nurse should use as much of the client's existing internal and external resources as possible to stabilize the system by strengthening the internal lines of resistance and reducing the degree of reaction to the stressors. Neuman suggested the nurse should collaborate with the client to establish relevant goals. The goals are derived only after synthesizing comprehensive client data and relevant theory in order to determine an appropriate nursing diagnostic statement. With the nursing diagnostic statement and goals in mind, appropriate interventions can be planned and implemented (Neuman, 1995).

Reconstitution represents the return and maintenance of system stability following nursing intervention for stressor reaction. The state of wellness may be higher, the same, or lower than the state of wellness before the system was stabilized. Death occurs when secondary prevention as intervention fails to protect the basic structure and thus fails to reconstitute the client (Neuman, 1995).

Tertiary prevention as intervention can begin at any point in the client's reconstitution. These actions are designed to "maintain" an optimal wellness level by supporting existing strengths and conserving client system energy. Tertiary preven-

tion tends to lead back to primary prevention in a circular fashion. Neuman pointed out that one or all three of these prevention modalities give direction to or may be used for nursing action with possible synergistic benefits (Neuman, 1995).

Nursing Tools for Model Implementation

Neuman has designed the Neuman nursing process format and the format for prevention as intervention to facilitate implementation of the Neuman model. These formats are presented in the third edition of Neuman's book (1995, pp. 18–20). The format demonstrates a process that guides information processing and goal-directed activities. Neuman used the nursing process within three categories: nursing diagnosis, nursing goals, and nursing outcomes. Comprehensive data are collected prior to formulating a nursing diagnosis. This process is facilitated using guides such as the assessment and intervention tool mentioned in Neuman's book (1995). Nursing goals are determined mutually with the caregiver–client-client system, along with mutually agreed upon prevention as intervention strategies. Nursing outcomes are determined by the accomplishment of the interventions and evaluation of goals following intervention. The Neuman nursing process format was validated in 1982 by doctoral students. The format's validity and social utility have been proven in a wide variety of nursing education and practice areas. Using the Neuman Systems Model, the nurse acquires significant and comprehensive client data to determine the impact or possible impact of environmental stressors upon the client system. Selected information is prioritized and related to relevant social science and nursing theories. Neuman suggested that the Neuman nursing process format has a unique component—that the client and caregiver perceptions are determined for relevant goal-setting. The nurse and the client mutually determine the client-intervention goals. Neuman pointed out that mutually agreed-upon goals and interventions are consistent with current mandates within the health-care system for client rights in health-care issues.

Neuman designed the format for prevention as intervention to convey appropriate nursing actions with each typology of prevention. Primary, secondary, and tertiary prevention nursing actions are listed in a table format in Neuman's book (1995, p. 20) to assist with model implementation. The nature of stressors and their threat to the client-client system are first determined for each type of prevention before any other nursing actions are initiated.

Global Applications of the Model

Because the model is flexible and adaptable to a wide range of groups and situations, people have used the model globally and for more than two decades. Neuman's first book, *The Neuman Systems Model: Application to Nursing Education and Practice,* was published in 1982 as a response to requests for data and support in applying the model. The third edition was published in 1995 in response to expanded use of the model globally and includes applications of the Neuman Systems Model to nursing education, practice, administration, and research. This edition is used as a primary resource for global applications highlighted in this chapter (Neuman, 1995).

APPLICATION OF THE NEUMAN SYSTEMS MODEL TO NURSING EDUCATION

Lowry, Walker, and Mirenda (1995) pointed out that in the 1980s, exploration and use of Neuman's model greatly accelerated in education at all levels of practice and in varied settings. These settings include the United States and locations such as Canada, Europe, Australia, and the Far East.

Many schools of nursing in the United States have chosen to use the Neuman Systems Model as a curriculum framework or for selected courses. Most schools surveyed indicated reasons they chose the Neuman model. These include consistency with the school's beliefs; philosophy; and concepts of humans, health, nursing, and environment. Sixteen community college and university nursing programs have used the model. Associate degree nursing programs that have used the model include Athens Area Technical Institute, Athens, Georgia; Cecil Community College, North East, Maryland; Central Florida Community College, Ocala, Florida; Los Angeles County Medical Center School of Nursing, Los Angeles Valley College, Van Nuys, California; Santa Fe Community College, Gainesville, Florida; and Yakima Valley Community College, Yakima, Washington. Baccalaureate nursing programs that have used the model include

California State University, Fresno; Indiana University, Indianapolis; Purdue University, Fort Wayne, Indiana; University of Tennessee; and the University of Texas, Tyler. Gustavus Adolphus College and St. Peter and St. Olaf College, Northfield, Minnesota, also have used the model (Glazebrook, 1995; Hilton & Grafton, 1995; Klotz, 1995; Lowry & Newsome, 1995; Stittich, Flores, & Nuttall, 1995; Strickland-Seng, 1995).

Educational programs in the United States reported benefits with using the model. The model (1) facilitated cultural considerations in the curriculum related to the populations the schools and graduates served (Stittich, Flores, & Nuttall, 1995), (2) provided a nursing focus as opposed to medical focus (Lowry & Newsome, 1995), (3) included the concept of clients as holistic beings (Lowry & Newsome, 1995), (4) allowed flexibility in arrangement of content and conceptualization of program needs (Lowry & Newsome, 1995), (5) was comprehensive and facilitated seeing the person as composites of the five variables, (6) provided a framework to study individual illness and reaction to stressors, (7) was broad enough to allow educational programs to consider family as the context within which individuals live or as the unit of care, and (8) considered the created environment.

Education programs have developed evaluation instruments to determine the effects of using the model as a framework for nursing knowledge. The curriculum evaluation instrument cited in the literature is the Lowry-Jopp Neuman Model Evaluation Instrument. This instrument was developed to examine the efficacy of using the model at Cecil Community College (Lowry & Newsome, 1995). The results of a five-year longitudinal study showed that the graduates used the model most of the time when fulfilling roles of care provider and teacher. All classes in the study claimed colleagues rarely knew, accepted, or encouraged model use. Therefore, colleagues in work settings tended to have a negative effect on the use of models.

The model is also being used internationally. Craig (1995b) reported on the experiences of 10 educational institutions in Canada in six Canadian provinces. These institutions include the University of Saskatchewan, University of Prince Edward Island, University of Calgary, Brandon University of New Brunswick, Université de Moncton, University of Western Ontario, University of Windsor, Okanagan College, University of Toronto, and University of Ottawa. Model strengths that were reported include the holistic approach, which addressed levels of prevention that guided the student to focus on the client in his or her own environment. The model also assisted the student to carry out in-depth assessments, to categorize comprehensive data, and to plan specific interventions with the client. Students reported some difficulty in understanding the complexity of the model and the developmental and spiritual variables. Students also reported that it was not always easy to differentiate between the lines of defense and resistance or to assess the degree of stressor penetration.

The Neuman Model is also being used in educational institutions in South Australia, the United Kingdom, and Sweden (Engberg, 1995; McCulloch, 1995; Vaughan & Gough, 1995). McCulloch (1995) reported that a survey of all Australian university programs showed that four undergraduate programs used the model as the major organizational curriculum framework, and another 16 programs introduced undergraduate and postgraduate students to the Neuman Model as one of several models. Vaughan and Gough (1995) found that many nursing and midwifery students chose to use the model in their own practice in the United Kingdom. They also reported that Avon and Gloucestershire College of Health used the model as the guiding principle behind curriculum development for child care. Engberg (1995) reported that most colleges throughout Sweden use the Neuman Systems Model as the theoretical framework in the module of primary health in nursing education.

APPLICATION OF THE NEUMAN SYSTEMS MODEL TO NURSING PRACTICE

The Neuman Systems Model is being used in diverse practice settings. In the United States, the model is used to guide practice with clients with cognitive impairment, meeting family needs of clients in critical care; to provide stable support groups for parents with infants in neonatal intensive care units; and to meet the needs of home caregivers, with emphasis on clients with cancer, HIV/AIDS, and head traumas. The model is used in psychiatric nursing, gerontological nursing, perinatal nursing, and occupational health nursing (Bueno & Sengin, 1995; Chiverton & Flannery, 1995; McGee, 1995; Peirce & Fulmer, 1995; Russell,

Hileman, & Grant, 1995; Stuart & Wright, 1995; Trepanier, Dunn, & Sprague, 1995; Ware & Shannahan, 1995).

Internationally, the model is being used in Canada, the United Kingdom, Sweden, the Netherlands, New Zealand, Australia, Jordan, Israel, Slovenia, and several East Asian countries (e.g., Japan, Korea, and Taiwan). Practice areas include community/public health care (Betty Neuman, personal communication, January 10, 1999; Beddome, 1995; Beynon, 1995; Craig, 1995a; Damant, 1995; Davies & Proctor, 1995; Engberg, Bjalming, & Bertilson, 1995; Felix, Hinds, Wolfe, & Martin, 1995; Vaughan & Gough, 1995; Verberk, 1995).

NURSING ADMINISTRATION AND THE NEUMAN SYSTEMS MODEL

The Neuman Systems Model has been used in diverse nursing administration settings in the United States. These settings include a community nursing center, psychiatric hospital, a continuing care retirement community, and Oklahoma State Public Health Nursing (Frioux, Roberts, & Butler, 1995; Rodriguez, 1995; Scicchitani, Cox, Heyduk, Maglicco, & Sargent, 1995; Walker, 1995a).

Poole and Flowers (1995) demonstrated how the model is used in case management of pregnant substance abusers. Kelley and Sanders (1995) presented an assessment tool that intertwines the management process, the Neuman Systems Model, and environmental dimensions. Walker (1995b) demonstrated how the model and total quality management are used to prepare health-care administrators for the future.

NURSING RESEARCH AND THE NEUMAN SYSTEMS MODEL

Gigliotti (1997) acknowledged that the Neuman Model's use as a guide in directing nursing education and clinical practice has received much national and international attention. However, the model's use as a guide to nursing research and the generation of nursing theory based on the research is in the early stages of development, although growing. To facilitate the use of nursing research with the Neuman Systems Model, Meleis (1995) has elaborated on principles and approaches that may be used to develop a futuristic agenda to validate the Neuman Systems Theory.

Fawcett (1995c) has offered guidelines for constructing Neuman Systems Model–based studies. Neuman revisited these guidelines in her 1996 article in *Nursing Science Quarterly.* She acknowledged that the Neuman model has guided a range of study designs, from qualitative descriptions of relevant phenomena to quantitative experiments that tested the effects of prevention interventions on a variety of client-system outcomes. She provided numerous examples of descriptive studies, correlational research, and experimental and quasiexperimental studies. Neuman elaborated on how to construct Neuman Model-based research.

Smith and Edgil (1995) have proposed a plan for testing middle-range theories with the model. Their plan involved the creation of an Institute for the Study of the Model to formulate and test theories through collaboration, including interdisciplinary and multisite efforts. They suggested directions for the work to be done, an organizing structure, and a task analysis of what and who would be appropriate to participate in task completion. Breckenridge (1995) has actually used the Neuman model to develop a middle-range theory based on nephrology practice. Gigliotti (1997) has identified conceptual and empirical concerns imposed upon her when she operationalized Neuman's lines of defense and resistance in her research. She concluded that the Neuman model offers an excellent and comprehensive framework from which to view the metaconcepts relevant to the discipline of nursing: person, environment, health, and nursing. Gigliotti says it is time to institute the comprehensive research program proposed by Smith and Edgil (1995).

Projections for Use of the Model in the Twenty-First Century

Neuman believes her model is "both concept and process relevant as a directive toward nursing and other health care activities in the challenging 21st Century" (Betty Neuman, personal communication, January 10, 1999). This model has been used to make projections about the future of nursing and health care. Procter and Cheek (1995) and Tomlinson and Anderson (1995) provided two examples of this use. Procter and Cheek used the model to project the role of the nurse in world catastrophic events, and Tomlinson and Anderson

used the model to project family health as a system. Procter and Cheek studied experiences of Serbian Australians at the time of the civil war in the former Yugoslavia using the Neuman model to understand the experiences. As a result of the study, the researchers came up with implications for the role of nursing in world catastrophic events. The researchers suggested that the goal of nursing in such worldwide events should be to assist individuals and communities to retain maximum wellness and system stability as they strive for a sense of inner peace and contentment against impossible odds.

Tomlinson and Anderson (1995) recognized that there is an increasing focus on the family system as a health entity. They acknowledged, however, that there is not a universally accepted definition of "family health" as a systems phenomenon. Tomlinson and Anderson proposed that the nurse who uses the broad concepts of the Neuman model along with a shared family health systems perspective, in which the whole family is the client in the health promotion enterprise, will be well prepared to meet future nursing challenges.

SUMMARY

The Neuman Systems Model has been used for over two decades; first as a teaching tool and later as a conceptual model to observe and interpret the phenomena of nursing and health care globally. Dr. Neuman (1997, p. 20) wrote: "[T]he future of the Neuman Systems Model looks bright." She believes her model can readily accommodate future changes in health-care delivery. The reader has been introduced to the model and some of the global applications of the model. The reader is also referred to additional citations compiled by Dr. Jacqueline Fawcett (1995a; 1995b).

References

Beddome, G. (1995). Community-as-client assessment. A Neuman-based guide for education and practice. In Neuman, B., *The Neuman Systems Model* (3rd ed., pp. 567–579). Norwalk, CT: Appleton & Lange.

Beynon, C. E. (1995). Neuman-based experiences of the Middlesex-London Health Unit. In Neuman, B., *The Neuman Systems Model* (3rd ed., pp. 537–547). Norwalk, CT: Appleton & Lange.

Breckenridge, D. M. (1995). Nephrology practice and directions for nursing research. In Neuman, B., *The Neuman Systems Model* (3rd ed., pp. 499–507). Norwalk, CT: Appleton & Lange.

Bueno, M. M., & Sengin, K. K. (1995). The Neuman Systems Model for critical care nursing. A framework for practice. In Neuman, B., *The Neuman Systems Model* (3rd ed., pp. 275–291). Norwalk, CT: Appleton & Lange.

Chiverton, P., & Flannery J. C. (1995). Cognitive impairment. Use of the Neuman Systems Model. In Neuman, B., *The Neuman Systems Model* (3rd ed., pp. 249–259). Norwalk, CT: Appleton & Lange.

Craig, D. M. (1995a). Community/public health nursing in Canada. Use of the Neuman Systems Model in a new paradigm. In Neuman, B., *The Neuman Systems Model* (3rd ed., pp. 529–535). Norwalk, CT: Appleton & Lange.

Craig, D. M. (1995b). The Neuman Systems Model Examples of its use in Canadian educational programs. In Neuman, B., *The Neuman Systems Model* (3rd ed., pp. 521–527). Norwalk, CT: Appleton & Lange.

Damant, M. (1995). Community nursing in the United Kingdom. A case for reconciliation using the Neuman Systems Model. In Neuman, B., *The Neuman Systems Model* (3rd ed., pp. 607–620). Norwalk, CT: Appleton & Lange.

Davies, P., & Proctor, H. (1995). In Wales: Using the model in community mental health. In Neuman, B., *The Neuman Systems Model* (3rd ed., pp. 621–627). Norwalk, CT: Appleton & Lange.

Engberg, I. B. (1995). Brief abstracts. Use of the Neuman Systems Model in Sweden. In Neuman, B., *The Neuman Systems Model* (3rd ed., pp. 653–656). Norwalk, CT: Appleton & Lange.

Engberg, I. B., Bjalming, E., & Bertilson, B. (1995). A structure for documenting primary health care in Sweden using the Neuman Systems Model. In Neuman, B., *The Neuman Systems Model* (3rd ed., pp. 637–651). Norwalk, CT: Appleton & Lange.

Fawcett, J. (1995a). *Analysis and evaluation of conceptual models of nursing.* Philadelphia: F. A. Davis.

Fawcett, J. (1995b). Bibliography. Citations compiled by Jacqueline Fawcett. In Neuman, B., *The Neuman Systems Model* (3rd ed., pp. 704–718). Norwalk, CT: Appleton & Lange.

Fawcett, J. (1995c). Constructing conceptual-theoretical-empirical structures for research. Future implications for use of the Neuman Systems Model. In Neuman, B., *The Neuman Systems Model* (3rd ed., pp. 459–471). Norwalk, CT: Appleton & Lange.

Felix, M., Hinds, C., Wolfe, C., & Martin, A. (1995). The Neuman Systems Model in a chronic care facility: A Canadian experience. In Neuman, B., *The Neuman Systems Model* (3rd ed., pp. 549–566). Norwalk, CT: Appleton & Lange.

Frioux, T. D., Roberts, A. G., & Butler, S. J. (1995). Oklahoma State public health nursing. In Neuman, B., *The Neuman Systems Model* (3rd ed., pp. 407–414). Norwalk, CT: Appleton & Lange.

Fulton, R. A. (1995). The spiritual variable. In Neuman, B., *The Neuman Systems Model* (3rd ed., pp. 77–91). Norwalk, CT: Appleton & Lange.

Gigliotti, E. (1997). Use of Neuman's lines of defense and resistance in nursing research: Conceptual and empirical considerations. *Nursing Science Quarterly, 10,* 136–143.

Glazebrook, R. S. (1995). The Neuman Systems Model in cooperative baccalaureate nursing education: The Minnesota Intercollegiate Nursing Consortium Experience. In Neuman, B., *The Neuman Systems Model* (3rd ed., pp. 227–230). Norwalk, CT: Appleton & Lange.

Hilton, S. A., & Grafton, M. D. (1995). Curriculum transition based on the Neuman Systems Model. Los Angeles County Medical Center School of Nursing. In Neuman, B., *The Neuman Systems Model* (3rd ed., pp. 163–174). Norwalk, CT: Appleton & Lange.

Kelley, J. A., & Sanders, N. F. (1995). A systems approach to the health of nursing and health care organizations. In Neuman, B., *The Neuman Systems Model* (3rd ed., pp. 347–364). Norwalk, CT: Appleton & Lange.

Klotz, L. C. (1995). Integration of the Neuman Systems Model into the BSN curriculum at the University of Texas at Tyler. In Neuman, B., *The Neuman Systems Model* (3rd ed., pp. 183–195). Norwalk, CT: Appleton & Lange.

Lowry, L. W., & Newsome, G. G. (1995). Neuman-based associate degree programs: Past, present, and future. In Neuman, B., *The Neuman Systems Model* (3rd ed., pp. 197–214). Norwalk, CT: Appleton & Lange.

Lowry, L. W., Walker, P. H, & Mirenda, R. (1995). Through the looking glass: Back to the future. In Neuman, B., *The Neuman Systems Model* (3rd ed., pp. 63–76). Norwalk, CT: Appleton & Lange.

McCulloch, S. J. (1995). Utilization of the Neuman Systems Model: University of South Australia. In Neuman, B., *The Neuman Systems Model* (3rd ed., pp. 591–597). Norwalk, CT: Appleton & Lange.

McGee, M. (1995). Implications for use of the Neuman Systems Model in occupational health nursing. In Neuman, B., *The Neuman Systems Model* (3rd ed., pp. 657–667). Norwalk, CT: Appleton & Lange.

Meleis, A. I. (1995). Theory testing and theory support: Principles, challenges, and a sojourn into the future. In Neuman, B., *The Neuman Systems Model* (3rd ed., pp. 447–457). Norwalk, CT: Appleton & Lange.

Neuman, B. (1982). *The Neuman Systems Model: Application to nursing education and practice.* Norwalk, CT: Appleton-Century-Crofts.

Neuman, B. (1995). *The Neuman Systems Model* (3rd ed.). Norwalk, CT: Appleton & Lange.

Neuman, B. (1996). The Neuman Systems Model in research and practice. *Nursing Science Quarterly, 9,* 67–70.

Neuman, B. (1997). The Neuman Systems Model: Reflections and projections. *Nursing Science Quarterly, 10,* 18–21.

Peirce, A. G., & Fulmer, T. T. (1995). Application of the Neuman Systems Model to gerontological nursing. In Neuman, B., *The Neuman Systems Model* (3rd ed., pp. 293–308). Norwalk, CT: Appleton & Lange.

Poole, V. L., & Flowers, J. S. (1995). Care management of pregnant substance abusers using the Neuman Systems Model. In Neuman, B., *The Neuman Systems Model* (3rd ed., pp. 377–386). Norwalk, CT: Appleton & Lange.

Procter, N. G., & Cheek, J. (1995). Nurses' role in world catastrophic events: War dislocation effects on Serbian Australians. In Neuman, B., *The Neuman Systems Model* (3rd ed., pp. 119–131). Norwalk, CT: Appleton & Lange.

Rodriguez, M. L. (1995). The Neuman Systems Model adapted to a continuing care retirement community. In Neuman, B.,

The Neuman Systems Model (3rd ed., pp. 431–442). Norwalk, CT: Appleton & Lange.

Russell, J., Hileman, J. W., & Grant, J. S. (1995). Assessing and meeting the needs of home caregivers using the Neuman Systems Model. In Neuman, B., *The Neuman Systems Model* (3rd ed., pp. 331–341). Norwalk, CT: Appleton & Lange.

Scicchitani, B., Cox, J. G., Heyduk, L. J., Maglicco, P. A., & Sargent, N. A. (1995). Implementing the Neuman model in a psychiatric hospital. In Neuman, B., *The Neuman Systems Model* (3rd ed., pp. 387–395). Norwalk, CT: Appleton & Lange.

Smith, M. C., & Edgil, A. E. (1995). Future directions for research with the Neuman Systems Model. In Neuman, B., *The Neuman Systems Model* (3rd ed., pp. 509–517). Norwalk, CT: Appleton & Lange.

Stittich, E. M., Flores, F. C., & Nuttall, P. (1995). Cultural considerations in a Neuman-based curriculum. In Neuman, B., *The Neuman Systems Model* (3rd ed., pp. 147–162). Norwalk, CT: Appleton & Lange.

Strickland-Seng, V. (1995). The Neuman Systems Model in clinical evaluation of students. In Neuman, B., *The Neuman Systems Model* (3rd ed., pp. 215–225). Norwalk, CT: Appleton & Lange.

Stuart, G. W., & Wright, L. K. (1995). Applying the Neuman Systems Model to psychiatric nursing practice. In Neuman, B., *The Neuman Systems Model* (3rd ed., pp. 263–273). Norwalk, CT: Appleton & Lange.

Tomlinson, P. S., & Anderson, K. H. (1995). Family health and the Neuman Systems Model. In Neuman, B., *The Neuman Systems Model* (3rd ed., pp. 133–144). Norwalk, CT: Appleton & Lange.

Trepanier, M., Dunn, S. I., & Sprague, A. E. (1995). Application of the Neuman Systems Model to perinatal nursing. In Neuman, B., *The Neuman Systems Model* (3rd ed., pp. 309–320). Norwalk, CT: Appleton & Lange.

Vaughan, B., & Gough, P. (1995). Use of the Neuman Systems Model in England. In Neuman, B., *The Neuman Systems Model* (3rd ed., pp. 599–605). Norwalk, CT: Appleton & Lange.

Verberk, F. (1995). In Holland: Application of the Neuman model in psychiatric nursing. In Neuman, B., *The Neuman Systems Model* (3rd ed., pp. 629–636). Norwalk, CT: Appleton & Lange.

Walker, P. H. (1995a). Neuman-based education, practice, and research in a community nursing center. In Neuman, B., *The Neuman Systems Model* (3rd ed., pp. 415–430). Norwalk, CT: Appleton & Lange.

Walker, P. H. (1995b). TQM and the Neuman Systems Model: Education for health care administration. In Neuman, B., *The Neuman Systems Model* (3rd ed., pp. 365–376). Norwalk, CT: Appleton & Lange.

Ware, L. A., & Shannahan, M. K. (1995). Using Neuman for a stable parent support group in neonatal intensive care. In Neuman, B., *The Neuman Systems Model* (3rd ed., pp. 321–330). Norwalk, CT: Appleton & Lange.

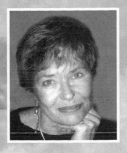

Jean Watson

CHAPTER 19

PART ONE: Jean Watson's Theory of Human Caring

Jean Watson

Introducing the Theorist
Introducing the Theory
Major Conceptual Elements
Implications of the Caring Model
Summary

Introducing the Theorist

Dr. Jean Watson is a distinguished professor of nursing and former dean of the School of Nursing at the University of Colorado. She is the founder of the Center for Human Caring in Colorado. She is also a member of the American Academy of Nursing and has served as president of the National League for Nursing.

Dr. Watson has earned undergraduate and graduate degrees in nursing and psychiatric-mental health nursing and holds a doctorate in educational psychology and counseling. She is a widely published author and is the recipient of several awards and honors, including an international Kellogg Fellowship in Australia; a Fulbright Research Award in Sweden; and six honorary doctoral degrees, including three international honorary doctorates: Sweden, United Kingdom, and Canada.

Dr. Watson's published works on the philosophy and theory of human caring and the art and science of nursing are used by clinical nurses and academic programs throughout the world. Her caring philosophy is used to guide new models of caring and healing practices in diverse settings and in several different countries. More recent clinical-research initiatives are underway in clinical agencies interested in transforming nursing practice from the inside out and heading toward caring-healing practices and models of caring, guided by Watson's theory and philosophy.

Dr. Watson's book, *Postmodern Nursing and Beyond,* reflects her most recent work on caring theory and nursing healing practices (Watson, 1999). In addition, her 2002 book on caring instruments (Watson, J. *Assessing and Measuring Caring in Nursing and Health Sciences.* New York: Springer. A critique and collation of 21 instruments for assessing and measuring caring) seeks to bridge modern and postmodern views of caring and healing in relation to current thinking, while pointing toward a new future beyond current practices. Her latest work is entitled *Caring Science as Sacred Science* (Watson, 2004/5), which makes a case for a deep moral-ethical, spirit-filled foundation for caring and healing that is based upon infinite love and an expanding cosmology. This view in turn elicits the finest of nursing as the art, science, and spiritual practice it is meant to be, as it is the highest form of compassionate service to society and humanity.

Introducing the Theory

The Theory of Human Caring was developed between 1975 and 1979 while I was teaching at the University of Colorado. It emerged from my own views of nursing, combined and informed by my doctoral studies in educational-clinical and social psychology. It was my initial attempt to bring meaning and focus to nursing as an emerging discipline and distinct health profession that had its own unique values, knowledge, and practices, and its own ethic and mission to society. The work was also influenced by my involvement with an integrated academic nursing curriculum and efforts to find common meaning and order to nursing that transcended settings, populations, specialty, sub-specialty areas, and so forth.

From my emerging perspective, I tried to make explicit that nursing's values, knowledge, and practices of human caring were geared toward subjective inner healing processes and the life world of the experiencing person. This required unique caring-healing arts and a framework called "carative factors," which complemented conventional medicine but stood in stark contrast to "curative factors." At the same time, this emerging philosophy and theory of human caring sought to balance the cure orientation of medicine, giving nursing its unique disciplinary, scientific, and professional standing with itself and its public.

MAJOR CONCEPTUAL ELEMENTS

The major conceptual elements of the original (and emergent) theory are:

- Ten carative factors (evolving toward "clinical caritas processes")
- Transpersonal caring relationship
- Caring moment/caring occasion
- Caring-healing modalities

Other dynamic aspects of the theory that have emerged or are emerging as more explicit components include:

- Expanded views of self and person (transpersonal mind-body-spirit unity of being, embodied spirit
- Caring-healing consciousness and intentionality to care and promote healing caring consciousness as energy within the human environment field of a caring moment
- Phenomenal field/unitary consciousness: unbroken wholeness and connectedness of all
- Advanced caring-healing modalities/nursing arts as future model for advanced practice of nursing qua nursing (consciously guided by one's nursing ethical-theoretical-philosophical orientation).

CARING SCIENCE

The latest emergence of the work is a more explicit development of caring science as a deep moral-ethical context of infinite and cosmic love. This view takes nursing and healing work beyond conventional thinking. The latest orientation is located within nursing at its finest while transcending nursing. Caring science as model for nursing allows nursing's caring-healing core to become both discipline-specific and transdisciplinary. Thus, nursing's timeless, enduring, and most noble contributions come of age through a caring science orientation—scientifically, aesthetically, and ethically.

Ten Carative Factors

The original (1979) work was organized around 10 carative factors as a framework for providing a format and focus for nursing phenomena. Although "carative factors" is still the current terminology for the "core" of nursing, providing a structure for the initial work, the term "factor" is too stagnant for my sensibilities today; I offer another concept that is more in keeping with my own evolution and future directions for the "theory." I offer now the concept of "clinical caritas" and "caritas processes" as consistent with a more fluid and contemporary movement with these ideas and my expanding directions.

Caritas comes from the Greek word meaning "to cherish and appreciate, giving special attention to, or loving." It connotes something that is very fine, that indeed is precious. The word "caritas" also is closely related to the original word "carative" from my 1979 book. At this time, I now make new connections between carative and caritas and without hesitation compare them to invoke love, which caritas conveys. This allows love and caring to come together for a new form of deep transpersonal caring. This relationship between love and caring connotes inner healing for self and others, extending to nature and the larger universe, unfolding and evolving within a cosmology that is both metaphysical and transcendent with the coevolving human in the universe. This emerging model of transpersonal caring moves from carative to caritas. This integrative expanded perspective is postmodern, in that it transcends conventional industrial, static models of nursing while simultaneously evoking both the past and the future. For example, the future of nursing is tied to Nightingale's sense of "calling," guided by a deep sense of commitment and a covenantal ethic of human service, cherishing our phenomena, our subject matter, and those we

> It is when we include caring and love in our work and in our life that we discover and affirm that nursing, like teaching, is more than just a job.

serve. It is when we include caring and love in our work and in our life that we discover and affirm that nursing, like teaching, is more than just a job; it is also a life-giving and life-receiving career for a lifetime of growth and learning. Such maturity and integration of past with present and future now require transforming self and those we serve, including our institutions and the profession itself. As we more publicly and professionally assert these

positions for our theories, our ethics, and our practices—even for our science—we also locate ourselves and our profession and discipline within a new, emerging cosmology. Such thinking calls for a sense of reverence and sacredness with regard to life and all living things. It incorporates both art and science, as they are also being redefined, acknowledging a convergence between art, science, and spirituality. As we enter into the transpersonal caring theory and philosophy, we simultaneously are challenged to relocate ourselves in these emerging ideas and to question for ourselves how the theory speaks to us. This invites us into a new relationship with ourselves and our ideas about life, nursing, and theory.

Original Carative Factors

The original carative factors served as a guide to what was referred to as the "core of nursing," in contrast to nursing's "trim." *Core* pointed to those aspects of nursing that potentiate therapeutic healing processes and relationships—they affect the one caring and the one being cared for. Further, the basic core was grounded in what I referred to as the philosophy, science, and even art of caring. Carative is that deeper and larger dimension of nursing that goes beyond the "trim" of changing times, setting, procedures, functional tasks, specialized focus around disease, and treatment and technology. Although the "trim" is important and not expendable, the point is that nursing cannot be defined around its trim and what it does in a given setting and at a given point in time. Nor can nursing's trim define and clarify its larger professional ethic and mission to society—its raison d'être for the public. That is where nursing theory comes into play, and transpersonal caring theory offers another way that both differs from and complements that which has come to be known as "modern" nursing and conventional medical-nursing frameworks.

The 10 carative factors included in the original work are the following:

1. Formation of a humanistic-altruistic system of values.
2. Instillation of faith-hope.
3. Cultivation of sensitivity to one's self and to others.
4. Development of a helping-trusting, human caring relationship.
5. Promotion and acceptance of the expression of positive and negative feelings.

6. Systematic use of a creative problem-solving caring process.
7. Promotion of transpersonal teaching-learning.
8. Provision for a supportive, protective, and/or corrective mental, physical, societal, and spiritual environment.
9. Assistance with gratification of human needs.
10. Allowance for existential-phenomenological-spiritual forces. (Watson, 1979/1985)

Although some of the basic tenets of the original carative factors still hold, and indeed are used as the basis for some theory-guided practice models and research, what I am proposing here, as part of my evolution and the evolution of these ideas and the theory itself, is to transpose the carative factors into "clinical caritas processes." For example, consider the following within the context of clinical caritas and emerging transpersonal caring theory.

From Carative Factors to Clinical Caritas Processes

As carative factors evolve within an expanding perspective, and as my ideas and values evolve, I now offer the following translation of the original carative factors into clinical caritas processes, suggesting more open ways in which they can be considered. For example:

1. Formation of humanistic-altruistic system of values becomes a practice of loving kindness and equanimity within the context of caring consciousness.
2. Instillation of faith-hope becomes being authentically present and enabling and sustaining the deep belief system and subjective life world of self and one being cared for.
3. Cultivation of sensitivity to one's self and to others becomes cultivation of one's own spiritual practices and transpersonal self, going beyond ego self, opening to others with sensitivity and compassion.
4. Development of a helping-trusting, human caring relationship becomes developing and sustaining a helping-trusting, authentic caring relationship.
5. Promotion and acceptance of the expression of positive and negative feelings becomes being present to, and supportive of, the expression of positive and negative feelings as a connection with deeper spirit of self and the one being cared for.

6. Systematic use of a creative problem-solving caring process becomes creative use of self and all ways of knowing as part of the caring process; to engage in artistry of caring-healing practices.
7. Promotion of transpersonal teaching-learning becomes engaging in genuine teaching-learning experience that attends to unity of being and meaning, attempting to stay within others' frames of reference.
8. Provision for a supportive, protective, and/or corrective mental, physical, societal, and spiritual environment becomes creating a healing environment at all levels (a physical and nonphysical, subtle environment of energy and consciousness, whereby wholeness, beauty, comfort, dignity, and peace are potentiated).
9. Assistance with gratification of human needs becomes assisting with basic needs, with an intentional caring consciousness, administering "human care essentials," which potentiate alignment of mind-body-spirit, wholeness, and unity of being in all aspects of care, tending to both embodied spirit and evolving spiritual emergence.
10. Allowance for existential-phenomenological-spiritual forces becomes opening and attending to spiritual-mysterious and existential dimensions of one's own life-death; soul care for self and the one being cared for.

What differs in the clinical caritas framework is that a decidedly spiritual dimension and an overt evocation of love and caring are merged for a new paradigm for this millennium. Such a perspective ironically places nursing within its most mature framework and is consistent with the Nightingale model of nursing—yet to be actualized but awaiting its evolution within a caring-healing theory. This direction, while embedded in theory, goes beyond theory and becomes a converging paradigm for nursing's future.

Thus, I consider my work more a philosophical, ethical, intellectual blueprint for nursing's evolving disciplinary/professional matrix, rather than a specific theory per se. Nevertheless, others interact with the original work at levels of concreteness or abstractness. The caring theory has been, and is still being, used as a guide for educational curricula, clinical practice models, methods for research and inquiry, and administrative directions for nursing and health-care delivery.

This work posits a value's explicit moral foundation and takes a specific position with respect to the centrality of human caring, "caritas," and love as now an ethic and ontology. It is also a critical starting point for nursing's existence, broad societal mission, and the basis for further advancement for caring-healing practices. Nevertheless, its use and evolution is dependent upon "critical, reflective practices that must be continuously questioned and critiqued in order to remain dynamic, flexible, and endlessly self-revising and emergent" (Watson, 1996, p. 143).

Transpersonal Caring Relationship

The terms *transpersonal* and *a transpersonal caring relationship* are foundational to the work. *Transpersonal* conveys a concern for the inner life world and subjective meaning of another who is fully embodied. But transpersonal also goes beyond the ego self and beyond the given moment, reaching to the deeper connections to spirit and with the broader universe. Thus, a transpersonal caring relationship moves beyond ego self and radiates to spiritual, even cosmic, concerns and connections that tap into healing possibilities and potentials.

> *Transpersonal caring seeks to connect with and embrace the spirit or soul of the other through the processes of caring and healing and being in authentic relation, in the moment.*

Transpersonal caring seeks to connect with and embrace the spirit or soul of the other through the processes of caring and healing and being in authentic relation, in the moment.

Such a transpersonal relation is influenced by the caring consciousness and intentionality of the nurse as she or he enters into the life space or phenomenal field of another person and is able to detect the other person's condition of being (at the soul or spirit level). It implies a focus on the uniqueness of self and other and the uniqueness of the moment, wherein the coming together is mutual and reciprocal, each fully embodied in the moment, while paradoxically capable of transcending the moment, open to new possibilities.

Transpersonal caring calls for an authenticity of being and becoming, an ability to be present to self and others in a reflective frame. The transpersonal nurse has the ability to center consciousness and intentionality on caring, healing, and wholeness, rather than on disease, illness, and pathology.

Transpersonal caring competencies are related to ontological development of the nurse's human competencies and ways of being and becoming. Thus, "ontological caring competencies" become as critical in this model as "technological curing competencies" were in the conventional modern, Western nursing-medicine model, which is now coming to an end.

Within the model of transpersonal caring, clinical caritas consciousness is engaged at a foundational ethical level for entry into this framework. The nurse attempts to enter into and stay within the other's frame of reference for connecting with the inner life world of meaning and spirit of the other. Together, they join in a mutual search for meaning and wholeness of being and becoming, to potentiate comfort measures, pain control, a sense of well-being, wholeness, or even a spiritual transcendence of suffering. The person is viewed as whole and complete, regardless of illness or disease (Watson, 1996, p. 153).

Assumptions of Transpersonal Caring Relationship

The nurse's moral commitment, intentionality, and caritas consciousness is to protect, enhance, promote, and potentiate human dignity, wholeness, and healing, wherein a person creates or cocreates his or her own meaning for existence, healing, wholeness, and living and dying.

The nurse's will and consciousness affirm the subjective-spiritual significance of the person while seeking to sustain caring in the midst of threat and despair—biological, institutional, or otherwise. This honors the I-Thou relationship versus an I-It relationship.

The nurse seeks to recognize, accurately detect, and connect with the inner condition of spirit of another through genuine presencing and being centered in the caring moment. Actions, words, behaviors, cognition, body language, feelings, intuition, thought, senses, the energy field, and so on, all contribute to transpersonal caring connection. The nurse's ability to connect with another at this transpersonal spirit-to-spirit level is translated via movements, gestures, facial expressions, procedures, information, touch, sound, verbal expressions, and other scientific, technical, aesthetic, and human means of communication, into nursing human art/acts or intentional caring-healing modalities.

The caring-healing modalities within the context of transpersonal caring/caritas consciousness potentiate harmony, wholeness, and unity of being by releasing some of the disharmony, the blocked energy that interferes with the natural healing processes. As a result, the nurse helps another through this process to access the healer within, in the fullest sense of Nightingale's view of nursing.

Ongoing personal-professional development and spiritual growth and personal spiritual practice assist the nurse in entering into this deeper level of professional healing practice, allowing the nurse to awaken to the transpersonal condition of the world and to actualize more fully "ontological competencies" necessary for this level of advanced practice of nursing. Valuable teachers for this work include the nurse's own life history and previous experiences, which provide opportunities for focused studies, the nurse having lived through or experienced various human conditions and having imagined others' feelings in various circumstances. To some degree, the necessary knowledge and consciousness can be gained through work with other cultures and the study of the humanities (art, drama, literature, personal story, narratives of illness journeys, etc.), along with an exploration of one's own values, deep beliefs, relationship with self and others, and one's world. Other facilitators include personal- growth experiences such as psychotherapy, transpersonal psychology, meditation, bioenergetics work, and other models for spiritual awakening. Continuous growth is ongoing for developing and maturing within a transpersonal caring model. The notion of health professionals as wounded healers is acknowledged as part of the necessary growth and compassion called forth within this theory/ philosophy.

Caring Moment/Caring Occasion

A caring occasion occurs whenever the nurse and another come together with their unique life histories and phenomenal fields in a human-to-human transaction. The coming together in a given moment becomes a focal point in space and time. It becomes transcendent, whereby experience and perception take place, but the actual caring occasion has a greater field of its own, in a given moment. The process goes beyond itself yet arises from aspects of itself that become part of the life history of each person, as well as part of some larger, more complex pattern of life (Watson, 1985, p. 59; 1996, p. 157).

A caring moment involves an action and choice by both the nurse and other. The moment of

> **A caring moment involves an action and choice by both the nurse and other.**

coming together presents the two with the opportunity to decide how to *be in the moment,* in the relationship—what to do with and in the moment. If the caring moment is *transpersonal,* each feels a connection with the other at the spirit level; thus, the moment transcends time and space, opening up new possibilities for healing and human connection at a deeper level than that of physical interaction. For example:

> [W]e learn from one another how to be human by identifying ourselves with others, finding their dilemmas in ourselves. What we all learn from it is self-knowledge. The self we learn about ... is every self. IT is universal—the human self. We learn to recognize ourselves in others ... [it] keeps alive our common humanity and avoids reducing self or other to the moral status of object. (Watson, 1985, pp. 59–60)

Caring (Healing) Consciousness

The dynamic of transpersonal caring (healing) within a caring moment is manifest in a field of consciousness. The transpersonal dimensions of a caring moment are affected by the nurse's consciousness in the caring moment, which in turn affects the field of the whole. The role of consciousness with respect to a holographic view of science has been discussed in earlier writings (Watson, 1992, p. 148) and include the following points:

- The whole caring-healing-loving consciousness is contained within a single caring moment.
- The one caring and the one being cared for are interconnected; the caring-healing process is connected with the other human(s) and with the higher energy of the universe.
- The caring-healing-loving consciousness of the nurse is communicated to the one being cared for.
- Caring-healing-loving consciousness exists through and transcends time and space and can be dominant over physical dimensions.

Within this context, it is acknowledged that the process is relational and connected. It transcends time, space, and physicality. The process is inter-subjective with transcendent possibilities that go beyond the given caring moment.

IMPLICATIONS OF THE CARING MODEL

The Caring Model or Theory can be considered a philosophical and moral/ethical foundation for professional nursing and is part of the central focus for nursing at the disciplinary level. A model of caring includes a call for both art and science. It offers a framework that embraces and intersects with art, science, humanities, spirituality, and new dimensions of mind-body-spirit medicine and nursing evolving openly as central to human phenomena of nursing practice.

I emphasize that it is possible to read, study, learn about, even teach and research the caring theory. However, to truly "get it," one has to experience it personally. The model is both an invitation and an opportunity to interact with the ideas, experiment with and grow within the philosophy, and to live it out in one's personal/professional life.

The ideas as originally developed, as well as in the current evolving phase (Watson, 1999, 2003, 2004), provide us with a chance to assess, critique, and see where or how, or even if, we may locate ourselves within a framework of caring science as a basis for the emerging ideas in relation to our own "theories and philosophies of professional nursing and/or caring practice." If one chooses to use the caring-science perspective as theory, model, philosophy, ethic, or ethos for transforming self and practice, or self and system, the following questions may help (Watson, 1996, p. 161):

- Is there congruence between the values and major concepts and beliefs in the model and the given nurse, group, system, organization, curriculum, population needs, clinical administrative setting, or other entity that is considering interacting with the caring model to transform and/or improve practice?
- What is one's view of "human"? And what does it mean to be human, caring, healing, becoming, growing, transforming, and so on? For example, in the words of Teilhard de Chardin: "Are we humans having a spiritual experience, or are we spiritual beings having a human experience?" Such thinking in regard to this philosophical

question can guide one's worldview and help to clarify where one may locate self within the caring framework.

- Are those interacting and engaging in the model interested in their own personal evolution: Are they committed to seeking authentic connections and caring-healing relationships with self and others?
- Are those involved "conscious" of their caring caritas or noncaring consciousness and intentionally in a given moment, at individual and system level? Are they interested and committed to expanding their caring consciousness and actions to self, other, environment, nature, and wider universe?
- Are those working within the model interested in shifting their focus from a modern medical science-technocure orientation to a true caring-healing-loving model?

This work, in both its original and evolving forms, seeks to develop caring as an ontological-epistemological foundation for a theoretical-philosophical-ethical framework for the profession and discipline of nursing and to clarify its mature relationship and distinct intersection with other health sciences. Nursing caring theory-based activities as guides to practice, education, and research have developed throughout the United States and other parts of the world. The caring model is consistently one of the nursing caring theories used as a guide. Nurses' reflective-critical practice models are increasingly adhering to a caring ethic and ethos.

SUMMARY

Nursing's future and nursing in the future will depend on nursing maturing as the distinct health, healing, and caring profession that it has always represented across time but has yet to actualize. Nursing thus ironically is now challenged to stand and mature within its own paradigm, while simultaneously having to transcend it and share with others. The future already reveals that all health-care practitioners will need to work within a shared framework of caring relationships and human-environment field modalities, pay attention to consciousness, intentionality, transformed mind-body-spirit medicine, and will need to embrace healing arts and caring practices and processes and the spiritual dimensions of care much more completely. Thus, nursing is at its own crossroad of possibilities, between worldviews and paradigms. Nursing has entered a new era; it is invited and required to build upon its heritage and latest evolution in science and technology but must transcend itself for a postmodern future yet to be known. However, nursing's future holds promises of caring and healing mysteries and models yet to unfold, as opportunities for offering compassionate caritas services at individual, system, societal, national, and global levels for self, for profession, and for the broader world community. Nursing has a critical role to play in sustaining caring in humanity and making new connections between caring, love, and peace in the world.

PART TWO:
Application of Jean Watson's Theory of Human Caring

Terri Kaye Woodward

Transpersonal Caring Theory and the caring model "can be read, taught, learned about, studied, researched and even practiced: however, to truly 'get it,' one has to personally experience it—interact and grow within the philosophy and intention of the model" (Watson, 1996, p.160). This section of the chapter provides a look into Transpersonal Caring Theory in action.

PRACTICE

October 2002 presented the opportunity for 17 interdisciplinary health-care professionals at the children's hospital in Denver, Colorado, to participate in a pilot study designed to (a) explore the effect of integrating Caring Theory into comprehensive pediatric pain management, and (b) examine the Attending Nurse Caring Model®[1] (ANCM) as a care delivery model for hospitalized children in pain. A three-day retreat launched the pilot study. Participants were invited to explore Transpersonal Human Caring Theory (Caring Theory), as taught and modeled by Dr. Jean Watson, through experiential interactions with caring-healing modalities. The end of the retreat opened opportunities for participants to merge Plie Caring Theory and pain theory into an emerging caring-healing praxis.

Returning from the retreat to the preexisting schedules, customs and habits of hospital routine was both daunting and exciting. We had lived Caring Theory, and not as a remote and abstract philosophical ideal; rather, we had experienced caring as the very core of our true selves, and it was the call that led us into health-care professions. Invigorated by the retreat, we returned to our 37-bed acute care inpatient pediatric unit, eager to apply Caring Theory to improve pediatric pain management. Our experiences throughout the retreat had accentuated caring as our core value. Caring Theory could not be restricted to a single area of practice.

Wheeler & Chinn (1991, p. 2) define praxis as "values made visible through deliberate action." This definition unites the ontology or the essence of nursing to nursing actions, to what nurses do. Nursing within acute care inpatient hospital settings is practiced dependently, collaboratively, and independently (Bernardo, 1998). Bernardo describes dependent practice as energy directed by and requiring physician orders, collaborative practice as interdependent energy directed toward activities with other health-care professionals, and independent practice as "where the meaningful role and impact of nursing may evolve" (p. 43). Although Bernardo's description of inpatient nursing captures the composite and fragmented role

---

[1] See Watson, J., & Foster, R. (2002). The Attending Nurse Caring Model® integrating theory, evidence and advanced caring-healing therapeutics for transforming professional practice. *Journal of Clinical Nursing, 12,* 360–365.

allotted to nurses within the current health-care hierarchy, it does not describe our vision of a caring praxis. Our vision is based in the caring paradigm of deep respect for humanity and all life, of wonder and awe of life's mystery, and the interconnectedness from mind-body-spirit unity into cosmic oneness (Watson, 1996). Gadow (1995) describes nursing as a lived world of interdependency and shared knowledge, rather than as a service provided. Caring praxis within this lived world is a praxis that offers "a combination of action and reflection . . . praxis is about a relationship with self, and a relationship with the wider community" (Penny & Warelow, 1999, p. 260). Caring praxis, therefore, is collaborative praxis.

Collaboration and cocreation are key elements in our endeavors to translate Caring Theory into practice. They reveal the nonlinear process and relational aspect of caring praxis. Both require openness to unknown possibilities, honor the unique contributions of self and other(s), and acknowledge growth and transformation as inherent to life experience. These key elements support the evolution of praxis away from predetermined goals and set outcomes toward authentic caring-healing expressions. Through collaboration and cocreation, we can build upon existing foundations to nurture evolution from what is to what can be.

Our mission, to translate Caring Theory into praxis, has strong foundational support. Building on this supportive base, we have committed our intentions and energies toward creating a caring culture. The following is not intended as an algorithm to guide one through varied steps until caring is achieved but is rather a description of our ongoing processes and growth toward an ever-evolving caring praxis. These processes are cocreations that emerged from collaboration with other ANCM participants, fellow health professionals, patients and families, our environment, and our caring intentions.

First Steps

One of our first challenges was to make the ANCM visible. Six tangible exhibits have been displayed on the unit as evidence of our commitment to caring values. First, a large, colorful poster titled "CARING" is positioned at the entrance to our unit. Depicting pictures of diverse families at the center, the poster states our three initial goals for theory-guided practice: (1) create caring-healing environments, (2) optimize pain management through pharmacological and caring-healing measures, and (3) prepare children and families for procedures and interventions. Watson's clinical caritas processes are listed, as well as an abbreviated version of her guidelines for cultivating caring-healing throughout the day (Watson, 2002). This poster, written in Caring Theory language, expresses our intention to all and reminds us that caring is the core of our praxis.

Second, a shallow bowl of smooth, rounded river stones is located in a prominent position at each nursing desk. A sign posted by the stones identify them as "Caring-Healing Touch Stones" inviting one to select a stone as "every human being has the ability to share their incredible gift of loving-healing. These stones serve as a reminder of our capacity to love and heal. Pick up a stone, feel its smooth cool surface, let its weight remind you of your own gifts of love and healing. Share in the love and healing of all who have touched this stone before you and pass on your love and healing to all who will hold this stone after you."[2]

Third, latched wicker blessing baskets have been placed adjacent to the caring-healing touch stones. Written instructions invite families, visitors, and staff to offer names for a blessing by writing the person's initials on a slip of paper and placing the paper in the basket. Every Monday through Friday, the unit chaplain, holistic clinical nurse specialist (CNS), and interested staff devote thirty minutes of meditative silence within a healing space to ask for peace and hope for all names contained within the baskets.

Fourth, signs picturing a snoozing cartoon-styled tiger have been posted on each patient's door announcing "Quiet Time." Quiet time is a midday, half-hour pause from hospital hustle-bustle. Lights in the hall are dimmed, voices are hushed, and steps are softened to allow a pause for reflection. Staff tries not to enter patient rooms unless summoned.

Fifth, a booklet has been written and published to welcome families and patients to our unit, to introduce health team members, unit routines, available activities, and define frequently used medical terms. This book emphasizes that patients, parents, and families are members of the health team. A description of our caring attending team is also included.

Sixth and most recently, the unit chaplain, child-life specialist, and social worker have organized a

---

[2] Written by Terri Woodward.

weekly support session called "Goodies and Gathering," offered every Thursday morning. It is held in our healing room—a conference room painted to resemble a cozy room with a beautiful outdoor view[3] and redecorated with comfortable armchairs, soft lighting, and plants. Goodies and Gathering extends a safe retreat within the hospital setting. Offering one hour to parents and another to staff, these professionals provide snacks to feed the body, a sacred space to nourish emotions, and their caring presence to nurture the spirit.

ACT

To honor the collaborative partnership of our ANCM participants, to include patients and families as equal partners in the health-care team, and open participations to all, we have adopted the name Attending Caring Team (ACT). The acronym ACT reinforces that our actions are opportunities to make caring visible. Care as the core of praxis differs from the centrality of cure in the medical model. To describe our intentions to others we compiled the following "elevator" description of ACT, a terse, thirty-second summary that renders the meaning of ACT in the time frame of a shared elevator ride:

> The core of the Attending Caring Team (ACT) is caring-healing for patients, families and ourselves. ACT co-creates relationships and collaborative practices between patients, families and health care providers. ACT practice enables health care providers to redefine themselves as caregivers rather than taskmasters. We provide **Health Care** not Health Tasks.

Large signs are currently being professionally produced and will be hung at various locations on our unit. These signs serve a dual purpose. The largest, posted conspicuously at our threshold, identifies our unit as the home of the Attending Caring Team. Smaller signs, posted at each nurse's station, spell out the above ACT definition, inviting everyone entering our unit to participate in the collaborative cocreation of caring-healing.

Giving ourselves a name and making our caring intentions visible contribute to establishing an identity, yet may be perceived as peripheral activi-

ties. In order for these expressions to be deliberate actions of praxis, the centrality of caring as our core value was clearly articulated. Caring Theory is the flexible framework guiding our unit goals and unit education and has been integrated into our implementation of an institutional customer service initiative.

Unit goals are written yearly. Reflective of the broader institutional mission statement, each unit is encouraged to develop a mission statement and outline goals designed to achieve that mission. In 2003, our mission statement was rewritten to focus on provision of quality *family centered care,* defined as "an environment of caring-healing recognizing families as equal partners in collaboration with all health care providers." One of the goals to achieve this mission literally spells out caring. We promote a caring-healing environment for patients, families, and staff through:

- Compassion, competence, commitment
- Advocacy
- Respect, research
- Individuality
- Nurturing
- Generosity

Education

Unit educational offerings have also been revised to reflect Caring Theory. Phase classes, a two-year curriculum of serial seminars designed to support new hires in their clinical, educational, and professional growth, now include a unit on self-care to promote personal healing and support self-growth. The unit on pain management has been expanded to include use of caring-healing modalities. A new interactive session on the caritas processes has been added that asks participants to reflect on how these processes are already evident in their praxis and to explore ways they can deepen caring praxis both individually and collectively as a unit. The tracking tool used to assess a new employee's progress through orientation now includes an area for reflection on growing in caring competencies. In addition to changes in phase classes, informal "clock hours" are offered monthly. Clock hours are designed to respond to the immediate needs of the unit and encompass a diverse range of topics, from conflict resolution, debriefing after specific events, and professional development, to health treatment plans, physiology of medical diagnosis, and in-

---

[3] Artwork created by and generously donated by artist Cynthia Telsey.

services on new technologies and pharmacological interventions. Offered on the unit at varying hours to accommodate all work shifts, clock hours provide a way for staff members to fulfill continuing educational requirements without impinging on their days off.

Customer Service

Caring Theory has provided depth to an institutional initiative to use FISH philosophy to enhance customer service (Lundin, Paul, & Christensen, 2000). Imported from Pike's Fish Market in Seattle, FISH advocates four premises to improve employee and customer satisfaction: presence, make their day, play, and choose your attitude. Briefly summarized, FISH advocates that when employees bring their full awareness through presence, focus on customers to make their day, invoke fun into the day through appropriate play, and through conscious awareness choose their attitude, work environments improve for all. When the four FISH premises are viewed from the perspective of transpersonal caring, they become opportunities for authentic human-to-human connectedness through I-Thou relationships. The merger of Caring Theory with FISH philosophy has inspired the following activities. A parade composed of patients, their families, nurses, and volunteers—complete with marching music, hats, streamers, flags, and noise makers—is celebrated two to three times a week right before the playroom closes for lunch. This flamboyant display lasts less than five minutes but invigorates participants and bystanders alike. In addition to being vital for children and especially appropriate in a pediatric setting, play unites us all in the life and joy of each moment. When our parade marches, visitors, rounding doctors, all present on the unit pause to watch, wave, and cheer us on. A weekly bedtime story is read in our healing room. Patients are invited to bring their pillows and favorite stuffed animal or doll and come dressed in pajamas. Night- and day-shift staff have honored one another with surprise beginning-of-the-shift meals, staying late to care for patients and families, and refusing to give off-going report until their oncoming coworkers had eaten. Colorful caring stickers are awarded when one staff member catches another in the ACT of caring, being present, making another's day, playing, and choosing a positive attitude.

ACT Guidelines

Placing Caring Theory at the core of our praxis supports practicing caring-healing arts to promote wholeness, comfort, harmony, and inner healing. The intentional conscious presence of our authentic being to provide a caring-healing environment is the most essential of these arts. Presence as the foundation for cocreating caring relationships has led to writing ACT guidelines. Written in the doctor order section of the chart, ACT guidelines provide a formal way to honor unique families' values and beliefs. Preferred ways of having dressing changes performed, most helpful comfort measures, home schedules, and special needs or requests are examples of what these guidelines might address. ACT members purposely selected the word *guideline* as opposed to *order* as more congruent with cocreative collaborate praxis and to encourage critical thinking and flexibility. Building practice on caring relationships has led to an increase in both the type and volume of care conferences held on our unit. Previously, care conferences were called as a way to disseminate information to families when complicated issues arose or when communication between multiple teams faltered and families were receiving conflicting reports, plans, and instructions. Now, these conferences are offered proactively as a way to coordinate team efforts and to ensure we are working toward the families' goals. Transitional conferences provide an opportunity to coordinate continuity of care, share insight into the unique personality and preferences of the child, coordinate team effort, meet families, provide them tours of our unit, and collaborate with families. Other caring-healing arts offered on our unit are therapeutic touch, guided imagery, relaxation, visualization, aromatherapy, and massage. As ACT participants, our challenge is to express our caring values through every activity and interaction. Caring Theory guides us and manifests in innumerable ways. Our interview process, meeting format, and a CNS role have been transfigured through Caring Theory. Our interview process has transformed from an interrogative threestep procedure into more of a sharing dialogue. Unit meetings have been conducted in a routine fashion with the committee chair in a lead position to open, run, and close the meeting, delegating tasks and responsibilities to committee members as the chair saw fit. The mutuality, transpersonal relationship, and caring consciousness of Caring Theory do not support this meeting format. We are adopting another meeting style that expresses caring values.

Our unit director had the foresight to budget a position for a CNS to support the cocreation of caring praxis. The traditional CNS roles—researcher, clinical expert, collaborator, educator, and change agent—have allowed the integration of Caring Theory development into all aspects of our unit program. The CNS role advocates self-care and facilitates staff members to incorporate caring-healing arts into their practice through modeling and hands-on support. In addition to providing assistance, searching for resources, acting as liaison with other health-care teams, and promoting staff in their efforts, the very presence of the CNS on the unit reinforces our commitment to caring praxis.

SUMMARY

Caring-healing cocreation is fluid, not static. Over 100 years ago, Florence Nightingale wrote, "I entirely repudiate the distinction usually drawn between the man of thought and the man of action" (Vivinus & Nergaard, 1990, p. 310). Nightingale rejected the separation of the ideal (theory) from action (practice). For Nightingale, nursing is not a profession or a job one performs, but is rather a calling. Dedicating her life toward achieving the ideal, she challenged others to "let the Ideal go if you are not trying to incorporate it in your daily life" (Vivinus & Nergaard, 1990, p. 310). We continue to work toward incorporating caring ideal in every action. Currently, we are modifying our competency-based guidelines to emphasize caring competency within tasks and skills. Building relationships for supportive collaborative practice is the most exciting and most challenging endeavor we are now facing as old roles are reevaluated in light of cocreating caring-healing relationships. Watson and Foster (2003, p. 361) describe the potential of such collaboration: "the new caring-healing practice environment is increasingly dependent on partnerships, negotiation, coordination, new forms of communication pattern and authentic relationships. The new emphasis

is on a change of consciousness, a focused intentionality towards caring and healing relationships and modalities, a shift towards a spiritualization of health vs. a limited medicalized view." Our ACT commitment is to authentic relationships and the creation of caring-healing environments.

References

Bernardo, A. (1998). Technology and true presence in nursing. *Holistic Nursing Practice, 12*(4), 40–49.

Gadow, S. (1995). Narrative and exploration: Toward a poetics of knowledge in nursing. *Nursing Inquiry, 2,* 211–214.

Lundin, S. C., Paul, H., & Christensen, J. (2000). *Fish! A remarkable way to boost morale and improve results.* New York: Hyperion.

Penny, W., & Warelow, P. J. (1999). Understanding the prattle of praxis. *Nursing Inquiry, 6*(4), 259–268.

Swanson, K. M. (1991). Empirical development of a middle range nursing theory. *Nursing Research, 40*(3), 161–166.

Vivinus, M., & Nergaard, B. (1990). *Ever yours, Florence Nightingale.* Cambridge: Harvard University Press.

Watson, J. (1996). Watson's theory of transpersonal caring. In Walker, P. H., & Newman, B. (Eds.), *Blueprint for use of nursing models: Education, research, practice and administration.* New York: National League for Nursing Press.

Watson, J. (1999). *Postmodern nursing and beyond.* New York: Churchill Livingstone.

Watson, J. (2001). Post-hospital nursing: Shortage, shifts and scripts. *Nursing Administration Quarterly, 25*(3), 77–82.

Watson, J. (2002). Intentionality and caring-healing consciousness: A practice of transpersonal nursing. *Holistic Nursing Practice, 16*(4), 12–19.

Watson, J., & Foster, R. (2003). The Attending Nurse Caring Model®: Integrating theory, evidence and advanced caring-healing therapeutics for transforming professional practice. *Journal of Clinical Nursing, 12,* 360–365.

Wheeler, C. E., & Chinn, P. L. (1991). *Peace and Power: A handbook of feminist process* (3rd ed.). New York: National League for Nursing Press.

Bibliography

PUBLICATIONS/AUDIOVISUALS

Bevis, E. O., & Watson, J. (1989). *Toward a caring curriculum. A new pedagogy for nursing* (reprinted 2000). Mass: Jones & Bartlett.

Chinn, P., & Watson, J. (Eds.). (1994). *Art and aesthetics of nursing.* NY: NLN.

Leininger, M., & Watson, J. (Eds.). (1990). *The caring imperative in education.* NY: NLN.

Taylor, R., & Watson, J. (Eds.). (1989). *They shall not hurt: Human suffering and human caring.* Boulder, CO: Colorado Associated University Press.

Watson, J. (1979). *Nursing: The philosophy and science of caring.*

Boston: Little, Brown and Company. (2nd printing, 1985. Boulder, CO: University Press of Colorado.) Translated into French and Korean.

Watson, J. (1985). *Nursing: Human science and human care.* CT: Appleton-Century-Crofts. (2nd printing, 1988; 3rd printing, 1999. NY: National League for Nursing (Jones and Bartlett: Mass.) Translated into Japanese, Swedish, Chinese, Korean, German, Norwegian, and Danish.

Watson, J. (Ed.). (1994). *Applying the art and science of human caring.* NY: National League for Nursing.

Watson, J. (1999). *Postmodern nursing and beyond* (Japanese translation, 2004). Edinburgh, Scotland, UK: Churchill Livingstone/WB Saunders.

Watson, J. (2002). *Instruments for assessing and measuring caring in nursing and health sciences.* NY: Springer. (AJN Book of the Year Award, 2002. Japanese translation 2003.)

Watson, J. (2004). *Caring science as sacred science.* Philadelphia: F. A. Davis.

Watson, J., & Ray, M. (Eds.). (1988). *The ethics of care and the ethics of cure: Synthesis in chronicity.* NY: NLN.

Journal Articles

Fawcett, J. (2002). The nurse theorists: 21st century updates—Jean Watson. *Nursing Science Quarterly, 15*(3), 214–219.

Fawcett, J., Watson, J., Neuman, B., & Hinton-Walker, P. (2001). On theories and evidence. *Journal of Nursing Scholarship, 33*(2), 121–128.

Quinn, J., Smith, M., Swanson, K., Ritenbaugh, C., Watson, J. (2003). The healing relationship in clinical nursing: Guidelines for research. *Journal of Alternative Therapies, 9*(3), A65–79.

Watson, J. (1988). Human caring as moral context for nursing education. *Nursing and Health Care, 9*(8), 422–425.

Watson, J. (1988). New dimensions of human caring theory. *Nursing Science Quarterly, 1*(4), 175–181.

Watson, J. (1990). The moral failure of the patriarchy. *Nursing Outlook, 28*(2), 62–66.

Watson, J. (1998). Nightingale and the enduring legacy of transpersonal human caring. *Journal of Holistic Nursing, 16*(2), 18–21.

Watson, J. (2000). Leading via caring-healing: The fourfold way toward transformative leadership. *Nursing Administration Quarterly* (25th Anniversary Edition), *25*(1), 1–6.

Watson, J. (2000). Reconsidering caring in the home. *Journal of Geriatric Nursing, 21*(6), 330–331.

Watson, J. (2000). Via negativa: Considering caring by way of non-caring. *Australian Journal of Holistic Nursing, 7*(1), 4–8.

Watson, J. (2001). Post-hospital nursing: Shortages, shifts, and scripts. *Nursing Administrative Quarterly, 25*(3), 77–82. Available online at http://www.dartmouth.edu/~ahechome/workforce.html, then click "The Nursing Shortage."

Watson, J. (2002). Guest editorial: Nursing: Seeking its source and survival. *ICU NURS WEB J 9,* 1–7. www.nursing.gr/J.W.editorial.pdf

Watson, J. (2002). Holistic nursing and caring: A values based approach. *Journal of Japan Academy of Nursing Science, 22*(2), 69–74.

Watson, J. (2002). Intentionality and caring-healing consciousness: A theory of transpersonal nursing. *Holistic Nursing Journal, 16*(4), 12–19.

Watson, J. (2002). Metaphysics of virtual caring communities. *International Journal of Human Caring, 6*(1).

Watson, J. (2003). Love and caring: Ethics of face and hand. *Nursing Administrative Quarterly, 27*(3), 197–202.

Watson, J., & Foster, R. (2003). The attending nurse caring model: Integrating theory, evidence and advanced caring-healing therapeutics for transforming professional practice. *Journal of Clinical Nursing, 12,* 360–365.

Watson, J., & Smith, M. C. (2002). Caring science and the science of unitary human beings: A trans-theoretical discourse for nursing knowledge development. *Journal of Advanced Nursing, 37*(5), 452–461.

Watson, J. (1994). A frog, a rock, a ritual: An eco-caring cosmology. In Schuster, E., & Brown, C. (Ed.), *Caring and environmental connection.* NY: NLN

Watson, J. (1996). Artistry and caring: Heart and soul of nursing. In Marks-Maran, D., & Rose (Eds.), *Reconstructing nursing: Beyond art & science* (pp. 54–63). London: Bailliere Tindall Ltd.

Watson, J. (1996). Poeticizing as truth on nursing inquiry. In Kikuchi, J., Simmons, H., & Romyn, D. (Eds.), *Truth in nursing inquiry* (pp. 125–139). Thousand Oaks, CA: Sage.

Watson, J. (1996). Watson's theory of transpersonal caring. In Walker, P. H., & Neuman, B. (Eds.), *Blueprint for use of nursing models: Education, research, practice, & administration* (pp. 141–184). NY: National League for Nursing Press.

Watson, J. (1999). Alternative therapies and nursing practice. In Watson, J. (Ed.), *Nurse's handbook of alternative and complementary therapies.* Springhouse, PA: Springhouse.

Watson, J., & Chinn, P. L. (1994). Art and aesthetics as passage between centuries. In Chinn, P. L., & Watson, J. (Eds.), *Art and aesthetics in nursing* (pp. xiii–xviii). NY: National League for Nursing.

AUDIOVISUAL OR MEDIA PRODUCTIONS

Watson FITNE. (1997). *The nurse theorists portraits of excellence. Jean Watson A theory of caring* [video and CD]. To obtain go to: www.fitne.net.

Watson (1988). *The Denver nursing project in human caring* [videotape]. University of Colorado Health Science Center, School of Nursing, Denver, CO. Contact: ellen.janasko@uchsc.edu.

Watson (1988). *The power of caring: The power to make a difference* [videotape]. Center for Human Caring Video, University of Colorado Health Sciences Center, School of Nursing, Denver, CO. Contact: ellen.janasko@uchsc.edu.

Watson, J. (1989). *Theories at work* [videotape]. National League for Nursing, New York, NY. In conjunction with University of Colorado HSC/SoN Chair in Caring Science. Contact ellen.janasko@uchsc.edu.

For complete publication citations of Watson and related publications and clinical-educational initiatives and contact information on Watson's *caring human theory*, please go to www.uchsc.edu/nursing/caring.

Watson, J. (1994). *Applying the art and science of human caring,* Parts I and II [videotape]. National League for Nursing, New York, NY. In conjunction with the University of Colorado HSC/SoN, Chair in Caring Science. Contact: Ellen. janasko@uchsc.edu.

Watson, J. (1999). *A meta-reflection on nursing's present* [audiotape]. American Holistic Nurses Association. Boulder, Colorado: SoundsTrue Production.

Watson, J. (1999). *Private psalms. A mantra and meditation for healing* [CD]. Music by Dallas Smith and Susan Mazer. To obtain: e-mail University of Colorado Health Sciences Center Bookstore at traci.mathis@uchsc.edu. (All pro-ceeds from bookstore CDs sales go to support activities of the Murchinson-Scoville Endowed Chair in Caring Science.)

Watson, J. (2001). *Creating a culture of caring* [audiotape]. At the Creative Healthcare Management 9th Annual CHCM, Minneapolis, MN.

Watson, J. (2000). *Importance of story and health care.* 2nd National Gathering on Relationship-Centered Caring. Fetzer Institute Conference, Florida.

Watson, J. (2001). *Reconnecting with spirit: Caring and healing our living and dying.* International Parish Nursing Conference. Westberg Symposium. September, 2001.

CHAPTER 20

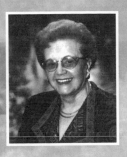

Madeleine M. Leininger

PART ONE: **Madeleine M. Leininger's Theory of Culture Care Diversity and Universality**

Madeleine M. Leininger

Introducing the Theorist

Madeleine Leininger is the founder and leader of the field of transcultural nursing, focusing on comparative human care theory and research, and she is founder of the worldwide Transcultural Nursing Society. Dr. Leininger's initial nursing education was at St. Anthony School of Nursing in Denver, Colorado. Her undergraduate degree is from Mt. St. Scholastic College in Atchison, Kansas, and her master's degree was earned at the Catholic University of America in Washington, D.C. She completed her PhD in social and cultural anthropology at the University of Washington. Dr. Leininger was dean and professor of nursing at the Universities of Washington and Utah where she helped initiate and direct the first doctoral programs in nursing. She facilitated the development of master degree programs in nursing at American and overseas institutions. Dr. Leininger is a fellow and distinguished living legend of the American Academy of Nursing. She is professor emeritus of the College of Nursing at Wayne State University and is adjunct professor at the University of Nebraska, College of Nursing.

Dr. Leininger is the author and/or editor of 30 books, has published over 250 articles, and has given more than 1,200 public lectures throughout the United States and abroad. Some of her well-known books include *Basic Psychiatric Concepts in Nursing* (Leininger & Hofling, 1960); *Caring: An Essential Human Need* (1981); *Care: The Essence of Nursing and Health* (1984); *Care: Discovery and Uses in Clinical and Community Nursing* (1988); *Care: Ethical and Moral Dimensions of Care* (1990d); and *Culture Care Diversity and Universality: A Theory of Nursing* (1991). Some of her books were the first in that area of nursing to be published. *Nursing and Anthropology: Two Worlds to Blend* (1970) was the first book to bring together nursing and anthropology. *Transcultural Nursing: Concepts, Theories, and Practices* (1978) was the first book on transcultural nursing. The *Qualitative Research Methods in Nursing* (1985) was the first qualitative research methods book in nursing.

Her published books and articles cover five decades of cumulative transcultural nursing and human care with many cultures throughout the world. In 1989, Dr. Leininger initiated the *Journal of Transcultural Nursing*, which was the first transcultural nursing journal in the world.

Dr. Leininger conducted the first field study of the Gadsup of the Eastern Highlands of New Guinea in the early 1960s, and since then has studied approximately 25 Western and non-Western cultures. Dr. Leininger led nurses to use qualitative ethnonursing research methods and developed the first nursing research method called *ethnonursing*. She also provided new ways to provide culturally competent health care and coined the phrase "culturally congruent care" in the 1960s. In 1987, she initiated the idea of worldwide certification of nurses prepared in transcultural nursing in order to protect and respect the cultural needs and lifeways of people of diverse cultures.

As a pioneering nurse educator, leader, theorist, and administrator, Dr. Leininger has been a risk taker, futurist, and innovator. She has never been afraid to bring forth new directions and practical issues in education and service. Her persistent leadership has made transcultural nursing and human care central to nursing and respected as formal areas of study and practice. She has been called the "Margaret Mead of the health field" and the "New Nightingale" by colleagues and students. Dr. Leininger's genuine interest and enthusiasm for whatever she pursues is contagious, inspiring, and challenging.

Introducing the Theory

One of the most significant and unique contributions of Dr. Leininger was the development of her Culture Care Diversity and Universality Theory. She introduced this theory in the early 1960s to provide culturally congruent and competent care (Leininger, 1991a, 1995). She believed that transcultural nursing care could provide meaningful and therapeutic health and healing outcomes. As she developed the theory, she identified transcultural nursing concepts, principles, theories, and research-based knowledge to guide, challenge, and explain nursing practices. This was a significant and new contribution to nursing and has been an important means to open the door to advance new scientific and humanistic dimensions of caring for people of diverse and similar cultures. The use of this culture care theory has greatly expanded nursings' knowledge base about people of diverse cultures in the world.

The Theory of Culture Care Diversity and Universality was developed in order to establish a substansive knowledge base to guide nurses in discovery and use of the knowledge in transcultural nursing practices. It was at this time that Dr. Leininger envisioned that nurses would need transcultural knowledge and practices to function with people of diverse cultures worldwide (Leininger, 1970, 1978). This was the post–World War II period, when many new immigrants and refugees were coming to America, and the world was becoming more multicultural. Leininger held

> *Caring for people of many different cultures was a critical and esssential need, yet nurses and other health professionals were not prepared to meet this global challenge.*

that caring for people of many different cultures was a critical and esssential need, yet nurses and other health professionals were not prepared to meet this global challenge. Instead, nursing and medicine were focused on using new medical technologies and treatment regimes. They were focused on studying biomedical diseases and symptoms. Shifting to a transcultural perspective was a major change but a critical need.

This part of the chapter presents an overview of the Theory of Culture Care Diversity and Universality, along with its purpose, goals, assumptions, theoretical tenets, predicted hunches, and related general features of the theory. The next part of the chapter discusses applications of the knowledge in clinical and community settings. For more in-depth reading of the theorist's perspectives, readers should consult primary literature on the theory (Leininger, 1970, 1981, 1989a, 1989b, 1990a, 1990b, 1991, 1995, 1997, 1998, 2002, and 2004).

FACTORS LEADING TO THE THEORY

A frequent question often posed to Dr. Leininger is, "What led you to develop your theory?" Her major motivation was the desire to discover unknown or little known knowledge about cultures and their core values, beliefs, and needs. The idea to develop the Culture Care Theory came to her while she was functioning as a clinical child nurse specialist in a child guidance home in a large Midwestern city (Leininger, 1970, 1991, 1995). From her focused observations and daily nursing experiences with the children, she became aware that the children in the guidance home were from many different cultures. Children were different in their behaviors, needs, responses, and care expectations. In the home were children who were Anglo-Caucasian, African American, Jewish American, Appalachian, and many other cultures. The children's parents responded to the children differently, and their expectations of care and treatment modes were different. The reality was a cultural shock to Leininger as she was not prepared to care for children of diverse cultures. Likewise, nurses, physicians, social workers, and health professionals in the guidance home were also not prepared to respond to such cultural differences. Because of this cultural shock, she felt helpless to care for the children and their parents. It soon became evident that she needed cultural knowledge to be helpful to the children. Her psychiatric and general nursing care knowl-

edge and experiences were woefully inadequate. She decided to pursue doctoral study in anthropology. While in the anthropology program, she discovered a wealth of potentially valuable knowledge that would be helpful within a nursing perspective. To care for children of diverse cultures and link such knowledge into nursing thought and actions was a major challenge. It was essential to incorporate new cultural knowledge into nursing. It was knowledge that went beyond the traditional physical and emotional needs of clients. Leininger was concerned whether it would be possible to incorporate such new knowledge, given the traditional norms of nursing and its orientation toward medical knowledge.

At that time, she had questioned what made nursing a distinct and legitimate profession. She declared in the mid-1950s that care is (or should be)

> *Care is (or should be) the essence and central domain of nursing.*

the essence and central domain of nursing. However, many nurses resisted this idea, because they thought care was not important and was too feminine, too soft, and too vague and that it would never explain nursing and be accepted by medicine (Leininger, 1970, 1977, 1981, 1984). Nonetheless, Leininger firmly held to the claim and began to teach, study, and write about care as the essence of nursing as its unique and dominant attribute (Leininger, 1970, 1981, 1988, 1991). From both anthropological and nursing perspectives, she held that care and caring were basic and essential human needs for human growth, development, and survival (Leininger, 1977, 1981). She argued that what humans need is human caring to survive from birth to old age, when ill or well. Nevertheless, care needed to be specific and appropriate to cultures.

Her next step in the theory was to conceptualize selected cultural perspectives and transcultural nursing concepts derived from anthropology. She developed assumptions of culture care in order to establish a new knowledge base for the new field of transcultural nursing. Synthesizing or interfacing culture care into nursing was a real challenge. The new Theory of Culture Care Diversity and Universality had to be soundly and logically developed (Leininger, 1976, 1978, 1990a, 1990b, 1991). Formulating such cultural care knowledge was essential to support the new discipline of transcultural nursing. Findings from the theory could be the knowledge to care for people of different cultures. The idea of providing care was largely taken for granted or assumed to be understood by nurses, clients, and the public (Leininger, 1981, 1984). Yet the meaning of "care" from the perspective of different cultures was unknown to nurses and not in the literature prior to establishing the nursing theory in the early 1960s. Care knowledge had to be discovered with cultures.

Prior to her work, there were no theories explicitly focused on care and culture in nursing environments, let alone research studies to explicate care meanings and phenomena in nursing (Leininger, 1981, 1988, 1990a, 1991, 1995). Theoretical and practice meanings of care in relation to specific cultures had not been studied, especially from a comparative cultural perspective. Leininger saw the urgent need to develop a whole new body of culturally based care knowledge to support transcultural nursing care. Shifting nurses' thinking and attitudes from medical symptoms, diseases, and treatments to that of knowing cultures and caring values and patterns was a major task. But nursing needed an appropriate theory to discover care, and she held that her theory could open many new knowledge doorways.

RATIONALE FOR TRANSCULTURAL NURSING: SIGNS AND NEED

The rationale and need for change in nursing in America and elsewhere (Leininger, 1970, 1978, 1984, 1989a, 1990a, 1995) was as follows:

1. There were increased numbers of global migrations of people from virtually every place in the world due to modern electronics, transportation, and communication. These people needed sensitive and appropriate care.
2. There were signs of cultural stresses and cultural conflicts as nurses tried to care for strangers from many Western and non-Western cultures.
3. There were cultural indications of consumer fears and resistance to health personnel as they used new technologies and treatment modes that did not fit their values and lifeways.
4. There were signs that some clients from different cultures were angry, frustrated, and misunderstood by health personnel due to cultural

ignorance of the clients' beliefs, values, and expectations.
5. There were signs of misdiagnosis and mistreatment of clients from unknown cultures because they did not understatnd the culture of the client.
6. There were signs that nurses, physicians, and other professional health personnel were becoming quite frustrated in caring for cultural strangers. Culture care factors of clients were largely misunderstood or neglected.
7. There were signs that consumers of different cultures, whether in the home, hospital, or clinic, were being treated in ways that did not satisfy them and this influenced their recovery.
8. There were many signs of intercultural conflicts and cultural pain among staff that led to tensions.
9. There were very few health personnel of different cultures caring for clients.
10. Nurses were beginning to work in foreign countries in the military or as missionaries, and they were having great difficulty understanding and providing appropriate caring for clients of diverse cultures. They complained that they did not understand the peoples' needs, values, and lifeways.

For these reasons and many others, it was clearly evident in the 1960s that people of different cultures were not receiving care that was congruent with their cultural beliefs and values (Leininger, 1978, 1995). Nurses and other health professionals urgently needed transcultural knowledge and skills to work efficiently with people of diverse cultures.

While anthropologists were clearly experts about cultures, many did not know what to do with patients, nor were they interested in nurses' work, in nursing as a profession, or in the study of human care phenomena in the early 1950s. Most anthropologists in those early days were far more interested in medical diseases, archaeological findings, and in physical and psychological problems of culture. So, Leininger took a leadership role in the new field she called *transcultural nursing*. She needed to develop educational programs to provide culturally safe and congruent care practices that could be beneficial to cultures, to teach nurses about cultures, and to fit the knowledge in with care practices. She initiated a number of transcultural nursing undergraduate and transcultural nursing graduate courses and programs by the mid 1970s and early 1980s. These offerings were gradually accepted by nurses and helped them to care for diverse cultures and enjoy the work with clients (Leininger, 1989a, 1995).

Nurses were the largest and most direct health-care providers, so great opportunities existed for them to change health care to incorporate culturally congruent care practices. Such was the ultimate goal of transcultural nursing. Nurses and those in other health-care disciplines urgently needed to become transculturally prepared to meet a growing multicultural world. Inadequate culturally based services were leading to client dissatisfaction and new sets of problems. In fact, some clients would not ever use health services because the staff were not culturally sensitive to their needs and care.

As more courses and programs in transcultural nursing were offered to educate nurses to learn basic concepts, principles, and practices, the interest of nurses began to grow. As more nurses began to study and use the Theory of Culture Care Diversity and Universality, the concept of transcultural nursing became meaningful. Leininger had defined transcultural nursing as an area of study and practice focused on cultural care (caring) values, beliefs, and practices of particular cultures. The goal was to provide culture-specific and congruent care to people of diverse cultures (Leininger, 1978, 1984, 1995). The central purpose

> *The central purpose of transcultural nursing was to use research-based knowledge to help nurses discover care values and practices and use this knowledge in safe, responsible, and meaningful ways to care for people of different cultures.*

of transcultural nursing was to use research-based knowledge to help nurses discover care values and practices and use this knowledge in safe, responsible, and meaningful ways to care for people of different cultures. Today the Culture Care Theory has led to a wealth of research-based knowledge to guide nurses in the care of clients, families, and communities of different cultures or subcultures.

MAJOR THEORETICAL TENETS

In developing the Theory of Culture Care Diversity and Universality, Leininger identified several predictive tenets or premises as essential for nurses and others to use with the theory.

Commonalities

A major principal tenet was that cultural care diversities and similarities (or commonalities) would be found within cultures. This tenet challenges nurses to discover this knowledge so that nurses could use cultural data in order to provide therapeutic outcomes. It was predicted there would be a gold mine of knowledge if nurses were patient and persistent to discover care values and patterns within cultures. It has been a major missing dimension of traditional nursing. Leininger has stated that human beings are born, they live, and they die with their specific cultural values and beliefs, as well as with their historical and environmental context and that care has been important for their survival and well-being. Leininger predicted that discovering which elements of care were culturally universal and which were different would drastically revolutionize nursing and ultimately transform the health-care systems and practices (Leininger, 1978, 1990a, 1990b, 1991).

Worldview and Social Structure Factors

Another major tenet of the theory was that worldview and social structure factors—such as religion (and spirituality), political and economic considerations, kinship (family ties), education, technology, language expressions, the environmental context, and cultural history—were important influences on health-care outcomes (Leininger, 1995). This broad and multifaceted view provided a holistic perspective to understand people and grasp their world and environment within a historical context. Data from this holistic research-based knowledge was predicted to guide nurses for the health and well-being of the individual or to help disabled or dying clients from different cultures. These social structure factors influencing human care from different cultures would provide new insights to provide culturally congruent care. They need, however, to be studied systematically by nurse researchers. Superficial knowledge would not be helpful with culture. These factors, plus the history of cultures and knowledge of their environmental factors, had to be discovered in order to create the theory and to bring new insights and new knowledge. This data would also disclose ways clients would remain well and prevent illnesses. Indeed, holistic cultural knowledge needed to be discovered, rather than small pieces of medical knowledge, in order to make decisions in arriving at culturally congruent care, which was the theory's goal (Leininger, 1991).

Discovering cultural care knowledge would necessitate entering the cultural world to observe, listen, and validate ideas. Transcultural nursing is an immersion experience not a "dip in and dip out" experience. No longer could nurses rely only on bits and pieces of partial or fragmented medical and psychological knowledge. Nurses needed to become aware of the social structure knowledge, cultural history, language uses, and environmental factors in which people lived. It was these factors that were important to understand cultural and care expressions. Thus, nurses had to be taught the philosophy of transcultural nursing, the culture care theory, and how to discover culture knowledge. It was the transcultural nursing courses and programs that provided such instruction and mentoring.

Professional and Generic Care

Another major and predicted tenet of the theory was that there were care differences and similarities with regard to two kinds of care, namely professional and generic (traditional or indigenous folk), and their practices (Leininger, 1991). These differences were also predicted to influence the health and well-being of clients. These differences would identify gaps in care, inappropriate care, and also beneficial care. Such findings would influence the recovery (healing), health, and well-being of clients of different cultures. Marked differences between generic and professional care ideas and actions could lead to serious client-nurse conflicts, potential illnesses, and even death (Leininger, 1978, 1995). These differences needed to be identified and resolved.

Three Modalities

Leininger also identified three new creative ways to attain and maintain culturally congruent care (Leininger, 1991). The three modalities postulated were (1) culture care preservation or maintenance, (2) culture care accommodation or negotiation, and (3) culture care restructuring or repatterning (Leininger, 1991, 1995). These three modes were very different from traditional nursing practices, routines, or interventions. They were focused on ways to use theory data creatively to facilitate congruent care to fit clients' particular cultural needs. To arrive at culturally appropriate care, the nurse had to draw upon fresh culture care research and discovered knowledge from the people, along with theory data findings. The care had to be tailored to or fit the client needs. Leininger believed that routine interventions would not always be appropriate and could lead to cultural imposition, cultural tensions, and cultural conflicts. Thus, nurses had to shift from relying on routine interventions and from focusing on symptoms to care practices derived from the clients' culture and from the theory. They had to use holistic care knowledge from the theory and not medical data. Most importantly, they had to use both generic and professional care data. This was a new challenge but a rewarding one for the nurse and the client if thoughtfully done. Examples of the use of the three modalites containing theory findings are in several published sources (Leininger, 1995, 1999, 2002) and are presented in the next part of this chapter.

Since this theory has been used, new kinds of transcultural nursing knowledge have been forthcoming. Culturally based care has been discovered to prevent illness and to maintain wellness. Ways to help people throughout the life cycle (birth to death) have been discovered. Cultural patterns of caring and health maintenance have also been discovered, with environmental and historical factors. Most importantly, cultural differences and simularities have been discovered with the theory.

THEORETICAL ASSUMPTIONS: PURPOSE, GOAL, AND DEFINITIONS OF THE THEORY

This next section discusses some of the major assumptions, definitions, and purposes of the theory. The theory's overriding purpose was to discover, document, analyze, and identify the cultural and care factors influencing human beings in health, sickness, and dying and to thereby advance and improve nursing practices.

The theory's goal was to use research-based knowledge in order to provide culturally congruent, safe, and beneficial care to people of diverse or similar cultures for their health and well-being or for meaningful dying. This goal of arriving at culturally congruent care was predicted to promote the health and well-being of clients or to help clients face disability or death in culturally meaningful and satisfying ways. Thus, the ultimate and primary goal of the theory was to provide culturally congruent care that was tailor-made for the lifeways and values of people (Leininger, 1991, 1995).

Theory Assumptions

Several assumptions or basic beliefs to the theory were constructed by the theorist. They are as follows (Leininger, 1970, 1977, 1981, 1984, 1991, 1997a):

1. Care is essential for human growth, development, and survival and to face death or dying.
2. Care is essential to curing and healing; there can be no curing without caring.
3. The forms, expressions, patterns, and processes of human care vary among all cultures of the world.

> *Forms, expressions, patterns, and processes of human care vary among all cultures of the world.*

4. Every culture has generic (lay, folk, or naturalistic) care and usually professional care practices.
5. Culture care values and beliefs are embedded in religious, kinship, social, political, cultural, economic, and historical dimensions of the social structure and in language and environmental contexts.
6. Therapeutic nursing care can only occur when client culture care values, expressions, and/or practices are known and used explicitly to provide human care.
7. Differences between caregiver and care receiver expectations need to be understood in order to provide beneficial, satisfying, and congruent care.
8. Culturally congruent, specific, or universal care modes are essential to the health or well-being of people of cultures.
9. Nursing is essentially a transcultural care profession and discipline.

Orientational Theory Definitions

Since the theory has been built with a qualitative focus, the definitions are orientational rather than highly restrictive:

1. *Culture care diversity:* Refers to variability and/or differences in meanings, patterns, values, lifeways, or symbols of care within or between cultures that demonstrate assistive, supportive, or enabling human care expressions (Leininger, 1991, p. 47).
2. *Culture care universality:* Refers to the common, similar, or dominant uniform care meanings, patterns, values, lifeways, or symbols that are manifest with cultures and reflect assistive, supportive, facilitative, or enabling ways to help people (Leininger, 1991, p. 47).
3. *Care:* Refers to abstract and concrete phenomena related to assisting, supporting, or enabling experiences toward or for others with evident or anticipated care needs to ameliorate or improve a human condition or lifeway. "Caring" refers generally to care actions and activities (Leininger, 1991, p. 46).
4. *Culture:* Refers to the learned, shared, and transmitted values, beliefs, norms, and lifeways of a particular group that guides their thinking, decisions, and actions in patterned ways (Leininger, 1991, p. 47).
5. *Culture care:* Refers to subjectively and objectively learned and transmitted values, beliefs, and patterned lifeways that assist, support, facilitate, or enable another individual or group to maintain well-being and health, to improve their human condition and lifeway, or to deal with illness, handicaps, or death (Leininger, 1991, p. 47).
6. *Professional care:* Refers to formally taught, learned, and transmitted professional care, health, illness, wellness, and related knowledge and skills that are found in professional institutions and held to be beneficial to clients (they are usually etic or outsiders' views) (Leininger, 1990, 1995, p. 106).
7. *Generic (folk and lay) care:* Refers to culturally learned and transmitted indigenous (or traditional, folk, lay, and home-based) knowledge or skills used to provide assistive, supportive, enabling, or facilitative acts toward or for another individual or group (they are largely emic or insiders' views) (Leininger, 1995, p. 106).
8. *Health:* Refers to a state of well-being that is culturally defined, valued, and practiced and reflects the ability of individuals (or groups) to perform their daily role activities in culturally

expressed, beneficial, and patterned ways (Leininger, 1993, 1995, p. 106).

9. *Culture care preservation or maintenance*: Refers to those assistive, supporting, facilitative, or enabling professional actions and decisions that help people of a particular culture to retain and/or preserve relevant care values so that they can maintain their well-being, recover from illness, or face handicaps and/or death (Leininger, 1991, p. 48).

10. *Culture care accommodation or negotiation*: Refers to those assistive, supporting, facilitative, or enabling creative professional actions and decisions that help people of a designated culture to adapt to, or to negotiate with, others for beneficial or satisfying health outcomes (Leininger, 1991, p. 48).

11. *Culture care repatterning or restructuring*: Refers to those assistive, supporting, facilitative, or enabling professional actions and decisions that help clients reorder, change, or greatly modify their own lifeways for new, different, and beneficial health-care patterns while respecting the client(s)' cultural values and beliefs to provide beneficial and healthy lifeways (Leininger, 1991, p. 49). (These patterns are mutually established between care givers and receivers.)

12. *Ethnohistory*: Refers to past facts, events, instances, and experiences of individuals, groups, cultures, and institutions that have been primarily experienced or known in the past and which describe, explain, and interpret human lifeways within a particular culture over short or long periods of time (Leininger, 1991, p. 48).

13. *Environmental context*: Refers to the totality of an event, situation, or particular experience that gives meaning to human expressions, interpretations, and social actions in particular physical, ecological, sociopolitical, and/or cultural settings (Leininger, 1991, p. 48).

14. *Worldview*: Refers to the way in which people tend to look out on the world or their universe to form a picture or value stance about their life or the world around them (Leininger, 1991, p. 47).

15. *Kinship and social factors*: Refers to family intergenerational linkages and social interactions based on cultural beliefs, values, and recurrent lifeways over time.

16. *Religion and spiritual factors*: Refers to the supernatural and natural beliefs and practices that guide individual and group thoughts and actions toward the good or desired ways to improve one's lifeways.

17. *Political factors*: Refers to authority and power over others that regulates or influences another's actions, decisions, or behavior.

18. *Technological factors*: Refers to the use of electrical, mechanical, or physical (nonhuman) objects used in the service of humans.

19. *Education factors*: Refers to formal and informal modes of learning or acquiring knowledge about specific ideas or diverse subject matter domains or phenomena.

20. *Economic factors*: Refers to the production, distribution, and use of negotiable material or consumable productions held valuable to or needed by human beings.

21. *Environmental factors*: Refers to the totality of factors within one's geographic or ecological living area.

22. *Culturally congruent care*: Refers to the use of culturally based care knowledge and action modes with individuals or groups in beneficial and meaningful ways to assist or improve one's health and well-being or to face illness, disabilities, or death (Leininger, 2002).

The above definitions are called *orientational* rather than *operational*, in order to permit the researcher to discover unknown phenomena or vaguely known ideas. Orientational terms allow discovery and are usually congruent with the client lifeways. They are important in using the qualitative ethnonursing discovery method, which is focused on how people know, understand, and experience their world using cultural knowledge and lifeways (Leininger, 1985, 1991, 1997a, 1997b, 1999, 2000).

The Sunrise Enabler: A Conceptual Guide to Knowledge Discovery

The sunrise enabler (Figure 20–1) was developed by Leininger to provide a holistic and comprehensive conceptual picture of the major factors influencing Culture Care Diversity and Universality (Leininger, 1995, 1997a; Leininger & McFarland, 2002). The model can be a valuable conceptual visual guide to discover multiple factors influencing

Leininger's Sunrise Enabler to Discover Culture Care

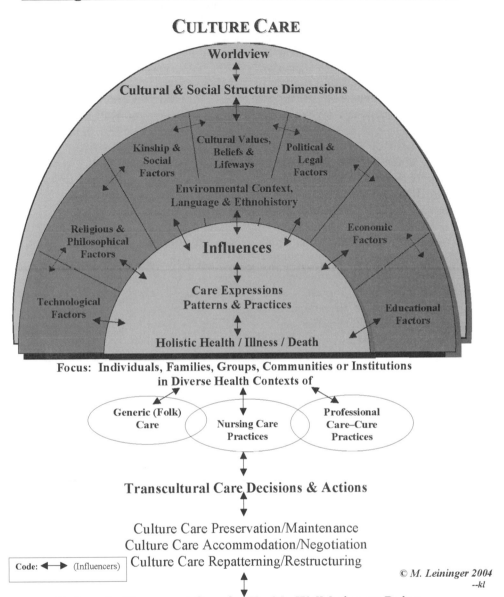

FIGURE 20–1   Leininger's sunrise enabler to discover culture care. © M. Leininger 2004.

human care and cultural lifeways of different cultures. The enabler serves as a cognitive guide for the researcher to visualize and reflect on different factors predicted to influence culturally based care.

> *The sunrise enabler can also be used as a valuable guide for doing culturalogical health-care assessment of clients.*

The sunrise enabler can also be used as a valuable guide for doing culturalogical health-care assessment of clients. As the researcher uses the model, the different factors alert him or her to discover culture care phenomena. Gender and sexual orientation, race, class factors, and biomedical condition are studied as part of the theory. These factors tend to be embedded in the worldview and in the social structure and take time to discover.

The care values and beliefs are usually lodged into environment, religion, kinship, and daily life patterns.

The nurse can begin the discovery at any place in the enabler and follow the informants' ideas and experiences about care. If one starts in the upper part of the enabler, one needs to reflect on all aspects depicted in order to obtain holistic or total care data. Some nurses like to start with generic and professional care, and then look at how religion, economics, and other factors influence these care modes. One always moves with the informants' interest and story rather than the researcher's interest. Flexibility in using the enabler will lead to a total or holistic view of care.

The three modes of action and decision (in the lower part) are very important to keep in mind. The nursing actions or decisions are studied until one realizes the care needed. The nurse discovers with the informant the appropriate actions, decisions, or plans for care. Throughout this discovery process, the nurse holds his or her own etic views, presuppositions, and biases in abeyance, so that the informants' ideas will come forth, rather than the researcher's views. Transcultural nurses are taught, guided, and mentored in ways to withhold their biases or wishes and to enter the client's worldview.

The nurse begins the study by stating a specific and explicit domain of inquiry. For example, the researcher may focus on a *domain of inquiry* (DOI) such as "culture care of Mexican American mothers caring for their children in their home." Every word in the domain statement is important and is studied with the sunrise enabler and the theory tenets. The nurse may have hunches about the domain and care, but until all data have been studied with the theory tenets, she cannot prove them. Full documentation of the informants' viewpoints, experiences, and actions is pursued. Generally, informants select what they like to talk about first, and the nurse accommodates their interest or stories about care. During the in-depth study of the domain of inquiry, all areas of the sunrise enabler are identified and confirmed with the informants. The informants become active participants throughout the discovery process and in a manner in which they feel comfortable and willing to share their ideas.

The real challenge is to focus care meanings, beliefs, values, and practices related to informants' culture, subtle and obvious, so differences and similarities about care are identified among key and general informants. The differences and similarities are important to document with the theory. Such differences may be with the historical, environmental, and social structure factors (differences about care with religion, family, and economic, political, legal, or other factors). If informants ask about the researcher's views, they must be carefully and sparsely shared. The researcher keeps in mind the fact that some informants may want to please the researcher by talking about their professional medicines and treatments in order to satisfy the researcher. Professional ideas, however, often cloud or mask the client's real interests and views. If this occurs, the researcher must be alert to such tendencies and keep the focus on the informants' ideas and on the domain of inquiry studied. The informants' knowledge is always kept central to the discovery process about culture care, health, and well-being. If factors are unfamiliar to the researcher, such as kinship, economics, and political and other considerations depicted in the model, the researcher should listen attentively to the informant's ideas. Getting the informant's emic (insider's) views, beliefs, and practices is central to studying the theory (Leininger, 1985, 1991, 1995, 1997a; Leininger & McFarland, 2002).

Throughout the study and use of the theory, the meanings, expressions, and patterns of culturally based care are important ideas to keep in mind. The nurse listens attentively to informants' accounts about care and then documents the ideas. What informants know and practice about care or caring in their culture is important. Documenting ideas from the informant's emic viewpoint is essential to arrive at accurate culturally based care. Unknown care meanings, such as the concepts of protection, respect, love, and many other care concepts, need to be teased out and explored in depth as they are the key words and ideas in understanding care. Such care meanings and expressions are not always readily known; informants ponder about care meanings and are often surprised that nurses are focused on care instead of medical symptoms. Sometimes informants may be reluctant to share social structure and factors such as religion and economical or political ideas as they fear they may not be accepted or understood by health personnel. Generic (folk or indigenous) knowledge often has rich care data and needs to be explored. Generic care ideas need to be appropriately integrated into the three modes of action and decision for congruent care outcomes. Both generic and professional care are integrated together so the clients benefit from both types of care.

The Sunrise Enabler was developed with the idea to "let the sun enter the researcher's mind" and discover largely unknown care factors of cultures. Letting the sun "rise and shine" is important and offers fresh and new insights about care practices. Generally, a wealth of new and unexpected nursing care knowledge is discovered that has never been known and used in present-day nursing and medical services.

Current Status of the Theory

Currently, the theory of culture care diversity and universality is being studied and used in many schools of nursing within the United States and other countries (Leininger & McFarland, 2002). The theory has grown in recognition and value for several reasons. First, the theory is the only nursing theory that focuses explicitly and in depth on discovering the meaning, uses, and patterns of culture care within and between specific cultures. Second, the theory provides comparative culture care differences and similarities among and within cultures. Thus, it has greatly expanded nurses' knowledge about care so essential for nurses to know and use in practices. Third, the theory has a "built-in" and tailor-made ethnonursing nursing research method that helps to realize the theory tenets. It is different from ethnography and other research methods. The ethnonursing method is a qualitative method and is valuable in discovering largely covert, complex, and generally hidden care knowledge in cultures or subcultures. It was the first specific research method designed so that the theory and method fit together. This has brought forth a wealth of new data. Quantitative data methods were not helpful to find hidden care data.

Fourth, the theory of culture care is the only theory that searches for comprehensive and holistic care data relying on social structure, worldview, and multiple factors in a culture in order to get a holistic knowledge base about care. The theory predicts the health and well-being of people and focuses on the totality of lifeways of individuals, families, groups, communities, and/or institutions related to culture and care phenomena. It gives a comprehensive picture of care knowledge and often in a historical and environmental context. Some nurse researchers have studied care with limited variables or in regard to medical symptoms and diseases—an approach that is too limited and fails to identify care beliefs and values from the informants' views. Discovering the totality of living with a caring ethos in a culture has provided a wealth of new knowledge about clients' lifeworld and care.

Fifth, the theory has both abstract and practical dimensions. This characteristic helps nurse researchers to discover what exists, or has the potential to be known and used for human caring and health practices. What exists and does not exist is important to discover, as is the potential for future discoveries. Some theories deal only with abstract phenomena, but this theory has both abstract and practical realities.

Sixth, the theory of culture care is a synthesized concept; integrated with the ethnonursing method, it has already provided a wealth of many new insights, knowledge areas, and valuable ways to work with people of diverse cultures (5 books and 250 articles), showing different ways to care for cultures. These transcultural nursing research findings are the new knowledge holdings that support the new discipline of transcultural nursing. These are the "gold nuggets" to change or transform health care to realize therapeutic outcomes for different cultures. Several transcultural nursing studies have been reported in the *Journal of Transcultural Nursing* and other transcultural nursing books and journals since 1980. They substantiate the theory (Leininger, 1991, 1995, 1997a, 1997b).

Seventh, the theory and its research findings are stimulating nursing faculty and clinicians to use culture specific care appropriate and safe for cultures. Thus, transcultural nursing knowledge is to be used in clinical and community settings. Nursing administrators in service and academia need to be active change leaders to use transcultural nursing findings. Nursing faculty members need to promote and teach ways to be effective with cultures (Leininger, 1998). Nurse consultants are using the theory findings for effective consultation services with cultures. The theory is being used a lot to do culturalogical–health care assessments. Today, transcultural nursing concepts, findings, policies, and standards of care are being developed and used from findings (Leininger, 1991). Interdisciplinary health personnel are finding the theory and transcultural nursing concepts and are finding help in their work.

Eighth, informants of diverse cultures are often very pleased to have their culture understood and have care made to fit their cultural values and beliefs. This has been the most rewarding benefit of the theory. The research is actually being used in people care. The consumer also likes the ethnonursing method as they can "tell their story" and guide health researchers to discover the truths about their culture. Informants speak of being more comfortable with researchers. They dislike narrowly focused studies on numbers, variables, and short instant responses.

Ninth, reflective thinking with the users of the theory and method are occurring and valued. The theory encourages the researcher or clinician to discover culture from the people and to let them be in control of their ideas and their accounts.

Tenth, nurse researchers who have been prepared in transcultural nursing and have used the theory and method commonly say things like, "I love the theory. It is the only theory that makes sense to help cultures. They grow in ideas and enjoy discovering new knowledge of the lifeways of people and their meanings." They dislike the return to traditional nursing ways.

Eleventh, nurses who have used the theory and findings over time often speak of how much they have learned about themselves and about new cultures and caring values and practices. Nurses discover their ethnocentric tendencies as well as radical biases. The findings are helpful to reduce cultural biases and prejudices that influence quality of care to people of different cultures. Ethnocentrism and racial biases and prejudices are being reduced with transcultural research. Many nurses also like to discover the differences and similarities among cultures as it expands their worldviews and deepens their appreciation of human beings of diverse cultures. Learning to become immersed in a culture has been a major benefit. Most of all, nurses are overwhelmed to discover care meaning and values from informants; they thought such research would not yield benefits.

Finally, the strength of the theory is that it can be used in any culture and at any time and with most disciplines. Other disciplines have to modify the theory slightly to fit their major and unique interest and goals of their discipline. Several disciplines, including dentistry, medicine, social work, and pharmacy, are now using the culturally congruent care theory or teaching it in their programs. Most encouraging is the fact that the concept of "culturally congruent care" (the term that was coined in the early 1960s) has now become a major goal for United States government and several states. The concept is growing in use and will become a global force.

In general, the theory of culture care is a theory of global interest and significance as we continue to understand cultures and their care needs and practices worldwide. Transcultural nursing concepts, principles, theory, and findings must become fully incorporated into professional areas of teaching, practice, consultation, and research. When this occurs, then one can anticipate true transcultural health practices and benefits to cultures. Unquestionably, the theory will continue to grow in relevance and use as our world becomes more intensely multicultural. Nurses and all health professionals will be expected in the near future to function competently with diverse cultures. The theory, along with many transcultural nursing concepts, principles, and research findings, will be used.

PART TWO:
Application of Leininger's Theory of Culture Care Diversity and Universality

Marilyn R. McFarland

The Ethnonursing Research Method

Culture Care Theory and Nursing Practice

Summary

References

$\mathcal{T}$he purpose of the second part of Chapter 20 is twofold. The first part will include an overview of the ethnonursing research method, which was designed to study the Theory of Culture Care Diversity and Universality. The second part will present a discussion of the implications of the culture care theory and related ethnonursing research findings for clinical nursing practice. Many nursing theories are rather abstract and do not focus on how practicing nurses might use the research findings related to a theory. However, with the Culture Care Theory, along with the ethnonursing method, there is a purposeful built-in means to discover and confirm data with informants in order to make nursing actions and decisions meaningful and culturally congruent (Leininger, 2002).

The Ethnonursing Research Method

The ethnonursing research method was specifically designed by Leininger (2002) to study the culture care theory. This was the first research method designed to study a nursing theory and related nursing phenomena. The method facilitates the discovery of people care knowledge and culturally based care related to the theory. Leininger has

> *Leininger has defined the ethnonursing research method as "a qualitative research method using naturalistic, open discovery, and largely inductively derived emic modes and processes with diverse strategies, techniques, and enabling tools to document, describe, understand, and interpret the people's meanings, experience, symbols, and other related aspects bearing on actual or potential nursing phenomena."*

defined the *ethnonursing research method* as "a qualitative research method using naturalistic, open discovery, and largely inductively derived emic modes and processes with diverse strategies, techniques, and enabling tools to document, describe, understand, and interpret the people's meanings, experience, symbols, and other related aspects bearing on actual or potential nursing phenomena" (1991b, p. 79).

Qualitative Paradigm and Quantitative Paradigm

In order to understand the qualitative ethnonursing research method, it is important to understand the major philosophical differences between the qualitative and quantitative paradigms. Leininger has described *qualitative paradigmatic research* as "characterized by naturalistic and open inquiry methods and techniques focused on systematically documenting, analyzing, and interpreting attributes, patterns, characteristics, and meanings of specific domains and gestaltic (or holistic) features of phenomena under study within designated environmental or living contexts" (Leininger, 1997, p. 43). She has described quantitative research as "characterized by a focus on an empirical and objective analysis of discrete and preselected variables that have been derived a priori and as theoretical statements or hypotheses in order to determine causal and measurable relationships among the variables being tested" (Leininger, 1997, p. 43). In qualitative research there is no control of informant's ideas or manipulation of data or variables by the researcher; open inquiry prevails to obtain data directly and naturally from informants in their own homes, communities, or other natural environmental contexts. In contrast, in quantitative research, precise measurements are obtained and specific causal relationships among variables are sought. Leininger has stated that the quantitative and qualitative paradigms should not be mixed, as they violate the philosophy, purposes, and integrity of each paradigm. The ethnonursing method is a unique and essential qualitative method to study caring and healing practices, beliefs, and values in diverse cultural and environmental contexts and is a major holistic method specifically designed to fit the culture care theory.

Purpose and Philosophical Features

Leininger developed the ethnonursing research method from a nursing and cultural care perspective to discover largely unknown phenomena held essential to practice nursing used (1985, 1991b). She has stated that the ethnonursing method is used to "systematically document and gain greater understanding and meaning of the people's daily life experiences related to human care, health, and well-being in different or similar environmental contexts" (Leininger, 1991b, p. 78). The central purpose of the ethnonursing research method is "to establish a naturalistic and largely emic open inquiry method to explicate and study nursing phenomena especially related to the Theory of Cultural Care Diversity and Universality" (Leininger, 1991b, p. 75). The term *ethnonursing* was purposefully coined for this method. The prefix *ethno* comes from the Greek word *ethos* and refers "to the people," while the suffix *nursing* is essential to focus the research on the phenomena of nursing, particularly human care, well-being, and health in different environments and cultural contexts (Leininger, 1991b).

The ethnonursing research method has philosophical and research features that fit well with the culture care theory. Philosophically, the ethnonursing method has been grounded with the people (Leininger, 1991b) and has supported the discovery of people truths in human living contexts (Leininger, 1988). This research method was de-

signed to tease out complex, elusive, and largely unknown nursing dimensions from the local people's viewpoints of human care, well-being, health, and environmental contexts. The terms *emic* and *etic* were important concepts chosen for foci with the ethnonursing method. Ethnonursing focuses largely on the importance of emic (insiders' or local peoples') views but does not neglect etic (the non-local or outsiders') views to obtain a holistic view. For instance, one ethnonursing researcher gathered emic data from elderly retirement home residents on their ideas and experiences with care but also gathered etic data focused on the professional perspectives of the nursing staff (McFarland, 1997). The culture care theory has been developed to be congruent with the ethnonursing method and requires the researcher to move into familiar and naturalistic people settings to discover human care and the related nursing phenomena of health (well-being), illness, and other phenomena within an environmental context (Leininger, 1991b, p. 85).

Domain of Inquiry

A *domain of inquiry* is the major focus of the ethnonursing researcher's interests. A domain of inquiry is broad and yet focused in order to obtain specific care and health outcomes of a culture within a nursing perspective. With the ethnonursing method, problem statements are not used because a researcher does not know whether there is a *people* problem or more of a researcher's problem of selected (and possibly biased) views of the people (Leininger, 1997). For example, some domains of inquiry in ethnonursing studies using the culture care theory have been: the care meanings and experiences of Lebanese Muslims living in the United States in a designated urban context (Luna, 1994); the cultural care of elderly Anglo and African American residents within the environmental context of a long-term care institution (McFarland, 1997); and the care of Mexican American women during pregnancy (Berry, 1999).

Key and General Informants

Key and general informants are important in the ethnonursing research method. The research using this method does not have subjects but works with informants. In an ethnonursing study of the culture care of Anglo and African American elderly residents of a retirement home, the researcher worked with the elders and nursing staff members as key and general informants (McFarland, 1997). The informants told the researcher about themselves and the cultural care within the environmental context of a retirement home. Key informants were carefully and purposefully selected, often by the people themselves (e.g., elderly residents suggested other residents for the researcher to observe, interview, and study about care, health, and well-being). These informants were most knowledgeable about the domain of inquiry and could give details to the nurse researcher. General informants usually are not as fully knowledgeable about the domain of inquiry as are key informants. They have general ideas about the domain, however, and can offer data from their emic and etic views. For instance, general informants can reflect on how similar and/or different their ideas are from those of the key informants when asked by the researcher.

Enablers

In order to discover the peoples' or insiders' (informants') emic views of care, Leininger (1991b) developed several enablers to tease out data bearing on cultural care related to specific domains of study. As the word denotes, enablers help tease out ideas from informants in meaningful and natural ways. Leininger (2002) specifically makes the point that enablers are different from tools, scales, or measurement instruments used in quantitative studies, which tend to cut off natural flow of informant ideas. Some of the enablers that serve as important guides to obtain data naturalistically and holistically are: Leininger's observation participation reflection enabler (Table 20–1); the stranger to trusted friend enabler (Table 20–2); Leininger's acculturation enabler (Leininger, 1991b); and specific enablers developed by the researcher to tap into ideas of informants related to

the specific domain of inquiry (Table 20–3). The sunrise enabler (see Part 1 of this chapter by Dr. Leininger, as well as the discussion under the three care modes later in this part of the chapter) assists and guides the researcher to tease out culture care and health data within each dimension of the enabler to discover holistic and yet specific cultural findings (Leininger, 2002).

The observation participation reflection enabler guides the nurse researcher to be an active observer and listener before being a participant in any research context. Researchers have found it most helpful to observe informants and their environmental contexts before and after the researcher becomes an active participant. This is quite different from the traditional participant observation method used in anthropology, because *the process is reversed* (Leininger, 1997).

The stranger to trusted friend enabler is extremely helpful when a researcher enters and remains in a strange and unfamiliar environment. The researcher moves from being a stranger to being a trusted friend and can eventually obtain accurate, honest, credible, and in-depth data from informants. Being a trusted friend leads to informants sharing their cultural secrets and their insights and experiences. For instance, the author used the stranger friend enabler to assess her relationship with elderly residents and the staff in a study of culture care in a retirement home. She used this enabler to enter the informant's world and get close to the people who were being studied (McFarland, 1997). Initially the researcher worked with a staff nurse while observing and interviewing the informants for the first few weeks she was at the institution. The staff nurse was friendly and acted as a guide but also watched the researcher and planned her day in a general way. The researcher

Table 20–1	**Leininger's Ethnonursing Observation-Participation-Reflection Phases**			
PHASES	1	2	3	4
Description	Primary observation and active listening (no active participation)	Primary observation with limited participation	Primary participation with continued observations	Primary reflection and reconfirmation of findings with informants

Source: Leininger, M. (1997). Overview and reflection of the Theory of Culture Care and the Ethnonursing Research Method. *Journal of Transcultural Nursing, 8*(2), 32–51.

Table 20–2	**Leininger's Stranger to Trusted Friend Enabler Guide**

The purpose of this enabler is to facilitate the researcher (or clinician, who can also use it) to move from a mainly distrusted stranger to a trusted friend in order to obtain authentic, credible, and dependable data or establish favorable relationships as a clinician. The user assesses himself or herself by reflecting on the indicators as he or she moves from stranger to friend.

INDICATORS OF STRANGER (LARGELY ETIC OR OUTSIDER'S VIEWS)	DATE NOTED	INDICATORS OF A TRUSTED FRIEND (LARGELY EMIC OR INSIDER'S VIEWS)	DATE NOTED
Active to protect self and others. They *are gatekeepers* and guard against outside intrusions. Suspicious and questioning.		Less active to protect self. More trusting of researchers (their *gatekeeping is down or less*). Less suspicious and less questioning of researcher.	
Actively watch and are attentive to what researcher does and says. Limited signs of trusting the researcher or stranger.		Less watching of the researcher's words and actions. More signs of trusting and accepting a new friend.	
Skeptical about the researcher's motives and work. May question how findings will be used by the researcher or stranger.		Less questioning of the researcher's motives, work, and behavior. Signs of working with and helping the researcher as a friend.	
Reluctant to share cultural secrets and views as private knowledge. Protective of local lifeways, values, and beliefs. Dislikes probing by the researcher or stranger.		Willing to share cultural secrets and private world information and experiences. Offers most local views, values, and interpretations spontaneously or without probes.	
Uncomfortable to become a friend or to confide in stranger. May come late, be absent, and withdraw from researcher at times.		Signs of being comfortable and enjoying friends and a sharing relationship. Gives presence, is on time, and gives evidence of being a *genuine friend*.	
Tends to offer inaccurate data. Modifies *truths* to protect self, family, community, and cultural lifeways. Emic values, beliefs, and practices are not shared spontaneously.		Wants research *truths* to be accurate regarding beliefs, people, values, and lifeways. Explains and interprets emic ideas so researcher has accurate data.	

Source: Leininger, M. (1991). *Culture care diversity and universality: A theory of nursing.* New York: National League for Nursing, p. 82.

Table 20–3	**Leininger's Phases of Ethnonursing Analysis for Qualitative Data**

FOURTH PHASE
MAJOR THEMES, RESEARCH FINDINGS, THEORETICAL FORMULATIONS, AND RECOMMENDATIONS

This is the highest phase of data analysis, synthesis, and interpretation. It requires synthesis of thinking, configurations, analysis, interpreting findings, and creative formulations from data of the previous phases. The researcher's task is to abstract and present major theses, research findings, recommendations, and sometimes theoretical formulations.

THIRD PHASE
PATTERN AND CONTEXTUAL ANALYSIS

Data are scrutinized to discover saturation ideas and recurrent patterns of similar or different meanings, expressions, structural forms, interpretations, or explanations of data related to the domain of inquiry. Data are examined to show patterning with respect to meaining-in-context and along with further credibility and confirmation of findings.

SECOND PHASE
IDENTIFICATION AND CATEGORIZATION OF DESCRIPTORS AND COMPONENTS

Data are coded and classified as related to the domain of inquiry and sometimes the questions under study. Emic or etic descriptors are studied within context and for similarities and differences. Recurrent components are studied for their meanings

FIRST PHASE
COLLECTING, DESCRIBING, AND DOCUMENTING RAW DATA (USE OF FIELD JOURNAL AND COMPUTER)

The researcher collects, describes, records, and begins to analyze data related to the purpose, domain of inquiry, or questions under study. This phase includes recording interview data from key and general informants; making observations and having participatory experiences; identifying contextual meanings; making preliminary interpretations; identifying symbols; and recording data related to the phenomena under study, mainly from an emic focus, but attentive to etic ideas. Field data from the condensed and full field journal are processed directly into the computer and coded.

Source: Leininger, M. (1991). *Culture care diversity and universality: A theory of nursing.* New York: National League for Nursing (p. 95).

---

knew she had moved from being a stranger to a trusted friend when the director of nursing said, "You are on your own today; you know, several residents really look forward to your visits." After the researcher had been at the research site for several months, an elderly Anglo American resident informant said to her, "I'm really revealing myself to you today," and then went on to describe her negative feelings about the increasing numbers of African Americans coming to live at the retirement home. The researcher had moved from a stranger to a trusted friend; the informant revealed meaningful and sensitive information to her, and the informant felt safe and trusted the researcher. This enabler is invaluable to gauge one's relationship with informants as the study progresses.

Leininger's acculturation enabler (Leininger, 1991b) has been used in many ethnonursing studies to identify traditional and nontraditional beliefs, values, and general lifeways of informants. This enabler is useful with all informants, but especially with immigrant groups undergoing rapid cultural changes. The Sunrise Enabler was also developed to help researchers discover multiple and diverse holistic lifeways related to culture care experiences and practices. It is unique as a guide for holistic yet specific factors influencing care in cultures under study within ethnohistorical, language, social structure, and environmental contexts (Leininger, 1991b, 1995, 1997).

In addition to the four enablers just discussed, the ethnonursing researcher develops a *special en-*

abler that fits with the specific domain of inquiry under study, such as the care meanings and experiences of Lebanese Muslims (Luna, 1989), the culture care of Anglo and African American elders (McFarland, 1997), and the culture care of pregnant Mexican American women (Berry, 1996). These enablers were specifically designed by the researchers to help tease out in-depth specific details of culture care phenomena related to the theoretical assumptions and the domain of inquiry of the study. Examples of special enablers can be found in the studies previously mentioned and in other ethnonursing research studies listed in the references at the end of this chapter and in the *Journal of Transcultural Nursing* (1989 to 1999). The complete text of an enabler, *The Experience of Mexican Americans Receiving Professional Nursing Care: An Ethnonursing Study,* has been published in the *Journal of Transcultural Nursing* (Zoucha, 1998, pp. 42–44).

Qualitative Criteria to Evaluate Ethnonursing Studies

Leininger (1991b, 1995) has developed specific criteria to evaluate qualitative research, including ethnonursing studies. Because qualitative studies have very different meanings and purposes, goals, and outcomes from quantitative studies, the nurse researcher is required to use qualitative criteria to evaluate ethnonursing research studies. Leininger's (1997) succinct definitions of qualitative criteria are as follows:

1. *Credibility:* Refers to direct evidence from the people and the environmental context as *truths* to the people.
2. *Confirmability:* Refers to documented verbatim evidence from the people who can firmly and knowingly confirm the data or findings.
3. *Meaning-in-context:* Refers to meaningful or understandable findings that are known and relevant to the people within their familiar and natural living environmental contexts.
4. *Recurrent patterning:* Refers to documented evidence of repeated patterns, themes, and acts over time, reflecting consistency in lifeways or patterned behaviors.
5. *Saturation:* Refers to in-depth evidence of taking in all that can be known or understood about phenomena or a domain of inquiry under study by the informants.
6. *Transferability:* Refers to whether the findings from the study will have similar (not identical) meanings and relevance in a similar situation or context (Leininger, 1997, p. 88).

Each of these criteria needs to be used thoughtfully and explicitly in a systematic and continuous process while obtaining data or observing informants over periods of time.

Four Phases of Ethnonursing Analysis for Qualitative Data

Leininger (2002) has developed the phases of ethnonursing qualitative data analysis (Table 20–3). The four phases provide for systematic ongoing data analysis, which occurs from the beginning of data collection until completion of the final analysis and written report of the research findings. The *QSR NUD*IST 4* (Qualitative Solutions and Research, 1997) computer analysis software program or similar ones can be used to assist the researcher with large-volume data analysis. The first two phases of data analysis are focused on obtaining raw data and beginning indicators of the phenomena under study. The third phase of data analysis requires that the researcher identify recurrent patterns. The fourth phase focuses on developing and synthesizing major themes derived from the previous sequential three phases. A research mentor skilled in the ethnonursing method can help the researcher reflect on the major phases and meet the qualitative evaluation criteria. Themes

must be clearly stated to provide guidance to assist nurses in providing culturally congruent and relevant care for people from diverse cultures or subcultures. Themes are the dominant finding from the analysis, and thematic statements require much critical and analytic thinking to accurately reflect the emic and etic raw data and holistic findings.

The Steps in the Ethnonursing Research Process

The general research process of conducting an ethnonursing study is presented as a guide. The process may be modified to fit with the research setting or context. The research process needs to be flexible so the researcher can move with the people and be open to make allowances or change plans in accord with naturalistic developments. As the researcher moves from stranger to friend in collecting and processing research data, modifications in the research plan often become necessary. The phases of the ethnonursing research method developed by Leininger (1991b, p. 105) are as follows:

1. Identify the general intent or purpose(s) of your study with a focus on the domain(s) of inquiry phenomenon under study, area of inquiry, or research questions being addressed.
2. Identify the potential significance of the study to advance nursing knowledge and practice.
3. Review available literature on the domain or phenomena being studied.
4. Conceptualize a research plan from the beginning to the end with the following general phases or sequence of factors in mind:
   a. Consider the research site, community, and people to study the phenomena.
   b. Deal with the informed consent expectations.
   c. Explore and gradually gain entry (with essential permissions and/or informed consent) to the community, hospital, or country where the study is being done.
   d. Anticipate potential barriers and facilitators related to gatekeepers' expectations, language, political leaders, location, and other factors.
   e. Select and appropriately use the ethnonursing enablers with the research process; for example, Leininger's stranger to trusted friend guide, observation participation reflection guide, and others. The researcher may also develop enablers as guides for their study.

f. Choose key and general informants.

g. Maintain trusting and favorable relationships with the people conferring with ethnonursing research experts to prevent unfavorable developments.

h. Collect and confirm data with observations, interviews, participant experiences, and other data. This is a continuous process from the beginning to the end and requires the use of qualitative research criteria to confirm findings and credibility factors.

i. Maintain continuous data processing on the computer and with field journals, depicting active analysis and reflections and discussions with research mentor(s). Computer-assisted data analysis with large volumes of qualitative data may be performed with *QSR NUD*IST 4* software as previously noted.

j. Frequently present and reconfirm findings with the people studied to check credibility and confirmability of findings.

k. Make plans to leave the field site, community, and informants in advance.

5. Do final analysis and writing of research findings soon after completing the study.

6. Prepare published findings in appropriate journals.

7. Help implement the findings with nurses interested in findings.

8. Plan future studies related to this domain or other new ones.

Again, flexibility exists with the ethnonursing data processing, but the above steps help to conceptualize the process and thus promote the researcher's ability to perform a systematic investigation that has credibility and meets other qualitative evaluation criteria.

Culture Care Theory and Nursing Practice

Over the past five decades, the culture care theory, along with the ethnonursing method, have been used by nurse researchers to discover knowledge that can be and has been used in nursing practice. Nurses can use such knowledge to care for individual clients and to focus on care practices that are beneficial for families, groups, communities, cul-

tures, and institutions. Our multicultural world has made it imperative that nurses understand different cultures to work and care for people who have diverse and similar values, beliefs, and ideas about nursing, health, caring, wellness, illness, death, and disabilities (Leininger, 1991a, 1995). As stated by Dr. Leininger in the first part of this chapter, the goal of the Theory of Culture Care Diversity and Universality is to improve or maintain health and well-being by providing culturally congruent care to people that is beneficial and fits with the lifeways of the client, family, or cultural group. The sunrise enabler serves as a cognitive map depicting the seven culture and social structure dimensions that influence care, which in turn influence the health and/or illness of clients. The culture care theory and the sunrise enabler include what is similar (universal) and different (diverse) between generic or folk care and professional care, and provides a focus on both types of care for the provision of culturally congruent care for clients in diverse nursing practice settings. Leininger (1991a) predicted that culturally congruent care would prevent cultural clashes, cultural illnesses, and other unfavorable human conditions under human control. These general ideas are kept in mind as one uses findings related to the theory in clinical practice.

THE THREE CARE MODES AND THE SUNRISE ENABLER

To provide a different focus from traditional nursing, Leininger developed the unique three modes of care to incorporate theory findings (refer to sunrise enabler, Figure 20–1). The three modes are: culture care preservation or maintenance; culture care accommodation or negotiation; and culture care repatterning or restructuring. The theorist has predicted that the researcher can use ethnoresearch findings to guide nursing judgments, decisions, and actions related to providing culturally congruent care (Leininger, 2002). Leininger prefers not to use

> *Leininger prefers not to use the phrase nursing intervention because this term often implies to clients from different cultures that the nurse is imposing his or her (etic) views, which may not be helpful.*

the phrase *nursing intervention* because this term often implies to clients from different cultures that the nurse is imposing his or her (etic) views, which may not be helpful. Instead, the term *nursing actions and decisions* is used, but always with the clients helping to arrive at whatever actions or decisions are planned and implemented. The modes fit with the clients' or peoples' lifeways and yet are therapeutic and satisfying for them. The nurse can draw upon scientific nursing, medical, and other knowledge with each mode.

Data collected from the upper and lower parts of the sunrise enabler provide culture care knowledge for nurse researchers to discover and establish useful ways to provide quality care practices. Active participatory involvement with clients is essential to arrive at culturally congruent care with one or all of the three action modes in order to meet clients' care needs in their particular environmental contexts. The use of these modes in nursing care is one of the most creative and rewarding features of transcultural and general nursing practice with clients of diverse cultures.

It is most important (and a shift in nursing) to carefully focus on the holistic dimensions, as depicted in the sunrise enabler, to arrive at therapeutic culture care practices. All the factors in the sunrise enabler (which include worldview and technological, religious, kinship, political-legal, economic, and educational factors, as well as cultural values and lifeways, environmental context, language, ethnohistory, and generic (folk) and professional care practices) must be considered to arrive at culturally congruent care (Leininger, 2002). Care generated from the culture care theory will only become safe, congruent, meaningful, and beneficial to clients when the nurse in clinical practice becomes fully aware of and explicitly uses knowledge generated from the theory and ethnonursing method whether in a community, home, or institutional context. The culture care theory, along with the ethnonursing method, are powerful means for new directions and practices in nursing. Incorporating culture specific care into client care is essential to practice professional care and to be licensed as registered nurses. Culture specific care is the safe means to ensure culturally based holistic care to fit the client's culture—a major challenge for nurses who practice and provide services in all health-care settings.

THE USE OF CULTURE CARE RESEARCH FINDINGS

Over the past five decades, Dr. Leininger and other research colleagues have used the culture care theory and the ethnonursing method to focus on the care meanings and experiences of 100 cultures (Leininger, 2002); they discovered 187 care constructs in Western and non-Western cultures (Leininger, 1998), as reported in the *Journal of Transcultural Nursing* (1989 to 1999). Leininger has listed the 11 most dominant constructs of care in priority ranking, with the most universal or frequently discovered first: respect for/about, concern for/about; attention to (details)/in anticipation of; helping-assisting or facilitative acts; active helping; presence (being physically there); understanding (beliefs, values, lifeways, and environmental); connectedness; protection (gender related); touching; and comfort measures (McFarland, 2002). These care constructs are the most critical and important universal or common findings to consider in nursing practice, but care diversities must also be considered. Although many of these dominant care constructs may be found in certain cultures, diversities will also be found. The ways in which culture care is applied and used in specific cultures will reflect both similarities and differences among (and sometimes within) different cultures. Next, three ethnonursing studies will be reviewed with focus on the findings, which have implications for nursing practice.

CULTURE CARE OF LEBANESE MUSLIMS IN THE UNITED STATES

In the late 1980s, Luna (1989), conducted an ethnonursing study of the culture care of Arab Muslim cultural groups in a large urban community in the Midwestern United States. In 1989, she published the findings relevant to the culture care of Lebanese Muslim Americans using Leininger's three modes of nursing decisions and actions to provide culturally congruent and responsible care. The study focused on the care for Lebanese Muslims in the hospital, clinic, and home-community contexts. She stated: "[An] understanding [of] the cultural context in which Lebanese Muslims attempt to adapt, survive, and practice their faith in America necessitates a look into the community into which they migrate" (Luna, 1994, p. 15). Luna's research findings and the nursing practice implications related to the home and community context in the late 1980s remain important as health care shifts from hospital care services to home or community settings. Luna discovered that attending a clinic in a Midwestern United States urban context was often a new and different approach to health care for Lebanese Muslim women, especially during pregnancy and childbirth. Luna's study revealed that many women relied on the traditional midwife in Lebanon for home deliveries. The routine of monthly and weekly visits to the prenatal clinic was incongruent with what these clients had experienced in their home country. In the United States, prenatal care in the clinic context involved long waiting periods with the husband missing work to take his wife to each appointment. Examination by a male physician was culturally incongruent for the women, so *culture care negotiation and repatterning* was essential for culturally congruent care. Luna described the clinic as *culturally decontextualized* for clients and their families because the prenatal care and the environmental clinic context in which the care was provided were not congruent with the clients' cultural values, beliefs, and practices (Luna, 1989). Luna discovered some dominant and universal care constructs for Lebanese Muslim men, which included surveillance, protection, and maintenance of the family. For Lebanese women, the dominant and universal care constructs included emphasizing the positive attributes of educating the children and maintaining a family caring environment according to the precepts of Islam. A number of generic or folk care practices were discovered relating to these care constructs that should be recognized, preserved, and maintained by nurses to enhance the health and well-being of clients. For instance, the female network in the Lebanese Muslim culture is very important at the time of birth; Lebanese women come together to care for one another and offer practical and emotional assistance for new immigrants who are struggling to survive in a new cultural context such as the United States. By recognizing the benefits of this network and by allowing women flexibility in their visiting and presence in the hospital and clinic contexts, the nurse would use culture care preservation to maintain these generic care practices for the health and well-being of clients.

Luna found that female modesty was an important cultural care value for Lebanese women; this was reflected in requests by female clients to have only female nurses, physicians, and other caregivers. Culture care accommodation of this generic care practice was accomplished by nurses negotiating for these women to have female caregivers whenever possible, which would promote health, well-being, and client satisfaction with care. By including Lebanese Muslim men in health teaching and discharge planning, Luna discovered a way to use culture care preservation that recognized the family as a unit, rather than focusing on the individual. Luna recognized that the patriarchal organization of the family should be preserved as a social structure feature, which acknowledges males for their roles in family care continuity rather than being narrowly interpreted as males always being in control. Negative stereotypes held by nurses about the Arab males' reluctance to participate in the birth process were also discovered, often presenting a barrier to giving nursing care. To counter this, Luna suggested the nurses use culture care preservation to maintain and support the generic culture care practices of men, which included surveillance, protection, and maintenance of the family.

Still another finding from Luna's study was the discovery of the importance of religious rituals to many Muslim clients as an essential component of providing care within their cultural context (Luna, 1989, 1994). Luna found that some Muslims pray three to five times a day, and others do not pray at all. During the culturalogical assessment (in the hospital context), Luna suggested the nurse should ask about the client's wishes regarding prayer. Culture care accommodation could be practiced by negotiating for an agreeable time and a private place for clients to pray, which for many Muslims is an important cultural expression for their health and well-being. She also suggested that nurses practice culture care accommodation for clients by negotiating with a social service organization that served Arab clients in order to gather written and video materials in the Arabic language related to health for use in the hospital and clinic settings. Luna (1989) identified approaches for culture care repatterning to improve attendance at the prenatal clinic for Lebanese Muslim women. Nurses should avoid direct confrontation and spend considerable time during the first clinic visit to educate women regarding the benefits of regular prenatal care, including emphasizing the health and well-being of both the mother and the baby.

In 1999, Wehbeh-Alamah conducted a two-year ethnonursing study using the culture care theory and studied the generic health-care beliefs, practices, and expressions of Lebanese American Muslim immigrants in two Midwestern U.S. cities. Her findings, which confirmed many of Luna's from 1989, included the discovery of specific generic folk care beliefs on practices that required culture care accommodation/negotiation in the home as well as in the hospital. These included providing for prayer while facing east five times a day; having large numbers of visitors when in the hospital or at home; and eating only halal meat. Many gender care findings were similar to those from Luna's study, revealing a persistence of many related care patterns over time as predicted in the culture care theory. However, the women in Wehbeh-Alamah's study believed the absence of extended family members in the United States had influenced male family members' thinking about the appropriateness of men caring for family members. The researcher reported that acculturation had changed men's view about providing care from the more traditional belief that the hands-on caring for the children, elderly, and sick belonged to women, to the more contemporary belief in cooperation and participation in direct caregiving by Muslim men (Wehbeh-Alamah, in press). Currently, Wehbeh-Alamah is conducting an ethnonursing study of the culture care of Syrian American Muslims living in a Midwestern U.S. city. In addition to discovering the culture care meanings, beliefs, and practices of this group, she will compare this study with her previous studies to arrive at universal and diverse care findings among Muslim immigrants from diverse cultures living in the United States.

CULTURE CARE OF ELDERLY ANGLO AND AFRICAN AMERICANS

In the mid 1990s, the theory of culture care was used to guide a study of the culture care of Anglo and African American elders in a long-term care institution (McFarland, 1997). This study revealed care implications for nurses who practice in retirement homes, nursing homes, apartments for the

aged, and other long-term care settings. Many residents from both cultural groups participated in the care of their fellow residents. Residents assisted other residents to the dining room, checked on others who did not appear for meals in the dining room (care as surveillance of others), and assisted in ambulation of those who were not able to walk independently. This focus on *other care* versus only *self care* was a form of culturally congruent care that residents desired in order to maintain healthy and beneficial lifeways in an institutional setting. Culture care preservation was practiced by nursing staff as these generic care practices were integrated into professional nursing care.

Within the retirement home, both Anglo and African American residents desired spiritual or religious care and had some diverse aspects of such care rooted in their respective cultures. The findings of both universality and diversity within the pattern of religious or spiritual care supported Leininger's theory, which states that "culture care concepts, meanings, expressions, patterns, processes, and structural forms of care are different (diversity) and similar (toward universality) among all cultures of the world" (Leininger, 1991a, p. 45). African American residents received care from church friends who ran errands, did banking and laundry, paid bills, visited, and brought communion to them. Anglo American residents received a more formal type of care from their churches, such as a minister coming to the retirement home to do a worship service or a church choir traveling to the retirement home to entertain the residents. The nurses at the retirement home practiced culture care preservation by maintaining the involvement of churches in the daily lives of both cultural groups to help residents face living in a retirement home with increasing disabilities related to aging and handicaps, and even dealing with the prospect of death. With an increase in the numbers of elderly from both the Anglo and African American cultural groups being admitted to long-term care institutions, the knowledge of culture specific care for both Anglo and African American elders is important for nurses who practice in these settings.

The generic care pattern of families helping their elderly relatives enhanced the health and lifeways of both Anglo and African American elders in the retirement home setting. Anglo American residents received help from their spouses and/or adult children. In contrast with the Anglo American findings, African American spouses, children, extended family members, and nonkin who were considered family reflected the care pattern of families helping elderly residents. Grandchildren, great grandchildren, nieces, nephews, grandnieces, and grandnephews, as well as church members or friends who were considered family and were referred to as brothers, sisters, or daughters, were involved in caring for African American elders. The nursing staff recognized the importance of family involvement in the care of residents and practiced culture care preservation to maintain culture specific family care practices for residents from each cultural group.

The care pattern of protection was important to African American residents but not to Anglo American residents. Most African American residents had left homes that were in unsafe neighborhoods and had moved into the facility partly for that reason. African American nursing staff recognized the importance of protective care and often accompanied African American residents when they wanted to go outside. The nursing staff made efforts to practice culture care accommodation by negotiating to take the residents outside to sit on the small grass strip around the perimeter of the parking lot of the home.

McFarland (1997) also discovered that the nursing care and the lifeways of elderly residents in the nursing home setting were less satisfying than in the apartment setting within the retirement home context. Professional nurses need to be more actively involved in culture care repatterning as *co-participants with elders* to restructure lifeway practices, care routines, and the environmental context of nursing homes (including room designs and privacy considerations). Culture care restructuring of these care-related concerns can only be accomplished when nurses assume an advocacy role for the elderly residents and work with governmental and private agencies that provide the funding and make the rules and regulations that affect long-term care. The culture care theory, with the ethnonursing method, assisted the researcher in this study in the discovery of action and decision modes that were culturally specific for Anglo and African American elders residing in a long-term care institution.

CULTURE CARE OF GERMAN AMERICANS

In 2000, McFarland & Zehnder (in press) conducted a two-year ethnonursing study of the culture care of German American elders living in a nursing home in a small Midwestern city in the United States. Their findings, which confirmed many of McFarland's (1997) earlier findings, included many care beliefs and practices that required culture care preservation. German American elder care practices included caring for fellow residents by assisting confused residents to find their assigned seat in the dining room or making items for the annual bazaar to raise money to buy flowers for the nursing home courtyard garden, thereby benefitting all of the residents. The finding of the important care of doing for others versus an emphasis on self-care was previously discovered in McFarland's earlier study in 1997 with Anglo American and African American elders and was confirmed in this German American study.

German American elders received spiritual care from the local German American church and pastor. The pastor conducted a worship service and a Bible class in German each week. Spiritual religious care, provided by connections with the Lutheran Church, was essential to German American elders in maintaining their traditional lifeways and health in the nursing home setting. This finding had also been discovered with Anglo American elders in McFarland's (1997) previous study and was confirmed with German American elders.

McFarland is currently conducting a comparative synthesis of culture care findings related to ethnonursing studies of elder care conducted by transcultural nurses with diverse cultures worldwide. This will hopefully lead to the discovery of universal and diverse care meanings, beliefs, and practices to meet the needs of the increasing numbers of elders worldwide who value generic culture-specific care to reaffirm their cultural identities in the latter phase of their lives.

SUMMARY

The purpose of the culture care theory (along with the ethnonursing method) has been to discover culture care with the goal of using the knowledge to combine generic and professional care. The goal is to provide culturally congruent nursing care using the three modes of nursing actions and decisions that is meaningful, safe, and beneficial to people of similar and diverse cultures worldwide (Leininger, 1991a, 1995). The clinical use of the three major care modes (culture care preservation or maintenance; culture care accommodation or negotiation; and culture care repatterning or restructuring) by nurses to guide nursing judgments, decisions, and actions is essential in order to provide culturally congruent care that is beneficial, satisfying, and meaningful to the people nurses serve. The studies of the four cultures just reviewed (Lebanese Muslim, Anglo American, African American, and German Americans) substantiate that the three modes are care centered and are based on the use of generic care (emic) knowledge along with professional care (etic) knowledge obtained from research using the culture care theory along with the ethnonursing method. This chapter has reviewed only a small selection of the culture care findings from ethnonursing research studies conducted over the past four decades. There is a wealth of additional findings of interest to practicing nurses who care for clients of all ages from diverse and similar cultural groups in many different institutional and community contexts around the world. More in-depth culture care findings along with the use of the three modes can be found in the *Journal of Transcultural Nursing* (1989 to 2004) and in the numerous books and articles by Dr. Madeleine Leininger. Nurses in clinical practice are advised to consult a list of research studies and doctoral dissertations conceptualized within the culture care theory for additional detailed nursing implications for clients from diverse cultures (Leininger & McFarland, 2002, in press).

The Theory of Culture Care Diversity and Universality is one of the most comprehensive yet practical theories to advance transcultural and general nursing knowledge with concomitant ways for practicing nurses to establish or improve care to people. Nursing students and practicing nurses have remained the strongest advocates of the culture care theory (Leininger, 2002). The theory focuses on a long-neglected area in nursing practice—culture care—that is most relevant to our multicultural world.

The Theory of Culture Care Diversity and Universality is depicted in the sunrise enabler as a rising sun. This visual metaphor is particularly apt as the future of the culture care theory shines brightly indeed, because it is holistic, comprehensive, and fits discovering care related to diverse and similar cultures, contexts, and ages of people in familiar and naturalistic ways. The theory is useful to nurses and to nursing and to professionals in other disciplines such as physical, occupational, and speech therapy, medicine, social work, and pharmacy. Health-care practitioners in other disciplines are beginning to use this theory because they also need to become knowledgeable about and sensitive and responsible to people of diverse cultures who need care (Leininger, 2002).

References

Berry, A. (1996). *Culture care expression, meanings, and experiences of pregnant Mexican American women within Leininger's culture care theory.* (UMI No. 9628875). Ann Arbor, MI: UMI Microfilm.

Berry, A. (1999). Mexican American women's expressions of the meaning of culturally congruent prenatal care. *Journal of Transcultural Nursing, 103,* 203–212.

Leininger, M. (1970). *Nursing and anthropology: Two worlds to blend.* New York: John Wiley and Sons.

Leininger, M. (1976). Transcultural nursing presents an exciting challenge. *The American Nurse, 5*(5), 6–9.

Leininger, M. (1977). Caring: The essence and central focus of nursing. *Nursing Research Foundation Report, 12*(1), 2–14.

Leininger, M. (1978). *Transcultural nursing: Concepts, theories, and practices.* New York: John Wiley and Sons.

Leininger, M. (1981). *Caring: An essential human need.* Thorofare, NJ: Slack.

Leininger, M. (1984). *Care: The essence of nursing and health.* Thorofare, NJ: Slack.

Leininger, M. (1985). *Qualitative research methods in nursing* (pp. 33–73). Orlando, FL: Grune & Stratton Co.

Leininger, M. (1988). *Care: Discovery and uses in clinical and community nursing.* Detroit: Wayne State University Press.

Leininger, M. (1989a). Transcultural nursing: Quo vadis (where goeth the field)? *Journal of Transcultural Nursing, 1*(1), 33–45.

Leininger, M. (1989b). Transcultural nurse specialists and generalists: New practitioners in nursing. *Journal of Transcultural Nursing, 1*(1), 4–16.

Leininger, M. (1990a). Transcultural nursing: A worldwide necessity to advance nursing knowledge and practices. In McCloskey, J., & Grace, H. (Eds.), *Current issues in nursing*. St. Louis: Mosby.

Leininger, M. (1990b). Culture: The conspicuous missing link to understand ethical and moral dimensions of human care. In Leininger, M. (Ed.), *Ethical and moral dimensions of care.* Detroit: Wayne State University Press.

Leininger, M. (1990c). Ethnomethods: The philosophic and epistemic basis to explicate transcultural nursing knowledge. *Journal of Transcultural Nursing, 1*(2), 40–51.

Leininger, M. (1990d). *Care: Ethical and moral dimensions of care.* Detroit: Wayne State University Press.

Leininger, M. (1991). *Culture care diversity and universality: A theory of nursing.* New York: National League for Nursing Press.

Leininger, M. (1991a). The theory of culture care diversity and universality. In Leininger, M. (Ed.), *Culture care diversity and universality: A theory of nursing* (pp. 5–68). New York: National League for Nursing Press.

Leininger, M. (1991b). Ethnonursing: A research method with enablers to study the theory of culture care. In Leininger, M. (Ed.), *Culture care diversity and universality: A theory of nursing* (pp. 73–118). New York: National League for Nursing Press.

Leininger, M. (1995). *Transcultural nursing: Concepts, theories, research, and practice.* Columbus, OH: McGraw Hill College Custom Series.

Leininger, M. (1995). *Transcultural nursing: Concepts theories, research, and practice.* Blacklick, OH: McGraw-Hill College Custom Series.

Leininger, M. (1997). Overview and reflection of the theory of culture care and the ethnonursing research method. *Journal of Transcultural Nursing, 8*(2), 32–51.

Leininger, M. (1997a). Overview of the theory of culture care with the ethnonursing research method. *Journal of Transcultural Nursing, 8*(2), 32–53.

Leininger, M. (1997b). Transcultural nursing research to transform nursing education and practice: 40 years. *Image: Journal of Nursing Scholarship, 29*(4), 341–347.

Leininger, M. (1998). Special research report: Dominant culture care (emic) meanings and practice findings from Leininger's theory. *Journal of Transcultural Nursing, 9*(2), 44–47.

Leininger, M., & Hofling, C. (1960). *Basic psychiatric concepts in nursing.* Philadelphia: Lippincott.

Leininger, M. M. (2002). Part I: The theory of culture care and the ethnonursing research method. In Leininger, M. M., & McFarland, M. R. (Eds.), *Transcultural nursing: concepts, theories, and practice* (3rd ed., pp. 71–98): Jones & Bartlett Publishers.

Leininger, M. M., & McFarland, M. R. (Eds.). (2002). *Transcultural nursing: Concepts, theories, and practice* (3rd ed.). New York: McGraw Hill, Medical Publishing Division.

Leininger, M. M., & McFarland, M. R. (Eds.) (in press). *Culture diversity & universality: A worldwide nursing theory* (2nd ed.). Sudbury, MA: Jones & Bartlett Publishers.

Luna, L. (1989). *Care and cultural context of Lebanese Muslims in an urban U.S. community: An ethnographic and ethnonursing study conceptualized within Leininger's theory.* (UMI No. 9022423). Ann Arbor, MI: UMI Microfilm.

Luna, L. (1994). Care and cultural context of Lebanese Muslim immigrants with Leininger's theory. *Journal of Transcultural Nursing, 5*(2), 12–20.

McFarland, M. R. (1995). *Cultural care of Anglo and African American elderly residents within the environmental context of a long-term care institution.* (UMI No. 9530568). Ann Arbor, MI: UMI Microfilm.

McFarland, M. R. (1997). Use of culture care theory with Anglo and African American elders in a long term care setting. *Nursing Science Quarterly, 10*(4), 186–192.

McFarland, M. R. (2002). Part II: Selected research findings from the culture care theory. In Leininger, M. M., & McFarland, M. R. (Eds.), *Transcultural Nursing: Concepts, theories, and practice* (3rd ed., pp. 99–116).

McFarland, M. R., & Zehnder, N. (in press). The culture care of German American elders within a nursing home context. In Leininger, M. M., & McFarland, M. R.(Eds.), *Culture care universality and diversity: A worldwide theory of nursing* (2nd ed.). Sudbury, MA: Jones & Bartlett.

Qualitative Solutions and Research. (1997). *QSR NUD*IST 4.* Thousand Oaks, CA: Sage Publication, Inc.

Wehbeh-Alamah, H. (in press). Generic care of Lebanese Muslim women in the Midwestern USA. In Leininger, M. M., & McFarland, M. R. (Eds.), *Culture care universality and diversity: A worldwide theory of nursing* (2nd ed.). Sudbury, MA: Jones & Bartlett.

Zoucha, R. (1998). The experiences of Mexican Americans receiving professional nursing care: An ethnonursing study. *Journal of Transcultural Nursing, 9*(2), 33–43.

CHAPTER 21

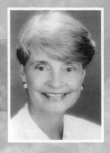

Anne Boykin

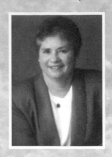

Savina O. Schoenhofer

Anne Boykin and Savina O. Schoenhofer's Nursing as Caring Theory

Anne Boykin & Savina O. Schoenhofer

Introducing the Theorists

Anne Boykin is dean and professor of the College of Nursing at Florida Atlantic University. She is director of the Christine E. Lynne Center for Caring, which is housed in the College of Nursing. This center was created for the purpose of humanizing care through the integration of teaching, research, and service. She has demonstrated a long-standing commitment to the International Association for Human Caring, holding the following positions: president-elect (1990 to 1993), president (1993 to 1996), and member of the nominating committee (1997 to 1999). As immediate past president, she served as coeditor of the journal *International Association for Human Caring* from 1996 to 1999.

Her scholarly work is centered in caring as the grounding for nursing. This is evidenced in her coauthored book, *Nursing As Caring: A Model for Transforming Practice* (1993), and the book *Living a Caring-based Program* (1994). The latter book illustrates how caring grounds the development of a nursing program from creating the environment for study through evaluation. She has also authored numerous book chapters and articles. She serves as a consultant locally, regionally, nationally, and internationally on the topic of caring.

Dr. Boykin is a graduate of Alverno College in Milwaukee, Wisconsin; she received her master's degree from Emory University in Atlanta, Georgia, and her doctorate from Vanderbilt University in Nashville, Tennessee.

Savina Schoenhofer's initial nursing study was at Wichita State University, where she earned undergraduate and graduate degrees in nursing, psychology, and counseling. She completed a PhD in educational foundations and administration at Kansas State University in 1983. In 1990, Schoenhofer cofounded *Nightingale Songs,* an early venue for communicating the beauty of nursing in poetry and prose. In addition to her work on caring, including coauthorship of *Nursing As Caring: A Model for Transforming Practice,* she has written on nursing values, primary care, nursing education, support, touch, personnel management in nursing homes, and mentoring. Her career in nursing has been significantly influenced by three colleagues: Lt. Col. Ann Ashjian (Ret.), whose community nursing practice in Brazil presented an inspiring model of nursing; Marilyn E. Parker, PhD, a faculty colleague who mentored her in the idea of nursing

as a discipline, the academic role in higher education, and the world of nursing theories and theorists; and Anne Boykin, PhD, who introduced her to caring as a substantive field of nursing study. Schoenhofer created and manages the Web site and discussion forum on the theory of nursing as caring (www.nursingascaring.com).

Introducing the Theory

This chapter is intended as an overview of the theory of nursing as caring, a general theory, framework, or disciplinary view of nursing. The theory of nursing as caring offers a view that permits a broad, encompassing understanding of any and all situations of nursing practice (Boykin & Schoenhofer, 1993). This theory serves as an organizing framework for nursing scholars in the various roles of practitioner, researcher, administrator, teacher, and developer.

Initially, we will present the theory in its most abstract form, addressing assumptions and key themes. We will then discuss the meaning of the theory in relation to practice and other nursing roles. In the second part of this chapter, Danielle Linden further describes the theory by illustrating its use as a guide to practice.

ASSUMPTIONS AND KEY THEMES

Certain fundamental beliefs about what it means to be human underlie the theory of nursing as caring. These assumptions, which will be illustrated later, reflect a particular set of values and key themes that provide a basis for understanding and explicating the meaning of nursing, listed as follows and detailed here:

- Persons are caring by virtue of their humanness.
- Persons are whole and complete in the moment.
- Persons live caring from moment to moment.
- Personhood is a way of living grounded in caring.
- Personhood is enhanced through participation in nurturing relationships with caring others.
- Nursing is both a discipline and a profession.

Caring

Caring is an altruistic, active expression of love and is the intentional and embodied recognition of value and connectedness. Caring is not the unique province of nursing. However, as a discipline and a profession, nursing uniquely focuses on caring as its central value, its primary interest, and the direct intention of its practice. The full meaning of caring cannot be restricted to a definition but is illuminated in the experience of caring and in the reflection on that experience.

Focus and Intention of Nursing

Disciplines as identifiable entities or "branches of knowledge" grow from the holistic "tree of knowledge" as need and purpose develop. A discipline is a community of scholars (King & Brownell, 1976) with a particular perspective on the world and what it means to be in the world. The disciplinary community represents a value system that is expressed in its unique focus on knowledge and practice.

> *The focus of nursing, from the perspective of the theory of nursing as caring, is person as living in caring and growing in caring.*

The *focus of nursing,* from the perspective of the theory of nursing as caring, is person as living in caring and growing in caring. The general *intention of nursing* as a practiced discipline is nurturing persons living caring and growing in caring.

Nursing Situation

The practice of nursing, and thus the practical knowledge of nursing, lives in the context of person-with-person caring. The *nursing situation* involves particular values, intentions, and actions of two or more persons choosing to live a nursing relationship. Nursing situation is understood to mean the shared lived experience in which *caring between* nurse and nursed enhances personhood. Nursing is created in the *caring between.* All knowledge of nursing is created and understood within the nursing situation. Any single nursing situation has the potential to illuminate the depth and complexity of nursing knowledge. Nursing situations are best communicated through aesthetic media to preserve the lived meaning of the situation and the openness of the situation as text. Storytelling, poetry, graphic arts, and dance are examples of effective modes of representing the lived experience and

allowing for reflection and creativity in advancing understanding.

Personhood

Personhood is understood to mean living grounded in caring. From the perspective of the theory of nursing as caring, personhood is the universal human call. A profound understanding of personhood communicates the paradox of person-as-person and person-in-communion all at once.

Call for Nursing

"A call for nursing is a call for acknowledgment and affirmation of the person living caring in specific ways in the immediate situation" (Boykin & Schoenhofer, 1993, p. 24). *Calls for nursing* are calls for nurturance through personal expressions of caring. Calls for nursing originate within persons as they live out caring uniquely, expressing personally meaningful dreams and aspirations for growing in caring. Calls for nursing are individually relevant ways of saying, "Know me as caring person in the moment and be with me as I try to live fully who I truly am." Intentionality (Schoenhofer, 2002) and authentic presence open the nurse to hearing calls for nursing. Because calls for nursing are unique situated personal expressions, they cannot be predicted, as in a "diagnosis." Nurses develop sensitivity and expertise in hearing calls through intention, experience, study, and reflection in a broad range of human situations.

Nursing Response

As an expression of nursing, "caring is the intentional and authentic presence of the nurse with another who is recognized as living caring and growing in caring" (Boykin & Schoenhofer, 1993, p. 25). The nurse enters the nursing situation with the intentional commitment of knowing the other as a caring person, and in that knowing, acknowledging, affirming, and celebrating the person as caring. The nursing response is a specific expression of caring nurturance to sustain and enhance the "other" as he or she lives caring and grows in caring in the situation of concern. Nursing responses to calls for caring evolve as nurses clarify their understandings of calls through presence and dialogue. Nursing responses are uniquely created for the moment and cannot be predicted or applied as preplanned protocols (Boykin & Schoenhofer,

1997). Sensitivity and skill in creating unique and effective ways of communicating caring are developed through intention, experience, study, and reflection in a broad range of human situations.

The "Caring Between"

The caring between is the source and ground of nursing. It is the loving relation into which nurse

> The caring between is the source and ground of nursing.

and nursed enter and cocreate by living the intention to care. Without the loving relation of the *caring between,* unidirectional activity or reciprocal exchange can occur, but nursing in its fullest sense does not occur. It is in the context of the *caring between* that personhood is enhanced, each expressing self and recognizing the other as caring person.

Lived Meaning of Nursing as Caring

Abstract presentations of assumptions and themes lay the groundwork and provide an orienting point. However, the lived meaning of nursing as caring can best be understood by the study of a nursing situation. The following poem is one nurse's expression of the meaning of nursing, situated in one particular experience of nursing and linked to a general conception of nursing.

I CARE FOR HIM

My hands are moist,
My heart is quick,
My nerves are taut,
He's in the next room,
I care for him.

The room is tense,
It's anger-filled,
The air seems thick,
I'm with him now,
I care for him.

Time goes slowly by,
As our fears subside,
I can sense his calm,
He softens now,
I care for him.

His eyes meet mine,
Unable to speak,
I feel his trust,
I open my heart,
I care for him.

It's time to leave.
Our bond is made,
Unspoken thoughts,
But understood,
I care for him!
—J. M. Collins (1993)

Each encounter—each nursing experience—brings with it the unknown. In Collins's reflections, he shares a story of practice that illuminates the opportunity to live and grow in caring.

In the nursing situation that inspired this poem, the nurse and nursed live caring uniquely. Initially, the nurse experiences the familiar human dilemma, aware of separateness while choosing connectedness as he responds to a yet-unknown call for nursing: "My hands are moist/my heart is quick/my nerves are taut . . . I care for him." As he enters the situation and encounters the patient as person, he is able to "let go" of his presumptive knowing of the patient as "angry." The nurse enters with the guiding perspective that all persons are caring. This allows him to see past the "anger-filled" room and to be "with him" (second stanza). As they connect through their humanness, the beauty and wholeness of other is uncovered and nurtured. By living caring moment to moment, hope emerges and fear subsides. Through this experience, both nurse and nursed live and grow in their understanding and expressions of caring.

In the first stanza, the nurse prepares to enter the nursing relationship with the formed intention of offering caring in authentic presence. Perhaps he has heard a report that the person he is about to encounter is a "difficult patient," and this is a part of his awareness; however, his nursing intention to care reminds him that he and his patient are, above all, caring persons. In the second stanza, the nurse enters the room, experiences the challenge that his intention to nurse has presented, and responds to the call for authentic presence and caring: "I'm with him now/I care for him." Patterns of knowing are called into play as the nurse brings together intuitive, personal knowing, empirical knowing, and the ethical knowing that it is right to offer care, creating the integrated understanding of aesthetic knowing that enables him to act on his nursing intention (Boykin, Parker, & Schoenhofer, 1994; Carper, 1978). Mayeroff's (1971) caring ingredients of courage, trust, and alternating rhythm are clearly evident.

Clarity of the call for nursing emerges as the nurse begins to understand that this particular man in this particular moment is calling to be known as a uniquely caring person, a person of value, worthy of respect and regard. The nurse listens intently and recognizes the unadorned honesty that sounds angry and demanding but is a personal expression of a heartfelt desire to be truly known and worthy of care. The nurse responds with steadfast presence and caring, communicated in his way of being and of doing. The caring ingredient of hope is drawn forth as the man softens and the nurse takes notice.

In the fourth stanza, the "caring between" develops, and personhood is enhanced as dreams and aspirations for growing in caring are realized: "His eyes meet mine...I open my heart." In the last stanza, the nursing situation is completed in linear time. But each one, nurse and nursed, goes forward, newly affirmed and celebrated as caring person, and the nursing situation continues to be a source of inspiration for living caring and growing in caring.

Assumptions in the Context of the Nursing Situation

In Collins's poem, the power of the basic assumption that all persons are caring by virtue of their humanness enabled the nurse to find the courage to live his intentions. The idea that persons are whole and complete in the moment permits the nurse to accept conflicting feelings and to be open to the nursed as a person, not merely as an entity with a diagnosis and superficially or normatively understood behavior. The nurse demonstrated an understanding of the assumption that persons live caring from moment to moment, striving to know self and other as caring in the moment with a growing repertoire of ways of expressing caring. Personhood, a way of living grounded in caring that can be enhanced in relationship with caring other, comes through in that the nurse is successfully living his commitment to caring in the face of difficulty and in the mutuality and connectedness that emerged in the situation. The assumption that

nursing is both a discipline and a profession is affirmed as the nurse draws on a set of values and a developed knowledge of nursing as caring to actively offer his presence in service to the nursed.

NURSING AS CARING: HISTORICAL PERSPECTIVE AND CURRENT DEVELOPMENT

The theory of nursing as caring developed as an outgrowth of the curriculum development work in the College of Nursing at Florida Atlantic University, where both authors were among the faculty group revising the caring-based curriculum. When the revised curriculum was in place, each of us recognized the potential and even the necessity of continuing to develop and structure ideas and themes toward a comprehensive expression of the meaning and purpose of nursing as a discipline and a profession. The point of departure was the acceptance that caring is the end, rather than the means, of nursing, and that caring is the intention of nursing rather than merely its instrument. This work led to the statement of focus of nursing as "nurturing persons living caring and growing in caring." Further work to identify foundational assumptions about nursing clarified the idea of the nursing situation, a shared lived experience in which the caring between enhances personhood, with personhood understood as living grounded in caring. The clarified focus and the idea of the nursing situation are the key themes that draw forth the meaning of the assumptions underlying the theory and permit the practical understanding of nursing as both a discipline and a profession. As critique of the theory and study of nursing situations progressed, the notion of nursing being primarily concerned with health was seen as limiting, and we now understand nursing to be concerned with human living.

Three bodies of work significantly influenced the initial development of nursing as caring. Roach's (1987/2002) basic thesis that caring is the human mode of being was incorporated into the most basic assumption of the theory. We view Paterson and Zderad's (1988) existential phenomenological theory of humanistic nursing as the historical antecedent of nursing as caring. Seminal ideas such as "the between," "call for nursing," "nursing response," and "personhood" served as substantive and structural bases for our conceptualization of nursing as caring. Mayeroff's (1971) work, *On Caring*, provided a language that facilitated the recognition and description of the practical meaning of caring in nursing situations. In addition to the work of these thinkers, both authors are long-standing members of the community of nursing scholars whose study focuses on caring and who are supported and undoubtedly influenced in many subtle ways by the members of this community and their work.

Fledgling forms of the theory of nursing as caring were first published in 1990 and 1991, with the first complete exposition of the theory presented at a theory conference in 1992 (Boykin & Schoenhofer, 1990, 1991; Schoenhofer & Boykin, 1993), followed by the work, *Nursing As Caring: A Model for Transforming Practice,* published in 1993 (Boykin & Schoenhofer, 1993) and re-released with an epilogue in 2001 (Boykin & Schoenhofer, 2001).

Research and development efforts at the time of this writing are concentrated on expanding the language of caring by uncovering personal ways of living caring in everyday life (Schoenhofer, Bingham, & Hutchins, 1998), reconceptualizing nursing outcomes as "value experienced in nursing situations" (Boykin & Schoenhofer, 1997; Schoenhofer & Boykin, 1998a, 1998b), and in consultation with graduate students, nursing faculties, and health-care agencies who are using aspects of the theory to ground research, teaching, and practice.

Applications

NURSING AS CARING IN NURSING PRACTICE

The commitment of the nurse practicing nursing as caring is to nurture persons living caring and growing in caring. This implies that the nurse comes to know the other as a caring person in the moment. "Difficult to care" situations are those that demonstrate the extent of knowledge and commitment needed to nurse effectively. An everyday understanding of the meaning of caring is obviously challenged when the nurse is presented with someone for whom it is difficult to care. In these extreme (though not unusual) situations, a task-oriented, nondiscipline-based concept of nursing may be adequate to assure the completion of certain treatment and surveillance techniques. Still, in our eyes, that is an insufficient response—it certainly is not the nursing we advocate. The theory of nursing as caring calls upon the nurse to reach deep within a well-developed knowledge base that has been structured using all available patterns of knowing, grounded in the obligations and intentionality inherent in the commitment to know persons as caring. These patterns of knowing may develop knowledge as intuition; scientifically quantifiable data emerging from research; and related knowledge from a variety of disciplines, ethical beliefs, and many other types of knowing. All knowledge held by the nurse that may be relevant to understanding the situation at hand is drawn forward and integrated as understanding that guides practice in particular nursing situations (aesthetic knowing). Although the degree of challenge presented from situation to situation varies, the commitment to know self and other as caring persons is steadfast.

The nursing as caring theory, grounded in the assumption that all persons are caring, has as its focus a general call to nurture persons in their unique ways of living caring and growing as caring persons. The challenge for nursing, then, is not to discover what is missing, weakened, or needed in another, but to come to know the other as caring person and to nurture that person in situation-specific, creative ways and to acknowledge, support, and celebrate the caring that is. We no longer understand nursing as a "process" in the sense of a complex sequence of predictable acts resulting in some predetermined desirable end product.

> *Nursing, we believe, is inherently processual, in the sense that it is always unfolding and is guided by intentionality and the commitment to care.*

Nursing, we believe, is inherently processual, in the sense that it is always unfolding and is guided by intentionality and the commitment to care.

The nurse practicing within the caring context described here will most often be interfacing with the health-care system in two ways: first, communicating nursing so that it can be understood with clarity and richness; and second, articulating nursing service as a unique contribution within the system in such a way that the system itself grows to support nursing.

NURSING AS CARING IN NURSING ADMINISTRATION

From the viewpoint of nursing as caring, the nurse administrator makes decisions through a lens in which the focus of nursing is on nurturing persons as they live caring and grow in caring. All activities in the practice of nursing administration are grounded in a concern for creating, maintaining, and supporting an environment in which calls for nursing are heard and nurturing responses are given (Boykin & Schoenhofer, 2001). From this point of view, the expectation arises that nursing administrators participate in shaping a culture that evolves from the values articulated within nursing as caring.

Although often perceived to be "removed" from the direct care of the nursed, the nursing administrator is intimately involved in multiple nursing situations simultaneously, hearing calls for nursing and participating in responses to these calls. As calls for nursing are known, one of the unique responses of the nursing administrator is to enter the world of the nursed either directly or indirectly, to understand special calls when they occur, and to assist in securing the resources needed by each nurse to nurture persons as they live and grow in caring (Boykin & Schoenhofer, 1993). All administrative activities should be approached with this goal in mind. Here, the nurse administrator reflects on the obligations inherent in the role in relation to the nursed. The presiding moral basis for determining right action is the belief that all persons are caring. Frequently, the nurse administrator may enter the world of the nursed through the stories of colleagues who are assuming another role, such as that of nurse manager. The nursing administrator assists others within the organization to understand the focus of nursing and to secure the resources necessary to achieve the goals of nursing.

The nurse administrator is subject to challenges similar to those of the practitioner and often walks a very precarious tightrope between direct caregivers and corporate executives. The nurse administrator, whether at the executive or managerial level of the organizational chart, is held accountable for "customer satisfaction" as well as for "the bottom line." Nurses who "move up the executive ladder"

may, on the one hand, be suspected of disassociating from their nursing colleagues, and, on the other hand, of not being sufficiently cognizant of the harsh realities of fiscal constraint. Administrative practice guided by the assumptions and themes of nursing as caring can enhance eloquence in articulating the connection between caregiver and institutional mission: the person seeking care. Nursing practice leaders who recognize their care role,

> *Nursing practice leaders who recognize their care role, indirect as it may be, are in an excellent position to act on their committed intention to promote caring environments.*

indirect as it may be, are in an excellent position to act on their committed intention to promote caring environments. Participating in rigorous negotiations for fiscal, material, and human resources and for improvements in nursing practice calls for special skill on the part of the nurse administrator—skill in recognizing, acknowledging, and celebrating the other (e.g., CEO, CFO, nurse manager, or staff nurse) as a caring person. The nurse administrator who understands the caring ingredients (Mayeroff, 1971) recognizes that caring is neither soft nor fixed in its expression. A developed understanding of the caring ingredients helps the nurse administrator mobilize the courage to be honest with self and other, to trust patience, and to value alternating rhythm with true humility while living a hope-filled commitment to knowing self and other as caring persons.

NURSING AS CARING IN NURSING EDUCATION

From the perspective of nursing as caring, all structures and activities should reflect the fundamental assumption that persons are caring by virtue of their humanness. Other assumptions and values reflected in the education program include: knowing the person as whole and complete in the moment and living caring uniquely; understanding that personhood is a way of living grounded in caring and is enhanced through participation in nurturing relationships with caring others; and affirming nursing as a discipline and profession.

The curriculum, the foundation of the education program, asserts the focus and domain of nursing as nurturing persons living caring and growing in caring:

> The model for organizational design of nursing education is analogous to the dancing circle. . . . Members of the circle include administrators, faculty, colleagues, students, staff, community, and the nursed. What this circle represents is the commitment of each dancer to understand and support the study of the discipline of nursing. The role of education administrators in the circle, represented by deans and department chairpersons is more clearly understood when the origin of the word is reflected upon. The term "administrator" derives from the Latin *ad ministrare,* to serve (according to Webster's, cited in Guralnik, 1976). This definition connotes the idea of rendering service. Administrators within the circle are by nature of [their] role obligated to ministering, to securing, and to providing resources needed by faculty, students, and staff to meet program objectives. Faculty, students, and administrators dance together in the study of nursing. Faculty support an environment that values the uniqueness of each person and sustains each person's unique way of living and growing in caring. This process requires trust, hope, courage, and patience. Because the purpose of nursing education is to study the discipline and practice of nursing, the nursed must be in the circle, and the focus of study must be the nursing situation, the shared lived experience of caring between nurse and nursed and all those who participate in the dance of caring persons. The community created is that of persons living caring in the moment and growing in personhood, each person valued as special and unique. (Boykin & Schoenhofer, 1993, pp. 73–74)

In teaching nursing as caring, faculty assist students to come to know, appreciate, and celebrate both self and other as caring persons. Students, as well as faculty, are in a continual search to discover greater meaning of caring as uniquely expressed in nursing. Examples of a nursing education program based on values similar to those of nursing as caring are illustrated in the book *Living a Caring-based Program* (Boykin, 1994).

Mentoring students as colearners and creating caring learning environments while concomitantly accepting responsibility for summative evaluation calls for the integrated foundation provided by the guiding intention to know and nurture persons as caring. This intention helps the nurse to transcend limiting historical practices while creatively inventing ways to inspire. The humility of unknowing, joined with courage and hope, helps the nurse educator to guide the study of nursing as a commitment to knowing and nurturing persons as caring. Many nurse educators are struck with the incongruity of instilling a commitment to nursing as an opportunity to care through means that seem to view the student as an object and view the discipline as a preexisting set of operating rules. Nursing education practiced from the perspective of nursing as caring opens the way for faculty to truly value the discipline and the student.

NURSING AS CARING IN RESEARCH AND DEVELOPMENT

The roles of researcher and developer in nursing take on a particular focus when guided by the theory of nursing as caring. The assumptions and focus of nursing explicated in the theory provide an organizing value system that suggests certain key questions and methods. Research questions lead to exploration and illumination of patterns of living caring personally (Schoenhofer, Bingham, & Hutchins, 1998) and in nursing practice (Schoenhofer & Boykin, 1998b). Dialogue, description, and innovations in interpretative approaches characterize research methods. Development of systems and structures (e.g., policy formulation, information management, nursing delivery, and reimbursement) to support nursing necessitates sustained efforts in reframing and refocusing familiar systems as well as creating novel configurations (Schoenhofer, 1995; Schoenhofer & Boykin, 1998a).

Nurses in research and development roles carry out their work facing environmental pressures similar to those experienced by the practitioner, the administrator, and the educator. Research and development in nursing require disciplinary-congruent values and perspectives, free-ranging thought, openness, and creativity. Institutional systems and structures often seem to favor values and practices that are incongruent with the values of the nursing discipline, in their overly patterned thought, rigidity, and conformity. Researchers and developers guided by the assumptions and themes of nursing as caring are empowered to create novel methods in the search for understanding and meaning and to articulate effectively the value, purpose, and relevance of their work (Schoenhofer, 2002).

Questions Nurses Ask about the Theory of Nursing as Caring

The following presents several common questions—and responses—that nurses ask about nursing as caring.

HOW DOES THE NURSE COME TO KNOW SELF AND OTHER AS CARING PERSONS?

Nursing practice guided by the theory of nursing as caring entails living the commitment to know self and other as living caring in the moment and growing in caring. Living this commitment requires intention, formal study, and reflection on experience. Mayeroff's (1971) caring ingredients offer a useful starting point for the nurse committed to knowing self and other as caring persons. These ingredients include knowing, alternating rhythm, honesty, courage, trust, patience, humility, and hope. Roach's (1987/2002) five Cs—commitment, confidence, conscience, competence, and compassion—offer another conceptual framework that is helpful in providing a language of caring. Coming to know self as caring is facilitated by:

- Trusting in self; freeing self up to become what one can truly become, and valuing self.
- Learning to let go, to transcend—to let go of problems, difficulties, in order to remember the interconnectedness that enables us to know self and other as living caring, even in suffering and in seeking relief from suffering.
- Being open and humble enough to experience and know self, to be at home with one's feelings.
- Continuously calling to consciousness that each person is living caring in the moment and that we are each developing uniquely in our personhood.
- Taking time to experience our humanness fully; for one can only truly understand in another what one can understand in self.
- Finding hope in the moment. (Schoenhofer & Boykin, 1993, pp. 85–86)

MUST I LIKE MY PATIENTS TO NURSE THEM?

The simple answer to this question is yes. In order to know the other as caring, the nurse must find some basis for respectful human connection with the person. Does this mean that the nurse must like everything about the person, including personal life choices? Perhaps not; however, the nurse as nurse is not called upon to judge the other, only to care for the other. A concern with judging or censuring another's actions is a distraction from the real purpose for nursing—that is, coming to know the other as caring person, as one with dreams and aspirations of growing in caring, and responding to calls for caring in ways that nurture personhood.

WHAT ABOUT NURSING A PERSON FOR WHOM IT IS DIFFICULT TO CARE?

Related to the previous dilemma, this question presents the crucible within which one's commitment to the assumptions and themes of nursing as caring is tested to the limit. The underlying question is, "Does the person to be nursed deserve or merit my care?" Again, as before, the simple answer is yes. All persons are caring, even when not all chosen actions of the person live up to the ideal to which we are all called by virtue of our humanness. In discussions of hypothetical situations involving child molesters, serial killers, and even political figures who have attempted mass destruction and racial annihilation, certain ethical systems permit and even call for making judgments. However, when such a person presents to the nurse for care, the nursing ethic of caring supersedes all other values. The theory of nursing as caring asserts that it is *only* through recognizing and responding to the other as a caring person that nursing is created and personhood enhanced in that nursing situation. This question and the previous one make it clear that caring is much more than "sweetness and light"; caring effectively in "difficult to care" situations is the most challenging prospect a nurse can face. It is only with sustained intentionality, commitment, study, and reflection that the nurse is able to offer nursing in these situations. Falling short in one's commitment does not necessitate self-deprecation nor does it warrant condemnation by others; rather, it presents an opportunity to care for self and other and to grow in personhood. Making real the potential of such an opportunity calls for seeing with clarity, reaffirming commitment, and engaging in study and reflection, individually and in concert with caring others.

IS IT IMPOSSIBLE TO NURSE SOMEONE WHO IS IN AN UNCONSCIOUS OR ALTERED STATE OF AWARENESS?

The key point here is the "caring between" that *is* the nursing creation: When nursing a person who is unconscious, the nurse lives the commitment to know the other as caring person. How is that commitment lived? It requires that all ways of knowing be brought into action. The nurse must make self as caring person available to the one nursed. The fullness of the nurse as caring person is called forth. This requires use of Mayeroff's caring ingredients: the alternating rhythm of knowing about the other and knowing the other directly through authentic presence and attunement; the hope and courage to risk opening self to one who cannot communicate verbally; patiently trusting in self to understand the other's mode of living caring in the moment; honest humility as one brings all that one knows and remains open to learning from the other. The nurse attuned to the other as person might, for example, experience the vulnerability of the person who lies unconscious from surgical anesthetic or traumatic injury. In that vulnerability, the nurse recognizes that the one nursed is living caring in humility, hope, and trust. Instead of responding to the vulnerability, merely "taking care of" the other, the nurse practicing nursing as caring might respond by honoring the other's humility, by participating in the other's hopefulness, and by steadfast trustworthiness. Creating caring in the moment in this situation might come from the nurse resonating with past and present experiences of vulnerability. Connected to this form of personal knowing might be an ethical knowing that power as a reciprocal of vulnerability has the potential to develop undesirable status differential in the nurse-patient role relationship. As the nurse sifts through a myriad of empirical data, the most significant information emerges—this is a *person* with whom I am called to care. Ethical knowing again merges with other pathways as the nurse forms the decision to go beyond vulnerability and engage the other as caring person, rather than as helpless object of another's concern. Aesthetic knowing comes in the praxis of caring, in living chosen ways of honoring humility, joining in hope, and demonstrating trustworthiness in the moment (Schoenhofer & Boykin, 1993, pp. 86–87).

HOW DOES THE NURSING PROCESS FIT WITH THIS THEORY?

Process, as it is understood in the term "nursing process," connotes a systematic and sequential series of steps resulting in a predetermined, specifiable product. Nursing process, as introduced into nursing by Orlando (1961), is a linear stepwise decision-making tool based on rational analysis of empirical data (known in other disciplines as the problem-solving process) and is a key structural theme of many nursing theories developed in past decades. Proponents of the theory of nursing as caring view nursing not as a process with an endpoint, but as an ongoing process; that is, as dynamic and unfolding, guided by intentionality although not directed by a preenvisioned outcome or product. Nursing responses of care arise in aesthetic knowing, in the creative and evolving patterns of appreciation and understanding, and in the context of a shared lived experience of caring. Instead of preselected and quantifiable outcomes, the value of nursing to the nursed and to others is that which is experienced as valuable arising in and evolving through the "caring between" of the nursing situation. Much of that value is neither measurable nor empirically verifiable. That which is measurable and empirically verifiable is relevant in the situation, however, and may be called upon at any time to contribute to and through the nurse's empirical knowing. Information that the nurse has available becomes knowledge within the nursing situation. Knowing the person directly is what guides the selection and patterning of relevant points of factual information in a nursing situation. That is, any fact or set of facts from nursing research or related bodies of information can be considered for relevance and drawn into the supporting knowledge base. This knowledge base remains open and evolving as the nurse employs an alternating rhythm of scanning and considering facts for relevance while remaining grounded in the nursing situation (Schoenhofer & Boykin, 1993, pp. 89–90).

In addition to empirical knowing, knowing for nursing purposes also requires personal knowing, including intuition and ethical knowing, all converging in aesthetic knowing within each unique nursing situation.

HOW PRACTICAL IS THIS THEORY IN THE REAL WORLD OF NURSING?

Nurses are frequently heard to say they have no time for caring, given the demands of the role. All nursing roles are lived out in the context of a contemporary environment. At the beginning of the twenty-first century, the environment for practice, administration, education, and research is fraught with many challenges, such as

- technological advancement and proliferation that can promote routinization and depersonalization on the part of the caregiver as well as the one seeking care;
- demands for immediate and measurable outcomes that favor a focus on the simplistic and the superficial;
- organizational and occupational configurations that tend to promote fragmentation and alienation; and
- economic focus and profit motive ("time is money") as the apparent prime institutional value.

Nurses express frustration when evaluating their own caring efforts against an idealized, rule-driven conception of caring. Practice guided by the theory of nursing as caring reflects the assumption that caring is created from moment to moment and does not demand idealized patterns of caring. Caring in the moment (and moment to moment) occurs when the nurse is living a committed intention to know and nurture the other as caring person (Boykin & Schoenhofer, 2000). No predetermined ideal amount of time or form of dialogue is prescribed. A simple example of living this intention to care is the nurse who goes to the IV or the monitor *through* the person, rather than going directly to the technology and failing to acknowledge the person. When the nurse goes *through* the person, it becomes clear that the use of technology is one way the nurse expresses caring *for the person* (Schoenhofer, 2001). In proposing his model of machine technologies and caring in nursing, Locsin (1995, 2001) distinguishes between mere technological competence and technological competence as an intentional expression of caring in nursing. Simply avowing an intention to care is not sufficient. The committed intention to care is supported by serious study of caring and ongoing reflection. As Locsin (1995, p. 203) so aptly states:

[A]s people seriously involved in giving care know, there are various ways of expressing caring. Professional nurses will continue to find meaning in their technological caring competencies, expressed intentionally and authentically, to know another as a whole person. Through the harmonious coexistence of machine technology and caring technology the practice of nursing is transformed into an experience of caring.

The practicality of the theory of nursing as caring is being tested in various nursing practice settings. Nursing practice models have been developed in acute and long-term care settings. In 2002, a two-year demonstration project was completed that focused on designing, implementing, and evaluating a theory-based practice model using nursing as caring. This project demonstrated that when nursing practice is intentionally focused on coming to know a person as caring and on nurturing and supporting those nursed as they live their caring, transformation of care occurs. Within this new model, those nursed could articulate the "experience of being cared for"; patient and nurse satisfaction increased dramatically; retention increased; and the environment for care became grounded in the values of and respect for person (Boykin, Schoenhofer, Smith, St. Jean, & Aleman, 2003).

At the time of this writing, a similar project is under development in the emergency department of a community hospital. Caring from the heart—a model for interdisciplinary practice in a long-term care facility and based on the theory of nursing as caring—was designed through collaboration between project personnel and all stakeholders. Foundational values of respect and coming to know grounded the model, which revolves around the major themes of: responding to that which matters; caring as a way of expressing spiritual commitment; devotion inspired by love for others; commitment to creating a home environment; and coming to know and respect person as person (Touhy, Strews, & Brown, 2003). The major building blocks of the nursing models for an acute care hospital and for a long-term care facility each reflect central themes of nursing as caring, but those themes are drawn out in ways unique to the setting and to the persons involved in each setting. The differences and similarities in these two practice models demonstrate the power of nursing as caring to transform practice in a way that reflects unity without conformity, uniqueness within oneness.

The Lived Experience of Nursing as Caring

By Danielle Linden

The application of nursing as caring in my practice has been fulfilling both professionally and personally. I have been invited to share this experience.

Nursing as caring requires the nurse to use many different ways of knowing to come to know "other" in the fullness of one's existence. Each domain contains a vast amount of knowledge. The nurse must be knowledgeable of each and artfully apply this knowledge in an effort to transcend the physical boundaries of the human body to come to know other's complex existence. Personally, this effort is rewarded by enhancing who I am as a person.

Current Practice as an Advanced Practice Nurse

As an advanced registered nurse practitioner (ARNP) in family practice, I see patients in a primary care setting. Grounded in nursing as caring, I borrow knowledge from other disciplines, such as pathophysiology, microbiology, pharmacology, and philosophy and use this knowledge to come to know other in each moment of our visit. Some patients have immediate acute needs. Others have chronic problems that require maintenance therapy. All of them need to be recognized as holistic and complex human beings with a unique existence in this world, living in caring and growing in caring. I am a facilitator of this process and risk entering into another's world with the intent of living caring in that nursing situation.

In practice, I emphasize wellness and prevention. Nursing as caring guides the nursing situation, serving as a framework in my patient encounters. I walk in the room with the intent of coming to know other as a holistic being with a body, mind, and spirit. The call for nursing then begins to unfold and reveals itself to me. My presence with other is authentic, and there exists a genuine responsiveness to come to know other. Authentic presence allows one to know that which is not spoken. A person can speak one's mind. A physical assessment can reveal an ailment. The spirit, however, must be attended to as well. Everything is revealed in one's spirit. When you are in authentic presence with other, the call for nursing unfolds before you. These are the profound encounters that never leave you.

Then there are the more frequent encounters where reflection becomes a useful tool to uncover the deeper meaning behind these chance nursing situations. Sometimes the patients' call for nursing is physical. I recognize it and treat accordingly. Reflection allows me to answer these questions: Was I nursing? What did I do differently from another health-care provider? My answer is the perspective from which I practice. I walked into the room with the willingness to come to know other, whatever may have been revealed in that moment. It was the way I touched the patient, my tone of voice, my unhurried pace, and my smile—all the tools I use to convey to other that I am there and that I care. The goal is to enhance other as he or she lives and grows in caring.

I take time regularly to reflect upon the profound and not-so-profound nursing situations in my life. Reflection uncovers those hidden meanings that are not readily apparent in the moment. It is also a time for self-growth and validation—a process of coming to know self and others as caring persons.

Sharing with Others

Another form of reflection is the sharing of nursing situations with others. There are many different ways one can present a nursing situation, such as case presentations, poems, projects, and various other art forms. When one shares a nursing situation with others, new possibilities for knowing other unfold exponentially. Each practitioner brings the wealth of his or her education and experiences. New revelations come to life.

I share with you here a nursing situation I encountered. First, I will present it in the traditional medical model, and then I will present the same story in a nursing perspective grounded in the nursing as caring theory. Through comparison, the lived experience of both of these models will make clearer the difference between practice perspectives.

Medical Model Case Presentation

E. S. was a 76-year-old white female patient who came to the office with the complaint of a lump in her abdomen. She remarked that she did not like going to the doctor and had neglected to have any checkups in quite a few years. A comprehensive history and physical exam was unremarkable with the exception of her abdomen, which revealed a small, palpable, nontender mass in the right lower quadrant. I ordered blood tests, all of which were unremarkable with the exception of the Ca125, which was 625, well above normal parameters. My suspicion for ovarian cancer was confirmed.

Three days after our initial visit, I asked her to return to the office so we could discuss the results. She did so, and with her she brought a gift. She said I had done so much for her in our visit, she wanted to share with me a precious gift the Lord had given her—her voice. There, in the office, I sat with her labs in my lap as she serenaded me with a song. I don't remember the name of the song, but the verse told me Jesus was calling her home and she was not afraid.

When she was done, we discussed the findings. I advised her that although the blood test was not diagnostic, the possibility of cancer did exist and she needed to see an oncological gynecologist. She cried and we hugged.

After a month of invasive testing at the family's prompting, exploratory surgery and biopsies confirmed the diagnosis of ovarian cancer with extensive metastasis. The patient underwent a total abdominal hysterectomy and bilateral salpingo-oophorectomy with debulking, and she died shortly thereafter.

There is a lot one can learn from a case presentation such as this one, but it does not reflect the essence of what occurred between the nurse and the one nursed. The reader is left wondering what the nurse did that prompted such a special present in return.

Nursing as Caring Case Presentation

As the morning rolled along, I began to dream. I dreamed I was a tree. My roots entwined deep within the foundation upon which I stood. I took from the Earth what I needed to nourish and strengthen me. My roots drank from the spring of knowledge beneath me. I felt strong. I grew tall. My arms outstretched, reached for the sun, found the sky, and in it, a gentle breeze that surrounded and calmed me. I stood in awe of the sun's beauty as its rays poured over me and warmed my spirit. I felt connected. I felt whole.

I saw a glow on the horizon, unlike the sun and different from the moon and stars. An ember, the residual of a fire that has burned through the night, tirelessly, to provide warmth. I was drawn to it. Unafraid that my branches might catch fire and burn, I reached for her abdomen. I searched. As my hands pressed on, I began to feel the Earth slipping from the sky. I reached upward, grasping for the restoration of harmonious interconnectedness, but in the sky, there is nothing to grab onto. You may grow into it, enjoy its beauty, bask in its breezes, and breathe in its life-giving oxygen, but you cannot hold on to it or possess it.

My arms grew weary, my leaves were wilted, so I drank from the spring beneath my foundation. My roots nourished me with courage, patience, trust, and humility. She reached for my hand. Her spirit filled me and strengthened me as she ascended toward the sky. I began to feel stronger and reached toward the sky, hoping to catch one last glimpse of her ember and saw her reflection in the sun. Her rays poured over me and warmed my spirit. I felt whole once again.

This nursing story is a reflection of a nursing situation grounded in caring. It demonstrates the perspective of enhancing other as one lives and grows in caring, which subsequently results in the enhancement of self as the nurse lives and grows in caring.

Ways of Knowing

I chose this story as the medium with which to share. Boykin and Schoenhofer encourage nurses to choose various art forms as media for sharing and reflection. This is aesthetic knowing. It is the artful integration of all the ways of knowing to create a meaningful, caring moment that is born in a nursing situation.

Personal knowing is that which is known intuitively by encountering self and other. Authentic presence is a key component for my intuitive experiences when I just know. The patient trusted me and humbled herself to ask me to validate her concern that the mass in her belly was of grave concern. The patient knew, intuitively, before I laid my hands on her. There is a lot to be gained by learning to trust our intuition, and we can "know" more by engaging in authentic presence. Authentic presence, for me, removes all physical boundaries to my coming to know other. It is a spiritual connectedness that has no time limits or physical boundaries. It is a feeling of interconnectedness with the patient that reverberates beyond the room, city, state, country, world, and galaxy. It brings with it the wisdom of the universe.

The first three basic assumptions inherent in nursing as caring facilitate the lived experience of authentic presence in this moment. The assumption that this person is a caring person by virtue of her humanness, complete in that moment, gave me the courage to enter into authentic presence to come to know her as a complete, caring person in that moment. As the moment unfolded, our mutual trust enhanced and supported who we were as we lived and grew in that caring encounter.

The patient's need to share with me a special gift was validation that she felt it, too. The fifth basic assumption of the theory of nursing as caring is personhood, which is enhanced through participation in nurturing relationships. As the patient demonstrated in the words of her song, she knew that her physical existence was coming to an end and she was not afraid. There was a mutual knowingness that was unspoken, even without the lab work or biopsies. Her lack of fear and her courage allowed her spirit to soar free in the open sky, giving me a glimpse of the spiritual existence.

This is not to devalue the importance of empirical knowledge. It, too, is an important part of coming to know other. Empirical knowledge is the information that is organized into laws and theories to describe, explain, or predict phenomena. This knowledge is acquired through the senses. Based in the sciences, it is our understanding of anatomy and physiology, diagnostic processes, and treatment regimens. For me, it is the concrete form of the foundation upon which my practice is built.

Empirical knowledge is essential to be recognized as a profession. The sixth assumption of nursing as caring is that nursing is both a discipline and a profession. The scientific evidence that lends theory-based knowledge to our profession gives us the diagnostic reasoning we need to address the physical needs that people have. In this particular situation, the laboratory findings confirmed that which we knew personally. Oftentimes the bereaved loved ones need a diagnosis to help cope with the grief of losing a family member.

This brings us to ethical knowing—the patience and compassion to be with grieving family members when they are not ready to let go of a loved one who is ready to die. Ethical knowing is also the recognition that these family members are caring persons as well, coping in the only way they know how, through their experiences. Humility has allowed me to come to know and respect the family's perspective. Patience is needed to allow other to come to know hope in the moment a loved one is diagnosed with a terminal illness. Hope for a spiritual existence beyond this world was revealed to me in this nursing situation.

Each of these patterns of knowing—aesthetic, personal, empirical, and ethical—is borrowed from Carper (1978). They serve as conceptual tools to help us understand and implement the theory of nursing as caring.

Broad Application for Advanced Practice Nursing: Summary

Nursing as caring provides a theoretical perspective with an organizing framework that guides practice and allows for the generation of new knowledge. In addition, it lends a methodological process to define, explain, and verify this knowledge. This theory reaches beyond the received view of traditional science. Nursing as caring guides the use of nursing knowledge and information from other disciplines in ways appropriate to nursing. Through the application of this theory, I have come to know new possibilities for nursing practice.

I believe now more than ever that, with the advancing roles of nurses, we need to be clear on what it is that we do that is different from other practitioners. As advanced practice nurses (APNs) and ARNPs assume more responsibilities and perform tasks that were traditionally reserved for those of the medical profession, the overlapping further blurs the boundaries of our professions. We need to maintain our nursing perspective. As nurse practitioners continue to be lumped into categories with other midlevel practitioners, we need to demonstrate to our patients that our profession was born of a need from society, a need that only nurses can fill. If there is no call to nursing, our profession will dissolve into the sea of midlevel practitioners.

Nursing theory sets apart what nurse practitioners do from any other profession. To ensure that our practice maintains its identity, the practice must be built upon research-based nursing theory. The theory of nursing as caring is one such theory.

References

Boykin, A. (Ed.). (1994). *Living a caring-based program*. New York: National League for Nursing Press.

Boykin, A., Parker, M. E., & Schoenhofer, S. O. (1994). Aesthetic knowing grounded in an explicit conception of nursing. *Nursing Science Quarterly, 7*, 158–161.

Boykin, A., & Schoenhofer, S. O. (1990). Caring in nursing: Analysis of extant theory. *Nursing Science Quarterly, 3*(4), 149–155.

Boykin, A., & Schoenhofer, S. O. (1991). Story as link between nursing practice, ontology, epistemology. *Image, 23*, 245–248.

Boykin, A., & Schoenhofer, S. O. (1993). *Nursing as caring: A model for transforming practice*. New York: National League for Nursing Press.

Boykin, A., & Schoenhofer, S. O. (1997). Reframing nursing outcomes. *Advanced Practice Nursing Quarterly, 1*(3), 60–65.

Boykin, A., & Schoenhofer, S. O. (2000). Invest in yourself. Is there really time to care? *Nursing Forum, 35*(4), 36–38.

Boykin, A., & Schoenhofer, S. O. (2001). *Nursing as caring: A model for transforming practice*. Sudbury, MA: Jones & Bartlett Publishers.

Boykin, A., & Schoenhofer, S. O. (2001). The role of nursing leadership in creating caring environments in health care delivery systems. *Nursing Administration Quarterly, 25*(1), 1–7.

Boykin, A., Schoenhofer, S. O., Smith, N., St. Jean, J., & Aleman, D. (2003). Transforming practice using a caring-based nursing model. *Nursing Administration Quarterly, 27*, 223–230.

Carper, B. A. (1978). Fundamental patterns of knowing in nursing. *Advances in Nursing Science, 1*(1), 13–24.

Collins, J. M. (1993). I care for him. *Nightingale Songs, 2*(4), 3. Retrieved March 28, 2004, at http://www.fau.edu/divdept/nursing/ngsongs/vol2num4.htm

Gaut, D., & Boykin, A. (Eds.). (1994). *Caring as healing: Renewal through hope.* New York: National League for Nursing Press.

Guralnik, D. (1976). *Webster's new world dictionary of the American language.* Cleveland: William Collings & World Publishing Co.

King, A., & Brownell, J. (1976). *The curriculum and the disciplines of knowledge.* Huntington, New York: Robert E. Krieger Publishing Co.

Locsin, R. C. (1995). Machine technologies and caring in nursing. *Image, 27*, 201–203.

Locsin, R. C. (2001). *Advancing technology, caring and nursing.* Westport, CT: Auburn House.

Mayeroff, M. (1971). *On caring.* New York: Harper & Row.

Orlando, I. (1961). *The dynamic nurse-patient relationship: Function, process and principles.* New York: G. P. Putnam's Sons.

Nursing as Caring Web site. www.nursingascaring.com

Paterson, J. G., & Zderad, L. T. (1988). *Humanistic nursing.* New York: National League for Nursing Press.

Roach, S. (1987/2002). *Caring, the human mode of being. A blueprint for the health professions.* Ottawa, Canada: CHA Press.

Schoenhofer, S. O. (1995). Rethinking primary care: Connections to nursing. *Advances in Nursing Science, 17*(4), 12–21.

Schoenhofer, S. O. (2001). A framework for caring in a technologically dependent nursing practice environment. In Locsin, R. C. (Ed.), *Advancing technology, caring and nursing* (pp. 3–11). Westport, CT: Auburn House.

Schoenhofer, S. O. (2002a). Choosing personhood: Intentionality and the theory of nursing as caring. *Holistic Nursing Practice, 16,* 36–40.

Schoenhofer, S. O. (2002b). Considering philosophical underpinnings of an emergent methodology for nursing as caring inquiry. *Nursing Science Quarterly, 15*(4), 275–281.

Schoenhofer, S. O., Bingham, V., & Hutchins, G. C. (1998). Giving of oneself on another's behalf: The phenomenology of everyday caring. *International Journal for Human Caring, 2*(1), 23–29.

Schoenhofer, S. O., & Boykin, A. (1993). Nursing as caring: An emerging general theory of nursing. In Parker, M. E. (Ed.), *Patterns of nursing theories in practice* (pp. 83–92). New York: National League for Nursing Press.

Schoenhofer, S. O., & Boykin, A. (1998a). The value of caring experienced in nursing. *International Journal for Human Caring, 2*(3), 9–15.

Schoenhofer, S. O., & Boykin, A. (1998b). Discovering the value of nursing in high-technology environments: Outcomes revisited. *Holistic Nursing Practice, 12*(4), 31–39.

Touhy, T., Strews, W., & Brown, C. (2003). *Caring from the heart.* CD-Rom available from Dr. Theris Touhy, Christine E. Lynn College of Nursing, Florida Atlantic University, 777 Glades Rd., Boca Raton, FL 33431-0991.

SECTION IV

Nursing Theory: Illustrating Processes of Development

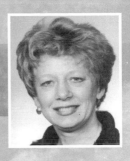

Kristen M. Swanson

CHAPTER 22

Kristen M. Swanson:
A Program of
Research on Caring

Kristen M. Swanson

*I*n this chapter, I provide answers to questions posed by students and practitioners who have wanted to know more about the origins and progress of my research and theorizing on caring. I have situated myself as a nurse and as a woman so that the context of my scholarship, particularly as it pertains to caring, may be understood. I consider myself to be a second-generation nursing scholar. I was taught by first-generation nurse scientists (that is, nurses who received their doctoral education in fields other than nursing). My struggles for identity as a woman and as an academician were, like many women of my era (the baby boomers), a somewhat organic and reflective process of self-discovery during a rapidly changing social scene (witness the women's movement, civil rights, etc.). Third-generation nursing scholars (those taught by nurses whose doctoral preparation is in nursing) may find my "yearning" somewhat odd. To those who might offer critique about the egocentricity of my pondering, I offer the defense of having been brought up during an era in which nurses dealt with such struggles as, "Are we a profession? Have we a unique body of knowledge? Are we entitled to a space in the full (i.e., PhD-granting) academy?" I fully appreciate that questions of uniqueness and entitlement have not completely disappeared. Rather, they have faded as a backdrop to the weightier concerns of making a significant contribution to the health of all, working collaboratively with consumers and other scientists and practitioners, embracing pluralism, and acknowledging the socially constructed power differentials associated with gender, race, poverty, and class.

Turning Point

In September 1982 I had no intention of studying caring; my goal was to study what it was like for women to miscarry. It was my dissertation chair, Dr. Jean Watson, who guided me toward the need to examine caring in the context of miscarriage. I am forever grateful for her foresight and wisdom.

> *I believe that the key to my program of research is that I have studied human responses to a specific health problem (miscarriage) in a framework (caring) that assumed from the start that a clinical therapeutic had to be defined.*

I believe that the key to my program of research is that I have studied human responses to a specific health problem (miscarriage) in a framework (caring) that assumed from the start that a clinical therapeutic had to be defined. So, hand in glove, the research has constantly gone back and forth between "what's wrong and what can be done about it," "what's right and how can it be strengthened," and "what's real to women (and most recently their mates) who miscarry and how might care be customized to that reality." The back-and-forth nature of this line of inquiry has resulted in insights about the nature of miscarrying and caring that might otherwise have remained elusive.

Predoctoral Experiences

My preparation for studying caring-based therapeutics from a psychosocial perspective began, ironically, in a cardiac critical care unit. After receiving my BSN at the University of Rhode Island, I was wisely coached by Dean Barbara Tate to pursue a job at the brand-new University of Massachusetts Medical Center (U. Mass.) in Worcester, Massachusetts. I was drawn to that institution because of the nursing administration's clear articulation of how nursing could and should be. It was so exciting to be there from day one. We were all part of shaping the institutional vision for practice. It was phenomenal witnessing myself and my friends (nurses, physicians, respiratory therapists, and housekeepers) make a profound difference in the lives of those we served. However, what I learned most from that experience came from the patients and their families. I realized that there was a powerful force that people could call upon to get themselves through incredibly difficult times. Watching patients move into a space of total dependency and come out the other side restored was like witnessing a miracle unfold. Sitting with spouses in the waiting room while they entrusted the heart (and lives) of their partner to the surgical team was awe-inspiring. It was encouraging to observe the inner reserves family members could call upon in order to hand over that which they could not control. I felt so privileged, humbled, and grateful to be invited into the spaces that patients and families created in order to endure their transitions through illness, recovery, and, in some instances, death.

After a year and a half at U. Mass., I was still a fairly new nurse and was very unclear about what all of these emotional insights had to do with nursing. I saw all of it as more of something about my spiritual beliefs and me than about my profession. At that point, what mattered most to me as a nurse was my emerging technological savvy, understanding complex pathophysiological processes, and conveying that same information to other nurses. Hence, I applied to graduate schools with the intention of focusing on teaching and on the care of the acutely ill adult. Approximately two years after completing my baccalaureate degree, I enrolled in the Adult Health and Illness Nursing program at the University of Pennsylvania.

While at Penn, I served as the student representative to the graduate curriculum committee and, as such, was invited to attend a two-day retreat to revise the master's program. I distinctly remember listening to Dr. Jacqueline Fawcett and being amazed at hearing her talk about health, environments, persons, and nursing and claiming that these four concepts were the "stuff" that really comprised nursing. It was like hearing someone give voice to the inner stirrings I had kept to myself back in Massachusetts. It really impressed me that there were actually nurses who studied in such arenas. Shortly after the retreat, I received my MSN and was hired at Penn on a temporary basis to teach undergraduate medical-surgical nursing. I immediately enrolled as a postmaster's student in Dr. Fawcett's new course on the conceptual basis of nursing. It proved to be one of the best decisions I had ever made, primarily because it helped me to figure out an answer to that constant question, "Why doesn't a smart girl like you enter medicine?" I finally knew that it was because nursing, a discipline that I was now starting to understand from an experiential, personal and academic point of view, was more suited to my beliefs about serving people who were moving through the transitions of illness and wellness. I suppose it is safe to say that I was beginning to understand that my "gifts" lie not in the diagnosis and treatment of illness but in the ability to understand and work with people going through transitions of health, illness, and healing.

Doctoral Studies

Such insights made me want more; hence, I applied for doctoral studies and was accepted into the graduate program at the University of Colorado. My area of study, psychosocial nursing, emphasized such concepts as loss, stress, coping, caring, transactions, and person-environment fit. Having been supported by a National Institute of Mental Health (NIMH) traineeship, one requirement of our program was a hands-on experience with the process of undergoing a health promotion activity. Our faculty offered us the opportunity to carry out the requirement by enrolling ourselves in some type of support or behavior-change program of our own choosing. Four weeks into the same semester in which I was required to complete that exercise, my first son was born. I decided to enroll in a cesarean birth support group as a way to deal with the class assignment and the unexpected circumstances surrounding his birth. It so happened that an obstetrician had been invited to speak to the group about miscarriage at the first meeting I ever attended. I found his lecture informative with regard to the incidence, diagnosis, prognosis, and medical management of spontaneous abortion. However, when the physician sat down and the women began to talk about their personal experiences with miscarriage and other forms of pregnancy loss, I was suddenly overwhelmed with the realization that there had been a one-in-six chance that I could have miscarried my son. Up until that point, it had never occurred to me that anything could have gone wrong with something so central to my life. I was 29 years old and believed, quite naively, that anything was possible if you were only willing to work hard at it.

Two profound insights came to me from that meeting. First, I was acutely aware of the American Nurses' Association social policy statement, namely, "Nursing is the diagnosis and treatment of human responses to actual and potential health problems" (1980, p. 9). It was so clear to me that whereas the physician had talked about the health problem of spontaneously aborting, the women were living the human response to miscarrying. Second, being in my last semester of course work, I was desperately in need of a dissertation topic. From that point on it became clear to me that I wanted to understand what it was like to miscarry. The problem, of course, was that I was a critical care nurse and knew very little about anything having to do with childbearing. An additional concern was that during the early 1980s, although there was a very strong emphasis on epistemology, ontology, and the methodologies to support multiple ways of understanding nursing as a human science, our methods courses were very traditionally quantitative. Luckily, two mentors came my way. Dr. Jody Glittenberg, a nurse anthropologist, agreed to guide me through a predissertation pilot study of five women's experiences with miscarriage in order that I might learn about interpretive methods. Dr. Colleen Conway-Welch, a midwife, agreed to supervise my trek up the psychology-of-pregnancy learning curve.

DISSERTATION: CARING AND MISCARRIAGE

Twenty women who had miscarried within 16 weeks of being interviewed agreed to participate in my phenomenological study of miscarriage and caring. These results have been published in greater depth elsewhere (Swanson-Kauffman, 1985, 1986b, Swanson, 1991). Through that investigation, I proposed that caring consisted of five basic processes:

> *Caring consisted of five basic processes: knowing, being with, doing for, enabling, and maintaining belief.*

knowing, being with, doing for, enabling, and maintaining belief. At that time, the definitions were fairly awkward and definitely tied to the context of miscarriage. In addition to naming those five categories, I also learned some important things about studying caring: (1) if you directly ask people to describe what caring means to them, you force them to speak so abstractly that it is hard to find any substance; (2) if you ask people to list behaviors or words that indicate that others care, you end up with a laundry list of "niceties"; (3) if you ask people for detailed descriptions of what it was like for them to go through an event (i.e., miscarrying) and probe for their feelings and what the responses of others meant to them, it is much easier to unearth instances of people's caring and noncaring responses; and finally, (4) I learned that although my intentions were to gather data, many of my informants thanked me for what I did for them. As it turned out, a side effect of gathering detailed accounts of the informants' experiences was that women felt, heard, understood, and attended-to in a nonjudgmental fashion. In later years, this insight would actually become the grist for a series of caring-based intervention studies.

I have often been asked if my research was an application of Jean Watson's Theory of Human Caring (Watson, 1979/1985, 1985/1988). Neither Dr. Watson nor I have ever seen my research program as an application of her work per se, but we do agree that the compatibility of our scholarship lends credence to both of our claims about the nature of caring. I have come to view her work as having provided a research tradition that other scientists and I have followed. Watson's research tradition asserts that caring (1) is a central concept in nursing, (2) values multiple methodologies for inquiry, and (3) honors the importance of nurses (and others) studying caring so that it may be better understood, consciously claimed, and intentionally acted upon to promote, maintain, and restore health and healing.

Postdoctoral Study

POSTDOCTORAL STUDY #1: PROVIDING CARE IN THE NICU

Approximately nine months after I completed the dissertation, my second son was born. This child had a difficult start in life and spent a few days in the newborn intensive care unit (NICU). Through this event, I became aware that in my later childbearing loss (having a not-well child at birth), I, too, wished to receive the kinds of caring responses that my miscarriage informants had described. Hence, my next study, an individually awarded National Research Service Award postdoctoral fellowship (1989 to 1990), was inspired. Dr. Kathryn Barnard, at the University of Washington, agreed to sponsor this investigation and ended up opening doors for me that still continue to open. With her guidance, I spent over a year "hanging out" in the NICU at the University of Washington Medical Center (the staff gave me permission to acknowledge them and their practice site when discussing these findings).

The question I answered through the NICU phenomenological investigation was, "What is it like to be a provider of care to vulnerable infants?" In addition to my observational data, I did in-depth interviews with some of the mothers, fathers, physicians, nurses, and other health-care professionals who were responsible for the care of five infants. The results of this investigation are published elsewhere (Swanson, 1990). With respect to understanding caring, there were three main findings:

1. Although the names of the caring categories were retained, they were grammatically edited and somewhat refined so as to be more generic.

2. It was evident that care in a complex context called upon providers to simultaneously balance *caring* (for self and other), *attaching* (to people and roles), *managing responsibilities* (self-, other-, and society-assigned), and *avoiding bad outcomes* (for self, other, and society).

3. What complicated everything was that each NICU provider (parent or professional) knew only a portion of the whole story surrounding the care of any one infant. Hence, there existed a strong potential for conflict stemming from misunderstanding others and second-guessing one another's motives.

While I was presenting the findings of the NICU study to a group of neonatologists, I received a very interesting comment. One young physician told me that it was the caring and attaching parts of his vocation that brought him into medicine, yet he was primarily evaluated on and made accountable for the aspects of his job that dealt with managing responsibilities and avoiding bad outcomes. Such a schism in his role-performance expectations and evaluations had forced him to hold the caring and attaching parts of doing his job inside. Unfortunately, it was his experience that those more person-centered aspects of his role could not be "stuffed" for too long and that they oftentimes came hauntingly into his consciousness at about 3 A.M. His remarks left me to wonder if the true origin of burnout is the failure of professions and care delivery systems to adequately value, monitor, and reward practitioners whose comprehensive care embraces *caring, attaching, managing responsibilities,* and *avoiding bad outcomes.*

POSTDOCTORAL STUDY #2: CARING FOR SOCIALLY AT-RISK MOTHERS

While I was still a postdoctoral scholar, Dr. Barnard invited me to present my research on caring to a group of five master's-prepared public health nurses. They became quite excited and claimed that the model captured what it had been like for them to care for a group of socially at-risk new mothers. As it turned out, about four years prior to my meeting them, these five advanced practice nurses had participated in Dr. Barnard's Clinical Nursing

Models Project (Barnard et al., 1988). They had provided care to 68 socially at-risk expectant mothers for approximately 18 months (from shortly after conception until their babies were 12 months old). The purpose of the intervention had been to help the mothers take control of themselves and their lives so that they could ultimately take care of their babies. As I listened to these nurses endorsing the relevance of the caring model to their practice, I began to wonder what the mothers would have to say about the nurses. Would the mothers (1) remember the nurses, and (2) describe the nurses as caring?

I was able to locate 8 of the original 68 mothers (a group of women with highly transient lifestyles). They agreed to participate in a study of what it had been like to receive an intensive long-term advanced practice nursing intervention. The result of this phenomenological inquiry was that the caring categories were further refined and a definition of caring was finally derived.

Hence, as a result of the miscarriage, NICU, and high-risk mothers studies, I began to call the caring model a middle-range theory of caring. I define

> *I define caring as a "nurturing way of relating to a valued 'other' toward whom one feels a personal sense of commitment and responsibility."*

caring as a "nurturing way of relating to a valued 'other' toward whom one feels a personal sense of commitment and responsibility" (Swanson, 1991, p. 162). "Knowing," striving to understand an event as it has meaning in the life of the other, involves avoiding assumptions, focusing on the one cared for, seeking cues, assessing thoroughly, and engaging the self of both the one caring and the one cared for. "Being with" means being emotionally present to the other. It includes being there, conveying availability, and sharing feelings while not burdening the one cared for. "Doing for" means doing for the other what he or she would do for him- or herself if it were at all possible. The therapeutic acts of doing for include anticipating needs, comforting, performing competently and skillfully, and protecting the other while preserving their dignity. "Enabling" means facilitating the other's passage through life transitions and unfamiliar events. It involves focusing on the event, informing, explaining, supporting, allowing and validating feelings, generating alternatives, thinking things through, and giving feedback. The last caring category is "maintaining belief," which means sustaining faith in the other's capacity to get through an event or transition and face a future with meaning. This means believing in the other and holding him or her in esteem, maintaining a hope-filled attitude, offering realistic optimism, helping find meaning, and going the distance or standing by the one cared for, no matter how his or her situation may unfold (Swanson, 1991, 1993, 1999a, 1999b).

The Miscarriage Caring Project

As my postdoctoral studies were coming to an end, Dr. Barnard challenged me and claimed, "I think you've described caring long enough. It's time you did something with it!" We discussed how data-gathering interviews were so often perceived by study participants as caring. Together we realized that, at the very least, open-ended interviews involved aspects of knowing, being with, and maintaining belief. We suspected that if doing-for and enabling interventions specifically focused on common human responses to health conditions were added, it would be possible to transform the techniques of phenomenological data gathering into a caring intervention. That conversation ultimately led to my design of a caring-based counseling intervention for women who miscarried.

The next thing I knew, I was writing a proposal for a Solomon four-group randomized experimental design (Swanson, 1999a, 1999b). It was funded by the National Institute of Nursing Research and the University of Washington Center for Women's Health Research. The primary purpose of the study was to examine the effects of three one-hour-long, caring-based counseling sessions on the integration of loss (miscarriage impact) and women's emotional well-being (moods and self-esteem) in the first year after miscarrying. Additional aims of the study were to (1) examine the effects of early versus delayed measurement and the passage of time on women's healing in the first year after loss, and (2) develop strategies to monitor caring as the intervention/process variable.

An assumption of the caring theory was that the recipient's well-being should be enhanced by receipt of caring from a provider who is informed about common human responses to a designated health problem (Swanson, 1993). Specifically, it was proposed that if women were guided through in-depth discussion of their experience and felt understood, informed, provided for, validated, and believed in, they would be better prepared to integrate miscarrying into their lives. Content for the three counseling sessions was derived from the miscarriage model—a phenomenologically derived model that summarized the common human responses to miscarriage (Swanson, 1999b; Swanson-Kauffman, 1983, 1985, 1986a, 1986b, 1988).

Women were randomly assigned to two levels of treatment (caring-based counseling and controls) and two levels of measurement ("early"—completion of outcome measures immediately, six weeks, four months, and one year postloss; or "delayed"—completion of outcome measures at four months and one year only). Counseling took place at one, five, and eleven weeks postloss. ANOVA was used to analyze treatment effects. Outcome measures included self-esteem (Rosenberg, 1965); overall emotional disturbance, anger, depression, anxiety, and confusion (McNair, Lorr, & Droppleman, 1981); and overall miscarriage impact, personal significance, devastating event, lost baby, and feeling of isolation (investigator-developed Impact of Miscarriage Scale).

A more detailed report of these findings is published elsewhere (Swanson, 1999a). There were 242 women enrolled, 185 of whom completed. Participants were within five weeks of loss at enrollment; 89 percent were partnered, 77 percent were employed, and 94 percent were Caucasian. Over one year, main effects included the following: (1) caring was effective in reducing overall emotional disturbance, anger, and depression; and (2) with the passage of time, women attributed less personal significance to miscarrying and realized increased self-esteem and decreased anxiety, depression, anger, and confusion.

In summary, the Miscarriage Caring Project provided evidence that, although time had a healing effect on women after miscarrying, caring did make a difference in the amount of anger, depression, and overall disturbed moods that women experienced after miscarriage. This study was unique in that it employed a clinical research model to determine whether or not caring made a difference.

I believe that its greatest strength lies in the fact that the intervention was based both on an empirically derived understanding of what it is like to miscarry and on a conscientious attempt to enact caring in counseling women through their loss. Of course, the greatest limitation of that study is that I derived the caring theory (developed from the intervention) and conducted most of the counseling sessions. Hence, it is unknown whether similar results would be derived under different circumstances. My work is further limited by the lack of diversity in my research participants. Over the years, I have predominantly worked with middle-class, married, educated Caucasian women. I am currently making a concerted effort to rectify this situation and to examine what it is like for diverse groups of women to experience both miscarriage and caring.

Monitoring caring as an intervention variable was the second specific aim of the Miscarriage Caring Project. Three strategies were employed to document that, as claimed, caring had indeed occurred. First, approximately 10 percent of the intervention sessions were transcribed. Analysis was done by research associate Katherine Klaich, RN, PhD, having also been one of the counselors in the study, found she could not approach analysis of the transcripts naively—that is, with no preconceived notions, as would be expected in the conduct of phenomenologic analysis. Hence, she employed both deductive and inductive content analytic techniques to render the transcribed counseling sessions meaningful. She began with the broad question, "Is there evidence of caring as defined by Swanson [1991] on the part of the nurse counselors?" The unit of analysis was each emic phrase that was used by the nurse counselor. Phrases were coded for which (if any) of the five caring processes were represented by the emic utterances. Each counselor statement was then further coded for which subcategory of the five processes was represented by the phrase. Twenty-nine subcategories of the five major processes were defined. With few exceptions (social chitchat), every therapeutic utterance of the nurse counselor could be accounted for by one of the subcategories.

The second way in which caring was monitored was through the completion of paper-and-pencil measures. Before each session, the counselor completed a Profile of Mood States (McNair, Lorr, & Droppleman, 1981) in order to document her presession moods (thus enabling examination of the association between counselor presession mood and self or client postsession ratings of caring). After each session, women were asked to complete the Caring Professional Scale (investigator-developed). Women, having been left alone to complete the measure, were asked to place the evaluations in a sealed envelope. In the meantime, in another room, the counselor wrote out her counseling notes and completed the Counselor Rating Scale, a brief five-item rating of how well the session went.

The Caring Professional Scale (2002) originally consisted of 18 items on a five-point Likert-type scale. It was developed through the Miscarriage Caring Project and was completed by participants in order to rate the nurse counselors who conducted the intervention and to evaluate the nurses, physicians, or midwives who took care of the women at the time of their miscarriage. The items included: "Was the health-care provider that just took care of you understanding, informative, aware of your feelings, centered on you, etc.?" The response set ranged from 1 ("yes, definitely") to 5 ("not at all"). The items were derived from the caring theory. Three negatively worded items (abrupt, emotionally distant, and insulting) were dropped due to minimal variability across all of the data sets. For the counselors at one, five, and eleven weeks postloss, Chronbach alphas were .80, .95, and .90 (sample sizes for the counselor reliability estimates were 80, 87, and 76). The lower reliability estimates were because the counselors' caring professional scores were consistently high and lacked variability (mean item scores ranged from 4.52 to 5.0).

Noteworthy findings include the following:

1. Each counselor had a full range of presession feelings, and those feelings/moods were, as might be expected, highly intercorrelated.
2. For the most part, counselor presession mood was not associated with postsession evaluations.
3. The caring professional scores were extremely high for both counselors, indicating that, overall, the clients were pleased with what they got and, as claimed, caring was "delivered" and "received."
4. One of the counselors was a psychiatric nurse by background. She knew very little about miscarriage prior to participating in this study and had

recently experienced a death in her family. The only time her presession moods (in this case, depression and confusion) were significantly associated ($p \leq .05$) with any of the postsession ratings (both client caring professional score and counselor self-rating) was in Session I. During Session I, women discussed in-depth what the actual events of miscarrying felt like. It is possible that the counselor was so touched by and caught up in the sadness of the stories that her own vulnerabilities were a bit less veiled.

5. Session II, in which the two topics addressed were relationship oriented (who the woman could share her loss with and what it felt like to go out in public as a woman who had miscarried), was the only session in which the other counselor's vulnerabilities came through. This counselor, having just gone through a divorce, was probably least able to hide her presession moods (depression, ($p \leq .05$) and low vigor, confusion, fatigue, and tension (all at $p \leq .01$), as was evident in the significant associations with her own postsession self-ratings. Also, most notably, there was an association between this counselor's presession tension and the client's caring professional rating ($p \leq .05$).

A Literary Meta-Analysis of Caring

Another recent project was an in-depth review of the literature. This literary meta-analysis is published elsewhere (Swanson, 1999). Approximately 130 data-based publications on caring were reviewed for this state-of-the-science paper. Developed was a framework for discourse about caring knowledge in nursing. Proposed were five domains (or levels) of knowledge about caring in nursing. I believe that these domains are hierarchical and that studies conducted at any one domain (e.g., Level III) assumes the presence of all previous domains (e.g., Levels I and II). The first domain includes descriptions of the capacities or characteristics of caring persons. Level II deals with the concerns and/or commitments that lead to caring actions. These are the values nurses hold that lead them to practice in a caring manner. Level III describes the conditions (nurse, patient, and organizational factors) that enhance or diminish the likelihood of caring occurring. Level IV summa-

rizes caring actions. This summary consisted of two parts. In the first part, a meta-analysis of 18 quantitative studies of caring actions was performed. It was demonstrated that the top five caring behaviors valued by patients were that the nurse (1) helps the patient to feel confident that adequate care was provided; (2) knows how to give shots and manage equipment; (3) gets to know the patient as a person; (4) treats the patient with respect; and (5) puts the patient first, no matter what. By contrast, the top five caring behaviors valued by nurses were: (1) listens to the patient, (2) allows expression of feelings, (3) touches when comforting is needed, (4) is perceptive of the patient's needs, and (5) realizes the patient knows himself/herself best. The second part of the caring actions summary was a review of 67 interpretive studies of how caring is expressed (the total number of participants was 2,314). These qualitative studies were classified under Swanson's caring processes, thus lending credibility to caring theory. The last domain was labeled "consequences." These are the intentional and unintentional outcomes of caring and noncaring for patient and provider. In summary, this literary meta-analysis clarified what "caring" means, as the term is used in nursing, and validated the generalizability or transferability of Swanson's caring theory beyond the perinatal contexts from which it was originally derived.

Couples Miscarriage Healing Project

I am currently principal investigator on an NIH-, NINR-funded randomized trial of three caring-based interventions against control to see if we can make a difference in men and women's healing after miscarriage. The purpose of this randomized trial is to compare the effects of nurse caring (three nurse counseling sessions), self-caring (three home-delivered videotapes and journals), combined caring (one nurse counseling plus three videotapes and journals), and no intervention (control) on the emotional healing, integration of loss, and couple well-being of women and their partners (husbands or male mates) in the first year after miscarrying. All intervention materials have been developed based on the Miscarriage Model and the Caring Theory. Our goal is to enroll 340 couples. This study is ongoing.

SUMMARY

Much work lies ahead. The profession has a long way to go to make a case for the education needed to support caring practices; the importance of nurses practicing in a caring manner; the essential contributions of caring to the well-being of all; and the costs of caring in terms of time, money, and personal energy expended. The discipline also has much work left to do. It is essential that nurse investigators frame nursing interventions under the framework of caring in order to tie together the essential contributions of the profession to the health of society. Finally, caring, in order to be effective, must be sensitive to those involved in caring transactions (nurses and clients), to the cultural contexts in which it is performed, and to the common responses that individuals, families, groups, and communities experience when living with conditions of wellness and illness.

References

American Nurses' Association. (1980). *Nursing: A social policy statement*. Kansas City, MO: American Nurses' Association.

Barnard, K. E., Magyary, D., Sumner, G., Booth, C. L., Mitchell, S. K., & Spieker, S. (1988). Prevention of parenting alterations for women with low social support. *Psychiatry, 51*, 248–253.

McNair, D. M., Lorr, M., & Droppleman, L. F. (1981). *Profile of mood states: Manual*. San Diego: Educational and Industrial Testing Service.

Rosenberg, M. (1965). *Society and the adolescent self-image*. Princeton: Princeton University Press.

Swanson, K. M. (1990). Providing care in the NICU: Sometimes an act of love. *Advances in Nursing Science, 13*(1), 60–73.

Swanson, K. M. (1991). Empirical development of a middle-range theory of caring. *Nursing Research, 40*, 161–166.

Swanson, K. M. (1993). Nursing as informed caring for the well-being of others. *Image, 25*, 352–357.

Swanson, K. M. (1999). What's known about caring in nursing science: A literary meta-analysis. In Hinshaw, A. S., Feetham, S., & Shaver, J. (Eds.), *Handbook of clinical nursing research*. Thousand Oaks, CA: Sage.

Swanson, K. M. (1999a). The effects of caring, measurement, and time on miscarriage impact and women's well-being in the first year subsequent to loss. *Nursing Research, 48*, 6, 288–298.

Swanson, K. M. (1999b). Research-based practice with women who miscarry. *Image: Journal of Nursing Scholarship, 31*, 4, 339–345.

Swanson, K. M. (2002). Caring Profession Scale. In Watson, J. (Ed.) *Assessing and measuring caring in nursing and health science*. New York: Springer.

Swanson-Kauffman, K. M. (1983). The unborn one: The human experience of miscarriage (Doctoral dissertation, University of Colorado Health Sciences Center, 1983). *Dissertation Abstracts International, 43*, AAT8404456.

Swanson-Kauffman, K. M. (1985). Miscarriage: A new understanding of the mother's experience. *Proceedings of the 50th anniversary celebration of the University of Pennsylvania School of Nursing, 63–78*.

Swanson-Kauffman, K. M. (1986a). A combined qualitative methodology for nursing research. *Advances in Nursing Science, 8*(3), 58–69.

Swanson-Kauffman, K. M. (1986b). Caring in the instance of unexpected early pregnancy loss. *Topics in Clinical Nursing, 8*(2), 37–46.

Swanson-Kauffman, K. M. (1988). The caring needs of women who miscarry. In Leininger, M. M. (Ed.), *Care: Discovery and uses in clinical and community nursing*. Detroit: Wayne State University Press.

Watson, M. J. (1979/1985). *Nursing: The philosophy and science of caring*. Boulder, CO: Colorado Associated Press.

Watson, M. J. (1985/1988). *Nursing: Human science and human care*. New York: National League for Nursing.

CHAPTER 23

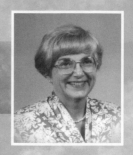

Marilyn Anne Ray

PART ONE: Marilyn Anne Ray's Theory of Bureaucratic Caring

Marilyn Anne Ray

Introducing the Theorist

Marilyn A. Ray, RN, PhD, CTN is a professor at Florida Atlantic University, College of Nursing, in Boca Raton, Florida. She holds a bachelor's of science in nursing and a master's of science from the University of Colorado in Denver, Colorado, a master's of arts in cultural anthropology from McMaster University in Hamilton, Canada, and a doctorate from the University of Utah in Transcultural Nursing. She retired as a colonel in 1999 after 30 years of service with the U.S. Air Force Reserve Nurse Corps. As a certified transcultural

nurse, she has published widely on the subjects of caring in organizational cultures, caring theory and inquiry development, transcultural caring, and transcultural ethics. She is a review board member of the *Journal of Transcultural Nursing*. Dr. Ray's research has revolved around cultural, technological, and economic issues related to caring in complex organizations. Her current research, which uses both qualitative and quantitative research methods, relates to the study of the complex nurse-patient relational caring process and its impact on economic and patient outcomes in hospitals. She is actively engaged in teaching doctoral students and guiding doctoral students' research that focuses on the administrative, ethical, and information technological practice of nursing and transcultural nursing.

Introducing the Theory

This chapter will present a discussion of contemporary nursing culture, share theoretical views related to the author's developmental theoretical vision of nursing, and discuss the Theory of Bureaucratic Caring as a grounded theory. After revisiting the theory in the contemporary age, the author will elucidate bureaucratic caring theory as a holographic theory to further the vision of nursing and organizations as relational, integrated, and complex. Theory is the intellectual life of nursing (Levine, 1995). "Scientific theories in the discipline of nursing have developed out of the choices and assumptions a particular theorist believes about nursing, what the basis of nursing's knowledge is, and what nurses do or how they practice in the real world" (Ray, 1998, p. 91). Van Manen (1982) refers to theory as "wakefulness of mind" or the pure viewing of truth. *Truth* in the Greek sense is not the property of consensus among theorists but the disclosure of the essential nature or the good of things. In essence, truth refers to contemplating the good (van Manen, 1982). Collectively, theories in nursing have focused on the good of nursing—what nursing is and what it does or should do. Based on the assumptions of nursing as serving the good, the locus of the discipline centers on caring for others, caring in the human health experience (Newman, 1992; Newman, Sime, & Corcoran-Perry, 1991). A theory of nursing actually must direct or enlighten the good. Theories such as the classical grand theories in nursing of Rogers, Leininger, Newman, Watson, and Parse demonstrate a diversity of integrated approaches to nursing based on the worldview and education of an individual theorist. Ongoing research through testing and evaluation has supported the validity and reliability of the theories. Grounded or middle-range theories, however, focus on particular aspects of nursing practice and are commonly generated from nursing practice. As such, some intellectuals view middle-range theories as more relevant and useful to nursing than the application of grand theories (Cody, 1996). However, rather than show partiality for one

theory over another, the diversity of nursing theories that emphasize holistic points of view actually support the new picture of reality in science. Revolutionary approaches to scientific theory development, such as the quantum theory, the science of wholeness, holographic and chaos theories, and fractals or the idea of self-similarity within the sciences of complexity (Bassingthwaighte, Liebovitch, & West, 1994; Battista, 1982; Briggs & Peat, 1984; Davidson & Ray, 1991; Harmon, 1998; Peat, 2003; Ray, 1998; Wheatley, 1999; Wilbur, 1982) illuminate the nature and creativity of science itself. The conception of the multiple interconnectedness and relational reality of all things, the interdependence of all human phenomena, and the discovery of order in a chaotic world demonstrate the pioneering story of twentieth-century science and how the insightful idea of relationality (a powerful nursing concept) is shaping the science of the twenty-first century.

Given the nature of nursing as expanded consciousness (Newman, in Parker, 2001) and the notion of theory as wakefulness, this author holds the position that nurses do need nursing theory to stimulate thinking and critique as they function in the complex world of nursing science, research, education, and practice. Theories, as the integration of knowledge, research, and experience, highlight the way in which scholars of nursing interpret their world and the context where nursing is lived. Theories in this sense are also philosophies or ideologies that serve a practical purpose. The Theory

> *The Theory of Bureaucratic Caring illuminated in this chapter is a theory with a practical purpose that emerged from the worldviews of health professionals and clients in practice.*

of Bureaucratic Caring illuminated in this chapter is a theory with a practical purpose that emerged from the worldviews of health professionals and clients in practice (Ray, 1981, 1989). By illustrating the significance of spiritual and ethical caring in relation to the structural dimensions of complex organizational cultures, such as political, economic, technological, and legal, bureaucratic caring theory invites us to view how a new model may facilitate understanding of how nursing can be practiced in modern health-care environments.

CONTEMPORARY NURSING PRACTICE

The practice of nursing occurs in organizations that are generally bureaucratic or systematic in nature. Although there has been much discussion about the end of bureaucracy to better cope with twenty-first-century innovation and worklife (Pinchot & Pinchot, 1994), bureaucracy remains a valuable tool to identify and understand the fundamentally different principles that undergird coordinated and relational organizational systems. Organizational culture has a rich heritage and has been studied both formally and informally since the 1930s in the United States (O'Grady & Malloch, 2003; Smircich, 1985). Informal organization or the integration of codes of conduct encompassing commitment, identity, character, coherence, and a sense of community was considered essential to the successful functioning or the administering of power and authority in the formal organization. Political, economic, legal, and technical systems comprise the formal organization. What distinguishes organizations as culture from other paradigms, such as organizations as machines, brains, or other images (Morgan, 1997), is its foundation in anthropology or the study of how people act in communities or formalized structures and the significance or meaning of work life (Ciulla, 2000; Louis, 1985). Organizational cultures, therefore, are viewed as social constructions, symbolically formed and reproduced through interaction (Smircich, 1985). The beliefs about work emerge in organizational mission and policy statements. A nation's prevailing tenets and expectations about the nature of work, leisure, and employment are pivotal to the work life of people; hence, there is an interplay between the macrocosm of a national/global culture and the microcosm of specific organizations (Eisenberg & Goodall, 1993). In recent years, economics has been a potent contestant in macro- and microcultures. There is an ever greater concentration of economic and political power in a handful of corporations, which separate their interests (usually profit-driven) from the interests of human beings, which are life-centered (Korten, 1995; Schroeder, 2003; Turkel & Ray, 2000).

Health care and its activities are tightly interwoven into the social and economic fabric of nations. As organizations were affected by issues of cost and profit, health-care systems underwent immense change, particularly in the United States. Confidence in major health-care institutions and their leaders fell so low as to put the legitimacy of executives at risk. Old rules of loyalty and commitment to employees, investment in the worker, fairness in pay, and the need to provide good benefits were in jeopardy. Health-care systems fell victim to the corporatization of the human enterprise. Consequently, the conflict between health care as a business and caring as a human need resulted in a crisis in nursing and health-care organizations (Page, 2004).

The actual work of nurses, while undervalued in terms of both cost and worth (Turkel & Ray, 2000, 2001), currently is being evaluated in terms of issues of patient safety (Page, 2004). Nursing education is highlighted as a bridge to quality (Long, 2003). Since the Institute of Medicine report (Page, 2004), a resurgence of interest is taking place in the meaningfulness of work, particularly in many hospitals. The language of trust and morally worthy work (Cuilla, 2000; Ray, Turkel, & Marino, 2002) is replacing the language of downsizing, restructuring, mergers, and acquisitions. Cuilla (2000) stated that "[t]he most meaningful jobs are those in which people directly help others or create products that make life better for people" (p. 225). Although the traditional work of nurses is defined as directly helping others, contemporary nurses' work is also defined by and in the organizational context—legal, ethical, economics, technological, and political. Urging nurses, physicians, and administrators to find cohesion among organizational phenomena and body, mind, and spirit integration for the sake of the patient calls for the reinvention of work (Fox, 1994). Incorporating business principles and the "work of the soul" or relational self-organization (Ray, Turkel, & Marino, 2002) means leading in a new way (O'Grady & Malloch, 2003). It is a witness to the power and depth of reseeing the good of nursing, searching for meaning in life, and finding new meaning in the complexities of work itself.

Organizational Cultures as Transformational Bureaucracies

The transformation of nurses toward relational self-organization is a new pursuit for the profession. Identifying professional nurse caring work as having value and an expression of one's soul or one's creative self at work replaces the notion of nursing as performing machinelike tasks.

Bureaucracy, considered by some as a machine-like metaphor, plays a significant role in the meanings and symbols of organizations (Ray, 1981, 1989). Weber (1999) actually predicted that the future belonged to the bureaucracy and not to the working class. Weber, who saw bureaucracy as an efficient and superior form of organizational arrangement, predicted that bureaucratization of enterprise would dominate the world (Bell, 1974; Weber, 1999). This, of course, is witnessed by the current globalization of commerce. Recent acquisitions and mergers of industrial firms and even health-care systems, especially in the United States, are larger and hold more power than some world governments. The concept of bureaucratization is thus a worldwide phenomenon (Ray, 1989). Although considered less effective than other forms of organization, Britain and Cohen (1980) stated that, "Like it or not, humankind is being driven to a bureaucratized world whose forms and functions, whose authority and power must be understood if they are ever to be even partially controlled" (p. 27).

The characteristics of bureaucracies are as follows:

- A division of labor
- A hierarchy of offices
- A set of general rules that govern performances
- A separation of the personal from the official
- A selection of personnel on the basis of technical qualifications
- Equal treatment of all employees or standards of fairness
- Employment viewed as a career by participants
- Protection of dismissal by tenure (Eisenberg & Goodall, 1993).

Bureaucracy, while condemned by some as associated with red tape and inflexibility, continues to provide the most reasonable way in which to view systems and facilitate the preservation of organizations. In the past two decades, there has been a call for decentralization and the "flattening" of organizational structures—to become less bureaucratic and more participative or heterarchical (O'Grady & Malloch, 2003). Many firms have begun to hold to new principles that honor creativity and imagination (Morgan, 1997). Even nursing has advanced in a more collaborative or decentralized manner by its focus on patient-centered nursing and more decentralized control from administration (Long, 2003; Nyberg, 1998). But creative views still need to be marked with understanding of bureaucracy as economics sweeps the globe. Leadership models, which are fundamentally hierarchical because of the need for order, continue to head the short-lived participative movement toward decentralization. Power is still in the hands of a few as global economics and the market rule (Korten, 1995). As a result, the concept of bureaucracy does not seem as bad as was once thought. It can be considered as much less radical than the business paradigm that focuses on competition and response to market forces, subsequently eradicating standards of fairness for human beings in the workplace.

Caring as the Unifying Focus of Nursing

Caring in nursing brings things into being. It is humane and rational. As such, caring is considered by many nurse scholars to be the essence of nursing (Boykin & Schoenhofer, 2001, Leininger, 1981, 1991, 1997; Morse, Solberg, Neander, Bottorff, & Johnson, 1990; Ray, 1989, 1994a, 1994b; Swanson, 1991; Watson, 1985, 1988, 1997). Although not uniformly accepted, Newman, Sime, and Corcoran-Perry (1991; Newman, 1992) characterized the social mandate of the discipline of nursing as caring in the human health experience. Caring thus is an influential concept, and the expression "caring" in the human health experience emphasizes the social mandate to which nursing has responded throughout its history and encompasses the scope of the discipline (Roach, 2002). Caring, however, is manifested in different and complex ways in the nursing discipline and profession (Morse et al., 1990; Newman, 1992). Various paradigms that enfold the care and caring ideal exist in nursing. The totality (Fawcett, 1993), the simultaneity (Parse, 1987), and the unitary-transformative (Newman, 1992) paradigms have been the prevailing worldviews in nursing and have directed nursing theories. The totality paradigm demonstrates that nursing, person, society, environment, and health characterize the nature of nursing. The simultaneity paradigm illuminates the human-environment integral nature of nursing. The unitary-transformative paradigm states that what constitutes nursing's reality is the view that the human being is unitary and evolving as a self-organizing field embedded in a larger self-organizing field identified by pattern and interaction with the larger whole. Health is considered expanded consciousness, and caring in the human health experience is the focus of the

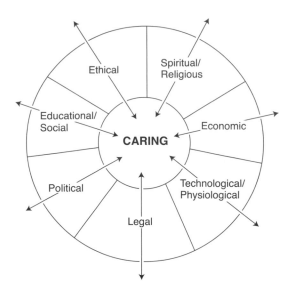

FIGURE 23–1 The grounded Theory of Bureaucratic Caring.

discipline (Newman, 1986, 1992; Newman, Sime, & Corcoran-Perry, 1991). Many caring theories correspond to one or all of these paradigms (Morse et al., 1990). The Theory of Bureaucratic Caring has its roots in all these paradigms by its synthesis of caring and the organizational context (see Figure 23–1).

BUREAUCRATIC CARING THEORY: EMERGENT GROUNDED THEORY

The Theory of Bureaucratic Caring originated as a grounded theory from a qualitative study of caring in the organizational culture and appeared first as the author's dissertation in 1981 and as articles in 1984 and 1989. In the qualitative study of caring in the institutional context, the research revealed that nurses and other professionals struggled with the paradox of serving the bureaucracy and serving human beings, especially clients, through caring. The discovery of bureaucratic caring resulted in both substantive and formal theories (Ray, 1981, 1984, 1989). The substantive theory emerged as differential caring and showed that caring in the complex organization of the hospital was complicated and differentiated itself in terms of meaning by its context—dominant caring dimensions related to areas of practice or units wherein professionals worked and clients resided. Differential Caring Theory showed that different

units espoused different caring models based on their organizational goals and values. The formal Theory of Bureaucratic Caring symbolized a dynamic structure of caring, which was synthesized from a dialectic between the thesis of caring as humanistic, social, educational, ethical, and religious/spiritual (elements of humanism and spirituality), and the antithesis of caring as economic, political, legal, and technological (dimensions of bureaucracy) (Ray, 1981, 1989).

Although the model demonstrates that the dimensions are equal, the research revealed that the economic, political, technical, and legal dimensions were dominant in relation to the social and ethical/spiritual dimensions. The theory reveals that nursing and caring are experiential and contextual and are influenced by the social structure or the culture (normative system) that is given in the organization. Interactions and symbolic systems of meaning are formed and reproduced from the constructions or dominant values held within the organization. In some respect, "we are the organization," which is analogous to Wittgenstein's (1969) adage, "we are our language."

The theory has been embraced by educators, researchers, nursing administrators, and clinicians who, after witnessing changes in health-care policy in the past decade, have begun to appreciate how the context—micro- and macrocultures—influences nursing. Moving away from centering on patient care to the economic justification of nursing and health-care systems has prompted professionals to desire a fuller understanding of how to preserve humanistic caring within the business or corporate culture (Miller, 1989; Nyberg, 1989, 1991, 1998). The theory also has been used in part as a foundation for additional research studies of the nurse-patient relationship (Ray, 1987; Turkel, 1997; Turkel & Ray, 2000, 2001).

Practice Theory Reviewed: Evolution of Theory Development

Facing the challenge of the crisis in health care and nursing, disillusionment of registered nurses about the disregard for their caring services, and the concern of the nursing profession and the public about the effects of the shortage of nurses (Page, 2004), working for the good of the whole is imperative. Running away from the chaos of hospitals or misunderstanding the meaning of work life cannot become the norm. Wherever nurses go, they will be haunted by bureaucracies, some functional, many problematic. What, then, is the deeper reality of nursing practice? The following is a presentation of theoretical views that relate to bureaucratic caring theory, culminating in a vision for understanding the deeper significance of nursing life.

SUBSTANTIVE AND FORMAL THEORY

Glaser and Strauss (1967; Glaser, 1978; Strauss & Corbin, 1998) were the first social scientists to present the perspective of social theory, both substantive and formal, discovered from inductive research processes. Substantive and formal theories emerge from in-depth qualitative studies of social cultural processes—action and interaction associated with the social world. The researcher considers evidence about how one event affects another and explains the things observed and recorded by developing theoretical relationships about the data. Theoretical sampling (Glaser, 1978) refines, elaborates, and exhausts conceptual categories so that an actual integration of descriptors and categories can facilitate the discovery of substantive theory. The discovery of a basic social process is the foundation for substantive theory. The formal theory is generated from both the inductive process, based on substantive knowledge/theory, and deductive approaches, which draw upon cumulative knowledge from the social world to examine the initial propositions advanced. A formal theory reflects the structure of both processes.

The Theory of Bureaucratic Caring integrated knowledge from data that is associated with researching the meaning and action of caring in the institutional culture of a hospital, which resulted in a substantive theory of differential caring. Narrative responses to the meaning of caring reported by different health-care professionals and patients produced varied beliefs and values, ranging from humanistic definitions, such as empathy, love, and ethical and religious delineations, to technological, legal, political, and economic descriptions. The formal theory evolved as a result of using the Hegelian dialectical process of examining and connecting codetermining polar opposites of the humanistic dimensions as the thesis of caring in relation to the dimensions of economics, politics, law, and technology of the bureaucracy as the antithesis of caring. The process was synthesized into a dialectical, formal Theory of Bureaucratic Caring. The laws of the dialectic—codetermination of polar opposites, negation of each of the separate codetermining opposites, and synthesis of conceptualizations toward transformation and change—demonstrated that the understanding of institutional caring as a whole, or the Theory of Bureaucratic Caring, is simply a representation of its integral nature in contemporary organizational culture. The theory shows that caring reached its completeness through the process of its own relevance in practice (Ray, 1981, 1989).

MIDDLE-RANGE THEORY

Middle-range theory deals with a relatively broad scope of phenomena but does not cover the full range of phenomena of a discipline, as do grand theories that encompass the fullest range or the most global phenomena in the discipline (Chinn & Kramer, 1995). As such, middle-range theories are generally considered narrower in scope than grand theories, and to some extent narrower than formal theory within the grounded theory tradition. There is a paradox in caring as middle-range theory. Caring in nursing, for example, may be considered by some intellectuals in the discipline as having a narrow scope or a foundation for a middle-range theory. However, others who have adopted Newman's (1992) paradigmatic view regarding the focus of the discipline of nursing as caring in the human health experience or who have seriously studied caring, may see it as a broad enough concept to capture the nature of nursing.

Is the Theory of Bureaucratic Caring a middle-range theory as well as a grounded theory? Middle-range theories are abstract enough to extend beyond data generated in a specific space, place, and time, but specific enough to allow for testing the theory in different arenas or permitting interventions for practice to transform nursing practice (Moody, 1990). The initial dialectical theory showed that "living caring in organizational life" with the meaning and symbols in an institutional culture reflects the culture of the macro or dominant culture. The meaning of "caring" in the organization showed that meaning was constituted within a larger pattern of significance.

Organizations are representations of our humanity (Smircich, 1985). Social forms and social arrangements reflect the interplay between cultural systems of thought and organization. The system reflected the symbols of political and economic power and authority, technology and the law, and the psychodynamics of caring in human experience. Middle-range theory embodies the perspective that these theories fall between the concrete world of practice and the grand theories that guide nursing research and practice (Moody, 1990). Bureaucratic caring reflects the concrete world of practice and responds to the caring ideal that is unique to nursing. Therefore, the Theory of Bureaucratic Caring is not only a grounded theory, but also a middle-range theory; it could also be considered a grand theory because of the ubiquitousness of the constructs of caring and culture.

HOLOGRAPHIC THEORY

The holographic paradigm in science recognizes that the ontology or "what is" of the universe or creation is the interconnectedness of all things, that the epistemology or knowledge that exists is in the relationship rather than in the objective world or subjective experience, that uncertainty is inherent in the relationship because everything is in process, and that information holds the key to grasping the holistic and complex nature of the meaning of holography or the whole (Battista, 1982; Harmon, 1998). *Holography* means that the implicit order

> *Holography means that the implicit order (the whole) and explicit order (the part) are interconnected, that everything is a holon in the sense that everything is a whole in one context and a part in another—each part being in the whole and the whole being in the part.*

(the whole) and explicit order (the part) are interconnected, that everything is a holon in the sense that everything is a whole in one context and a part in another—each part being in the whole and the whole being in the part (Harmon, 1998; Peat, 2003; Wilbur, 1982). It is the relational aspect of information that makes it a holistic rather than a mechanistic construct.

Ray (1998) states that "complexity theory is a scientific theory of dynamical systems collectively referred to as the sciences of complexity" (p. 91). Complexity theory has replaced other theories, such as Newtonian physics and even Einstein's beliefs that the physical world is governed by law and order. New scientific views state that phenomena that are antithetical actually coexist—determinism with uncertainty and reversibility with irreversibility (Nicolis & Prigogine, 1989). Thus, both linear and nonlinear and simple (e.g., gravity) and complex (economic and cultural) systems exist together. One of the tools in the studies of complexity is chaos theory. Chaos deals with life at the edge, or the notion that the concept of order exists within disorder at the system communication or choice point phases or where old patterns disintegrate or new patterns evolve (Davidson & Ray, 1991; Ray, 1994a, 1998). This new science, which signifies interrelationship of mind and matter, interconnectedness and choice, carries with it a moral responsibility and the quest toward wisdom, which includes awareness and creativity (Fox, 1994). Certain nursing theorists have embraced the notion of nursing as complexity in which consciousness, caring, and choice making are central to nursing (Davidson & Ray, 1991; Newman, 1986, 1992; Ray, 1994, 1998).

The Theory of Bureaucratic Caring as Holographic Theory

Can the Theory of Bureaucratic Caring be viewed as a holographic theory? The theory arose initially from the decisions that were made about the structure of organization (consciousness), the caring transactions that were engaged in (caring), and the effective negotiations or ability to make choices and reconcile the system demands with the humanistic client care needs (choice making). The theoretical processes of awareness of viewing truth or seeing the good of things (caring), and communication, are central to the theory. The dialectic of caring (the implicit order) in relation to the various structures (the explicit order) illustrates that there is room to consider the theory as holographic.

> *The synthesis of Bureaucratic Caring Theory shows that everything is interconnected—humanistic and spiritual caring and the organizational system— the whole is in the part and the part is in the whole, a holon.*

The synthesis of Bureaucratic Caring Theory shows that everything is interconnected—humanistic and spiritual caring and the organizational system—the whole is in the part and the part is in the whole, a holon.

How can knowledge of caring interconnectedness motivate nursing to continue to embrace the human dimension within the current economic and technologic environment of health care? Can higher ground be reclaimed for the twenty-first century? Higher ground requires that we make excellent choices. It is therefore imperative that spiritual and ethical caring thrive in complex systems. Figure 23–2, the holographic Theory of Bureaucratic Caring, illustrates that through spiritual/ethical caring as the choice point for communication in relation to the complexity of the sociocultural system, nursing can reclaim higher ground.

Reflections on the Theory as Holographic

Freeman (in Appell & Triloki, 1988) pointed out that human values are a function of the capacity to make choices and called for a paradigm giving recognition to awareness and choice. As noted, a revision toward this end is taking place in science based on the new holographic scientific worldview. Nursing has the capacity to make creative and moral choices for a preferred future. Nursing theory can focus on the capacity to continue to direct the good. Nursing is being shaped by the historical revolution going on in science, social sciences, and theology (Harmon, 1998; Newman, 1992; Ray, 1998; Reed, 1997; Watson, 1997; Wheatley, 1999). In these new approaches, constructs of consciousness and choice are central and demonstrate that phenomena of the universe, including society, arise from the choices that are or are not made (Freeman cited in Appell & Triloki, 1988; Harmon, 1998). In the social sciences, the critical task is to comprehend the relationship between what is given in culture (the jural order) and what is chosen (the moral and spiritual) between destiny and decision. In nursing, the unitary-transformative paradigm and the various theories of Newman, Leininger, Parse, Rogers, and the holographic Theory of Bureaucratic Caring are challenging nursing to comprehend a similar relationship. The unitary-transformative paradigm of nursing and their holographic tenets are consistent with the changing images of the new science despite the reality that nursing continues to be threatened by the business model over its long-term human interests for facilitating health and well-being (Davidson & Ray, 1991; Ray, 1994a, 1998; Reed, 1997; Vicenzi, White, & Begun, 1997). The creative, intuitive, ethical, and spiritual mind is unlimited, however. Through "authentic conscience" (Harmon, 1998) we must find hope in our creative powers.

In the revised theoretical model, everything is infused with spiritual/ethical caring (the center of the model) by its integrative and relational connection to the structures of organizational life (relational self-organization). Spiritual/ethical caring is both a part and a whole, and every part secures its purpose and meaning from each of the parts that can also be considered wholes. In other words, the model shows how spiritual/ethical caring is involved with qualitatively different processes or systems; for example, political, economic, technological, and legal. The systems, when integrated and presented as open and interactive, are a whole and must operate as such by conscious choice, especially by the choice making of nursing, which always has, or should have, the interest of humanity at heart.

The model presents a vision but it is based on the reality of practice. The model emphasizes a direction toward the unity of experience. Spirituality involves creativity and choice and refers to genuineness, vitality, and depth. It is revealed in

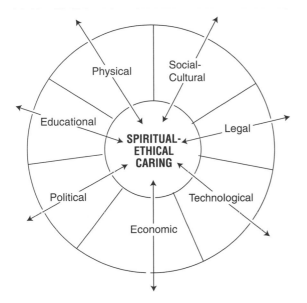

FIGURE 23–2   The holographic Theory of Bureaucratic Caring.

attachment, love, and community and comprehended within as intimacy and spirit (Harmon, 1998; Secretan, 1997). Secretan (p. 27) states: "Most of us have an innate understanding of soul, even though each of us might define it in a very different and personal way."

Fox (1994) calls for the theology of work—a redefinition of work. Because of the crisis of our relationship to work, we are challenged to reinvent it. For nursing, this is important because work puts us in touch with others, not only in terms of personal gain, but also at the level of service to humanity or the community of clients and other professionals. Work must be spiritual, with recognition of the creative spirit at work in us. Thus, nurses must be the "custodians of the human spirit" (Secretan, 1997, p. 27).

The ethical imperatives of caring that join with the spiritual relate to questions or issues about our moral obligations to others. The ethics of caring as edifying the good through communication and interaction involve never treating people simply as a means to an end or as an end in themselves, but rather as beings who have the capacity to make choices about the meaning of life, health, and caring. Ethical content—as principles of doing good, doing no harm, allowing choice, being fair, and promise-keeping—functions as the compass in our decisions to sustain humanity in the context of political, economic, and technological situations within organizations. Roach (2002) pointed out that ethical caring is operative at the level of discernment of principles, in the commitment needed to carry them out, and in the decisions or choices to uphold human dignity through love and compassion. Furthermore, Roach (2002) remarked that health is a community responsibility, an idea that is rooted in ancient Hebrew ethics. The expression of human caring as an ethical act is inspired by spiritual traditions that emphasize charity. Spiritual/ ethical caring for nursing does not question whether or not to care in complex systems but intimates how sincere deliberations and ultimately the facilitation of choices for the good of others can or should be accomplished. The scientist Sheldrake (1991, p. 207) remarks:

The recognition that we need to change the way we live [work] is gaining ground. It is like waking up from a dream. It brings with it a spirit of repentance, seeing in a new way, a change of heart. This conversion is intensified by the sense that the end of the age of oppression is at hand.

SUMMARY

As the twenty-first century is evolving, nursing in complex organizations has to evolve as well. As the Theory of Bureaucratic Caring has demonstrated, caring is the primordial construct and consciousness of nursing. Reenvisioning the theory as holographic shows that through creativity and imagination, nursing can build the profession it wants. Nurses are calling for expression of their own spiritual and ethical existence. The new scientific and spiritual approach to nursing theory as holographic will have positive effects. The union of science, ethics, and spirit will engender a new sense of hope for transformation in the work world. This transformation toward relational caring organization can occur in the economic and politically driven atmosphere of today. Nurses can reintroduce the spiritual and ethical dimensions of caring. The deep values that underlie choice to do good for the many will be felt both inside and outside organizations. We must awaken our consciences and act on this awareness and no longer surrender to injustices and oppressiveness of systems that focus primarily on the good of a few. "Healing a sick society [work world] is a part of the ministry of making whole" (Fox, 1994, p. 305). The holographic Theory of Bureaucratic Caring—idealistic, yet practical; visionary, yet real—can give direction and impetus to lead the way.

This transformation toward relational caring organization can occur in the economic and politically driven atmosphere of today. Nurses can reintroduce the spiritual and ethical dimensions of caring.

PART TWO:
Applications of Marilyn Ray's Theory of Bureaucratic Caring

Marian C. Turkel

Current Context of Health-Care Organizations

Review of the Literature: Political and Economic Constraints of Nursing Practice

---

Economic Implications of Bureaucratic Caring Theory: Research in Current Atmosphere of Health-Care Reform

---

Economic/Political Implications of Bureaucratic Caring

Summary

References

$\mathcal{R}$ay (1989, p. 31) warned that the "transformation of America and other health care systems to corporate enterprises emphasizing competitive management and economic gain seriously challenges nursing's humanistic philosophies and theories, and nursing's administrative and clinical policies." Approximately 15 years later, in the current managed care environment, there is an intense focus on operating costs and the bottom line, and caring is often not valued within the organizational culture. However, nurse researchers, nurse administrators, and nurses in practice can use the political and/or economic dimensions of the Theory of Bureaucratic Caring as a framework to guide practice and decision making. Use of these dimensions of the theory integrates the constructs of politics, economics, and caring within the health-care organization.

The purpose of this chapter is to illuminate the notion of political/economic caring in the current health-care environment. Ray's (1989) original Theory of Bureaucratic Caring included political and economic entities as separate and distinct structural caring categories. The revised Theory of Bureaucratic Caring, however, is represented as a complex holographic theory. Given this philosophical framework, the political and economic dimensions of bureaucratic caring as portrayed in this chapter are illuminated as interrelated constructs.

The political and economic dimensions of bureaucratic caring encompass not only health-care reform at the national level, but also refer to the political and economic impact of these changes at the organizational level. Through sections on the current context of health-care organizations, review of the literature related to the political and economic constraints of nursing practice, economic caring research, political and economic implications of bureaucratic caring, and visions for the future, we learn how the Theory of Bureaucratic Caring applies.

Current Context of Health-Care Organizations

In the wake of the controversial health-care reform process that is currently being debated in the United States, the central thesis in today's economic health-care milieu in both the for-profit and not-for-profit sectors is managed care (Williams & Torrens, 2002). Managed care is an economic concept based on the premise that purchasers of care, both public and private, are unwilling to tolerate the substantial growth of the last several years in health-care costs. Managed care involves managed competition and is based on the assumption that health-care prices will fall if hospitals and providers are forced to compete on the basis of cost and quality, like other industries (Williams & Torrens,

2002). Within traditional complex health-care organizations, community or public health agencies, or alternative health systems such as health maintenance organizations, financing in relation to managed care and managed competition is becoming a topic of heated discussion in the development of operational goals. This new form of health-care financing, based on the ratio of benefits over costs or the "highest quality services at the lowest available cost" (Prescott, 1993, p. 192), challenges the old ways of competing for and paying for health-care services. Cost-saving measures integrating patient outcomes are paramount to health-care organizational survival and the economic viability of professional nursing practice.

As the United States is in the midst of radical health-care changes, the entire debate focuses on the concept of economics. From an economic perspective, health-care organizations are a business. The competition for survival among organizations is becoming stronger, cost controls are becoming tighter, and reimbursement is declining. However,

> *The human dimension of health care is missing from the economic discussion.*

the human dimension of health care is missing from the economic discussion.

In the economic debate, the belief in caring for the patients as the goal of health-care organizations has been lost. Ray (1989) questioned how economic caring decisions are made related to patient care in order to enhance the human perspective within a corporate culture. When patients are hospitalized, it is the caring and compassion of the registered nurse that the patients perceive as quality care and making a difference in their recovery (Turkel, 1997). The concerns of patients themselves are not about costs or health-care finance. Yet, in a climate increasingly focused on economics, it has become difficult to quantify the economic value of caring. Consequently, newer cost systems, such as managed care, do not look at human caring or the nurse-patient relationship when allocating resource dollars for reimbursement.

Historically, nursing care delivery has not been financed or costed out in terms of reimbursement as a single entity. The prospective payment system of diagnostic related groups (DRGs) connected

nursing services to the bed rate for patients (Shaffer, 1985). The current reimbursement systems, including health maintenance organizations (HMOs), managed care, Medicare, Medicaid, and private insurers, are reimbursing hospitals at a flat capitated rate. Subsequently, it is hospital administrators who must determine how these resource dollars will be allocated within their respective institutions.

Thus, it is necessary for caring nursing interactions to be viewed as having value as an economic resource. When professional nursing salary dollars are viewed as an economic liability that limits the potential profit margins of organizations, they are examined closely, and in many instances the number of registered nurses has been significantly reduced (Ketter, 1995). Hospital executives attribute these workforce reductions to the declining reimbursements of a managed care environment. It is imperative to the future of professional nursing practice that the economic value of caring be studied and documented, so human caring is not subsumed by the economics of health care.

Review of the Literature: Political and Economic Constraints of Nursing Practice

In order to use the economic dimension of the Theory of Bureaucratic Caring to guide research, nursing administration, and clinical practice, it is necessary to understand both the way in which health care has been financed and the current reimbursement system. Nurses, who understand the economics of health-care organizations, will be able to synthesize this knowledge into a framework for practice that integrates the dimensions of economics and human caring.

Nursing had its origins in poorly paid domestic work and charitable religious organizations (Dolan, 1985). Prior to the establishment of Medicare and Medicaid in 1965, the health-care system was not profitable for hospitals. Nursing students subsidized hospitals, and hospital-based nursing care was not considered a reimbursable expense or source of revenue (Lynaugh & Fagin, 1988).

Nursing students provided the labor, and hospital administrators made no attempt to identify the real cost of nursing care. As nursing education moved away from the hospital setting to universities in the late 1950s and as the role of the student nurse was reformed, hospital administrators began to examine the actual cost and revenue of hospital nursing care (Lynaugh & Fagin, 1988). However, the retrospective reimbursement of Medicare and Medicaid in 1965 allowed for hospital profitability and the issue of nursing care costs was not confronted.

During this era of retrospective reimbursement (1965 to 1983), the actual cost of nursing care was unknown because it was embedded in the daily hospital room charge. However, acute care hospitals had been under scrutiny because of the rapidly escalating costs of health care. A 1976 report from the National Council on Wage and Price Stability reported that during the period of 1965 to 1976, hospital costs and physicians' fees rose more than 50 percent faster than the overall cost of living (Walker, 1983). Hospital administrators were under considerable pressure to control costs.

Nursing service represented the largest hospital department and was singled out as a major cost in operating expenditures (Porter-O'Grady, 1979). It was assumed that the rising costs of health care were due to nurses' salaries and the number of registered nurses (Walker, 1983). Yet nursing costs as a percent of hospital charges could not be identified, because historically they had been tied to the room rate.

During the late 1970s and early 1980s, health-care costs continued to rise and did not follow traditional economic patterns. Cost-based reimbursement altered the forces of supply and demand. In the traditional economic marketplace, when the price of a product or service goes up, the demand decreases and consumers seek alternatives at lower prices (Mansfield, 1991). However, in the health-care marketplace, consumers did not seek an alternative as the price of hospital-based care continued to rise (DiVestea, 1985). This imbalance of the supply-and-demand curve occurred because consumers paid little out-of-pocket expense for health care. Government expenditure for the cost-based reimbursement system was predicted to bankrupt Social Security by 1985 unless changes were made (Gapenski, 1993). In an attempt to control hospital costs, the government instituted a prospective payment system based on DRGs.

As a result of the prospective payment system, hospital administrators were pressured to increase efficiency, reduce costs, and maintain quality. Consequently, nursing administrators needed to develop systems to gather information relative to nursing costs and productivity. Research was conducted in order to examine the costs associated with nursing (Bargagliotti & Smith, 1985; Curtin, 1983; McCormick, 1986; Walker, 1983). Common to all these studies was the use of a patient classification system that was time-based and was a predictor of the level of care needed for each class of patient. Data derived from these studies were used to calculate nursing costs per DRG to predict expenditures and to determine nursing productivity.

These studies identified the amount of time nurses spent doing specific interventions but underrepresented the wide variations and clinical complexity of nursing care. This cost-accounting process did not include the humanistic, caring behaviors of nurses, so the costs associated with the humanistic caring behaviors were not determined.

Foshay (1988) investigated 20 registered nurses' perceptions of caring activities and the ability of patient classification systems to measure these caring activities. Findings from this study revealed that patient classification systems could not address the emotional needs of patients, the needs of the elderly, or unpredictable events that required intensive nursing interventions (Foshay, 1988). Specific caring behaviors that could not be measured included giving a reassuring presence, attentive listening, and providing information.

Other research of this time period focused on the cost and outcomes of all registered nurse staffing patterns (Dahlen & Gregor, 1985; Glandon, Colbert, & Thomasma, 1989; Halloran, 1983; Minyard, Wall, & Turner, 1986). These studies showed that nursing units staffed with more registered nurses had decreased costs per nursing diagnosis, increased patient satisfaction, and decreased length of stay.

Helt and Jelinek (1988) examined registered nurse staffing in five different hospitals over two years. During this time period, the hospitals had increased their nursing skill mix from 60 percent to

70 percent registered nurses. It was shown that, although the acuity of hospitalized patients increased, the average length of stay dropped from 9.2 to 7.3 days (Helt & Jelinek, 1988). Nursing productivity improved and quality of care scores increased with the increased registered nurse staffing. The higher costs of employing registered nurses was offset by the productivity gains, and the hospitals netted an average of 55 percent productivity savings (Helt & Jelinek, 1988).

Hospital administrators had made budgeting and operating decisions based on the undocumented belief that nursing care accounted for 30 percent to 60 percent of patient charges. However, documented nursing research showed this assumption to be in error. A study conducted at Stanford University Hospital found that actual nursing costs constituted only 14 percent to 21 percent of total hospital charges (Walker, 1983). Similarly, the Medicus Corporation funded a study in which data were collected from 22 hospitals and 80,000 patient records. Direct nursing care costs represented, on average, only 17.8 percent of the Medicare reimbursement for each of the top 40 DRGs (McCormick, 1986). In a study of Medicare reimbursement and operating room nursing costs, nursing represented only 11 percent of the total operating costs (Jennings, 1991).

By the time nursing researchers had demonstrated the difficulty of costing out caring activities with patient classification systems and the effectiveness of registered nurse staffing on patient outcomes, patient satisfaction, and mortality, the move toward managed care had already started. With the introduction of managed care and increased corporatization of health care, the economic environment was changing faster than nurse researchers could document the impact of these changes on clinical practice. In a managed care environment, reimbursement to hospitals had been further constrained. As a response to shrinking operating budgets, many hospital administrators have instituted registered nurse staff reductions or used unlicensed nursing assistants to replace registered nurses. As a result of these actions, the health-care industry is now faced with a shortage of registered nurses. According to statistics provided by the Division of Nursing of the U.S. Department of Health and Human Services (2000), over the next ten years the demand for nurses will continue to outpace the supply.

Economic Implications of Bureaucratic Caring Theory: Research in Current Atmosphere of Health-Care Reform

Investigation of the economic dimension of bureaucratic caring is being explicated in part in nursing research studies. Findings from these research studies have been valuable when linking the concepts of politics, economics, caring, cost, and quality in the new paradigm of health-care delivery. Although caring and economics may seem paradoxical, contemporary health-care concerns emphasize the importance of understanding the cost of caring in relation to quality.

Miller (1989, 1995), Nyberg (1989, 1990, 1991), Ray (1981, 1987, 1989), Ray and Turkel (2000, 2001, 2003), Turkel (1997, 2001), and Valentine (1989, 1991, 1993) have examined the paradox between the concepts of human caring and economics. It was a challenge for nurses to combine the science and art of caring within the economic context of the health-care environment. However, any efforts to reshape the health-care system in our country must take into account the value of caring.

Nyberg's (1990) research findings indicated that nurses were extremely frustrated over the economic pressures of the past five years but that human care was present in nurses' day-to-day practice. According to Nyberg (1989, p. 17), "[T]oday's economic environment constrains human care, but nurses see human care as their responsibility and goal." Nurse executives agreed that care and economics must be viewed as interdependent. One nurse administrator proposed "caring as the mission of the hospital with economic and management as supporting facets" (Nyberg, 1989, p. 14). Although human care is the goal of nursing, economics cannot be ignored.

Miller (1995, p. 30) used Nyberg's Caring Assessment Tool to evaluate nurses' ability to care on eight different pediatric nursing units in seven Colorado hospitals. Although there were organizational differences, results showed a high correlation of caring attributes among the various settings. Interviews conducted with nurses indicated a concern that their "ability to be caring was in jeopardy." Some of the responses they gave included "financial pressure on the hospital distracts us from our mission of caring" and "managed care emphasizes the efficiency of nursing tasks over caring" (Miller, 1995, p. 30). These nurses felt that the practice of caring was being seriously threatened by the economic pressure associated with health-care changes.

Ray (1997) interviewed six nurse administrators to study the art of caring in nursing administration. The theme—economic-political-ethical valuing and its three attributes of exchanging commodity values, negotiating the politics, and valuing the ethic of caring—showed that the caring expressions of nurse administrators are bound to the economics and politics of the organization (Ray, 1997). Narrative examples of the attribute, exchanging commodity values, were "making caring tangible" and "patient care is a commodity (economic good or value)." Narrative examples of the attribute negotiating the politics were "the nurse administrator is a system coordinator, nurses are the system and know what impinges on them," and "nurses are political beings (powerful in the organization)." Narrative examples of the attribute, valuing the ethics of caring, were "the nurse administrator needs to be caring and shouldn't be like other administrators," and "value of nursing is to care holistically." Findings from this research study validate the interwoven relationship among caring, economics, and politics within organizational culture.

A recent nursing study demonstrated that high-quality care is located in the reciprocal actions of the interpersonal nurse-patient relationship (Hoggard-Green, 1995). Turkel (1993) used an ethnographic approach to study nurse-patient interactions in the critical care environment. The subsequent theme generated among all categories of interaction was the nurse-patient relationship. In a qualitative study, Price (1993) examined the meaning of quality nursing care from the perspective of parents of hospitalized children. A key category that emerged from the data was a positive relationship between quality of care and parents' perspectives. In the wake of workplace restructuring as a result of health-care reform and managed care, nurses are finding themselves in a period of transition, moving from traditional in-patient hospital practice to community-based practice. In a research study conducted by Turkel, Tappen, and Hall (1999), the development of a positive nurse-patient relationship was shown to be seen as a reward for nurses undergoing change in practice roles.

The foregoing studies identified the critical nature of the nurse-patient relationship. However, these studies did not merge economic concepts into nursing research or theory. As the nursing practice environment has continued to change, new research is needed to explore how nurses can continue to provide humanistic care with limited economic resources.

CHALLENGE TO RESEARCHERS

The challenge to articulate the economic value of the nurse-patient relationship as a commodity, just as goods, money, and services are viewed in traditional economics, is imperative. Foa (1971), an exchange theorist, designed an economic theory that could bridge the gap between economic and noneconomic resources. In this model, noneconomic resources (love, status, and information) were correlated with economic resources (money, goods, and services). According to Ray (1987, p. 40), "[T]he inclusion of these resources is necessary and will require a major effort on the part of nurses and patients to see that they become an integral part of the health-care economic analysis."

In order to appraise the nurse-patient relationship as an economic interpersonal resource, it is necessary to conduct qualitative and quantitative research studies to describe this unique relationship as an economic exchange process and economic resource. The philosophical framework of the economic dimension of bureaucratic caring has served in part as the basis for this type of needed nursing research. Turkel (1997) interviewed nurses, patients, and administrators from the for-profit sector to examine the process involved in the development of the nurse-patient relationship as an economic resource. This research was conducted as managed care penetration was having an enormous impact on the current health-care delivery system.

Turkel found that diminishing health-care resources was the basic social problem encountered by nurses, patients, and administrators. The basic

The basic social process of the nurse-patient relationship as an economic resource was struggling to find a balance, which referred to sustaining the caring ideal in a new reality controlled by costs.

social process of the nurse-patient relationship as an economic resource was struggling to find a balance, which referred to sustaining the caring ideal in a new reality controlled by costs.

In a study conducted by Ray and Turkel (1999), qualitative interviews were accomplished in not-for-profit and military sectors of the health-care delivery system. The purpose of this research was to continue the study of the nurse-patient relationship as an economic interpersonal resource. Findings from this study identified that the nurse-patient relationship was both outcome and process. Categories, which emerged during data analysis, included relationships, caring, and costs.

In the study, a formal theory of the nurse-patient relationship as an economic resource was generated from the qualitative research. The formal theory of relational caring complexity illustrated that the caring relationship between the nurse, the patient, and the administrator is complex and cocreative, is both process and outcome, and is a function of a set of economic variables and a set of nurse-patient relational caring variables. Economic variables are depicted as time, technical, and organizational resources. Nurse-patient relational caring variables are caring, relationships, and education (Turkel & Ray, 2000).

CONTINUED RESEARCH ON ECONOMICS AND CARING

In order to measure caring as an economic resource and to further test the theory, Ray and Turkel (1999) developed and tested a professional and patient questionnaire designed to measure organizational caring. The Organizational Caring questionnaire is a 26-item professional and an 18-item patient questionnaire designed from qualitative research (Ray & Turkel, 1995, 1997, 1999) and validated and established as reliable through quantitative research (Ray & Turkel, 2003). The three subscales are caring, trust, and economics. The questionnaire has been distributed in five different hospitals to over 500 participants.

The qualitative data showed how critical the partnership among nurses, patients, and administrators is to the success of an organization. Hospital administrators have identified that nursing is key to their economic well-being and that they must invest in nursing and value the caring associated with the practice of professional nursing.

Findings from this research in process used regression analysis to determine whether or not there was a correlation between caring within the context of the nurse-patient relationship and patient and economic outcomes. The research's long-term goal is to establish caring as an economic interpersonal resource. The researchers' objective was to show, through empirical nursing research, that hospitals with a higher organizational caring score have increased patient and economic outcomes.

Economic/Political Implications of Bureaucratic Caring

Findings from current nursing research on the economic dimension of bureaucratic caring can be used to guide administrative practice within health-care organizations. As a dimension of her research, Turkel (1997) interviewed eight top-level hospital and corporate-level administrators to gain an understanding of how they viewed the experiences of nurses and patients in the hospital setting. Administrators were chosen to be interviewed because they make the ultimate decision on how to allocate scarce human and economic resources within the organizational setting.

Administrator participants explained the value and importance of the nurse-patient relationship. They discussed receiving letters from patients, scoring high on surveys, and getting positive verbal feedback from patients as indicators of caring nurse-patient interactions. One administrator shared the following with the researcher:

> Lying in a bed like that, people feel vulnerable and are vulnerable, and they want to know that someone is there for them and will share with them what's going on. And it has to do with the caring. I hear [patients say] that my nurse cared, she listened, and she kept me informed. I would say that more than half of the positive comments I receive from patients have to do with the nurses being caring. What comes back to me is they cared about me, they took time to talk to me, they were kind to me.

HEALTH CARE AND NURSING ADMINISTRATION

The results of ongoing research conducted by Turkel and Ray (2000, 2001, 2003) showed that administrators value caring and high-quality care.

However, their actions and the action of other administrators must then reflect these values to ensure that the caring philosophy of the hospital remains in the forefront of organizational profit-making or economics. The issue of time constraints and inadequate staffing has been identified as problematic. Nurses and patients view lack of time as a hindrance to forming a caring nurse-patient relationship. This points out the need for administrators to restructure the organization so that the maximum of nursing time is focused on direct nurse-patient interactions. Hospital administrators desire high levels of quality care and see financial benefits from return business when patients are satisfied with nursing care. To maintain this standard, administrators must maintain adequate staffing ratios in order to allow time for nurses to be with their patients.

In the research conducted by Turkel and Ray (2000, 2001, 2003), administrator participants confirmed the above but also discussed the concomitant need for maintaining care and quality. The challenge facing administrators in a managed care environment is the simultaneous management of costs, care, and quality. Ray (1989) asserted that this can be accomplished if administrators consider both the tangible and intangible benefits of services provided within the organization.

Administrators need to recognize caring as a value-added interaction. From this point of view, the benefits of the interaction outweigh the expense of the registered nurse. Caring can be viewed as an "opportunity cost" or the cost of doing it right. This concept is applicable to contemporary health-care organizations. If people don't come back to a hospital (because of poor care), "you've lost an opportunity."

NURSING PRACTICE

The economic and political dimensions of bureaucratic caring can be used to guide practice. Now is the time for professional nurses to become proactive and use theory-based practice to shape their future instead of having the future dictated by others outside the discipline. Staff nurses can hold close their core value that caring is the essence of nursing and can still retain a focus on meeting the bottom line.

Empirical studies have firmly established a link between caring and positive patient outcomes.

Positive patient outcomes are needed for organizational survival in this competitive era of health care. Given this, professional nursing practice must embrace and illuminate the caring philosophy.

Staff nurses describe the essence of nursing as the caring relationship between nurse and patient (Trossman, 1998). However, nurses are practicing in an environment where the economics and costs of health care permeate discussions and clinical decisions. The focus on costs is not a transient response to shrinking reimbursement; instead, it has become the catalyst for change within corporate health-care organizations.

Nurses are continuing to struggle with economic changes. With a system goal of decreasing length of stay and increasing staffing ratios, nurses need to establish trust and initiate a relationship during their first encounter with a patient. As this relationship is being established, nurses need to focus on being, knowing, and doing all at once (Turkel, 1997) and being there from a patient perspective. For the nurses, this means completing a task while simultaneously engaging with a patient. This holistic approach to practice means viewing the patient as a person in all his or her complexity and then identifying the needs for professional nursing as they arise.

Changes that incorporated the human caring dimension and the critical nature that human relationships play in hospital organizations were identified by Ray over two decades ago. Ray (1987) described the problems associated with economic changes in health care and the negative impact economics would have on nurse caring.

Current research (Turkel & Ray, 2000, 2001, 2003) on the economics of the nurse-patient relationship showed that the preservation of this relationship and humanistic caring was continuing to grow despite the heavy emphasis by administrators and insurance companies on cost control. The researchers recommend that administrators recognize and respect the contributions nursing could make in developing hospital organizations as politically moral, caring organizations.

FUTURE CHALLENGES

The political dimension of bureaucratic caring is reflective of the organizational climate in many of the current health-care environments. Relationships grounded in trust, respect, and mutual caring have not been established among executives, nursing leaders, and members of the nursing staff (Ray, Turkel, & Marino, 2002). As a result of this lack of trust within the organization, many nurses question both their own loyalty to the organization and if executive decisions are motivated by political considerations rather than a concern for the practice environment.

A grounded theory study conducted by Ray, Turkel, and Marino (2002) identified losing trust as a care category. Consequences of losing trust in the organization included nurses becoming disillusioned with nursing practice and experiencing decreased loyalty to the organization. Strategies for rebuilding the loss of trust in order to transform nursing within organizations included respecting the nursing staff, communicating with the nursing staff, maintaining visibility, and engaging in participative decision making. Administrators need to focus on rebuilding in order to create a better working environment for the nursing staff. Registered nurses view the rebuilding of trust as the key component to the recruitment and retention of nursing staff.

SUMMARY

The foundation for professional caring is the blending of the humanistic and empirical aspects of care. In today's environment, the nurse needs to integrate caring, knowledge, and skills all at once. Given political and economic constraints, the art of caring cannot occur in isolation from meeting the physical needs of patients. When caring is defined solely as science or as art, it is not adequate to reflect the reality of current practice.

Nurses must be able to understand and articulate the politics and the economics of nursing practice and health care. Classes that examine the environment of practice generally, and the politics and the economics of health care in relation to caring, must be integrated into staff-development curricula. Nurses need to search continually for different approaches to professional practice that will incorporate caring in an increasingly technical and cost-driven environment. Doing more with less no longer works; nurses

must move outside of the box to create innovative practice models based on nursing theory.

Administrative nursing research needs to continue to study the relationship among staff nursing caring, patient outcomes, and organizational economic outcomes. Further research is required to firmly establish the nurse-patient relationship as an economic resource in the new paradigm of evidence-based practice of health-care delivery (1999). Findings from these research studies will continue to validate the Theory of Bureaucratic Caring as a middle-range holographic practice theory.

Nurses need repeated exposure to the economics and costs associated with health care. Lack of knowledge in this area means others outside of nursing will continue to make the political and economic decisions concerning the practice of nursing. Having an in-depth knowledge of the economics of health care will allow nurses to challenge and change the system. A new theory-based model can be created for nursing practice that supports human caring in relation to the organization's economic and political values. The political and economic dimensions of bureaucratic caring serve as a philosophical/theoretical framework to guide both contemporary and futuristic research and theory-based nursing practice.

> *Having an in-depth knowledge of the economics of health care will allow nurses to challenge and change the system.*

References

Appell, G., & Triloki, N. (Eds.). 1988. *Choice and morality in anthropological perspective.* Albany: State University of New York Press.

Bargagliotti, L. A., & Smith, M. (1985). Patterns of nursing costs with capitated reimbursement. *Nursing Economics, 3*(5), 270–275.

Bassingthwaighte, J., Liebovitch, L., & West, B. (1994). *Fractal physiology.* New York: Oxford University Press.

Battista, J. (1982). The holographic model, holistic paradigm, information theory, and consciousness. In Wilber, K. (Ed.), *The holographic paradigm and other paradoxes* (pp. 143–150). Boulder, CO: Shambhala.

Bell, D. (1974). *The coming of post-industrial society.* New York: Basic Books.

Boykin, A., & Schoenhofer, S. (2001). *Nursing as caring: A model for transforming practice.* Sudbury, CT: Jones & Bartlett Publishers.

Britain, G., & Cohen, R. (1980). *Hierarchy and society: Anthropological perspectives on bureaucracy.* Philadelphia: ISHI.

Chinn, P., & Kramer, M. (1995). *Theory and nursing: A systematic approach* (4th ed.). St. Louis: Mosby.

Cody, W. (1996). Drowning in eclecticism. *Nursing Science Quarterly, 9,* 96–98.

Cuilla, J. (2000). *The working life: The promise and betrayal of modern work.* New York: Times Books/Random House.

Curtin, L. (1983). Determining costs of nursing service per DRG. *Nursing Management, 14*(4), 16–20.

Dahlen, A. L., & Gregor, J. R. (1985). Nursing costs by DRG with an all RN staff. In Shaffer, F. A. (Ed.), *Costing out nursing: Pricing our product* (pp. 113–122). New York: National League for Nursing Press.

Davidson, A., & Ray, M. (1991). Studying the human-environment phenomenon using the science of complexity. *Advances in Nursing Science, 14*(2), 73–87.

Dawes, M., Davies, P., Gray, A., Mant, J., Seers, K., & Snowball, R. (1999). *Evidence-based practice.* Edinburgh: Churchill-Livingstone.

DiVestea, N. (1985). The changing health care system: An overview. In Shaffer, F. A. (Ed.), *Costing out nursing: Pricing our product* (pp. 29–36). New York: National League for Nursing Press.

Dolan, J. (1985). *Nursing in society: A historical perspective.* Philadelphia: W. B. Saunders.

Eisenberg, E., & Goodall, H. (1993). *Organizational communication.* New York: St. Martin's Press.

Fawcett, J. (1993). From a plethora of paradigms to parsimony in worldviews. *Nursing Science Quarterly, 6,* 56–58.

Foa, U. (1971). Interpersonal and economic resources. *Science, 171*(29), 345–351.

Foshay, M. C. (1988). *Professional nurses' perceptions of their caring activities and their perceptions of the ability of patient classification systems to measure their caring activities.* Unpublished master's thesis, University of Southern Maine, Portland.

Fox, M. (1994). *The reinvention of work.* San Francisco: Harper.

Gapenski, L. (1993). *Understanding health care financial management: Text, cases, and models.* Ann Arbor, MI: Health Administration Press.

Glandon, G., Colbert, K., & Thomasma, M. (1989). Nursing delivery models and RN mix: Cost implications. *Nursing Management, 20*(5), 30–33.

Glaser, B. (1978). *Theoretical sensitivity.* Mill Valley, CA: The Sociology Press.

Glaser, B., & Strauss, A. (1967). *The discovery of grounded theory: Strategies for qualitative research.* Hawthorne, NY: Aldine de Gruyter.

Halloran, E. J. (1983). Nursing workload, medical diagnosis related groups, and nursing diagnosis. *Research in Nursing and Health, 8*(4), 421–433.

Harmon, W. (1998). *Global mind change* (2nd ed.). San Francisco: Berrett-Koehler Publishers, Inc.

Helt, E., & Jelinek, R. (1988). In the wake of cost cutting, nursing productivity, and quality improvement. *Nursing Management, 19*(6), 36–38, 42, 46–48.

Hoggard-Green, J. (1995). *A phenomenological study of a consumer's definition of quality health care.* Unpublished doctoral dissertation, University of Utah, Salt Lake City.

Jennings, T. (1991). Medicare reimbursement deficits: Are nursing care costs to blame? *Today's OR Nurse, 13*(9), 13–17.

Ketter, J. (1995). Re-engineering the workforce. *The American Nurse, 27*(3), 1, 14.

Korten, D. (1995). *When corporations rule the world.* San Francisco: Berrett-Koehler Publishers, Inc.

Leininger, M. (1981). The phenomenon of caring: Importance, research questions and theoretical considerations. In Leininger, M. (Ed.), *Caring: An essential human need* (pp. 3–15). Thorofare, NJ: Slack.

Leininger, M. (Ed.). (1981). *Caring: An essential human need.* Thorofare, NJ: Slack.

Leininger, M. (1991). *Culture care diversity and universality: A theory of nursing.* New York: National League for Nursing Press.

Leininger, M. (1997). Transcultural nursing research to transform nursing education and practice: 40 years. *Image: Journal of Nursing Scholarship, 29,* 341–354.

Levine, M. (1995). The rhetoric of nursing theory. *Image: Journal of Nursing Scholarship, 27,* 11–14.

Long, K. (2003). The Institute of Medicine Report, health profession education: A bridge to quality. *Policy, Politics & Nursing, 4*(4), 259–262.

Louis, M. (1985). An investigator's guide to workplace culture. In Frost, P., Moore, L., Louis, M., Lundberg, C., & Martin, J. (Eds.), *Organizational culture* (pp. 73–93). Beverly Hills: Sage.

Lynaugh, J., & Fagin, C. (1988). Nursing comes of age. *Image, 20*(4), 184–190.

Mansfield, E. (1991). *Microeconomics* (7th ed.). New York: Norton.

Matteson, M., & Ivancevich, J. (Eds.). *Management and organizational behavior classics* (7th ed.). Chicago: Irwin McGraw-Hill.

McCormick, B. (1986). What's the cost of nursing care? *Hospitals, 60,* 48–52.

Miller, K. (1989). The human care perspective on nursing administration. *Journal of Nursing Administration, 25*(11), 29–32.

Miller, K. (1995). Keeping the care in nursing care. *Journal of Nursing Administration, 25*(11), 29–32.

Minyard, K., Wall, J., & Turner, R. (1986). RNs may cost less than you think. *Journal of Nursing Administration, 16*(5), 29–34.

Moody, L. (1990). *Advancing nursing science through research.* Newbury Park, CA: Sage.

Morgan, G. (1997). *Images of organization* (2nd ed.). Thousand Oaks, CA: Sage.

Morse, J., Solberg, S., Neander, W., Bottorff, J., & Johnson, J. (1990). Concepts of caring and caring as a concept. *Advances in Nursing Science, 13,* 1–14.

Newman, M. (1986). *Health as expanding consciousness.* St. Louis: Mosby.

Newman, M. (1992). Prevailing paradigms in nursing. *Nursing Outlook, 40,* 10–14.

Newman, M., Sime, A., & Corcoran-Perry, S. (1991). The focus of the discipline of nursing. *Advances in Nursing Science, 14*(1), 1–6.

Nicolis, G., & Prigogine, I. (1989). *Explaining complexity.* New York: W. H. Freeman.

Nightingale, F. (1860/1969). *Notes on nursing: What it is and what it is not.* New York: Dover.

Nyberg, J. (1989). The element of caring in nursing administration. *Nursing Administration Quarterly, 13,* 9–16.

Nyberg, J. (1990). The effects of care and economics on nursing practice. *Journal of Nursing Administration, 20*(5), 13–18.

Nyberg, J. (1991). Theoretical explanations of human care and economics: Foundations of nursing administration practice. *Advances in Nursing Science, 13*(1), 74–84.

Nyberg, J. (1998). A caring approach in nursing administration. Niwot, CO: University Press of Colorado.

O'Grady, T. & Malloch, K. (2003). *Quantum leadership.* Boston: Jones and Bartlett Publishers.

Page, A. (Ed.). (2004). *Keeping patients safe: Transforming the work environment of nurses.* (Institute of Medicine Report). Washington, DC: The National Academies Press.

Parse, R. (1987). *Nursing science: Maps, paradigms, theories, and critiques.* Philadelphia: Saunders.

Peat, F. D. (2003). *From certainty to uncertainty: The story of science and ideas in the twentieth century.* Washington, DC: Joseph Henry Press.

Perrow, C. (1986). *Complex organizations: A critical essay* (2nd ed.). Glenview, IL: Scott, Foresman.

Pinchot, G., & Pinchot, E. (1994). *The end of bureaucracy & the rise of the intelligent organization.* San Francisco: Berrett-Koehler Publishers.

Porter-O'Grady, T. (1979). Financial planning: Budgeting for nurses, part I. *Supervisor Nurse, 10,* 35–38.

Prescott, P. (1993). Nursing: An important component of hospital survival under a reformed health care system. *Nursing Economics, 11*(4), 192–199.

Price, P. (1993). Parents' perceptions of the meaning of quality nursing care. *Advances in Nursing Science, 16*(1), 33–41.

Ray, M. (1981). *A study of caring within the institutional culture.* Unpublished doctoral dissertation. Salt Lake City, UT: University of Utah.

Ray, M. (1984). The development of a nursing classification system of caring. In Leininger, M. (Ed.), *Care, the essence of nursing and health* (pp. 95–112). Thorofare, NJ: Slack.

Ray, M. (1987). Health care economics and human caring: Why the moral conflict must be resolved. *Family and Community Health, 10*(1), 35–43.

Ray, M. (1989). The Theory of Bureaucratic Caring for nursing practice in the organizational culture. *Nursing Administration Quarterly, 13*(2), 31–42.

Ray, M. (1994a). Complex caring dynamics: A unifying model of nursing inquiry. *Theoretic and applied chaos in nursing, 1*(1), 23–32.

Ray, M. (1994b). Communal moral experience as the starting point for research in health care ethics. *Nursing Outlook, 41,* 104–109.

Ray, M. (1998). Complexity and nursing science. *Nursing Science Quarterly, 11,* 91–93.

Ray, M., & Turkel, M. (1999). *Econometric Analysis of the Nurse-Patient Relationship.*

Ray, M., & Turkel, M. (2000). Economic and Patient Outcomes of the Nurse-Patient Relationship. Grant funded by the Department of Defense, Tri-Service Nursing Research Council, August, 2000 ($429,255 for 3 years).

Ray, M., & Turkel, M. (2001). *Economic and Patient Outcomes of the Nurse-Patient Relationship.*

Ray, M., & Turkel, M. (2002). *Economic and Patient Outcomes of the Nurse-Patient Relationship.*

Ray, M., & Turkel, M. (2003). *Economic and Patient Outcomes of the Nurse-Patient Relationship.*

Ray, M., Turkel, M., & Marino, F. (2002). The transformative process for nursing in workforce redevelopment. *Nursing Administration Quarterly, 26*(2), 1–14.

Reed, P. (1997). Nursing: The ontology of the discipline. *Nursing Science Quarterly, 10,* 76–79.

Roach, M. S. (2002). *The human act of caring.* (rev. ed.). Ottawa, Canada: Canadian Hospital Association Press.

Secretan, L. (1997). *Reclaiming higher ground.* New York: McGraw-Hill.

Shaffer, F. (1985). *Costing out nursing: Pricing our product.* New York: National League for Nursing Press.

Sheldrake, R. (1991). *The rebirth of nature.* New York: Bantam.

Smircich, L. (1985). Is the concept of culture a paradigm for understanding organizations and ourselves? In Frost, P., Moore, L., Louis, M., Lundberg, C., & Martin, J. (Eds.), *Organizational culture.* Beverly Hills: Sage.

Strauss, A., & Corbin, J. (1998). *Basics of qualitative research* (2nd ed.). Newbury Park, CA: Sage.

Swanson, K. (1991). Empirical development of a middle-range theory of caring. *Nursing Research, 40,* 161–166.

Trossman, S. (1998). The human connection: Nurses and their patients. *The American Nurse, 30*(5), 1, 8.

Turkel, M. (1993). *Nurse-patient interactions in the critical-care setting.* Unpublished research findings.

Turkel, M. (1997). *Struggling to find a balance: A grounded theory study of the nurse-patient relationship in the changing health care environment.* Unpublished doctoral dissertation, University of Miami, Florida. Microfilm #9805958.

Turkel, M. (2001). Struggling to find a balance: The paradox between caring and economics. *Nursing Administration Quarterly, 26*(1), 67–82.

Turkel, M., & Ray, M. (2000). Relational complexity: A theory of the nurse-patient relationship within an economic context. *Nursing Science Quarterly, 13*(4), 307–313.

Turkel, M., & Ray, M. (2001). Relational complexity: From grounded theory to instrument development and theoretical testing. *Nursing Science Quarterly, 14*(4), 281–287.

Turkel, M., & Ray, M. (2003). A process model for policy analysis within the context of political caring. *International Journal For Human Caring, 7*(3), 26–34.

Turkel, M., Tappen, R., & Hall, R. (1999). Moments of excellence. *Journal of Gerontological Nursing, 25*(1), 7–12.

U.S. DHHS (2000). The registered nurse population: Findings from the national sample survey of registered nurses. U.S. DHHS/Division of Nursing. Washington, DC. Retrieved from www.bhpr.hrsa.gov/healthworkforce/reports/rnproject

Valentine, K. (1989). Caring is more than kindness: Modeling its complexities. *Journal of Nursing Administration, 19*(11), 28–34.

Valentine, K. (1991). Comprehensive assessment of caring and its relationship to outcome measures. *Journal of Nursing Quality Assurance, 5*(2), 59–68.

Valentine, K. (1993). Development of a nurse compensation system. In Gaut, D. A. (Ed.), *A global agenda for caring* (pp. 329–345). New York: National League for Nursing Press.

van Manen, M. (1982). Edifying theory: Serving the good. *Theory Into Practice, 31*, 45–49.

Vicenzi, A., White, K., & Begun, J. (1997). Chaos in nursing: Make it work for you. *American Journal of Nursing, 97*, 26–32.

Walker, D. (1983). The cost of nursing care in hospitals. *Journal of Nursing Administration, 13*(3), 13–18.

Watson, J. (1985). *Human science, human care: A theory of nursing.* Norwalk, CT: Appleton & Lange.

Watson, J. (1988). New dimensions of human caring theory. *Nursing Science Quarterly, 1,* 175–181.

Watson, J. (1997). The theory of human caring: Retrospective and prospective. *Nursing Science Quarterly,* 175–181.

Weber, M. (1999). The ideal bureaucracy. In Matteson, M., & Ivancevich, J. (Eds.), *Management and organizational behavior classics* (7th ed.). Chicago: Irwin McGraw-Hill.

Wheatley, M. (1999). *Leadership and the new science.* 2nd ed. San Francisco: Berrett-Koehler Publishers, Inc.

Wilbur, K. (Ed.). (1982). *The holographic paradigm and other paradoxes.* Boulder, CO: Shambhala.

Williams, S., & Torrens, P. (2002). *Introduction to health services* (6th ed.). Albany, NY: Delmar.

Wittgenstein, L. (1969). *On certainty.* New York: Harper & Row.

CHAPTER 24

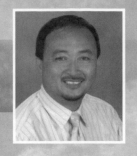

Rozzano C. Locsin

Technological Competency as Caring and the Practice of Knowing Persons as Whole

Rozzano C. Locsin

Introducing the Theory

Summary

References

---

*T*here is a great demand for a practice of nursing that is based on the authentic intention to know human beings fully as persons rather than as objects of care. Nursing intends and desires to use creative, imaginative, and innovative ways of affirming, appreciating, and celebrating human beings as whole persons. Often, the best way to realize these intentions is through expert and competent use of nursing technologies (Locsin, 1998).

Oftentimes perceived as the practice of using machine technologies in nursing (Locsin, 1995), technological competency as caring in nursing is the practice of knowing persons as whole (Locsin, 2001), frequently with the use of varying technologies. Contemporary definitions of technology include a means to an end, an instrument, a tool, or a human activity that increases or enhances efficiency (Heidegger, 1977). Conceptualizing technology and caring in nursing practice as a dichotomy continues to invigorate the debate that their coexistence is crucial to the understanding of technological competency as an expression of caring in nursing.

The purpose of this chapter is to describe and explain "knowing persons as whole," a framework of nursing guiding its practice and grounded in the theoretical construct of *technology competency as caring in nursing* (Locsin, 2004). This framework of practice illuminates the harmonious relationship between technology competency and caring in nursing. In this model, the focus of nursing is the person, a human being whose hopes, dreams, and aspirations are to live life fully as a caring person (Boykin and Schoenhofer, 2001).

Introducing the Theory

As a model of practice, *technological competency as caring in nursing* (Locsin, 2004) is as valuable today as it has been and will continue to be in the future. Advancing technologies in health care demand expertise with technologies. Often, such expertise is perceived as noncaring. It is the view of this chapter, however, that being technologically competent is being caring. As such, in appreciating this practice model, the following assumptions are posited:

- Persons are whole or complete in the moment (Boykin and Schoenhofer, 2001).
- Knowing persons is a process of nursing that allows for continuous appreciation of persons moment to moment (Locsin, 2005).
- Nursing is a discipline and a professional practice (Boykin and Schoenhofer, 2001)
- Technology is used to know persons as whole moment to moment (Locsin, 2004).

The ultimate purpose of technological competency in nursing is to acknowledge that wholeness of persons is a focus of nursing and that various

> *The ultimate purpose of technological competency in nursing is to acknowledge that wholeness of persons is a focus of nursing.*

technological means can and should be used in nursing in order for nursing to realize the wholeness of person more fully. This acknowledgment brings together the relatively abstract concept of wholeness of person with the more concrete concept of technology. Such acknowledgment compels the redesigning of processes of nursing—ways of

expressing, celebrating, and appreciating the practice of nursing as continuously knowing persons as whole moment to moment. In this practice of nursing, technology is used not to know "what is the person?" but rather to know "who is the person?" Appropriately, answers to the former question alludes to an expectation of knowing empirical facts about the composition of the person; the latter question requires the understanding of an unpredictable, irreducible person who is more than and different from the sum of his or her empirical self. The former question alludes to the idea of persons as objects; the latter addresses the uniqueness and individuality of persons as human beings who continuously unfold and therefore require continuous knowing (Locsin, 2004).

PERSONS AS WHOLE AND COMPLETE IN THE MOMENT

One of the earlier definitions of the word *person* was evident in Hudson's 1988 publication claiming that the "emphasis on inclusive rather than sexist language has brought into prominence the use of the word 'person'" (p. 12). The origin of the word *person* is from the Greek word *prosopon*, which means the actor's mask of Greek tragedy; in Roman origin, *persona* indicated the role played by the individual in social or legal relationships. Hudson (1988) also declares that "an individual in isolation is contrary to an understanding of 'person'" (p. 15). A necessary appreciation of persons is the view that human beings are whole or complete in the moment. As such, there is no need to fix them or to make them complete again (Boykin and Schoenhofer, 2001). There is no lack or anything missing that requires nurses' intervening to make persons "whole or complete" again, or for nurses to assist in this completion. Persons are complete in the moment. Their varying situations of care demand calls for creativity, innovation, and imagination from nurses so that they may come to know the persons as "whole" persons. The uniqueness of the person is relative to the response called forth in particular situations.

Inherent in humans as unpredictable, dynamic, and living beings is the regard for self-as-person. This appreciation is like the human concern for security, safety, self-esteem, and actualization popularized by Maslow (1943) in his quintessential theoretical model on the "hierarchy of needs." More important, however, is the understanding that being human is being a person, regardless of biophysical parts or technological enhancements.

Because the future may require relative appreciation of persons, today, if the ultimate criterion of being human is that humans are only those who are all natural, organic, and functional, being human may not be so easy to determine. The purely natural human being may not exist anymore. The understanding that technology-supported life is artificial and therefore is not natural stimulates discussions among practitioners of nursing (Locsin and Campling, 2004), particularly when the subject of concern is technology-dependent care and technology competency as an expression of caring in nursing. Other than the theological perspective offered by Hudson (1988) that "false comfort may be offered whenever it is implied that this life and this body are significantly less important than the 'spiritual body' and the 'next life,'" it may be necessary to

appreciate the understanding that the time has come to enhance an awareness of the posthuman or spiritual future" (p. 13). What structural requirements will the posthuman possess? Today, there are some human beings who have anatomic and/or physiologic components that are already electronic and/or mechanical; for example, mechanical cardiac valves, self-injecting insulin pumps, cardiac pacemakers, or artificial limbs, all appearing as excellent facsimiles of the real. Yet, the idea of a "whole person" and being natural continues to persist as a requirement of what a human being should be (Figure 24–1).

THE PROCESS OF KNOWING PERSONS

In appreciating persons as whole moment to moment, persons possess the prerogative and the choice whether or not to allow nurses to know them fully. Entering the world of the other is a

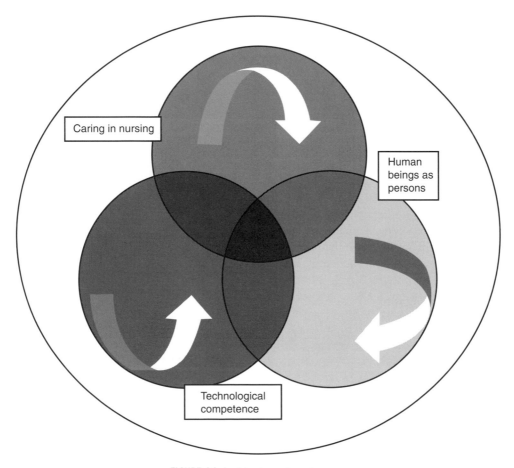

FIGURE 24–1   Nursing as knowing persons.

critical requisite to knowing as a process of nursing. Establishing rapport, trust, confidence, commitment, and the compassion to know others fully as persons is integral to this crucial positioning.

Wholeness is the idealized condition or situation about the one who is nursed. This idealization is held within the nurse's understanding of persons as complete human beings "in the moment." Expressions of this completeness vary from moment to moment. These expressions are human illustrations of living and growing. Oftentimes, using technology alone and focusing on the received technological data rather than on continually "knowing" the other fully as person, provides the nurse the understanding of persons as objects who need to be completed and made whole again. Paradoxically, because of the idea that human beings are unpredictable, it is not entirely possible for the nurse to fully know another human being—except in the moment and only if the person allows the nurse to know him or her by entering into his or her world.

In this perspective, the condition in which the nurse and the other allow each other to know each

> *The condition in which the nurse and the nursed allow each one to know each other exists as the nursing situation, the shared lived experience.*

other exists as the nursing situation, the shared lived experience between the nurse and nursed (Boykin and Schoenhofer, 2001). In this relationship, trust is established that the nurse will know the other fully as person; the trust that the nurse will not judge the person or categorize the person as just another human being or experience, but rather as a unique person who has hopes, dreams, and aspirations that are uniquely his or her own.

It is the nurse's responsibility to know the person's hopes, dreams, and aspirations. Technological competency as caring allows for this understanding. In doing so, the nurse also sanctions the other (the nursed) to know him or her as person. The expectation is that the nurse is to use multiple ways of knowing competently in the fullness of possibilities in using technologies in order to know the other fully as person. The nurse's responsibility is immeasurable in creating conditions that demand technological competency and care, much like the

wish to create a computerized human facsimile. In creating a nursing situation of care, there is a requisite competency to know persons fully, to understand, and to appreciate the important nuances of the person's hopes, dreams, and aspirations.

There are many ways of interpreting the concept of "person as whole." Three of the popular interpretations are derivations of the concept of person from dominant perspectives, those views that shape the popular understanding of the concept. Some of these interpretations delineating the exclusivity of disciplinary constructs influencing nursing care practices include the mind-body dualism popularly ascribed to Descartes, which supplies the continuing citation of the connection between mind and body. At least in nursing, the mind-body-spirit connection is popularized by Jean Watson in her theory of transpersonal caring. The simultaneity paradigm categorized the human environment mutual connection as the relationship that best serves human science nursing perspective and grounds theoretical frameworks and models of practice, including those of the caring sciences. These contemporary and popular elucidations create conceptions of human beings as the focus of nursing and of knowing persons in their wholeness as the practice of nursing.

The process of nursing is a dynamic unfolding of situations encompassing knowledgeable practices. The meaning of the process is characterized by listening, knowing, being with, enabling, and maintaining belief (Swanson, 1991). The following occurrences exemplify the process:

- Knowing and appreciating uniqueness of persons
- Designing participation in caring
- Implementation and evaluation (a simultaneous illustration and exercise of conjoining relationships crucial to knowing persons by using nursing technologies)
- Verifying knowledge of person through continuous knowing

In this model of practice, knowing is the primary process. "Knowing nursing means knowing in the realms of personal, ethical, empirical, and aesthetic—all at once" (Boykin and Schoenhofer, 2001, p. 6). The continuous, circular process demonstrates the ever-changing, dynamic, cyclical nature of knowing in nursing. Knowledge about the person that is derived from assessing, intervening, evaluating, and further assessing additionally informs the nurse that in knowing persons, one comes to understand the condition of more knowing about the person and about his or her being, in order for affirmation, support, and celebration of his or her hopes, dreams, and aspirations in the moment to occur. Supporting this process of knowing is the understanding that persons are unpredictable and simultaneously conceal and reveal themselves as persons from one moment to the

> *The nurse can only know the person fully in the moment. This knowing occurs only when the person allows the nurse to enter his or her world.*

next moment. The nurse can only know the person fully in the moment. This knowing occurs only when the person allows the nurse to enter his or her world. In this occurrence, the nurse and nursed become vulnerable as they move toward further continuous knowing.

Vulnerability allows participation, so that the nurse and nursed continue knowing each other moment to moment. In such situations, Daniels (1998) explains that "nurse's work is to ameliorate vulnerability" (p. 191). The embodiment of vulnerability in caring situations enables its recognition in others, participating in mutual vulnerability conditions, and sharing in the humanness of being vulnerable. Further, Daniels declares that "vulnerable individuals seek nursing care, and nurses seek those who are vulnerable" (p. 192). Allowing the nurse to enter the world of the one nursed is the mutual engagement of "power with" rather than having "power over" through a created hierarchy (Daniels, 1998). The nurse does not know more about the person than the person knows about himself or herself. No one knows the experience better than the person who encounters the situation.

Nonetheless, there is the possibility that the nurse will be able to predict and prescribe for the one nursed. When this occurs, these situations forcibly lead nurses to appreciate persons more as objects than as person. Such a situation can only occur when the nurse has assumed to "have known" the one nursed. While it can be assumed that with the process of "knowing persons as whole," opportunities to continuously know the other become limitless, there is also a much greater

likelihood that having "already known" the one nursed, the nurse will predict and prescribe activities or ways for the one nursed, causing objectification of person to ultimately occur (Figure 24–2).

To Know and Knowing

It is interesting to read the 10 definitions of the word *know* as a verb listed in the 1987 *Reader's Digest Illustrated Encyclopedic Dictionary* (p. 932). Of the 10 definitions, nine appropriately describe the intended use of the word, facilitating its understanding for the purpose and process of competently using technologies in nursing. These descriptions are:

- To perceive directly with the senses or mind
- To be certain of, regard, or accept as true beyond doubt
- To be capable of, have the skills to
- To have thorough or practical understanding of, as through experience of
- To be subjected to or limited by
- To recognize the character or quality of
- To be able to distinguish, recognize
- To be acquainted or familiar with
- To see, hear, or experience

While the action word *know* sustains the notion that nursing is concerned with activity and that the one who acts is knowledgeable (in the sense of understanding the rationales behind the activities), the word *knowing* is a key concept that alludes to the focus of an action from a cognitive perspective requiring description. Surprisingly, the encyclopedic dictionary attributes the definition of knowing as an adjective. Described here are the four descriptions of knowing:

- Possessing knowledge, intelligence, or understanding
- Suggestive of secret or private information
- Having or showing clever awareness and resourcefulness
- Planned; deliberate

Yet, "knowing" perfectly describes the ways of nursing—transpiring continuously as explicated from the framework of "knowing persons." It is the use of the word "knowing" in which the process of nursing as "knowing persons" is lived. The framework for practice clearly shows the circuitous and continuous process of knowing persons as a practice of nursing.

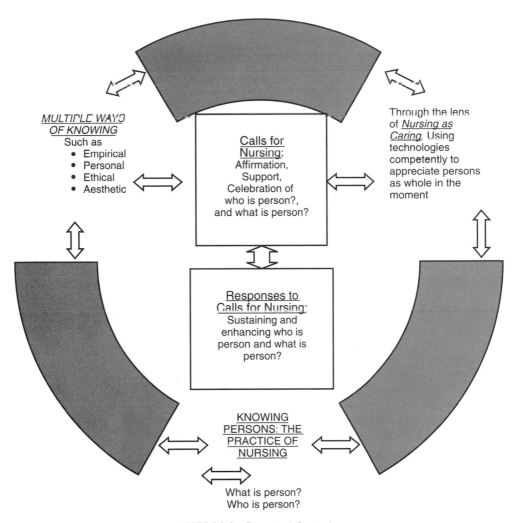

FIGURE 24–2   Framework for nursing.

While it is appreciated that nurses practice nursing from a theoretical perspective rather than from tradition or from blind obedience to instructions and directions, nevertheless, processes of nursing that are derived from extant theories of nursing continue to dictate and prescribe how a nurse should nurse. Contrary to this popular conception, "knowing persons" as a model of practice using technologies of nursing achieves for the nurse an appreciation of expertise and the knowledge of persons in the moment. Technologies allow nurses to know about the person only as much as what the person permits the nurse to know. It can be true that technologies detect the anatomical, physiological, chemical, and/or biological conditions of a person. This identifies the person as a living human being. However, with knowing persons, the nurse is allowed to understand and anticipate the ever-changing person from moment to moment.

> *The purpose of 'knowing the person' is derived from the nurse's intention to nurse, and the continuing appreciation of persons as ever-changing, never static, and who are dynamic human beings.*

The purpose of knowing the person is derived from the nurse's intention to nurse (Purnell and Locsin, 2000)—a continuing appreciation of the person as ever-changing, never static, and one who is a dynamic human being. The information derived from knowing the person is only relevant for the moment, for the persons' "state" can change moment to moment, a realization of a person as a dynamic, living, unpredictable human being. Importantly, knowing the "who or what" of persons helps nurses realize that a person is more than simply the physiochemical and anatomical being. Knowing persons allows the nurse to know "who and what" is the person.

Knowing When Using Technology

From such a view, it may be a perception that the process of knowing is only possible when using technologies in nursing. This is not necessarily true. This perception is supported by the idea that nursing is technology when technology is appreciated as anything that creates efficiency, be this an instrument or a tool, such as machines, or the activity of nurses when nursing. Sandelowski (1993) has argued about the metaphorical depiction of nursing as technology, or with technology as nursing, and the semiotic relationship of these concepts. Regardless, the idea of knowing persons guiding nursing practice is novel in the sense that there is no prescription or direction that is the ideal; rather there is the wholesome appreciation of an informed practice that allows the use of multiple ways of knowing such as described by Phenix (1964) and expanded by Carper (1978). These ways of knowing involve the empirical, ethical, personal, and aesthetic. Aesthetic expressions document, communicate, and perpetuate the appreciation of nursing as transpiring moment to moment. Popular aesthetic expressions include storytelling, poetry, visual expressions as in drawings, illustrations, and paintings, and aural renditions such as vocal and instrumental music. Encountering aesthetic expressions again allows the nurse and the nursed to relive the occasion anew. Reflecting on these experiences using the fundamental patterns of knowing (Carper, 1978) enhances learning, motivates the furtherance of knowledgeable practice, and increases the valuing of nursing as a professional practice grounded in a legitimate theoretical perspective of nursing.

The use of technologies in nursing is consequent to the contemporary demands for nursing actions requiring technological proficiency. There is no letting up, because advancing technology currently encompasses the bulk of functional activities that nurses are expected to perform, particularly when the practice is in a clinical setting. Clinical nursing is firmly rooted in the clinical health model (Smith, 1983) in which the organismic and mechanistic views of human beings as persons convincingly dictate the practice of nursing. Nevertheless, the process of knowing persons will prevail, for the model of technological competency as caring in nursing provides the nurse the fitting stimulation and motivation, and the prospected autonomy to judge critically a mode of action that desires an appreciation of persons as whole.

The model articulates continuous knowing. Continuing to know persons deters objectification,

> *Continuing to know persons deters objectification of persons, thus inhibiting the process that ultimately regards human beings as "stuff" to care about. As such persons are knowledgeable participants of their care.*

a process that ultimately regards human beings as "stuff" to care about, rather than as knowledgeable participants of their care. Participating in his or her care frees the person from having to be "assigned" a care that he or she may not want or need. This relationship signifies responsiveness (Hudson, 1988). Continuous knowing results from the contention that findings or information appreciated through consequent knowing further informs the desire to know "who is" and "what is" the person. Doing so inhibits substantiation as the ultimate reason for nursing. Continuous knowing overpowers the motivation to prescribe and direct the person's life. Rather, it affirms, supports, and celebrates his or her hopes, dreams, and aspirations as a participating human being.

CALLS AND RESPONSES FOR NURSING

Calls for nursing are illuminations of the persons' hopes, dreams, and aspirations. Calls for nursing are individual expressions by persons who seek ways toward affirmation, support, and celebration as person. The nurse appreciates the uniqueness of persons in his or her nursing. In doing so, the nurse sustains and enhances the wholeness of the human being, while facilitating the realization of the persons' completeness through "acting for or with" the person. This is a way of affirming, supporting, and celebrating the person's wholeness.

The nurse relies on the person for calls for

nursing. These calls are specific mechanisms that persons use while allowing the nurse to respond with authentic intentions to know them fully as persons in the moment. Calls for nursing may be expressed in various ways, oftentimes as hopes and dreams, such as hoping to be with friends while recuperating in the hospital, or desiring to play the piano when his or her fingers are well enough to function effectively, or simply the ultimate desire to go home, or the wish to die peacefully. As uniquely as these calls for nursing are expressed, the nurse knows the person continuously moment to moment. Communicating the created nursing responses may be as patterns of relating information, such as those derived from machines like the EKG monitor, in order to know the physiological status of the person in the moment or to administer life-saving medications, institute transfer plans, or refer patients for services to other health-care

> **The entirety of nursing is to direct, focus, attain, sustain, and maintain the person.**

professionals. The entirety of nursing is to direct, focus, attain, sustain, and maintain the person. In doing so, hearing calls for nursing is continuous and momentarily complete.

Knowing persons allows the nurse to use technologies in articulating calls for nursing. The empirical, personal, ethical, and aesthetic ways of knowing that are fundamental to understanding persons as whole increase the likelihood of knowing persons in the moment. As unpredictable and

> **As unpredictable and dynamic, human beings are ever-changing moment to moment.**

dynamic, human beings are ever-changing moment to moment. This characteristic challenges the nurse to know persons continuously as wholes, discouraging and ceasing the traditional conception of possibly knowing persons completely at once, in order to prescribe and predict their expressions of wholeness. In continuously knowing persons as whole through articulated technologies in nursing, the nurse can perhaps intervene to facilitate patients' recognition of the person's wholeness in the moment.

SUMMARY

The purpose of this chapter is to describe and explain "knowing persons as whole," a framework of nursing guiding a practice grounded in the theoretical construct of *technological competency as caring in nursing* (Locsin, 2004). This framework of practice illuminates the harmonious relationship between technology competency and caring in nursing. In this model, the focus of nursing is the person.

Critical to understanding the phenomenon of technological competency as caring in nursing are the conceptual descriptions of technology, caring, and nursing. Assumptions about human beings as persons, nursing as caring, and technological competency are presented as foundational to the process of knowing persons as whole in the moment—a process of nursing grounded in the perspective of technological competency as caring in nursing.

The process of knowing persons as whole is explicated as technological efficiency in nursing practice. The model of practice is illustrated through the understanding of technology and caring as coexisting in nursing. The process of knowing persons is continuous. In this process of nursing, with calls and responses, the nurse and nursed come to know each other more fully as persons in the moment. Grounding the process is the appreciation of persons as whole and complete in the moment, of human beings as unpredictable, of technological competency as an expression of caring in nursing, and of nursing as critical to health care.

References

Boykin, A., & Schoenhofer, S. (2001). *Nursing as caring: A model for transforming practice.* New York: Jones and Bartlett, National League for Nursing Press.

Carper, B. (1978). Fundamental patterns of knowing in nursing. *Advances in Nursing Science, 1*(1), 13–24.

Daniels, L. (1998). Vulnerability as a key to authenticity. *Image: Journal of Nursing Scholarship, 30*(2), 191–192.

Heidegger, M. (1977). *The question concerning technology.* New York: Harper and Row.

Hudson, R. (1988). Whole or parts—a theological perspective

on 'person.' *The Australian Journal of Advanced Nursing, 6*(1), 12–20.

Hudson, G. (1993). Empathy and technology in the coronary care unit. *Intensive Critical Care Nursing, 9*(1), 55–61.

Locsin, R. (1995). Machine technologies and caring in nursing. *Image: Journal of Nursing Scholarship, 27*(3), 201–203.

Locsin, R. (1998). Technologic competence as expression of caring in critical care settings. *Holistic Nursing Practice, 12*(4), 50–56.

Locsin, R. (2001). Practicing nursing: Technological competency as an expression of caring in nursing. In Locsin, R. (2001). *Advancing Technology, Caring, and Nursing.* Connecticut: Auburn House, Greenwood Publishing Group.

Locsin, R. (2005). *Technological competency as caring in nursing: A model for practice.* Indianapolis, IN: Sigma Theta Tau International.

Locsin, R., and Campling, A. (2005). Techno sapiens and posthumans: Nursing, caring and technology. In Locsin, R. (2005). *Technological competency as caring in nursing: A model for practice.* Indianapolis, IN: Sigma Theta Tau International.

Maslow A. H. (1943). A theory of human motivation. *Psychological Review, 50,* 370–396.

Phenix, P. H. (1964). *Realms of meaning.* New York: McGraw Hill.

Purnell, M., and Locsin, R. (2000). Intentionality: Unification in nursing. Unpublished manuscript. Florida Atlantic University College of Nursing, Boca Raton, Florida.

Reader's Digest Association. (1987). *Reader's Digest Illustrated Encyclopedic Dictionary* (p. 932). Pleasantville, New York: The Reader's Digest Association.

Sandelowski, M. (1993). Toward a theory of technology dependency. *Nursing Outlook, 41*(1), 36–42.

Smith, J. (1983). *The idea of health: Implications for the nursing professional.* New York: Teachers College Press.

Swanson, M. (1991). Dimensions of caring interventions. *Nursing Research, 40,* 161–166

CHAPTER 25

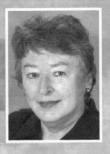

Marilyn E. Parker

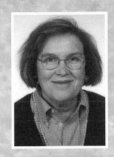

Charlotte D. Barry

Developing a Community Nursing Practice Model

Marilyn E. Parker and Charlotte D. Barry

Introducing the Theorists

Marilyn E. Parker is a professor at the Christine E. Lynn College of Nursing at Florida Atlantic University, where she is founding director of the Quantum Foundation Center for Innovation in School and Community Well-Being. She earned degrees from Incarnate Word College (BSN), the Catholic University of America (MSN), and Kansas State University (PhD). Her overall career mission is to enhance nursing practice and education through nursing theory, using both innovative and traditional means to improve care and advance the discipline.

As principal investigator for a program of grants to create and use a new Community Nursing Practice Model, Dr. Parker has provided leadership to develop transdisciplinary school-based wellness centers devoted to health and social services for children and families from underserved multicultural communities, teaching university students from several disciplines, and developing research and policy to promote community well-being. In 2002, Dr. Parker received the President's Leadership Award at Florida Atlantic University, recognizing exemplary service to the university and to the community.

Dr. Parker's active participation in nursing education and health care in several countries led to her 2001 Fulbright Scholar Award to Thailand. It is there that she continues to teach, consult, and participate in research with Thai colleagues in developing a Thai nursing practice model based on perspectives of practicing nursing in Thailand. Her commitment to caring for underserved populations and to health policy evaluation led to being named a National Public Health Leadership Institute Fellow and to being elected a distinguished practitioner in the National Academies of Practice—Nursing. Dr. Parker is a fellow in the American Academy of Nursing.

Charlotte D. Barry is an associate professor and associate director at the Quantum Foundation Center for Innovation in School and Community Well-Being at the Florida Atlantic University Christine E. Lynn College of Nursing. Dr. Barry serves on the Education Committee of the National Association of School Nurses. She has been active in the Florida Association of School Nurses since 1996 and has served as president, treasurer, and board member. Taking the lead with school nursing education in Florida, she has developed academic courses that have been conducted online as well as in the classroom. One course has been adapted to a continuing education (CE) program preparing school nurses for national certification. Workshops have been developed and conducted on critical thinking and competency skills for school nurses.

The focus of Dr. Barry's scholarship and teaching has been caring for persons in schools and communities. Her writings include nursing values, inquiry groups for community assessments, and cultural caring. Her current research includes the study of adiposity in children, health-care provider's cultural competence, and multisite studies with school nurses throughout Florida.

Dr. Barry has had leadership roles in many organizations, including the International Association of Human Caring (IAHC). She attended her first IAHC conference in Texas in the early '90s and during a poetry workshop became inspired to write a poem entitled "I Am Nurse." Since that time she has been an active member of IAHC, holding various leadership positions, and has served as a manuscript reviewer for the International Journal of Human Caring.

Dr. Barry graduated from Brooklyn College where she earned an associate degree in nursing; she holds a bachelor's degree in health administration, a master's degree in nursing from Florida Atlantic University in Boca Raton, and a doctoral degree from the University of Miami, Florida. She is nationally certified in school nursing.

Developing a Community Nursing Practice Model: The Ideal and the Practical

Developing the Community Nursing Practice Model described herein began with, and continues to be a blend of, the ideal and the practical. The ideal was the commitment of one of the authors to developing and using nursing concepts to guide nursing practice, education, and scholarship, and of a desire to develop a nursing practice as an essential component of a nursing college. The practical was the added commitment of the other author in bringing this model to life. The added efforts of faculty, staff and students contributed to the development model intended to reflect the concept of nursing held by the faculty of nursing, *nursing is nurturing wholeness of persons and environments through caring,* and the mission of the Christine E. Lynn College of Nursing (Florida Atlantic University College of Nursing Philosophy and Mission, 1994/2003).

The model's initial conceptual framework also grew out of the political reality that some concepts that were readily understood and valued by persons in the wider community must be used in order to secure funding. The result was a proposal for a demonstration project to develop a framework for nursing as primary health care and early intervention (Parker, 1996). This proposal expressed the ideal, or the major components of the faculty nursing focus statement, and the political and practical, which are the principals of the World Health Organization (WHO) principles of primary health care (1978). Another blend of ideal and practical was the political reality and hope that such a demonstration project, if successful, would be embraced by the administration and the faculty of the College of Nursing as well as the community being served.

The concepts and relationships of the model briefly set forth as part of the proposal for funding have continued to be the guiding force for the community practice. Through various participatory-action approaches, including ongoing shared reflection, intuitive insights, and discoveries, the Community Nursing Practice Model has evolved and continues to develop. The education of university students and the conduct of student and faculty research are integrated with nursing and social work practice. Throughout the early development and ongoing refinement of the model, there has been nurturing of collaborative community partnerships, evaluation and development of school and community health policy, and development of enriched community.

The model has been used as a framework for curriculum development for a master's program in advanced community nursing at Naresuan University, Phitsanulok, Thailand. The faculty of nursing at Mbarara University of Science and Technology, Mbarara, Uganda, has used the model to develop study of advanced community nursing and to design and operate the first school-based community nursing center in Uganda. Today, ten years after the initial proposal for the demonstration project was funded, the Community Nursing Practice Model guides a diverse, complex, and transdisciplinary practice of nursing and social work in four school-based community wellness

centers serving children and families from diverse multicultural communities and is accepted by local communities and providers as essential to the health care system. In 2004, more than 10,000 persons received primary health care and an additional 12,000 participated in various health-promotion activities. This year also more than 100 undergraduate, master's, and doctoral students studied nursing practice and research and eight nursing faculty practiced and conducted research guided by the model. An academic center, The Quantum Foundation Center for Innovation in School and Community Well-Being that provides a home for this integrated practice is also an outcome, as are ongoing proposals to fund integrated practice and scholarship. The model is featured in a major community nursing text (Clark, 2003). The practice received the 2001 award for Outstanding Faculty Practice from the National Organization of Nurse Practitioner Faculties.

The Community Nursing Practice Model

Essential values that form the basis of the model are 1) respect for person; 2) persons are caring, and caring is understood as the essence of nursing; 3) persons are whole and always connected with one another in families and communities. These essential or transcendent values area always present in nursing situations, while other actualizing values guide practice in certain situations.

The principles of primary health care from the World Health Organization (1978) are the actualizing values. These additional concepts of the model are 1) access; 2) essentiality; 3) community participation; 4) empowerment, and 5) intersectoral collaboration. These also guide health care and social service practice. Concepts of practice that have emerged include transitional care and enhancing care. The model illuminates these values and each of the concepts in four interrelated themes: nursing, person, community, and environment, along with a structure of interconnecting services, activities, and community partnerships (Parker and Barry, 1999). An inquiry group method has been

An inquiry group method has been designed and is the primary means of ongoing assessment and evaluation.

designed and is the primary means of ongoing assessment and evaluation (Parker, Barry, & King, 2000; Ryan, Hawkins, Parker, & Hawkins, 2004).

NURSING

The unique focus of nursing is nurturing the wholeness of persons and environments through

> *The focus of nursing is nurturing wholeness of persons and environment through caring.*

caring (FAU, 1994/2003). Nursing practice, education, and scholarship require creative integration of multiple ways of knowing and understanding through knowledge synthesis within a context of value and meaning. Nursing knowledge is embedded in the nursing situation, the lived experience of caring between the nurse and the one receiving care. The nurse is authentically present for the other, to hear calls for caring and to create dynamic nursing responses. The school-based community wellness centers and satellite sites in the community become places for persons and families to access nursing and social services where they are: in homes, work camps, schools, or under trees in a community gathering spot. Nursing is dynamic and portable; there is no predetermined nursing and often no predetermined access place (Parker, 1997; Parker & Barry, 1999).

Nursing practice is further described within the context of transitional care and enhancing care. Transitional care is that in which clients and families are provided essential health care while being enrolled in a local insurance plan that will partially support that care. Over several weeks, clients are assisted to enroll in long-term forms of health-care insurance and related benefits and are referred to a more permanent source of health care in the community. Transitional care, an ideal for nursing and social work practice, is sometimes not possible due to immigration status, a complex and confounding application process, or other issues of the family.

> *Enhancing care describes nursing and social work that is intended to assist the client and family who need care in addition to that provided by a local health-care provider.*

Enhancing care describes nursing and social work that is intended to assist the client and family who need care in addition to that provided by a local health-care provider.

PERSON

Respect for person is present in all aspects of nursing, with clients, community members, and colleagues. Respect includes a stance of humility that the nurse does not know all that can be known about a person and a situation, acknowledging that the person is the expert in his/her own care and knowing his/her experience. Respect carries with it an openness to learn and grow. Values and beliefs of various cultures are reflected in expressions of respect and caring. The person as whole and connected with others, not the disease or problem, is the focus of nursing.

Persons are empowered by understanding choices, how to choose, and how to live daily with choices made. The person defines what is necessary to well-being and what priorities exist in daily life of the family. Nursing and social work practice based on practical, sound, culturally acceptable, and cost-effective methods are necessary for well-being and wholeness of persons, families, and communities.

Early on, Swadener & Lubeck's (1995) work on deconstructing the discourse of risk was a major influence on practice. "At risk" connotes a deficiency that needs fixing; a doing to rather than collaborating with. Thinking about children and families "at promise" instead of "at risk" inspires an approach to knowing the other as whole and filled with potential.

> *Respect and caring in nursing require full participation of persons, families, and communities in assessment, design, and evaluation of services.*

Respect and caring in nursing require full participation of persons, families, and communities in assessment, design, and evaluation of services. Based on this concept, an inquiry group method is used for ongoing appraisal of services. This method is defined as a "route of knowing" and "a route to other questions." Each person is a coparticipant, an expert knower in their experience; the facilitator is expert knower of the process. The facilitator's role is to encourage expressions of knowing so calls for nursing and guidance for nursing responses can be heard. In this way, the essential care for persons and families can be known, and care designed, offered, and evaluated (Barry, 1998; Parker, Barry, & King, 2000).

COMMUNITY

Community, as understood within the model, was formed from the classical definition offered by Smith and Maurer (1995) and from the Peck's existential, relational view (1987). According to Smith and Maurer, a community is defined by its members and is characterized by shared values. This expanded notion of community moves away from a locale as a defining characteristic and includes self-defined groups who share common interests and concerns and who interact with one another.

Community, offered by Peck (1987), is a safe place for members and ensures the security of being included and honored. His work focuses on building community through a web of relationships grounded in acceptance of individual and cultural differences among faculty and staff and acceptance of others in the widening circles, including: colleagues within the practice and discipline, other health-care colleagues from varied disciplines, grant funders, and other collaborators. The notion of a transdisciplinary care is an exemplar of this approach to community. Another defining characteristic of community, according to Peck, is willingness to risk and to tolerate a certain lack of structure. The practice guided by the model reflects this in fostering a creative approach to program development, implementation, evaluation, and research.

Practice in the model, whether unfolding in a clinic or under a tree where persons have gathered, provides a welcoming and safe place for sharing stories of caring. The intention to know others as experts in their self-care while listening to their hopes and dreams for well-being creates a communion between the client and provider that guides the development of a nurturing relationship. Knowing the other in relationship to their communities, such as family, school, work, worship, or play, honors the complexity of the context of persons' lives and offers the opportunity to understand and participate with them.

ENVIRONMENT

The notion of environment within this model provides the context for understanding the wholeness of interconnected lives. The environment, one of the oldest concepts in nursing described by Nightingale (1859/1992), is not only immediate effects of air, odors, noise, and warmth on the reparative powers of the patient, but also indicates the social settings that contribute to health and illness. Another nursing visionary, Lillian Wald, witnessed the hardships of poverty and disenfranchisement on the residents of the lower Manhattan immigrant communities; she developed the Henry Street Settlement House to provide a broad range of care that included direct physical care up to and including finding jobs, housing, and influencing the creation of child labor laws (Barry, 2003).

Chooporian (1986) reinspired nurses to expand the notion of environment to include not only the immediate context of patients' lives, but also to think of the relationship between health and social issues that "influence human beings and hence create conditions for heath and illness" (p. 53). Reflecting on earth caring, Schuster (1990) urged another look at the environment, inviting nurses to consider a broader view that included nonhuman species and the nonhuman world. Acknowledging the interrelatedness of all living things energizes caring from this broader perspective into a wider circle. Kleffel (1996) described this as "an ecocentric approach grounded in the cosmos. The whole environment, including inanimate elements such as rocks and minerals, along with animate animals and plants, is assigned an intrinsic value" (p. 4). This directs thinking about the interconnectedness of all elements, both animate and inanimate. Teaching, practice, and scholarship require a caring context that respects, explores, nurtures, and celebrates the interconnectedness of all living things and inanimate objects throughout the global environment.

Structure of Services and Activities

The model is envisioned as three concentric circles around a core. Envisioning the model as a water color representation, one can appreciate the vibrancy of practice within the model, the amorphous interconnectedness of the core and the

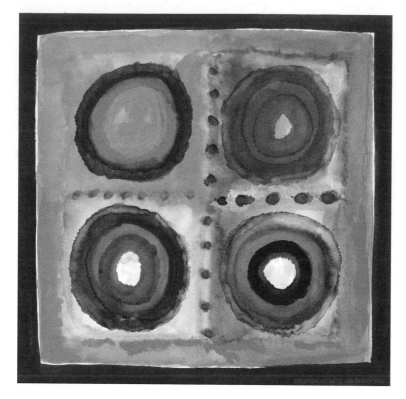

FIGURE 25–1 Community Nursing Practice Model

circles, and the "certain lack of structure" draws attention to the beauty in creating as well as the beauty in differences. Represented in Fig. 25–1, the model calls into the circles others to create programs and environments to nurtured well being.

CORE SERVICES

Core services are provided at each practice site and illuminate the focus of nursing: nurturing wholeness of persons and environments through caring. The unique experiences of staff and faculty with those receiving care create the substance of the core: respecting self-care practice, honoring lay and indigenous care, inviting participation and listening to clients' stories of health and well-being, providing care that is essential for the other, supporting caring for self, family and community, providing care that is culturally competent and collaborating with others for care. These services, provided to children, students, school staff, and families from the community, occur in the following and frequently overlapping categories of care: (a) *design and coordinate care:* examples are making and receiving referrals, navigation to other health services, and insurance enrollment, home visits, and pro-

grams such as the Celebrity Chef Cooking Club, Senior Health Program, or Yoga for Children; the concepts of transitional and enhancing care are illuminated here through the development of collaborative relationships; (b) *primary prevention and health education:* examples include child-development milestones, pre- and postnatal wellness, breast health, testicular height, stress reduction, chronic illness management, car safety, and administration of immunizations; (c) *secondary prevention/health screening/early intervention:* examples include hearing and vision, height/weight/BMI, cholesterol, blood sugar, blood pressure, clinical breast exams, lead levels, assessment, and early management of health issues; (d) *tertiary prevention/primary care:* assessment, diagnosis, treatment, and care management for chronic health issues, crisis intervention and behavioral support, and collaborating with others for transitional and enhancing care.

FIRST CIRCLE

The first circle of the model depicts a widening circle of concern and support for well being of persons and communities. This circle includes persons and groups in each school and community who share concern for the well-being of persons served at the centers. This includes participants in inquiry groups, parents/guardians, school faculty, and non-instructional staff, after-school groups, parent/teacher organizations, and school advisory councils. The services provided within this circle might include: (a) *consultation and collaboration:* building relationships and community, answering inquiries on matters of health and well-being, providing in-service and health education, serving on school committees, reviewing policies and procedures; (b) *appraisal and evaluation:* conducting community assessments, appraising care provided, evaluating outcomes, and promoting programs that enhance well-being for individuals and communities.

SECOND CIRCLE

The second circle draws attention to the wider context of concern and influence for well being and includes structured and organized groups whose members also share concern for the education and well-being of the persons served at the centers but within a wider range or jurisdiction such as a district or county. Examples of these policy-making or advising groups include the school district and county public health department, the county health-care district, Children's Service Council, American Lung Association, and the American Red Cross. Local funders who offer support for use of the model include the Health Care District of Palm Beach County, which offered initial support, and the Quantum Foundation, the ongoing sustaining funder. The services provided in this circle include (a) *consultation and collaboration:* building relationships and community with members of these groups, contributing to policy appraisal, development, and evaluation, leading and serving on teams and committees responsible for overseeing the care of students and families, and providing school nurse education; (b) *research and evaluation:* assessing school health services, describing research findings for best practices related to school and community health, and designing research projects focused on school/community health issues and or school/community nursing practice.

THIRD CIRCLE

The third circle includes state, regional, national, and international organizations with whom we are related in various ways. Services within this circle are focused on (a) *consultation and collaboration:* building relationships and community with members and collaborating about scholarship, policy, outcomes, practice, research, educational needs of school nurses and advanced practice nurses, and sustainability through ongoing and additional funding; (b) *appraisal and evaluation:* school nursing and advanced practice faculty organizations offer a milieu for discussion and appraisal of the services provided at the centers. Organizations in this circle include Florida Department of Health: Office of School Health, Florida Association of School Nurses, Florida Association of School Health, National Association of School Nurses, National Assembly of School-Based Health Centers, and the National Nursing Centers Consortium.

CONNECTION OF CORE TO CONCENTRIC CIRCLES

Connections of the core to the concentric circles of services illuminate the appreciation of the complexity of the practice within the Community Nursing Practice Model. The core service of *consultation and collaboration* is a primary focus of practice, beginning with nursing and social work colleagues and extending to participating clients, families, policy makers, funders, and legislators. This value-laden service has been essential to the viability and sustainability of this model. It promotes the stance of humility that guides the respectful question throughout the circles: How can we be helpful to you? The answer directs the creation of respectful individualized care and program development. Essential health-care services are created within the core and extend into the first circle.

Connections to the second circle unfold from the collaborating relationships with colleagues in the health department, school district, health-care district, and other groups taking the lead with school and community health. Committees on which center administrators and staff serve meet regularly to discuss school and community health issues and to seek consensus on possible solutions. These committees include the School Health Task Force and Advisory Groups and the Access Palm Beach County collaboration. The health department provides consultation on health and practice matters; the school district provides the physical space for the centers, and through a collaborative agreement with the health-care district, many of our clients without health insurance can be enrolled in a safety-net program of health services. Physicians are consultants for medical questions and referrals. School nurse education is also provided for nurses in the local county and in surrounding areas of this state.

Like the other circles, the third circle depicts the breadth of relationships developed at meetings, and through publications and presentations at local, regional, national, and international conferences. Administration and faculty have been recognized for the contribution made to the health and well-being of children and families. Faculty, staff, and students participate on panels, sharing their experiences in caring for underinsured and uninsured persons.

SUMMARY

The fundamental beliefs and commitment to the discipline and unique practice of nursing provided for both creating and sustaining this Community Nursing Practice Model. This model provides the environment in which nursing is practiced from the core beliefs of respect, caring, and wholeness. The centers, developed and managed by nurses, have demonstrated the integration of the mission and philosophy of the College of Nursing. Members of the faculty and center staff are encouraged to practice from these beliefs and to reach out and through the concentric circles, strengthening and widening the web of relationships with colleagues, clients, and community members. Through use of this model, the ideals of the discipline are brought into reality of care for wholeness and well being of persons and families in multicultural communities.

References

Barry, C. (1994). Face painting as metaphor. In Schuster, E., & Brown, C. (Eds.), *Exploring our environmental connections* (pp. 279–286). New York: National League for Nursing Press.

Barry, C. (1998). The celebrity chef cooking club: A peer involvement feeding program promoting cooperation and community building. *Florida Journal of School Health, 9*(1), 17–20.

Barry, C. (2003). *A retrospective: Looking back on Linda Rogers and the history of school nursing.* Paper presented at the 8th annual Florida Association of School Nurses Conference: Past, Present and Future: Continuing the Vision. Orlando, Florida, January 2003.

Barry, C., Bozas, L., Carswell, J., Hurtado, M., Keller, M., Lewis, E., Poole, K., & Tipton, B. (1998). Nursing a school-aged child provides an insight to the Guatemalan culture. *Florida Journal of School Health, 9*(1), 29–36.

Chooporian, T. (1986). Reconceptualizing the environment. In Mocia, P. (Ed.), *New approaches to theory development* (pp. 39–54). New York: National League for Nursing Press.

Clark, M. J. (2003). *Community health nursing: Caring for populations.* Saddle River, NJ: Prentice Hall.

Florida Atlantic University Christine E. Lynn College of Nursing. (1994/2003). Mission and philosophy. In *Faculty Handbook,* Boca Raton, FL: Florida Atlantic University Christine E. Lynn College of Nursing.

Kleffel, D. (1996). Environmental paradigms: Moving toward an ecocentric perspective. *Advances in Nursing Science, 18*(4), 1–10.

Nightingale, F. (1859/1992) Notes on nursing: Commemorative edition with commentaries by contemporary nursing leaders. Philadelphia. J. B. Lippincott.

Peck, S. (1987). *The different drum: Community making and peace.* New York: Simon & Schuster.

Parker, M. E. (1996). Designing a nursing model of primary health care and early intervention. Proposal funded by the health care district of Palm Beach County, FL.

Parker, M. E. (1997). Emerging innovations: Caring in action. *International Journal for Human Caring, 1*(2), 9–10.

Parker, M. E., & Barry, C. D. (1997, June). Love and suffering at the margins. Paper presented at the International Association of Human Caring Research Conference, the Primacy of Love and Existential Suffering, Helsinki, Finland.

Parker, M. E., & Barry, C. D. (1999). Community practice guided by a nursing model. *Nursing Science Quarterly, 12*(2), 125–131.

Parker, M. E., Barry, C. D., & King, B. (2000). Use of inquiry method for assessment and evaluation in a school-based community nursing project. *Family and Community Health, 23*(2), 54–61.

Ryan, E., Hawkins, W., Parker, M. E., & Hawkins, M. (2004). Perceptions of access to U. S. health care of Haitian immigrants in South Florida. *Florida Public Health Review, 1,* 36–43.

Schuster, E. (1990). Earth caring. *Advances in Nursing Science, 13*(1), 25–30.

Smith, C. & Mauer, F. (1995). Community health nursing: theory and practice. Philadelphia: W.B. Saunders.

Swadener, B. & Lubeck, S. (1995). Children and families "at promise." Deconstructing the discourse on risk. Albany: State University of New York Press.

World Health Organization, Alma-Ata. (1978). *Primary health care.* Geneva, Switzerland: World Health Organization.

Index

Page numbers followed by *f* indicate figures; page numbers followed by *t* indicate tables.